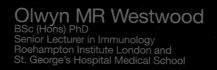

Olwyn MR Westwood
BSc (Hons) PhD
Senior Lecturer in Immunology
Roehampton Institute London and
St. George's Hospital Medical School

The Scientific Basis for Health Care

M Mosby

London Philadelphia St Louis Sydney Tokyo

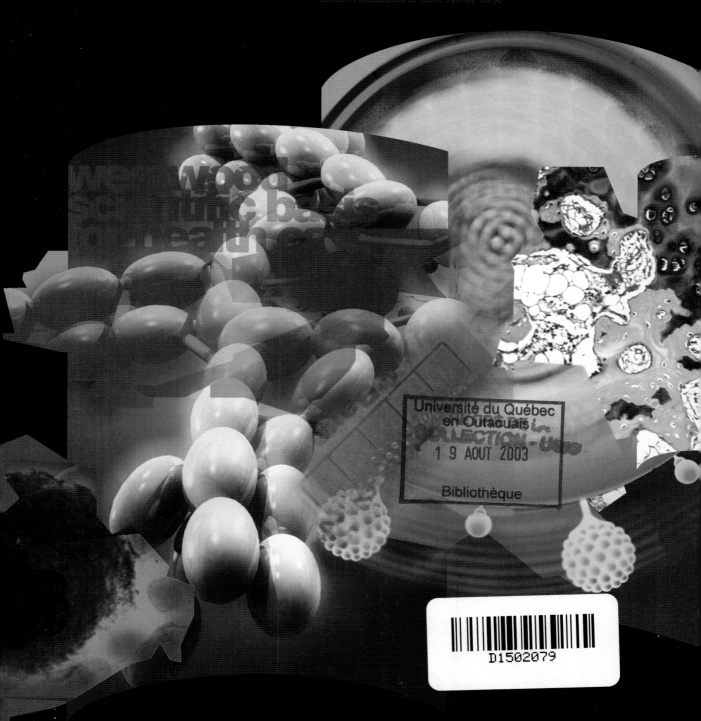

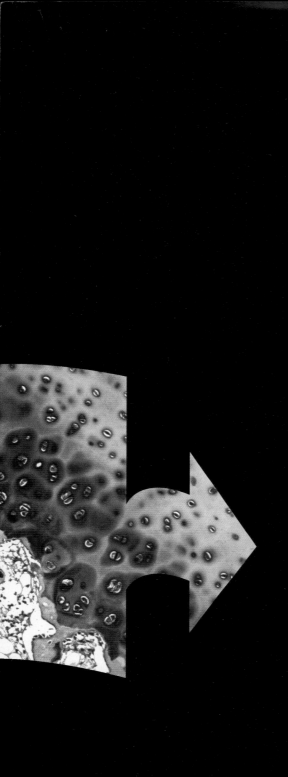

Publisher	**Jill Northcott**
Development Editor	**Gillian Harris, Natasha DuPont**
Project Manager	**Ian MacQuarrie**
Design	**Paul Phillips**
Cover Design	**Greg Smith**
Illustration Manager	**Danny Pyne**
Illustrators	**Mike Saiz**
	Robin Dean
	Paul Bernson
Production	**Ewan Halley**
Indexer	**Anita Reid**

Mosby

An imprint of Harcourt Brace and Company Limited

Copyright © Harcourt Brace and Company Limited 1999

ISBN 0 7234 24403

Printed by Printer Trento, Italy.

A CIP catalogue record for this book is available from the British Library.

The publisher and author have undertaken reasonable endeavours to check drugs, dosages, adverse effects and contraindications in this book. We recommend that the reader should always check the manufacturer's instructions and information in the British National Formulary (BNF) or similar publication before administering any drug.

CONTENTS

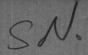

CONTENTS

The education and training of health care professionals is going through a period of major change, not least the transfer from hospital-based schools into multi-disciplinary higher education. Recent Health Service reforms have resulted in a reorganisation of the way that health care is delivered and has included a shift to primary care from the acute sector. Accompanying these changes has been an extension of the role of many health care professionals which places on them the need for a wide understanding of their subject, and the ability to relate their own work to that of others.

It is against this background of change that *The Scientific Basis for Health Care* was conceived. We identified the need for a single volume text that would bring together essential concepts in cell biology, pharmacology, microbiology, immunology and basic pathology, within a clinical context for students on health care courses. The intention of the authors has been to present complex topics in a straightforward way, but encourage the reader to pursue topics in more depth where appropriate through further reading.

The book will be suitable for students following courses in biomedical sciences, medicine, nursing, midwifery, and other professions allied to medicine such as physiotherapy and radiography. It will provide students with a broad overview and the underpinning knowledge that they will hopefully relate to other studies in their particular discipline. It has been deliberately written to meet the needs of a multi-professional audience providing information on common core material for these professions. In addition to health care students, the book will be of interest to students of more general biology courses who wish to gain an understanding of pathological processes.

The team of authors are experts in their own fields and all of them are involved with the Health Service either in the delivery of health care or through teaching undergraduate and postgraduate students. Throughout the book, concepts are often explained with anecdotal evidence from first-hand experience in clinical practice. There is cross-referencing throughout the text because a key strength is the inter-relationships that are developed across the core subjects.

It is our hope that this book will form a robust foundation for health care students helping them to extend and develop their own areas of expertise whilst being mindful of the responsibilities of others. If *The Scientific Basis for Health Care* makes even a small contribution to better patient care by future generations of health care professionals, it will have served its purpose well.

Dr Olwyn MR Westwood
Senior Lecturer in Immunology
Roehampton Institute London & St. George's Hospital
Medical School

ACKNOWLEDGEMENTS

Many grateful thanks must go to the team of authors for their contributions to this project, in an ethos where the research assessment exercise seems to place more value in the writing of research papers than other scholarly activities, such as preparing textbooks for students. Though it is with sadness that we record the recent death of one of the authors, Dr Ian M James.

I would like to express my sincere gratitude to the following experts for their help and advice. To colleagues at St. George's Hospital Medical School including: Professor Frank Hay (Vice Principal), Dr. Gerald Levin (Consultant in Clinical Biochemistry); Gillian Chumbley (Clinical Nurse Specialist in Pain Management); Susan Gove and her team of librarians, Andrew Rolland and Joseph Morton (Audiovisual Services), and Deborah Bunyan (Dean's office, Faculty of Healthcare Sciences). Also to Dr. Cristina Navarrete (Consultant Clinical Scientist & Head of Histocompatibility and Immunogenetics, National Blood Service, London & South East), Professor Christopher McGuigan (Welsh School of Pharmacy), and my students of health care, in particular Sue Reid, and the tutors who read so many of the chapters. Lastly to all the Mosby team, past and present, whose vision, support and enthusiasm has meant this book is now in your hands.

Habakkuk 2: v2.

CONTRIBUTORS

Dr Emma H. Baker
Clinical Pharmacology Unit
Dept. of Pharmacology
St George's Hospital Medical School
London

Dr Dilip K. Banerjee
Dept. of Medical Microbiology
St George's Hospital Medical School
London

Dr Carol M. Blow
Fairacre (Surgery)
Fetcham
Surrey

Dr Clive Bullock,
School of Life Sciences
Roehampton Institute London
London

Dr John M. Gibbons
Dept of Pharmaceutical Chemistry
University of London School of Pharmacy
London

Dr Andrew P. Jewell
School of Life Sciences
Kingston University
Surrey

Dr Ian M. James
Academic Dept. of Medicine
Royal Free Hospital School of Medicine
London

Nicola C. McBride
Dept. of Haematology
St Bartholomew's and Royal London School
of Medicine and Dentistry
London

Professor R. Michael Pittilo
Joint Faculty of Healthcare Sciences of
Kingston University and
St George's Hospital Medical School
London

Dr Christopher D. Rodger
School of Life Sciences
Roehampton Insititute London
London

Professor Carol A. Seymour
Division of Cardiological Sciences
St George's Hospital Medical School
London

Dr Michael E. Shipley
Bloomsbury Rheumatology Unit
University College London Hospitals
The Middlesex Hospital
London

Dr Olwyn MR Westwood
School of Life Sciences
Roehampton Insititute London
London

Dr Kwee L. Yong
Academic Department of Haematology
Royal Free and University College Medical
School
London

Cell Biology

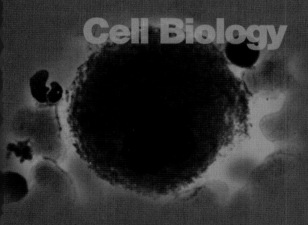

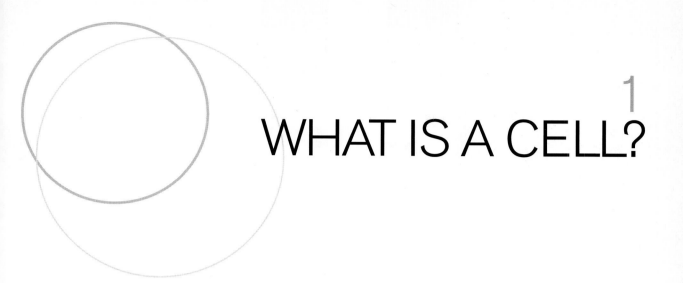

WHAT IS A CELL?

LEARNING OBJECTIVES

After studying this chapter students should have a clearer understanding of:
- overall structure and function of cellular components (organelles)
- mechanisms of transport in and out of cells
- different kinds of human tissues

It is expected that you should have a basic understanding of human anatomy, physiology and cell biology.

INTRODUCTION TO CELL ORGANIZATION

All living organisms are composed of individual units called cells, but they show two distinct levels of cellular organization. The earliest cells evolved around 3.5 billion years ago; these were prokaryotes – single-celled organisms, represented today by bacteria. Prokaryotic cells have a simple internal structure with no well-defined nucleus or nuclear membrane, and their deoxyribonucleic acid (DNA) is usually in the form of a single circular strand. They often contain small circular pieces of DNA known as plasmids.

Eukaryotic cells evolved later, around 1.2 billion years ago, probably as a result of an association between earlier cell types, and are found in plants, animals and fungi (including yeasts). Eukaryotic cells have a well-defined nucleus that is bounded by a nuclear membrane, and their DNA is organized into chromosomes. Around the nucleus is the cytosol, which contains numerous membrane-based structures, the cellular organelles.

Both prokaryocytes and eukaryocytes are enclosed by a limiting membrane. Plant cells and bacteria have a cell wall outside the membrane, and this prevents the cell from swelling and bursting under unfavourable osmotic conditions by providing a physical restraint on cell expansion. The cell wall is composed of cellulose fibrils in plants and sugar–protein polymers in bacteria. Gram-negative bacteria have an additional outer membrane containing sugar–lipid polymers (lipopolysaccharides) to protect them (Figure 1.1).

Although these two cell types show some differences in their cellular functions, the key difference lies in the way in which they divide and multiply. Prokaryotic cells rely on a relatively simple fission (splitting) process, while eukaryotes divide and separate their genetic material by the processes of meiosis and mitosis, leading to genetic variation through recombination, in which genetic material is exchanged between chromosomes.

Not all 'living' systems have a cell-based structure. For example, viruses are not cells – they are much smaller particles composed of DNA or ribonucleic acid (RNA) enclosed in a protein capsid. They lack ribosomes for protein synthesis and are unable to synthesize adenosine triphosphate (ATP) for energy. Consequently they are parasitic on the cells that they invade and rely on the biochemical machinery of the infected host cell.

Much simpler still are prions, tiny infectious particles composed entirely of protein. They are believed to be responsible for degenerative disorders of the brain such as scrapie in sheep, bovine spongiform encephalopathy (BSE) in cattle, and kuru and Creutzfeldt–Jakob disease (CJD) in humans. It is uncertain whether these particles can reproduce themselves (see Chapter 38).

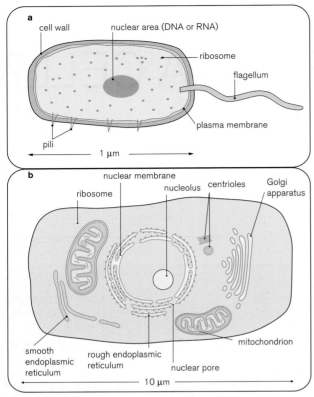

Figure 1.1 Prokaryotes and eukaryotes.
(a) A generalized bacterial cell (prokaryote).
(b) A generalized mammalian cell (eukaryote).

THE STRUCTURE OF EUKARYOTIC CELLS

CELL MEMBRANES

Cell membranes are composed mainly of phospholipid molecules that have a hydrophilic ('water-loving') head and a hydrophobic ('water-hating') tail. These molecules are arranged in two layers, known as a bilayer, and their hydrophilic heads face the outer and inner surfaces, with a central core of hydrophobic tails. Bulky cholesterol molecules are also present in the membrane to stabilize it and to prevent the phospholipids from crystallizing and stiffening the membrane. In electron micrographs produced from a transmission electron microscope, membranes have a 'tramline' or three-layered sandwich appearance (Figure 1.2).

All eukaryotic cells are bounded by a plasma membrane, which maintains the integrity of the cell by acting as a selectively permeable barrier. It also acts as the site for communication with the external environment and with other cells. Similarly, the membranes that surround cellular organelles separate metabolic activity into distinct compartments within the cell.

Membrane molecules are in continuous motion, giving a fluid structure. The phospholipids circulate rapidly within each layer and occasionally between layers, a phenomenon known as 'flip-flop motion'. Although the bilayer forms a continuous fluid film over the cell surface, this layer is momentarily breached many times each second as the cell flexes and moves, producing temporary pores that allow small molecules such as water to cross the membrane.

Membrane proteins move around like icebergs in the lipid bilayer and fulfil a variety of important functions. They may act as channels or carriers, allowing the selective transport of solutes across the lipid bilayer. Proteins on the outside of the plasma membrane may act as receptor sites for specific molecules which convey information between cells, particularly hormones (e.g. insulin) and neurotransmitters (e.g. acetylcholine).

Enzyme proteins are commonly associated with membranes. For example, the enzyme adenylate cyclase, which is present in the plasma membrane of many cells, catalyses the conversion of ATP to cyclic adenosine monophosphate (cyclic AMP). Cyclic AMP is known as a 'second messenger'; it passes on the stimulus when hormones such as adrenaline or glucagon bind to the surface of their target cells. Another important example is acetylcholinesterase, which is found in the membranes of skeletal muscle cells at muscle–nerve junctions. This enzyme catalyses the breakdown of the neurotransmitter, acetylcholine, after it has stimulated a muscle contraction. Proteins protruding on to the outer surface may act as cell-adhesion molecules that link to adjacent cells or to collagen fibres found in connective tissue; these functions are considered in more detail later.

Some of the most significant proteins in the immunological defence system are found on the surfaces of mammalian nucleated cells – they are called the 'major histocompatibility complex' (MHC); the human equivalent is referred to as the 'human leukocyte antigen' (HLA) system. The HLA molecules are the tissue type antigens that are tested and matched between a patient undergoing an organ or tissue transplantation and the prospective donor (see Chapters 24 and 29). They fulfil an important part of immune function by acting as a 'signboard' to indicate the presence of intracellular infections and abnormalities such as malignancy. Similarly, cancer cells show changes in their cell surface markers, enabling them to be recognized and destroyed at an early stage (see Chapters 5 and 30).

Carbohydrates are found on the outer surface of plasma membranes and are associated either with membrane proteins or with lipids. Some carbohydrates act as cell surface markers, defining the 'tissue type' of an

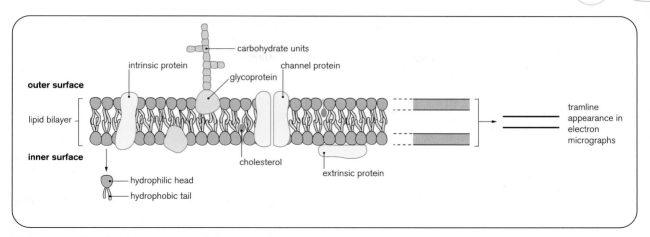

Figure 1.2 The fluid mosaic model of membrane structure. A membrane composed of a bilayer made up of phospholipids.

individual. They may have a role in anchoring membrane proteins and limiting cellular growth. Important carbohydrates found on the surface of red blood cells include the ABO blood group system. Matching the blood group of donor and recipient is necessary before a blood transfusion is given, since giving incompatible blood is potentially life-threatening (see Chapter 31).

The nuclear envelope has a double bilayer membrane structure, with the inner and outer layers fused at certain points to form permanent nuclear pores, which allow the passage of large molecules, such as RNA, out of the nucleus. The nucleus is the site of most of the genetic information of the cell. It contains a discrete area known as the nucleolus, which is not enclosed by a membrane but is detectable because of its high density. The nucleolus contains large numbers of granules that are rich in RNA, and it is the site of ribosome synthesis. Ribosomes, the sites for protein synthesis, are often found on the outer face of the nuclear envelope.

CELLULAR JUNCTIONS

Adjacent cells may be linked via specialized structures in the plasma membrane. These structures play a vital role in holding the cells of tissue systems together. The three main types are illustrated in Figure 1.3.

The plasma membranes of adjacent cells may be pulled together by bands of junctional proteins, which fix together like Velcro. These are known as tight junctions. The proteins are firmly anchored into each cell by protein fibres, forming a 'seam weld' between the cells. Tight junctions form an impermeable barrier between cells; they are found in epithelium that lines the gut and the kidney nephrons, where leakage of materials between cells must be avoided so that transport across the epithelium is controlled by the permeability properties of the cells themselves.

Gap junctions are permanent pores in the plasma membrane. They join neighbouring cells. They are formed by proteins that assemble to form connecting 'pipes' with a pore diameter of 2 nm. This allows small molecules to move freely between connected cells. Gap junctions are found in tissues where a close co-ordination between cells is needed, such as in muscle cells lining the gut (for peristalsis) and cardiac muscle cells (for atrial and ventricular contraction). A tissue that is composed of cells that are interconnected in this way is called a syncytium. Damage to a cell in a syncytium leads to an influx of calcium, which causes the proteins of the junction to twist, thereby sealing the gap and protecting the other linked cells.

Desmosomes fix neighbouring cells together through base plates on the inner face of each membrane. These are anchored with protein 'roots' that run into the cytosol of each cell. Desmosomes occur in tissues that are subject to expansion and contraction, in order to spread the forces throughout the tissue – typical examples include the skin and muscular organs such as the heart and uterus. The adjacent plasma membranes are separated by a gap filled with a dense fibrous material.

MEMBRANE RECEPTORS

Some proteins on the outer surface of plasma membranes act as receptor sites for hormones such as insulin, glucagon, and adrenaline – the first messengers. When these hormones bind, they trigger the production or release of a second messenger that will stimulate a response inside the cell. Binding may allow an ion such

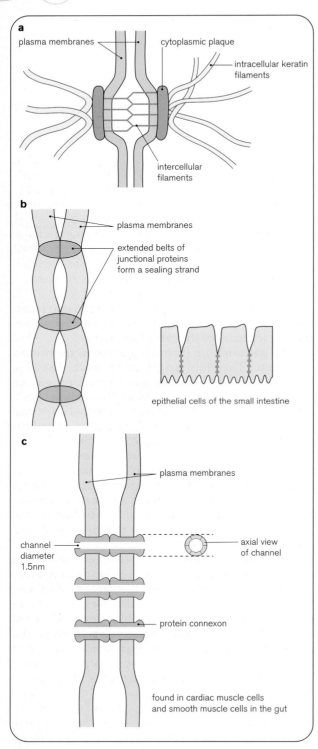

Figure 1.3 Cellular junctions. (a) Desmosome, found in cardiac muscle, skin epithelium, and neck of uterus. (b) Tight junction, found in epithelial cells of the small intestine. (c). Gap junction, found in cardiac muscle and smooth muscle cells in the gut.

as calcium to move into the cell, where it acts as a second messenger. In other cases, cyclic AMP is produced (see above). An example of the cyclic AMP system in action is the rapid breakdown of glycogen to form glucose for energy that happens in response to the release of the hormone adrenaline (e.g. in response to fear or anxiety).

MEMBRANE TRANSPORT

The plasma membrane acts as a selectively permeable barrier to the movement of substances in and out of the cell. Since the bilayer structure presents an essentially lipid (hydrophobic) barrier, lipid-soluble substances are transported more readily than water-soluble ones. Water solubility is associated with charged (ionic) species (also known as electrolytes), whereas uncharged species tend to be lipid soluble and hydrophobic. The terms 'polar' and 'non-polar' are commonly used to describe the presence or absence of charge. Hence sodium chloride, which is composed of sodium ions (Na^+) and chloride ions (Cl^-), is very water soluble and polar, whereas fats contain long, non-polar hydrocarbon chains and so are insoluble in water.

The other important property in membrane permeability is molecular size – small molecules such as water (H_2O) and ammonia (NH_3) can permeate membranes even though they are not lipid soluble. The presence of proteins in the plasma membrane provides another important route for the selective transport of specific solutes. The transport of any substance may occur by 'pinching off' sections of membrane to form packages or vesicles by the processes of exocytosis and endocytosis.

EXOCYTOSIS AND ENDOCYTOSIS

Large molecules and particles move across membranes by the processes of exocytosis and endocytosis. In exocytosis, the materials are packaged into vesicles, which fuse with the plasma membrane and release their contents. In endocytosis, a section of the membrane is internalized to form a vesicle containing solutes and fluid (pinocytosis) or solid particles such as micro-organisms, inorganic materials, or cellular debris (phagocytosis).

Pinocytosis occurs continuously in the cells that line the blood capillaries, where it is used to transport serum from the blood to the fluid surrounding the capillaries. The most important phagocytic cells are the neutrophils and the macrophages (meaning, literally, 'big eaters'), which make up around 70 per cent of circulating white cells. Carbohydrates on the surface of cells act as recognition sites for phagocytes and may activate or inhibit

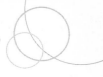

phagocytosis. Red blood cells are rapidly broken down in the spleen if the sugar (i.e. sialic acid) is removed from their surface, while some bacteria, such as *Streptococcus pneumoniae*, are protected from attack by immune cells by their polysaccharide capsule. Macrophages readily ingest solids such as carbon, silica, and lead particles, and they play a major role in protecting the alveoli in the lungs from particulate matter. In most cells the vesicles formed from phagocytosis fuse with lysosomes to allow digestion of their contents (see Chapter 22). Macrophages that phagocytose and become overloaded with fat have been implicated in the thickening and fat deposition that is found in blood vessel walls of patients with atheroma (see Chapter 32).

Exocytosis leads to an increase in the surface area of the plasma membrane; this is normally balanced by the opposite process of endocytosis, in which membrane sections are pinched off to form internal vesicles. Consequently, there is a constant turnover of all membrane components. In lactation, the balance is achieved by a neat, alternative mechanism. The milk protein casein is secreted by exocytosis from mammary gland cells, but the lipid droplets are released enclosed in a vesicle that is pinched off from the plasma membrane, so that the total plasma membrane area is maintained.

PASSIVE TRANSPORT ACROSS MEMBRANES
Simple Diffusion

All ions and molecules are in a state of continuous motion and tend to move in order to equalize their concentration, a process known as simple diffusion. The molecules move from an area of high concentration to an area of low concentration in order to achieve a state of equilibrium. Where there is a plasma membrane separating two fluids (e.g. cells immersed in blood), the rate of diffusion is limited by the properties of the membrane. Thus small molecules (such as oxygen and carbon dioxide in the alveoli) and non-polar solutes diffuse rapidly, whereas polar solutes diffuse only slowly, if at all.

Osmosis

Osmosis is the diffusion of water across a selectively permeable membrane from an area of higher water concentration to an area of lower water concentration. This happens where a non-penetrating dissolved solute (e.g. sugar or salt) is present in a higher concentration on one side of the membrane than the other:

The movement of water represents a force known as osmotic pressure; the amount of movement is related

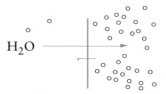

H_2O

o = dissolved solute

to the difference in concentration of dissolved solute on either side of the membrane. Some solutes (e.g. sodium chloride) are composed of two ions (Na^+ and Cl^-) and will therefore exert twice the osmotic pressure of a solute like glucose, which does not break up into ions.

Body fluids have the same osmotic concentration as 0.9 g sodium chloride dissolved in 100 ml water (0.9% saline (w/v = weight in volume)). This solution is sometimes referred to as isotonic saline. Isotonic dextrose solution, on the other hand, has a concentration of 5% (w/v). Therefore, solutions given as an intravenous infusion generally have the same osmotic concentration as the body fluids themselves and this concentration will depend on the solute or solutes present in the infusion. When blood proteins (e.g. serum albumin) are lost as a result of starvation, the osmotic pressure of the blood falls, so water moves by osmosis from the blood into the interstitial fluid, which bathes the tissues. This results in fluid accumulation and swelling, known as oedema (see also Box 1.1 and Chapter 2).

Carrier-Mediated Diffusion

In carrier-mediated diffusion, the presence of a carrier molecule aids the diffusion of a substance that is unable to penetrate the lipid bilayer membrane because of its size or solubility. The simplest carriers, known as uniports, transport just one type of molecule or ion. Symport carriers transport two molecules across the membrane in one direction. Antiport carriers can transport them in both directions – in or out of the cell (Figure 1.4).

A difference in concentration on either side of the membrane is the driving force for membrane transport. In the case of glucose, cells use a uniport system to absorb glucose from the blood, where the concentration of glucose is higher. However, glucose absorption from the gut and kidney tubules occurs together with sodium ions by means of a symport carrier. In this way, the high concentration of sodium ions in the gut or kidney tubule is used to aid the uptake of glucose, which is present at much lower concentrations. Antiport carriers are important in maintaining the correct pH (hydrogen ion concentration) inside cells. As the levels of hydrogen ions (H^+) in the cell rise and the pH falls, hydrogen ions are exchanged for sodium ions to bring the level of hydrogen ions down to within normal physiological limits. An example of an antiport carrier is found in the plasma membrane of red blood cells, which exchanges chloride ions for bicarbonate ions (HCO_3^-). The removal of bicarbonate ions in exchange for chloride ions is stimulated when pH levels in the red blood cell rise above normal. This carrier plays an important role in the transport of carbon dioxide, most of which is converted to bicarbonate in these red blood cells.

When cells need to accumulate or expel solutes across the plasma membrane against a concentration gradient, energy is expended; this is known as active transport. In situations where carrier-mediated transport relies on existing concentration gradients it may be regarded as a passive process – facilitated diffusion – in which no additional energy expenditure is involved. In some cases, however, the concentration gradient may have been generated by an active process requiring energy expenditure. A good example of this is the absorption of glucose into the intestinal epithelium, which requires a symport driven by sodium ions for uptake and which is then transported into the blood by facilitated diffusion. The process relies on a sodium ion concentration gradient being maintained by an active pump that expels sodium ions into the extracellular fluid in exchange for potassium ions (K^+). The epithelial cells of the gut are linked by tight junctions to prevent leakage between cells and to retain the membrane proteins in the correct zone on the cell surface.

This example illustrates the importance of sodium ions in absorption from the gut, since loss of electrolytes (ions) from the gut as a result of diarrhoea will reduce glucose uptake. The use of solutions of glucose and important electrolytes (oral rehydration therapy) is a cheap and effective method for restoring gut absorption processes in this situation.

Filtration

Filtration is a process by which hydrostatic pressure forces small-sized molecules through a selectively permeable membrane. It happens when the pressure on one side of the membrane is greater than the other side. However, it is still a passive process, since ATP is not involved in the filtration process. Filtration occurs in capillary beds where there are permeable blood vessel walls (e.g. in the glomeruli of the kidney). In health, large plasma proteins do not pass across capillary walls. However, where there is damage to the capillary bed, larger molecules are allowed to pass through; hence in patients with glomerulonephritis, protein and antibody molecules may be detected in the urine.

Dialysis

Dialysis is a process whereby smaller molecules and particles are allowed to pass across an artificial selectively permeable membrane while larger molecules and particles are retained. Dialysis does not occur naturally in the body, but it is the mechanism used in renal dialysis for patients with renal failure (see Person-Centred Study: Renal Dialysis).

ACTIVE TRANSPORT

Active transport is mediated by carriers that are directly linked to an energy source such as the metabolism of ATP to adenosine diphosphate (ADP) and phosphate.

BOX 1.1 EXCESS WATER IN THE LUNGS

It has been observed if fresh water is inhaled as a result of accidental submersion, there is more cellular damage to the lungs than there is if sea water is inhaled. The water molecules in fresh water permeate the cell membrane and burst the alveolar cells more rapidly because of the greater concentration gradient of dissolved salts present inside the cells compared to outside. An additional problem is the failure of the alveoli to reinflate as a result of the loss of lung surfactant, so water molecules stick to each other, collapsing the alveoli instead of wetting the lung surfaces. The use of artificial lung surfactant compounds are sometimes of benefit here. Surfactants are also often used to improve lung function in preterm babies, in whom a failure to produce sufficient surfactant creates a similar problem.

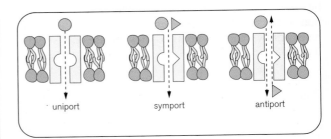

Figure 1.4 Carrier-mediated transport. This can be via a uniport (providing transport in one direction), a symport (providing transport of two molecules on one direction), and an antiport (providing transport of two molecules in two directions, e.g. exchange).

A favourable concentration gradient (high to low) is not required and transport normally occurs in one direction. A prime example of active transport is that mediated by the enzyme sodium–potassium ATPase, commonly known as the sodium pump.

The sodium pump is found in the plasma membrane and acts as a carrier and an enzyme. The pump consumes 30 per cent of a cell's energy expenditure, which is an indication of its metabolic significance. The main function of the sodium pump is to maintain an osmotic balance between the intracellular fluid and the extracellular fluid. As a result of metabolic activity, cells accumulate large amounts of amino acids, sugars, and other small molecules that are polar and attract oppositely charged ions. In addition, cells contain large numbers of protein molecules, which also carry electrical charges. Overall, an excess of osmotically active substances accumulates inside the plasma membrane, so water will tend to enter the cell by osmosis (because there are more water molecules outside the cell than inside it). The sodium pump actively expels sodium ions, thereby helping to maintain an equal concentration of osmotically active species inside and outside of the cell in order to limit water uptake and to control cell volume.

Plant and bacterial cells cope with osmotic problems in a much simpler way; they have an external cell wall, which physically restrains any increase in cell volume. Inhibitors of the sodium pump can cause animal cells to swell up and burst (lysis of the cell).

A well-studied sodium pump inhibitor is ouabain, a drug that strengthens heart contraction and has been used in the treatment of congestive cardiac failure. Largely as a result of the activity of the sodium pump, intracellular levels of sodium ions are relatively low (15 mmol/l) compared to extracellular levels (150 mmol/l), whereas intracellular levels of potassium ions are relatively high (150 mmol/l) compared to extracellular levels (5 mmol/l). The sodium and potassium levels in blood are maintained within strict limits by the homeostatic mechanisms of the body. Inadequate functioning of these mechanisms can lead to adverse consequences. For instance, with hyperkalaemia (raised serum potassium), abdominal cramps, gastrointestinal disturbances, and even cardiac arrest may occur (see Chapter 6).

A closely related enzyme carrier is the calcium pump, calcium ATPase, which is found in the membrane of the sarcoplasmic reticulum (a specialized form of internal membrane that stores calcium in muscle cells). The calcium pump couples the hydrolysis of ATP to the transport of calcium ions. Similar systems are used to control cytosol levels of calcium in other cell systems.

PERSON-CENTRED STUDY: RENAL DIALYSIS

Abdul was in chronic renal failure and required a kidney transplant. While waiting for a suitable graft, renal dialysis was necessary to filter his blood in order to remove nitrogenous wastes and maintain a normal fluid and electrolyte balance. There was a choice: was it to be haemodialysis or continuous ambulatory peritoneal dialysis (CAPD)? In both instances the blood would be allowed to make contact with a selectively permeable membrane, with a fluid of suitable osmotic concentration and solute composition on the other side. Then the passive processes of diffusion and osmosis would allow the blood composition to return to within normal limits (see Chapter 36).

In haemodialysis the blood is pumped through cellophane tubing with the dialysate solution flowing on the other side of the membrane. It requires patients either to attend a haemodialysis unit regularly, which is time-consuming, or to have a room specially designated in their home for the equipment. But Abdul had a large family and could not spare the space in his house, and he also had to continue working. Accordingly, CAPD was considered the most appropriate form of dialysis. In this method, the peritoneal membrane lining the abdominal cavity is used to act as the selectively permeable membrane. The dialysis fluid (dialysate) is introduced into the abdominal cavity via a Tenkoff catheter. Waste solutes and excess electrolytes diffuse across into the dialysate. Excess water is removed from the plasma by osmosis, for the dialysate solution is hypertonic. The CAPD method of dialysis allows a more regular clearing of waste products while maintaining normal daily activity, but it carries a risk of peritonitis.

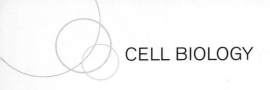

CELL BIOLOGY

Ion Channels

Plasma membranes of plant and animal cells contain ion channels, which are water-filled pores. Their primary function is to allow the selective transport of ions (mainly sodium, potassium, calcium, and chloride) without the expenditure of energy. Transport through ion channels requires a favourable concentration gradient (high to low) and can be up to 100 times faster than using carriers. A feature of most animal cells is the so-called potassium-leak channels, which make the plasma membrane much more permeable to potassium than to other ions. Some ion channels have gates that open and close in response to a variety of stimuli, and therefore there is a difference in the electrical charges between the inside and outside of the membrane. This occurs, for example, when nerve impulses are being transmitted along an axon (see Chapter 10).

CELLULAR ORGANELLES

Cellular organelles and examples of types of cells in which they are found are listed in Box 1.2.

Ribosomes and Protein Synthesis

The organization and function of ribosomes is remarkably uniform in all prokaryotic and eukaryotic cells. Ribosomes are large complexes of ribosomal RNA (rRNA) and protein, and they provide the catalytic site for protein synthesis. The ribosomes of eukaryotic cells are composed of one large unit and one small unit, giving them a 'cottage loaf' appearance. Free ribosomes are found in the cytosol, where they produce proteins that are destined for use inside the cell and are especially abundant in cells such as the reticulocytes. Here, for example, they produce the oxygen-carrying protein haemoglobin as the reticulocytes (immature red blood

---

BOX 1.2 CELLS AND ORGANELLES

Mitochondria are most abundant in cells with a high energy expenditure:
> adjacent to the contractile elements of muscle cells
> at the base of the sperm flagellum
> in liver cells
> in the epithelium of the proximal convoluted tubule in the nephron

Ribosomes, rough endoplasmic reticulum, and Golgi are abundant in cells concerned with protein synthesis and secretion:
> liver cells
> the cell body of nerve cells, where the neurotransmitters are synthesized
> zymogenic cells of the stomach, pancreatic acinar cells, and other enzyme-secreting cells
> intestinal absorptive cells
> goblet (mucus-secreting) cells

Smooth endoplasmic reticulum and Golgi are common in cells concerned with lipid synthesis and secretion and with detoxification:
> adrenal cortex
> interstitial cells of the testis
> liver cells
> intestinal absorptive cells

> parietal cells in the gastric mucosa, which secrete hydrochloric acid (HCl) and intrinsic factor for vitamin B12 absorption

Lysosomes are common in phagocytic cells:
> white blood cells such as macrophages
> osteoclasts

Tight junctions and desmosomes are common in epithelial cells and prevent leakage of substances between cells and hold tissues together:
> gastric mucosal cells, which prevent penetration of hydrochloric acid
> intestinal mucosal cells
> cells lining the kidney tubules
> cardiac cells

Gap junctions allow communication between cells in a tissue system:
> cardiac muscle cells
> smooth muscle cells of the gut lining

Cells lacking internal organelles are those with little active metabolic activity:
> red blood cells

cells with some nuclear material) develop into red blood cells (mature blood cells with no nucleus).

Bound ribosomes are attached to membranes inside the cell to form rough endoplasmic reticulum (RER). Most of the proteins produced here are either destined for export from the cell or are incorporated into a membrane (e.g. cell surface receptor molecules). These proteins pass into the endoplasmic reticulum (ER) and remain packaged inside membrane vesicles until they leave the cell via a distinct pathway (see below).

Liver cells use bound ribosomes to produce large amounts of blood proteins such as albumin, which are secreted into the blood, but they also have many free ribosomes, which the cells use to produce the proteins that are needed to support their active metabolism.

The synthesis of proteins from the individual amino acids takes place on the ribosome. Each ribosome has three binding sites – one binding site is for messenger RNA (mRNA), which bears the coding information for the order of the amino acids; and two further binding sites are for transfer RNA (tRNA) molecules, which bring specific amino acids for addition to the growing chain of amino acids (peptide). Ribosomes move along the mRNA, 'reading' the genetic code, thus ensuring that the amino acids are added in the correct order. If the amino acids were not added in the correct order, a mutant, non-functional protein could be produced (see Chapter 7). The ribosome becomes detached from the mRNA when the peptide chain is complete. Several ribosomes can use a mRNA molecule at once, rather like a production line, forming a polysome (i.e. a 'string' of ribosomes):

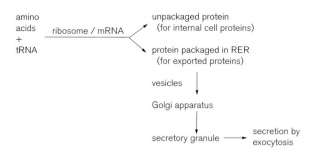

Endoplasmic Reticulum

Endoplasmic reticulum is composed of a series of interconnecting membranous tubes and flattened sacs (lamellae). The outer surfaces of the flattened areas may be studded with ribosomes, and this is known as rough endoplasmic reticulum (RER). The tubular areas without ribosomes are known as smooth endoplasmic reticulum (SER). ER is constantly synthesized and turned over, and the total amount can increase or decrease according to the needs of the cell. RER is concerned primarily with the synthesis of proteins destined for the plasma membrane (e.g. receptor proteins) or for export from the cell (e.g. secreted proteins such as enzymes). For example, the cytosol of the acinar cells of the pancreas, which produce and secrete digestive enzymes, is packed with RER. Secretory proteins pass into the lumen of the RER, where the polypeptide chains become folded and sugar residues may be added, a process known as glycosylation. Membrane and secretory proteins are then budded off in transport vesicles that fuse with the Golgi apparatus.

Regular intake of alcohol can lead to a rapid proliferation of ER in human liver cells (hepatocytes), since the liver is the primary site for ethanol metabolism (see Chapter 2). SER is concerned mainly with lipid synthesis, and hence extensive SER is found in cells of the adrenal cortex, where steroid hormones are synthesized from cholesterol. In the hepatocytes, the SER is involved in the mobilization of stored glucose and in a variety of reactions for the detoxification of foreign substances in the body (e.g. drugs) (see Chapter 9).

The Golgi Apparatus and Secretory Vesicles

The Golgi is composed of a series of flattened membranous sacs or cisternae, (typically between four and six in number), arranged into a fairly regular stack like a pile of saucers. Vesicles from the ER join the Golgi on one side and vesicles containing products for export are pinched off from the opposite side. The Golgi is particularly abundant in secretory cells that synthesize and release lipoproteins into the blood (e.g. liver cells) – the main lipid transport mechanism, and cells such as the goblet cells within the gut lining which secrete mucous (a polysaccharide–protein complex). In the Golgi, sugar residues (mainly galactose, fructose, and sialic acid) may be added to incoming molecules to synthesize glycoproteins and proteoglycans (compounds that are predominantly polysaccharide, with some protein). Polysaccharides are also produced here and secreted in vesicles, including hyaluronic acid found in connective tissue, and chondroitin sulphate, a component of cartilage. Two routes may be taken by secreted proteins, they may be either:
- packaged in vesicles and secreted continuously; or
- stored in secretory vesicles and released only in response to a specific stimulus (e.g. pancreatic enzymes released following a meal).

Calcium ions are involved in the mediation of many secretory processes; the degranulation of mast cells to release histamine in the allergic response is a well-studied example (see Chapter 26). Similarly, a rise in blood glucose concentrations stimulates a rise in intracellular calcium ion levels in the beta-cells of the pancreas, with the subsequent release of insulin by exocytosis (see

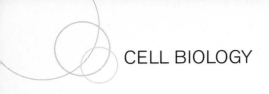

Chapter 35). Vesicles formed when materials are taken into the cell by endocytosis fuse with enzyme-filled vesicles from the Golgi to form endolysosomes. The endolysosomes then undergo membrane changes and lower their pH to form mature lysosomes, where the digestion of the absorbed materials takes place.

Lysosomes

Lysosomes are vesicles that contain around 40 hydrolytic enzymes. These enzymes work best at around pH 5. The pH of the cytosol, at 7.2, is different from that of the lysosome, and thus the enzymes would have a low activity if they were released. This is a safety mechanism to prevent cell autolysis. The acidic conditions of the lysosome are maintained by an ATP-dependent pump in the lysosome membrane. Lysosomal enzymes possess a chemical marker, mannose 6-phosphate, which enables them to be recognized, sorted, and packaged into lysosomes.

Lysosomes are involved in the recycling of cellular organelles, which is a continuous process; in extreme cases following cell damage or death, it is known as autophagy. Whole organelles are enclosed in a membrane to form an isolation vesicle, which then fuses with a lysosome to form an autophagic vesicle where breakdown occurs (see Box 1.3).

In liver cells, the life span of a mitochondrion is 10–12 days, and the life span of a ribosome is around 10 days. During starvation and the repair which follows injury, these recycling processes proceed even faster.

Osteoclasts, the giant multinucleated cells responsible for the breakdown and resorption of bone, use lysosomes to carry out their functions (see Chapter 39).

Specialized cells such as phagocytes e.g. macrophages, engulf foreign bodies such as micro-organisms and are degraded by lysosome action. The lysosomes in these cells contain the enzyme lysozyme, which degrades the carbohydrate component of bacterial cell walls. Hydrogen peroxide is also an effective agent against micro-organisms, for when immune cells do not produce it effectively there is an increased incidence of bacterial and fungal infections. This is amply demonstrated in children who suffer from chronic granulomatous disease, which is an inherited immunodeficiency disease (see Chapter 28).

Some materials ingested by lysosomes are not degradable, and as cells age, inactive debris-filled lysosomes called residual bodies may accumulate. In long-lived cells, such as nerve and muscle cells, these are known as lipofuscin granules. It is questionable whether these play a significant role in the ageing process (see Chapter 4).

Peroxisomes

Peroxisomes are small vesicles bounded by a single membrane. They are the site of reactions that require molecular oxygen. Such reactions are potentially toxic since they may involve the formation of hydrogen peroxide, a powerful oxidant and a precursor of chemically reactive species known as free radicals. An enzyme called catalase is present, and this removes hydrogen peroxide by converting it to water and oxygen. Free radicals attack biological molecules, particularly lipids, as they become degraded via a process called peroxidation. The toxicity of organic solvents (e.g. chloroform and carbon tetrachloride, as used by laboratories, in dry-cleaning fluids) and the tissue destruction associated with the disease rheumatoid arthritis also involve free radical reactions (see Chapters 4 and 27). It is noteworthy that peroxisomes also play a minor role in the oxidation of foreign substances such as ethanol.

Mitochondria

Mitochondria are large membranous organelles, about the same size as many bacteria. They are the centre for energy metabolism and oxygen use in the cell, and they are abundant in metabolically active cells such as muscle fibres. The smooth outer membrane is half protein and half lipid, and it is separated from the inner membrane by the intermembrane space. The inner membrane is folded to form cristae that increase the surface area for their associated enzymes.

The most intense metabolic activity occurs in the central matrix, which is the site of the citric acid cycle. The inner membrane (which is 80 per cent protein) is the site of oxidative phosphorylation (the production of ATP from ADP and phosphate, using oxygen). In the mitochondrion, pyruvate (a metabolite formed from the breakdown of glucose), is converted to carbon dioxide and water in a process that is coupled to the

---

BOX 1.3 INHERITED DISORDERS OF LYSOSOMAL FUNCTION

Disorders of lysosome function may present when lysosomal enzymes are missing. Tay–Sach's disease is an inherited disorder in which the enzyme hexosaminidase A is absent, causing substances called gangliosides to accumulate in brain cells and nerve axons. This leads to progressive degeneration of the nervous system and death by the age of 3 years.

production of ATP. In this way, cells convert the energy locked in glucose to a more usable chemical form. When ATP is broken down into ADP and phosphate, the energy released is used to drive energy-requiring processes such as the synthesis of proteins, fats, and polysaccharides, from simple biological molecules. (see Chapter 2).

Brown fat is most abundant in the neonate and in mammals that hibernate. It is composed of cells that contain many very large mitochondria. Therefore, the energy production of these cells becomes separated from ATP production, and the energy is released as heat (thermogenesis). Thus, brown fat plays an important part in maintaining body temperature in neonates and may be involved in maintaining body weight in adults by 'burning off' excess energy as heat.

The Cytoskeleton

A complex network of proteins called the cytoskeleton permeates the cytosol of the cell and provides a framework for cellular structure and function. Microtubules are the largest components of the cytoskeleton. They consist of hollow filaments made of the protein tubulin. These filaments are important in maintaining cell shape and providing channels for the transport of substances throughout the cell. They have a key role in the structure and movement of cilia and flagellae, and in the formation of the mitotic spindle for the separation of chromosomes during cell division. Cellular organelles and the plasma membrane are associated with a fine network of interlinked filaments known as the microtrabecular lattice, which limits their movement and orientation. Cytosolic enzymes are linked to the lattice to allow ordered sequences of biochemical reactions within the cell.

Twisted strands of the protein actin, which have contractile properties, form microfilaments that allow cells to change shape – the amoeboid movement of leukocytes in the blood is a good example of this. Similarly, muscle cells contain myosin microfilaments, which together with the actin microfilaments provide the basis of muscular contraction. Microfilaments are also found as the structural element of microvilli, which increase the surface area for absorption of the epithelia lining the kidney tubules and the small intestine. A single epithelial cell in this part of the gut can have as many as 3000 microvilli.

MEMBRANE POTENTIALS

Ions and other charged molecules are present inside cells and outside in the extracellular fluid that bathes the cells. Positive and negative charges are not usually evenly distributed on either side of the cell membrane, and this leads to a charge difference across the membrane – the membrane potential. This potential is the key to the function of specialized tissues such as muscle and nerve.

Why do cells have this uneven charge distribution on either side of the plasma membrane? Partly because the sodium pump ejects three sodium ions for every two potassium ions taken into the cell, but mainly because potassium ions continuously leak out of cells from a higher concentration inside the cell to a lower concentration outside. This means that there are bound to be more positive charges outside the plasma membrane than inside it.

Resting Membrane Potential

Where there is an equal distribution of positive and negative charges on either side of a membrane, then there will be no charge difference across the membrane. However, a tiny excess of positive ions on one side and negative ions on the other will produce a charge difference known as a resting membrane potential. This charge difference is usually between -20 mV and -200 mV, with the positive charge on the outside of the plasma membrane. Nerve and muscle cells have a resting potential of around -70 mV. Although this voltage seems very low, because cell membranes are so thin, the membrane proteins are exposed to powerful electrical fields, which affect their shape, and in turn affect the movement of ions across the membrane.

Action Potentials

Non-stimulated nerve cells have a resting membrane potential as a result of the uneven distribution of charges inside and outside of the membrane. Excitation of these cells leads to brief changes in their membrane potential (depolarization) and this change in membrane potential moves quickly along the plasma membrane and may be passed on to neighbouring cells. These changes are known as action potentials, and sodium and potassium ions move in and out of the cell in a well defined sequence of events.

First, sodium ions move into the cell through voltage-gated ion channels, reversing the membrane potential from -70 mV to around $+50$ mV, and the membrane becomes depolarized. These ion channels are closed when the membrane is in its resting state, but open up as the membrane depolarizes; this lets in even more sodium ions. However, as the membrane depolarizes further, the channels close, blocking any further entry of sodium ions. Now it is the turn for potassium ions to diffuse out from a higher concentration inside the cell to a lower concentration outside through leak channels, which slowly open as the membrane depolarizes. This movement of potassium ions restores the original membrane potential so the voltage-gated channels return to their resting form (i.e. repolarization). Until this happens (an elapsed time of several milliseconds) the membrane cannot be depolarized again and an action potential cannot therefore be generated. This delay is known as the refractory period. In the longer term, the action of the sodium pump restores the original distribution of sodium and potassium ions, which was upset by the action potential.

Depolarization of one area of a membrane triggers the depolarization of neighbouring areas, so that a wave of depolarization (the action potential) sweeps along the cell membrane. Nonetheless, the stimulus must be of sufficient strength to set off depolarization; below this point (the threshold), the axon will not be excited. However, if a weak stimulus (below the threshold) is repeated multiple times, the effect can be cumulative, so ultimately the nerve will react and transmit an impulse. Although the size of the response by the axon is independent of the intensity of one stimulation, the stimulus must be strong enough for a nerve impulse to be transmitted (i.e. it is an all-or-none phenomenon).

Myelinated nerves propagate action potentials around 50 times faster than unmyelinated nerves because their axons are surrounded by a myelin sheath derived from glial cells. These wrap around the axon concentrically, forming a fatty insulating layer in sections about 1 mm long, leaving exposed the sections of axon in between. These exposed areas are the nodes of Ranvier. The nerve impulse generated in a nodal region triggers a new action potential at the next node, so it is rapidly transmitted along the axon because it jumps from node to node. The symptoms of neurodegenerative disorders such as multiple sclerosis may result from loss of myelin and the consequent impairment of nerve conduction (see Chapter 38).

Synapses

Synapses are specialized cell junctions for the transmission of a nerve impulse between adjacent nerve cells or between nerve cells and other tissues such as muscle cells or glands. Unlike action potential, the transmission at the synapse is a chemical one, which is much slower and uses calcium ions and neurotransmitters. The end of the axon is expanded to form a synaptic knob containing synaptic vesicles, which store neurotransmitter molecules (e.g. acetylcholine) that have been synthesized in the presynaptic neurone. The presynaptic membrane contains calcium ion channels, which open in response to changes in membrane potential (i.e. they are voltage gated). The postsynaptic membrane contains receptors for the neurotransmitter as well as specific ion channels. A synaptic gap separating the two membranes is too wide for the action potential to jump across to the next cell.

When an action potential reaches the synaptic knob, calcium channels in the membrane open and calcium ions move in, increasing the calcium levels inside and triggering the vesicles to release the neurotransmitter into the synapse. The neurotransmitter binds to the receptors in the postsynaptic membrane, altering their shape. This opens up the ion channels there, generating a new action potential in the postsynaptic cell. Calcium levels are rapidly restored by the action of the calcium pump and uptake by cell organelles.

All synapses must have a mechanism to remove the neurotransmitter to switch off the stimulus. At muscle–nerve junctions, the enzyme acetylcholine esterase rapidly removes the neurotransmitter, acetylcholine. A number of toxins (including nerve gases, lead, and certain organophosphate pesticides) affect the nervous system by inhibiting the action of acetylcholinesterase. Inhibitors of this enzyme are also employed clinically to relieve the symptoms of myasthenia gravis sufferers, who have a reduced number of available acetylcholine receptors (see Chapter 27). The receptors for acetylcholine (also known as nicotinic receptors) are blocked by the drugs used as a muscle relaxant during surgery.

CELLS AND TISSUES

Tissues are groups of cells with a common structure and function. The cells are often bound together by extracellular materials, which may be rigid (as in bone), flexible (as in cartilage), or even liquid (as in blood). Tissues may associate to form organs, which are organized for their physiological functions. The four primary groups of tissues that make up organs are epithelia, connective tissue, muscle, and nerve. The gut, for example, is composed of several tissues: it has an epithelial lining and contains connective tissues (including blood), nervous tissue, and muscle layers.

EPITHELIAL TISSUES

The shapes and arrangements of epithelial cells are illustrated in Figure 1.5.

Simple Squamous Epithelium

Simple squamous epithelium consists of a single layer of flattened cells; this layer is very thin and smooth. This type of epithelium is found lining the blood capillaries and the alveoli of the lungs, where it permits the rapid diffusion of solutes and gases.

Stratified Squamous Epithelium

Stratified squamous epithelium has multiple layers of

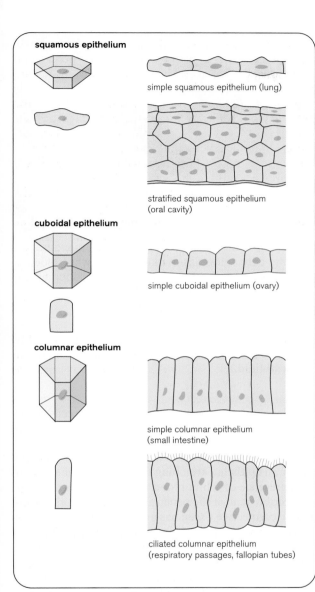

Figure 1.5a Epithelial tissues. Diagramatic representation of types of epithelial cells.

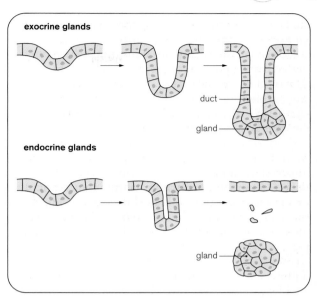

Figure 1.5b Epithelial tissues. An exocrine gland forms from invagination of membranous epithelial cells that remain connected to each other. An endocrine gland forms when this connection is lost, and they secrete substances directly into the blood.

Simple Cuboidal Epithelium

Simple cuboidal epithelium is found lining the cavities of secretory glands such as salivary glands and the thyroid.

Columnar Epithelium

Columnar epithelium contains a single layer of rectangular cells. It is characteristic of the gut lining. In the small intestine, the cells possess projections known as villi, and their membranes have extensions known as microvilli, which increase the surface area for the absorption of digested food and the secretion of digestive enzymes. Some columnar cells have cilia on their surface; these are found, for example, in the Fallopian tubes, where the cilia waft the ovum towards the uterus. Similarly, the cells lining the respiratory passages sweep mucous towards the mouth. Mucus-secreting goblet cells, found in the epithelia of the gut and respiratory passages, are also columnar epithelial cells. Mucus provides protection by trapping particulate matter, such as dust and microbes, which could otherwise enter the lungs. In the stomach it also acts as a barrier against attack by the stomach acid.

Glandular Epithelia

Glandular epithelia form during embryonic development when an epithelial layer becomes invaginated

cells which become increasingly flattened towards the surface of the tissue. The lower layers undergo cell division, while the surface layers may be dead, as in the skin, or remain living, as in the lining of the mouth, oesophagus, and vagina. In each of these, the tissue presents an effective barrier to the penetration of microorganisms. A specialized form known as transitional epithelium is found in the bladder. Here, the rounded surface cells are able to flatten as the bladder fills with urine, allowing its surface area and volume to increase without damage.

and develops its secretory function. The two main types of gland are exocrine and endocrine.

Exocrine glands remain connected to the epithelium by a narrow duct (e.g. sweat glands of the skin, salivary glands of the buccal cavity). During the development of endocrine (ductless) glands, the connection with the epithelium is lost, so the secretory products (in this case hormones) are secreted and diffuse into the extracellular spaces and then into the circulation. The pancreas is unique in that it has both exocrine and endocrine functions: alpha-amylase, lipases, and proteases are secreted into the duodenum via the pancreatic duct, while the endocrine cells of the islets of Langerhans secrete insulin, glucagon, and other hormones that diffuse into the bloodstream (see Chapter 35).

Epithelial Membranes

Epithelia may be organized into membranes covering or lining organ systems. These membranes may also secrete a fluid that aids their protective function. Serous membranes are composed of squamous epithelium that lines enclosed body cavities and surrounds the organs. Pleural membranes line the thorax and surround the lungs, protecting them from abrasion against the ribcage. The visceral pericardia are serous membranes that protect the heart. In both cases, serous fluid is secreted by the membranes to reduce friction. Perforation of the pleural membranes (pneumothorax or collapsed lung) allows air to enter the fluid-filled pleural cavity, causing partial or complete collapse of the affected lung. Pneumothorax may result from broken ribs, or it may occur spontaneously. The peritoneum lines the abdominal cavity, and the mesentery (visceral peritoneum) surrounds the abdominal organs. Again, serous fluid reduces friction between the organs (see Box 1.4).

CONNECTIVE TISSUE

Connective tissues are always composed of cells embedded in an extracellular matrix, often referred to as the 'glue' that binds cells and tissues together (Figure 1.6).

Like epithelial tissue, connective tissue may be organized to form membranes around organ systems. The sac around the heart is the fibrous pericardium, which anchors and limits its expansion within the thorax. The periosteum is a connective tissue membrane covering bones; it contains blood vessels and provides an area of attachment for tendons and ligaments. Skeletal muscles are surrounded by a fascia that anchors the tendons. The superficial fascia are connective tissue membranes containing fat cells; these membranes form a layer between the skin and the muscles. Joints require

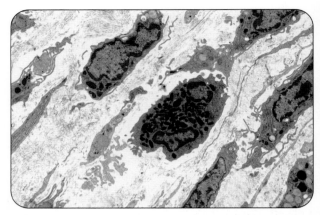

Figure 1.6 Connective tissue. Electron micrograph showing connective tissue that contains white blood cells. The connective tissue matrix and collagen fibres are produced by fibroblasts (× 2000).

lubrication to aid movement, and this is provided by the synovial membranes, which secrete and contain the synovial fluid.

Areolar Connective Tissue

Areolar connective tissue contains fibroblast cells, which produce protein fibres made of collagen and elastin to provide strength and elasticity respectively. 'Loose' areolar connective tissue is found beneath the skin and under all epithelia, attaching them to the tissues below. The presence of white blood cells in the matrix offers protection against the penetration of micro-organisms. Dense connective tissue has a much higher proportion of densely packed fibres. In the fibrous form, these are

BOX 1.4 PERITONITIS

Peritonitis erupts when the peritoneal membranes become inflamed owing to an infection or chemical irritation. A number of clinical conditions can precipitate this; for example, breaching of the gut wall as a result of a perforated peptic ulcer, an inflamed appendix, abdominal wounds, or surgery. Exchange of fluids between the gut and peritoneal cavity occurs, but the peritoneum secretes a viscous fluid that helps to seal off the perforated area. Peritonitis remains a possible cause of mortality following surgery.

mainly collagen; this form is generally found in tendons and ligaments, in the dermis of the skin, and in the outer layers of the larger arteries. In the elastic form, the fibres are mainly elastin, and this accounts for the natural elasticity of the lungs and the larger arteries such as the aorta.

The remaining specialized connective tissues are adipose tissue, cartilage, bone and blood. All the cells in these tissues (as well as in smooth muscle cells) are formed by the differentiation of fibroblast cells.

Adipose Tissue

Adipose tissue consists largely of fat cells (adipocytes), which store triglyceride (fat) in the form of lipid droplets, set in a matrix of collagen fibres. The lipid droplets in the adipocytes may occupy almost the whole cell volume. Adipose tissue is found beneath the dermis of the skin and around body organs. It constitutes the body's main energy store. Furthermore, it provides some thermal insulation and physical protection, particularly in the case of the eyes, the kidneys, and bony protrusions. Fat storage is typically greater in females (around 27 per cent of body mass) than in males (around 15 per cent) but these values are variable and may be markedly reduced in elite athletes and exceeded in obese subjects.

Cartilage

Cartilage consists of cells called chondrocytes set in spaces called lacunae. Chondrocytes secrete a fairly dense matrix that contains fibres but no blood vessels. However, most cartilage is surrounded by a connective tissue layer, the perichondrion, which contains capillaries that supply nutrients to the cartilage. These nutrients have to diffuse through the matrix to the cells. It is a slow process, and consequently damaged cartilage (common in sports injuries) heals very slowly. Softening of cartilage in the joints is known as chondromalacia; this commonly occurs on the inner surface of the patella as a result of overuse in sporting activities and causes pain when climbing or sitting. Rest and isometric exercise are recommended treatments, but surgical removal of the softened tissue may be necessary. Sometimes small pieces of bone or cartilage become detached as a result of injury or excessive use, and surgical removal is required to prevent further abrasion and wear and tear on the articulating surfaces of the joints.

Hyaline cartilage contains mainly collagen fibre. It is found as a cushion on the ends of bones, and in the trachea, nose, and larynx as well as in the embryonic skeleton. Elastic cartilage, found in the ear lobes, contains mainly elastin fibres. Fibrocartilage, which forms the outer layer of the intervertebral discs, is composed mainly of bundles of collagen with fewer chondrocytes. When this band of fibrocartilage gives way, a 'slipped disc' may result as the disc bulges outwards and presses against spinal nerves.

Bone

Bone consists of cells set in an extensive matrix of collagen fibre (to give strength and shock-absorbing properties), together with needle-like crystals of hydroxyapatite (a complex salt of calcium and phosphate), which make bone hard and dense. There are two forms of bone tissue – compact bone and spongy bone. Compact bone contains osteocytes set in concentric rings that surround central canals containing nerves and blood vessels. Osteocytes link to these canals via their cellular extensions, which run through small channels. Spongy bone is made up of calcified collagen and has a less regular structure.

Osteoblasts, which produce the collagen, change and develop into osteocytes when the matrix is calcified. Osteoclast cells degrade spongy bone, releasing calcium into the blood under the influence of parathyroid hormone (see Chapters 35 and 39). Both osteoblasts and osteoclasts are needed in the remodelling of bone during growth and in the repair processes following a fracture. When a bone breaks, blood from nearby injured tissues moves around and into the fracture, producing a haematoma. This provides a framework in which connective tissue cells and capillaries can grow and form granulation tissue, which replaces the clot. Osteoblasts then multiply and make a flexible bridge across the structure. The bridge then develops into a sticky callus and minerals are deposited. As calcification continues, mature bone is formed and it is then the job of the osteoclasts to resorb the callus and finally remove any extra bony callus in order to return the bone to its former shape (remodelling).

Osteoclasts are also responsible for the formation of bone marrow canals during embryonic and fetal life. These canals then become invaded by blood vessels to form red bone marrow, the site where stem cells divide and differentiate into red blood cells, white blood cells, and platelets (see Chapter 31). In adults, red bone marrow remains in the sternum, the vertebrae, the ribs, the base of the skull, and the ends of the long bones; elsewhere, it is replaced by adipocytes to form yellow bone marrow.

Blood

Although blood is a fluid, it is a connective tissue composed of red blood cells (erythrocytes), white blood cells (leukocytes), and platelets (thrombocytes) suspended in a liquid matrix (plasma). Cells occupy 45 per cent of the blood volume in healthy adult males and 42 per cent in healthy adult females; plasma occupies the remaining volume (see Chapter 31). Plasma is mostly water and serves as a solvent and transport medium for the distribution of electrolytes, hormones, and gases around the body.

The most abundant ions are sodium, potassium, and chloride, as well as bicarbonate, which arises from carbon dioxide being dissolved in plasma for its transport to the lungs from the tissues. Other solutes include glucose and amino acids; nitrogenous wastes such as urea; bilirubin (derived from haemoglobin); and creatinine. Proteins are an essential functional constituent of the plasma and are classified into albumins, globulins, and fibrinogen (a component of the blood clotting system). They contribute to the osmotic concentration of plasma, and they control its acidity by acting as buffering agents. Additionally, specialized transport operates for hydrophobic substances including fats, cholesterol, drugs, hormones, and the antibodies of the specific immune system. Some proteins (e.g. angiotensinogen) are hormone precursors, and others (e.g. lipoprotein lipase) are enzymes active in the blood.

Red blood cells are simple, disc-shaped cells with no nucleus or internal organelles. Their primary purpose is to contain the oxygen-carrying protein haemoglobin, which, like the other blood proteins, acts as a buffering agent. Red blood cells also contain the enzyme carbonic anhydrase, which speeds up the interconversion of carbon dioxide and bicarbonate for carbon dioxide transport.

White blood cells are part of the immune system. They are concerned with the destruction of invading micro-organisms, the surveillance and destruction of cancer cells, and the removal of cellular debris from the blood by phagocytosis. Platelets are small cellular fragments that have broken off from huge bone marrow cells called megakaryocytes. They have no nucleus, but unlike red blood cells they are metabolically active cells with internal organelles, and they contain muscle proteins, which enable them to contract. Platelets help to prevent blood loss by plugging damaged blood vessels (see Chapters 22 and 31 and Appendix 2).

MUSCLE

Muscle is a specialized tissue found in almost every organ of the body. All muscles contain two contractile protein filaments, actin and myosin, which are responsible for their contractile properties. There are three types of muscle in humans, which vary in structure depending on their physiological role (Figure 1.7):

- skeletal muscle (also known as striated or voluntary muscle);

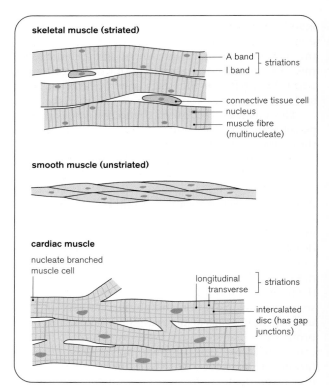

Figure 1.7 Skeletal, smooth, and cardiac muscle.

- smooth muscle (also known as involuntary muscle); and
- cardiac muscle.

Skeletal muscle is composed of long cylindrical cells, and when viewed microscopically, clear bands or striations are evident as a result of the arrangement of actin and myosin filaments. Smooth muscle, which lacks striations, allows the gut, blood vessels, uterus, and iris (in the eye) to have contractile functions. Cardiac muscle is unique to the heart, consisting of columns of highly branched and cross-linked cells, with striations that are fainter than in skeletal muscle. Cardiac and smooth muscle systems are linked by gap junctions (see above), allowing a progressive and controlled contractile response.

NERVOUS TISSUE

Nerve cells or neurones are elongated cells that generate and transmit waves of electrical excitation in the form of action potentials. They generally possess a cell body, which contains the nucleus and intracellular organelles. From the cell body emanate projections called dendrites, which are short, branched processes carrying impulses into the cell. A long, single axon transmits the nerve impulses to the synapses where they are passed on to other cells at the synapses by a chemical process. The axon of a large neurone may be as much as 15 000 nm in diameter and as long as 1 m. Although the cell body has many ribosomes, both free and associated with RER, to synthesize neurotransmitters, there are no ribosomes in the axon. Thus, the cell body must synthesize proteins for the whole cell; for instance, the neurotransmitter molecules are packaged into membrane vesicles that roll along the axon to the synapse.

All neurones are associated with supporting glial cells, which fill the spaces between them. Glial cells are not generally electrically excitable, and unlike neurones they remain capable of dividing throughout their life. Schwann cells wrap themselves around the axon of myelinated nerve fibres to form an insulating sheath; this increases the rate of nerve conduction and fulfils a vital role in the regeneration of damaged nerve cells. In the central nervous system, oligodendrocyte cells can wrap around several different axons, but in the absence of Schwann cells no regeneration of neurones is possible.

KEY POINTS

- Cell membranes are composed of a bilayer of phospholipids, which have a hydrophilic (water-loving) head and a hydrophobic (water-hating) tail.
- Cell membranes act as a selectively permeable barrier and a site for communication with the external environment and the other cells.
- Adjacent cells may be linked via specialized structures in the plasma membrane. These structures play a vital role in holding the cells of tissue systems together and in communication between cells.
- Some proteins on the outer surface of plasma membranes act as receptor sites for hormones such as insulin, glucagon, and adrenaline – the first messengers. When these hormones bind, they trigger the production or release of second messengers, which stimulate a response inside the cell.
- Large molecules and particles move across membranes by the processes of exocytosis and endocytosis. In exocytosis, the materials are packaged into vesicles that fuse with the plasma membrane, releasing their contents. In endocytosis a section of the membrane is internalized to form a vesicle containing solutes and fluid (pinocytosis) or solid particles such as micro-organisms, inorganic materials, or cell debris (phagocytosis).
- Membranes act as a selectively permeable barrier to the movement of substances in and out of the cell. Some mechanisms are passive and do not need an energy source e.g. simple diffusion, osmosis; but active transport requires energy.
- Positive and negative charges are not usually evenly distributed on either side of the cell membrane, and this leads to a charge difference across the membrane called the membrane potential.
- Tissues are groups of cells with a common structure and function. The cells are often bound together by extracellular materials, which may be rigid (as in bone), flexible (as in cartilage). or liquid (as in blood).

FURTHER READING

Alberts B, Bray D, Lewis J, Raff M, Roberts K, Watson JD (1996) Molecular Biology of the Cell, 3rd edition. Garland Publishing Inc, New York, London.

Burkitt HG, Stevens A, Lowe JS, Young B (1996) Wheater's Basic Histopathology: a Colour Atlas and Text, 3rd edition. Churchill Livingstone, Edinburgh.

Majno G, Joris I (1996) Cells, Tissues and Disease. Principles of General Pathology. Blackwell Science, Oxford.

Sherwood L (1995) Fundamentals of Physiology – a Human Perspective, 2nd edition. West publishing Co, New York.

Winsberghe D, Noback GR, Carola R (1995) Human Anatomy and Physiology, 3rd edition. McGraw Hill, New York.

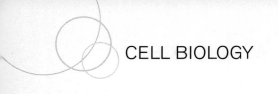

CELL BIOLOGY

CELLULAR ENERGY AND METABOLISM

LEARNING OBJECTIVES

After studying this chapter you will have a clearer understanding of:
- the metabolic processes for the release of usable forms of energy
- the sources of energy in the diet and their sequential use and storage
- the effects of starvation and exercise on the use of energy resources

INTRODUCTION

Metabolism refers to all the biochemical processes occurring within the body. The reactions leading to the biosynthesis of large and complex molecules from simple molecules are collectively known as anabolism (hence the association of anabolic steroids with body building). Conversely, the breakdown of complex biomolecules into their basic chemical components is referred to as catabolism.

A balance must be maintained between all these reactions in order to maintain normal physiological function and a steady body mass – this is termed homeostasis. However, preservation of homeostasis may be disturbed by such things as:
- changes in dietary intake;
- changes in energy expenditure;
- pathological states such as an infection;
- trauma, including surgery.

For instance, a natural response to infection is a rise in body temperature, which results from an increased catabolism; trauma and shock may produce similar dramatic effects (see Chapter 25). In these situations, metabolism adjusts to cope with changing demands.

When the mechanisms that maintain homeostasis are impaired or lost, abnormal metabolic states result. In the case of diabetes mellitus, a failure to produce the hormone insulin (as occurs in insulin-dependent dia-

betes mellitus) or a failure of body cells to respond to insulin (as in non-insulin-dependent diabetes mellitus) means that cells are unable to take in their primary energy source, glucose, from the blood. As a result, fats are catabolized, leading to weight loss and abnormally high levels of compounds called ketones in the blood (ketosis) as metabolism adjusts to provide alternative energy sources to glucose (Figure 2.1).

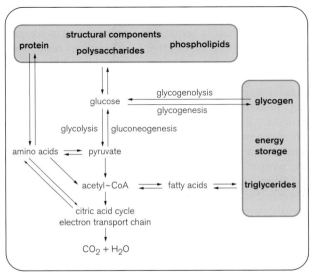

Figure 2.1 Major metabolic pathways.

CELL BIOLOGY

ENERGY METABOLISM

Energy transfer is an important aspect of metabolic pathways, since all chemical processes lead to energy changes. Anabolic processes require energy, which becomes incorporated into large storage molecules such as glycogen (a glucose polymer) and triglycerides (fats). These storage molecules represent the main energy stores in the body. When these compounds are catabolized, they release heat and generate more usable chemical forms of energy. The most significant of these are adenosine triphosphate (ATP), nicotinamide adenine dinucleotide (NAD) and its close relative, nicotinamide adenine dinucleotide phosphate (NADP). NAD and NADP incorporate niacin, one of the B vitamins, in their structures. These molecules are then used to drive anabolic reactions. They have a pivotal role in virtually all biological systems and metabolic pathways, for they are involved in many important energy-transfer reactions.

$$\text{ATP} \rightleftarrows \text{ADP} + \text{phosphate} + \text{energy released}$$
high energy form — for cellular metabolism

The chemical energy stored in ATP is released in this reaction and is used for energy-consuming processes such as muscular contraction. ATP is also required as part of the anabolic reactions that synthesize the body's proteins, fats, carbohydrates, and other components. In cellular respiration, the process is reversed, and the body's energy stores are broken down to provide energy to build up supplies of the ATP. Most ATP is produced in the mitochondria (see Chapter 1).

NAD and NADP also occur in higher and lower energy forms, but the energy is used to carry out the chemical processes of oxidation and reduction occurring inside cells. In oxidation, molecules gain oxygen or lose hydrogen or electrons, whereas in reduction, molecules lose oxygen or gain hydrogen or electrons.

The energy for all body processes comes from the main dietary constituents, carbohydrates (sugars), fats, and proteins. Carbohydrate and protein each yield around 4 kilocalories (kcal) per gram, while a gram of fat contains around 9 kcal. (The kilocalorie is a measure of energy – 1 kcal is the energy needed to raise the temperature of 1 kg of water by 1°C.)

Glucose, the primary energy source for cells, is absorbed into the blood from the small intestine. When supplies are plentiful, it is converted to glycogen (glycogenesis), and stored in the liver (about 100 g) to act as a reservoir in replenishing blood glucose as it is used by the cells. Muscle cells store more glycogen (about 400 g), but they lack the enzyme to release glucose into the blood, so this store can only be used by muscle cells. Fats and proteins can also be metabolized for energy.

Fats are stored in specialized adipose cells (see Chapter 1), but when fats are required as an energy source they are mobilized and released into the blood as fatty acids. The fatty acids are broken down to a molecule called acetyl coenzyme A, releasing usable energy in the form of ATP. From then on, the breakdown of fat and glucose follow a common pathway. Surplus amino acids are also broken down and fed into the cellular respiration pathway.

When energy is required, stored glycogen is broken down to glucose by an enzyme glycogen phosphorylase. This process is called glycogenolysis and may be activated by hormones, for instance by glucagon, the hormone released into the blood by the islets of Langerhans in the pancreas as blood glucose levels fall). Similarly, glycogenolysis can be stimulated by adrenaline released when a sudden increase in energy use is anticipated – the so-called 'flight or fight response'. The overall effect is the release of glucose into the blood from the liver, which acts as a glucose reservoir for other body cells.

CELLULAR RESPIRATION—AEROBIC

When carbohydrates like glucose are catabolized in the presence of oxygen, carbon dioxide and water are formed and energy is released:

$$(CH_2O) + \text{inspired } O_2 \rightarrow \text{expired } CO_2 + H_2O + \text{energy}$$

Like most catabolic processes in metabolism, respiration is, overall, an oxidation process. In practice, cellular respiration involves a complex series of chemical reactions, which can be divided into four distinct stages:
- glycolysis;
- pyruvate decarboxylase complex;
- the citric acid cycle;
- the electron transport chain.

Glycolysis

Glucose (a six-carbon 6C sugar) is broken down into two molecules of pyruvate (i.e. two three-carbon molecules). This pathway is anaerobic (no oxygen is involved) and takes place in the cytosol of the cell. It produces energy in a form that other body systems can use. Thus, every molecule of glucose metabolized generates two molecules of ATP (from ADP and phosphate). In addition, two molecules of NADH (the reduced form of NAD) are also released; these are subsequently diverted along the electron transport chain to generate more ATP.

Pyruvate Decarboxylase Complex

Although this is a single reaction, nevertheless it is a crucial stage in respiration. Pyruvate (a three-carbon molecule) is taken to the mitochondria and broken down to release carbon dioxide (a one-carbon molecule); the remainder of the molecule becomes linked to another molecule, coenzyme A, to form acetyl coenzyme A (acetyl CoA; a two-carbon carrier molecule). The carbon dioxide produced passes into the blood to be expired from the lungs.

The formation of acetyl CoA is a point of convergence in metabolism because it is also formed when fatty acids are broken down for energy. Consequently, glucose and fat catabolism follow a common pathway from this point onwards. Some amino acids are also degraded to pyruvate or acetyl CoA. If a person fasts for more than 24 hours, liver glycogen stores become exhausted and fats become a more important energy source.

As fatty acids are broken down, acetyl CoA accumulates; this triggers its conversion to simple carbon compounds called ketone bodies, which circulate in the blood as another energy source. This is the metabolic state known as ketosis, and the appearance of ketones in the urine is known as ketonuria. The smell of acetone on the breath of ketotic patients is a common feature – it is most commonly noted in people with diabetes and in women during prolonged labour. Several common amino acids, such as tryptophan and lysine, are broken down directly to ketones, contributing to ketosis when proteins are being used as a significant energy source, as is the case in extreme starvation.

Citric Acid Cycle

In a well-nourished person, acetyl CoA (with its two carbons) generally enters the cyclical pathway known as the citric acid cycle (or the Krebs' cycle). This occurs in the centre of the mitochondrion. The two carbons are each converted to carbon dioxide, which is expired from the lungs. The energy released in the cycle is incorporated into the coenzymes NAD and flavin adenine dinucleotide (FAD) which are then converted to higher energy forms (NADH and $FADH_2$) by the addition of hydrogen. These are subsequently diverted into the electron transport chain. [FAD is yet another coenzyme; it is derived from vitamin B2 (riboflavin), an essential dietary component.]

Electron Transport Chain

The energy from metabolism of fuels (carbohydrate, fat, or protein) is locked up in the higher energy forms of the coenzymes NADH and $FADH_2$. This energy needs to be converted into ATP, which is the most usable form of chemical energy, but as there is so much

energy present, it must be released in stages. A series of carrier proteins called cytochromes, found on the inner membrane of the mitochondria, ensure that the transfer is efficient.

Cytochromes have a structure that is rather similar to that of the haemoglobin subunits. They contain either iron or copper. These proteins are an essential component of the electron transport chain. In this process of energy transfer from NADH and $FADH_2$, the hydrogens are removed from the coenzymes to regenerate NAD and FAD which may be reused by the cell. The hydrogen atoms are then split into a hydrogen ion (H^+) plus an electron. Next, the electrons pass along the series of cytochromes, which act as electron carriers. The energy changes associated with the electron transport chain are used to convert ADP (with phosphate) into ATP – this is sometimes referred to as oxidative phosphorylation.

Like most metabolic reactions, the production of ATP from ADP is catalysed by an enzyme, and in this case it is ATP synthase. Each molecule of NADH passing along the electron transport chain leads to formation of three molecules of ATP, and each molecule of $FADH_2$ produces two molecules of ATP. At the end of this pathway, the final electron carrier (called cytochrome a_3) passes on two electrons to an oxygen atom (derived from inspired air), which combines with two hydrogen ions to makes water. This metabolic water (water made in the body) contributes to water balance.

The Need for Oxygen

Both blood haemoglobin and cytochrome a_3 have a high affinity for oxygen, but an even higher affinity for carbon monoxide, which is therefore a potent inhibitor of respiration. In blood, carbon monoxide displaces oxygen from haemoglobin, reducing the delivery of oxygen to the tissues, while inside the respiring cells it will block the electron transport chain and ATP formation by blocking the use of oxygen.

Car exhaust fumes and cigarette smoke are unavoidable environmental sources of carbon monoxide, but severe carbon monoxide poisoning usually results from faulty gas appliances in poorly ventilated areas. The increased risk of heart disease associated with smoking has been attributed to chronic exposure to carbon monoxide. Cyanide poisoning, which typically results from exposure to hydrogen cyanide fumes released in fires, also blocks the electron transport chain by binding chemically to cytochromes, and a number of chemicals (notably nitrophenols) inhibit cellular respiration by uncoupling electron transport from ATP formation.

Overall, 38 molecules of ATP are generated for each molecule of glucose consumed during aerobic respiration, which means that the efficiency of energy transfer from glucose to ATP is about 40%. This process relies on an adequate supply of oxygen at the end of the pathway to maintain the breakdown of pyruvate to carbon dioxide and water, and the production of ATP. Not all cells use oxygen; red blood cells have no mitochondria and therefore no citric acid cycle or electron transport chain, even though they are the cells that carry oxygen to the respiring tissues. There may be a lack of oxygen if the blood circulation to cells is poor or interrupted (see Chapter 3), or if the demand for oxygen exceeds the supply. This can happen during short periods of intense exercise (such as a 100 m sprint) or during prolonged exercise in unfit subjects, who use carbohydrate as their main fuel. In these situations, the much less efficient process of anaerobic respiration takes place. For example, elite athletes use oxygen more efficiently in the muscles and use more fat and less carbohydrate as fuels.

CELLULAR RESPIRATION—ANAEROBIC

When oxygen supplies are inadequate, the electron transport chain and citric acid cycle slow down, so pyruvate tends to accumulate. Therefore, respiration is diverted along another pathway to produce lactate. This is a simple reaction that uses the reduced NAD (NADH) formed earlier in glycolysis. NADH is regenerated back to NAD in the process so it can be used again to keep glycolysis going.

Anaerobic respiration has drawbacks, however. First, only two molecules of ATP are generated for each molecule of glucose converted to lactate (compared to 38 in aerobic respiration). Second, lactic acid is acidic and diffuses out into the blood, causing blood pH to fall, a condition known as lactic acidosis.

Buffer systems in the blood keep the pH within a range that is compatible with life (7.2–7.7; the normal pH range is 7.35–7.45). Increased acidity stimulates central chemoreceptors in the brain stem to prompt an increase in breathing rate. The pH of the blood is closely linked to the ratio of bicarbonate (alkali) to carbon dioxide (acid) that is present in the blood. Breathing more quickly removes carbon dioxide, pushing the pH back up to normal; this is known as compensated lactic acidosis.

Lactic acidosis also occurs in chronic alcoholics, in whom excess NADH is formed as a result of alcohol metabolism; this excess NADH converts pyruvate to lactate.

Lactic acid stimulates nerve endings, causing the muscle pain which accompanies prolonged exercise (cramp). As oxygen levels rise again, some lactate may be converted back to pyruvate, but most of it passes to the liver where it is converted back to glucose (Figure 2.2 and Box 2.1).

BOX 2.1 CRAMP

High levels of lactate are typically found in muscle tissue during strenuous exercise, when energy utilization exceeds the oxygen supply. The surplus pyruvate is diverted along another metabolic pathway, and when lactate is synthesized it results in the sensation of cramp. The process is reversible (indicated by the double arrows) and lactate can be oxidized back to pyruvate as pyruvate is used again.

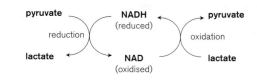

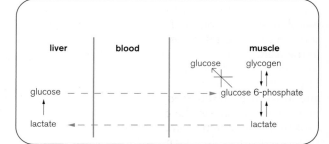

Figure 2.2 The Cori cycle. Lactate in muscle is converted to glucose in the liver.

ENZYMES

Nearly all metabolic reactions are catalysed by enzymes, which function optimally at body temperature (see also Table 2.1). Most enzymes are proteins, but some have prosthetic groups chemically bound to them, such as the iron-containing haem group found on cytochrome P_{450}, the drug-metabolizing enzyme found in liver cells.

In many enzyme systems, cofactors are an essential component of the catalytic process. Coenzymes, derived from the B vitamins, are often required. NAD is the most common coenzyme, and it is involved in many oxidation–reduction reactions, such as the interconversion of pyruvate and lactate by the enzyme lactate dehydrogenase, and the metabolism of alcohol by the enzyme alcohol dehydrogenase.

About one-quarter of enzymes need specific metal ions as cofactors for full activity. Over 100 zinc metallo-

Some Common Clinical Enzyme Assays

Enzyme	Disease Area
acid phosphatase	prostate cancer
alanine aminotransferase	liver, heart
alkaline phosphatase	liver, bone
amylase	pancreas
aspartate aminotransferase	liver, heart
creatine kinase	brain, heart, muscle
glucose 6-phosphate dehydrogenase	red blood cells (genetic deficiency)
lactate dehydrogenase	red blood cells, heart, liver
lipoprotein lipase	hyperlipoproteinaemia

Table 2.1 **Some common clinical enzyme assays.** See Chapter 6 for details of the uses of estimating serum enzymes levels in the diagnosis and treatment of diseases.

enzymes have been recorded, including carbonic anhydrase, which catalyses the carbon dioxide–bicarbonate equilibrium reaction in red blood cells. Copper is another mineral utilized by numerous enzymes, including superoxide dismutase, which removes free radicals from the body. Free radicals are atoms or molecules with an unpaired electron, which makes them intensely chemically reactive and energetic (see Chapters 1 and 4). They have been implicated in many destructive processes, including the breakdown of membrane lipids (peroxidation), and they may also be involved in the formation of atheroma formation in coronary artery disease (see Chapter 32) and in the inflammation that is associated with rheumatoid arthritis (see Chapter 27).

Severe dietary deficiency of these trace metals can cause dramatic symptoms. Zinc deficiency is commonly found in chronic alcoholics. It is characterized by dermatitis and poor wound healing. Copper deficiency may result in anaemia and demineralization of bone, though it is exceedingly rare.

Like all catalysts, enzymes speed up chemical processes by changing the reaction pathway. Most reactions have an energy barrier that must be overcome (the activation energy of the reaction). By changing the reaction route, catalysts avoid the energy barrier, so the reaction proceeds more easily. For instance, an

important protective enzyme found in red blood cells is catalase, which degrades the powerful oxidant hydrogen peroxide into the harmless products of water and oxygen. This reaction is essential because peroxides are a potent source of free radicals. It must be appreciated that enzymes can only speed up a process that is already energetically favourable (higher to lower energy); they are not a source of energy. However, an energetically unfavourable process may be made favourable by incorporating ATP into the reaction as a source of energy.

ENZYME STRUCTURE

Because most enzymes are proteins, they have a highly complex structure. Proteins are composed of a primary chain of amino acids; this chain is coiled to give a helical secondary structure, and this in turn may be folded to give a regular three-dimensional, tertiary structure.

This complex folding provides one or more pockets that are active sites, which are designed either to accommodate one specific substrate molecule (absolute specificity) or a range of substrates of similar size and shape (group specificity). The enzyme structures are held in place by relatively weak attractive forces (charge interactions, hydrogen bonding), which make them susceptible to changes in their environment, particularly to variations in temperature and pH. Because enzyme activity usually demands that they are folded into a precise structure, substances that bind to an enzyme or that interfere with it and change its shape can also affect its activity.

Most enzymes work fastest slightly above body temperature (37°C), so if body temperature rises (as a response to infection, for example), metabolism speeds up. Similarly enzymes can only maintain their active shape over a limited pH range. The destructive enzymes enclosed in lysosomes (see Chapter 1) work optimally at pH 5 and become much less active if released into the cell, where conditions are less acidic. Likewise the digestive enzyme, pepsin (optimum pH 1.5 to 2.5) breaks down proteins in the acid conditions of the stomach but is unstable if placed in water (pH 7). Yet trypsin, which also digests proteins, has an optimum pH of 7.5–8.5 and works in the small intestine.

Lead binds strongly to cysteine, an amino acid found in many enzymes, and permanently inactivates these enzymes by changing their shape. This accounts for many of the symptoms of lead poisoning. Lead inhibits the enzyme ferrochelatase and so blocks the incorporation of iron into haemoglobin. Lead also increases levels of the neurotransmitter acetylcholine by inhibiting acetylcholinesterase in the nerve synapses (see

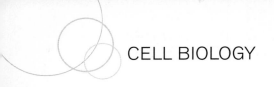
Chapter 1). This enzyme normally metabolizes the neurotransmitter, so lead as its inhibitor causes hyperactivity as the effects of acetylcholine persist.

ENZYME INHIBITORS

Some molecules bind to the active site of the enzyme and inhibit its activity. When the enzyme substrate and inhibitor are of a similar size and shape, both compete (reversibly) for a place in the active site (competitive inhibition).

When the enzyme picks up the inhibitor, this is a 'dead end' because the inhibitor hinders the uptake of substrate and slows the reaction. Alternatively, an inhibitor may bind to a nearby site and block the entrance of the substrate in or out of the active site. This is known as non-competitive inhibition and may be reversible or non-reversible. These mechanisms have been exploited by drug manufacturers for suitable therapies (see Chapter 11).

One of the earliest classes of antibiotics (the sulphonamides) inhibited bacterial growth by competing for an essential enzyme used by the bacteria to synthesize folic acid. The bacteria are not killed by the antibiotic; they simply cannot multiply as folic acid is necessary for the manufacture of DNA. Sulphonamides are selectively toxic to bacteria because humans do not have the capacity to synthesize folic acid (hence it is a dietary requirement). This selectivity is an important feature of successful antibiotics (see Chapter 19).

The drug methotrexate is a competitive inhibitor of the enzyme dihydrofolate reductase; it has been used to treat childhood leukaemia by blocking DNA synthesis in leukaemic cells (see Chapter 31). However, in this case the reaction is not specific to the abnormal cells, and hence some of the adverse side-effects of this treatment are bone marrow suppression, skin rashes, and gastrointestinal disturbances.

The utilization of enzyme inhibitors in drug design has been used to good effect in the treatment of alcoholic misuse – the drug disulfiram (Antabuse) is a non-competitive inhibitor of the enzyme aldehyde dehydrogenase. This enzyme metabolizes alcohol and leads to the accumulation of acetaldehyde, a toxic metabolite, which causes flushing and choking sensations. Similarly, monoamine oxidase inhibitors (MAOIs), such as phenelzine and isocarboxazid, used in the treatment of depression are non-competitive inhibitors. However they are irreversible inhibitors, so their therapeutic effects are present for weeks, even if treatment has been discontinued. Unfortunately, MAOIs also metabolize amines ingested in food. For this reason, foods rich in amines, such as tyramine must be avoided or severe hypertension may result (see Chapter 10).

Inhibition is also important in controlling the rate at which enzymes work. Take, for instance, this hypothetical metabolic pathway: as the final product D accumulates, it inhibits enzyme 2, and slows down the whole pathway.

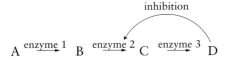

Product D may be the same shape as the enzyme substrate B (competitive inhibition). Alternatively D might be an allosteric enzyme inhibitor (allosteric means 'different shape' and allosteric enzymes occur at key points in metabolic pathways and act as 'stopcocks' which slow or speed up the flow of the whole pathway). Cellular respiration is controlled in this way in response to the demand for energy in the form of ATP.

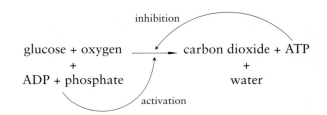

METABOLISM AND NUTRITION

The macronutrients of the human diet are protein, lipid (fat), and carbohydrate. These come from a variety of complex plant and animal materials. They must be broken down into simpler molecules that are small enough to be absorbed through the gut lining. This is achieved by the digestive processes that hydrolyse food (i.e. that break bonds by adding water) using enzymes as catalysts. Proteins therefore enter the body from the gastrointestinal tract as amino acids, carbohydrates enter the body as glucose and other simple sugars, and lipids (because of their fat solubility) are absorbed as larger units such as fatty acids, monoglycerides, and cholesterol. In addition to these macronutrients, a large number of other essential nutrients are required in the diet. These are minerals and vitamins, molecules that are essential in metabolism but that humans are unable to synthesize (see Appendix 1).

ENERGY SOURCES

Although glucose is the primary energy source for cellular respiration, all three macronutrients make an important contribution to energy supply because the breakdown pathways for carbohydrate, fat, and protein converge. Both glucose and fats are broken down to acetyl CoA, which is then used to build up energy supplies as ATP via the citric acid cycle and the electron transport chain. It is also possible to reverse the process and to use acetyl CoA to synthesize fats and (if necessary) glucose. So, to a large extent, carbohydrate and fat are interchangeable as energy sources. However, at least 20% of energy intake should come from carbohydrate in order to avoid the problem of ketosis (see below). Amino acids that are surplus to body requirements are also broken down for energy and are fed into cellular respiration at a number of points. Nitrogen is lost in this process and is then either used for the synthesis of other nitrogen compounds or excreted as urea. Although it appears that a lot of energy is available from protein, there is no storage of surplus protein in the body; all protein is either functional or being processed, mainly by the liver.

Basal Metabolic Rate

The energy needed for the body to maintain itself at rest is known as the basal metabolic rate (BMR). BMR declines with age and is normally lower in females than males. The reason behind the sex difference is that females have a higher proportion of fat per unit body mass than males, and fat consumes less energy than other tissues. Another way of putting this is that males have a higher lean body mass than females. As a rough guide,

BMR = body weight (kg) × 0.9 (for females) (kcal/hour)
BMR = body weight (kg) × 1.0 (for males) (kcal/hour)

The BMR is regulated by the thyroid gland, which in turn is controlled by the hypothalamus in the brain, where the body's 'thermostat' is set. Any additional energy intake as food must be matched by energy expenditure through physical exercise, or the body mass will increase. For instance, walking uses up to 270 kcal/hour, running around 720 kcal/hour, and swimming around 600 kcal/hour. Strenuous brain activity does not consume any additional energy above BMR!

BMR increases after a meal, a phenomenon known as dietary-induced thermogenesis. The decline in BMR in response to fasting or a reduced calorie intake is a means of conserving body fuels. For this reason, weight regulation is more reliably achieved through additional exercise than by eating less, though a combination of both is even more effective. Certain clinical conditions can affect the BMR, and it is increased when the presence of an infection evokes a fever response (see Chapters 23 and 25).

Respiratory Quotient

It is possible to determine the extent to which carbohydrates, fats, and proteins are being used for energy by measuring the composition of gases in inspired and expired air. Each type of fuel consumes different amounts of oxygen as it is broken down. This can be summarized as the respiratory quotient (RQ):

$$RQ = \frac{\text{carbon dioxide formed}}{\text{oxygen consumed}}$$

It has already been noted that for glucose, one molecule of carbon dioxide is produced for each molecule of carbohydrate used, giving an RQ of 1.0. The RQ value for fat is 0.7; the RQ value for protein is 0.8. Subjects on an average mixed diet show an RQ of around 0.8, but after a 24-hour fast, this would be expected to fall to around 0.75 as carbohydrate stores become depleted and stored fat is used as the main source of energy.

Carbohydrate and Gluconeogenesis

Carbohydrate enters the circulation as single unit sugars (monosaccharides), mainly glucose, after absorption from the small intestine. All body cells can absorb glucose, which is converted to glucose-6-phosphate, and metabolized via glycolysis and the citric acid cycle to release energy. Alternatively, it may be converted into glycogen, which is a large molecule composed of highly branched glucose chains, similar to starch, the plant polysaccharide.

Glycogen is stored primarily in liver cells and muscle. In liver cells, four enzymes are involved in the breakdown of glycogen to glucose, which may be released to replenish glucose levels in the blood. Liver cells are unique in being freely permeable to glucose. When blood glucose levels fall below 8.5 mmol/l, the liver is a net exporter of glucose. Conversely, if levels rise above this, it becomes a net importer and the glucose is converted to storage glycogen. Muscle cells lack the enzyme that converts glucose-6-phosphate back into glucose for release into the blood. This means that glycogen mobilized there can be used to fuel respiration within the muscle cell but is not available as a direct source of blood glucose. Glycogen breakdown is stimulated by the hormones glucagon and adrenaline, and inhibited by insulin. These hormones act in this way primarily through their influence on the activity of the enzyme glycogen phosphorylase. Insulin also increases the permeability of body cells to glucose. Hence, insulin and glucagon work together to control blood glucose levels by controlling the processes by which glucose enters and is removed from the blood (see Chapter 35).

Liver glycogen stores provide sufficient glucose for a few hours; however after this, if no glucose is eaten, it must be manufactured by alternative routes. Processes other than the breakdown of glycogen which lead to the synthesis of glucose are collectively known as gluconeogenesis (literally 'formation of glucose from new'). Fats and amino acids may both be used, but they have to be metabolized to acetyl CoA or pyruvate in order to enter the cellular respiration pathway. Fasting leads to a temporary rise in amino acid breakdown because glycogen stores are soon depleted. Certain amino acids (particularly alanine) have to be converted to lactate as an intermediate metabolite before pyruvate can be produced. Following pyruvate production, glycolysis can proceed in reverse to make glucose. The disadvantage of this is that the process demands some different enzymes to those used in normal glycolysis and requires an energy source (i.e. two molecules of ATP for each molecule of pyruvate converted to glucose).

Gluconeogenesis persists in the liver as feeding recommences following fasting because the liver preferentially uses the newly available glucose to replenish glycogen stores rather than to provide blood glucose. After a few hours, liver metabolism returns to the normal well-fed state – gluconeogenesis declines, glycolysis increases, and blood glucose is used to maintain glycogen stores. Peripheral tissues take up the glucose, the glucose is converted to lactate, and the liver can ultimately convert the lactate to glycogen (see also Box 2.2).

BOX 2.2 GLYCOGEN METABOLISM DISORDERS

There are a number of disorders of glycogen metabolism that involve deficiencies in the enzymes required for converting glycogen to glucose. In Type 1 glycogen storage disease (von Gierke's disease), a deficiency of the enzyme glucose-6-phosphatase in liver cells results in excessive deposition of glycogen in the liver.

Consequently, severe hypoglycaemia results after only short periods of fasting because the liver is unable to release glucose. In Pompe's disease type II, there is a deficiency of an enzyme that breaks down maltose to glucose. As a result, glycogen accumulates in the heart and central nervous system leading to learning disabilities and death from heart failure in infancy. Fortunately these are rare conditions.

Fat

Fat represents the body's major energy resource. It is stored in specialized fat cells (or adipocyte), which are found in the areolar connective tissue below the dermis and around the main body organs. Storage fats are triglycerides, which may be mobilized by an enzyme called hormone-sensitive lipase. Adrenaline and glucagon stimulate fat mobilization for immediate energy needs (e.g. the increased energy requirements of exercise). Conversely, thyroxine and growth hormone stimulate fat breakdown for longer-term energy needs (e.g. the energy requirements for the maintenance of body temperature and growth). Triglycerides are hydrolysed to fatty acids and glycerol, which are released into the blood stream. They are useful energy sources which are absorbed by cells; glycerol can be fed into glycolysis, and metabolized fatty acids release energy and acetyl CoA, which is fed into the citric acid cycle.

Dietary triglycerides are digested to monoglycerides and fatty acids via the action of gut lipases. These products can be absorbed by passive diffusion and reconstituted into triglycerides within the gut lining. Triglycerides are hydrophobic (water-hating) molecules; therefore they need to be physically combined into lipid–protein complexes (lipoproteins) in order to be soluble in the blood for transport to the liver and adipose tissue. Conversely, free fatty acids are bipolar (i.e. they have both hydrophilic and hydrophobic parts), so they can be transported directly by associating with plasma proteins. Commercially prepared glycerides containing medium-chain length fatty acids are used to feed patients with disorders affecting the digestion and transport of fats, because they are absorbed intact. Subsequently, within the gut mucosa, they are hydrolysed to glycerol and free fatty acids to be released and transported to the tissues via the bloodstream.

Some fatty acids cannot be synthesized by humans and are therefore an essential dietary requirement. Linoleic acid is one of the essential fatty acids; it is an important constituent of cell membranes and a precursor of prostaglandins. Prostaglandins are hormone-like molecules that stimulate the contraction of smooth muscle. They are involved in the control of blood pressure and, because they have a wide range of clinical uses, drug companies have produced them for treating hypertension, induced pregnancy terminations, and relief of nasal congestion. Other unsaturated fatty acids act as prostaglandin precursors and sources of gamma-linoleic acid; these fatty acids (notably primrose oil) are promoted on this basis as treatments for hangovers, premenstrual syndrome, and other conditions.

Brown fat is a specialized form of adipose tissue. Its cells possess many large mitochondria and it is served by a good blood supply. These specialized mitochondria are extremely active in dissipating energy as heat by uncoupling cellular respiration from ATP formation. This is particularly useful to neonates and hibernating mammals because it plays an important role in temperature regulation and heat generation when the body starts to cool. It is controlled by the hypothalamus, which regulates body temperature. Brown fat has also been implicated in controlling body mass by 'burning off' excess calories, (see Chapter 1). Although many environmental and behavioural factors are involved in weight regulation, some obese subjects seem to have less brown fat than normal.

Body Mass Index

Body mass index (BMI) is a measurement that is used as an alternative to height–weight tables for evaluating the possible health risks linked with under-nutrition and over-nutrition. A person's BMI is calculated from the height and weight:

BMI = body weight (kg)/height^2 (m^2)

For example, a woman who weighs 59 kg and is 1.62 m tall has a BMI of 22.5:

BMI = $59/1.62^2$ = 22.5

The acceptable ranges of BMIs for men and women, and the levels above which a person may be considered obese, are shown in Box 2.3.

The disadvantage of this index is that, although the body height and weight is known, it does not take into account the nature of the person's body composition. For instance, a body builder may have a high BMI as a result of a large muscle mass, rather than a lower proportion of body fat.

Protein

Proteins are composed of chains of amino acids linked by peptide bonds formed between the amino (–NH$_2$) group on one amino acid and the carboxyl acid (–COOH) group on another amino acid. They are the body's main source of nitrogen, and proteins that contain the amino acid cysteine also contain sulphur. There

are eight essential amino acids, which adults are unable to synthesize; therefore these are required in the diet. In addition to these eight amino acids, two more amino acids (arginine and histidine) are needed in infancy (see Person-Centred Study: Phenylketonuria).

Proteins are continually degraded and synthesized in metabolism, a process referred to as protein turnover. A 70 kg man who is taking in and excreting equal amounts of nitrogen (i.e. in nitrogen balance) will turn over approximately 400 g of protein each day. Nitrogen equilibrium occurs when nitrogen intake in the form of protein is balanced by the loss of nitrogenous waste products, such as urea in the urine. A positive nitrogen balance occurs when the body gains more nitrogen than it loses (e.g. during growth, pregnancy, or the recovery of tissues following injury). Conversely, where the nitrogen intake is less than nitrogen output the patient is said to be in negative nitrogen balance (e.g. during prolonged fasting or as a result of a low protein diet with inadequate energy intake).

Unlike carbohydrates, the amino acids that make up the proteins are not stored but are part of a dynamic pool (equivalent to the blood glucose reservoir). This pool is used for the synthesis of proteins (e.g. haem, albumin, and other nitrogen-containing biomolecules), but in extreme circumstances proteins are broken down for energy. Before the energy can be released however, the nitrogen must first be removed. This may be achieved in two ways:

- by deamination, in which the nitrogen is released as ammonia, a toxic product that is converted to urea in the liver for excretion by the kidneys; or
- by transamination, which involves the transfer of the amino group from an amino acid to another organic acid in order to make a different amino acid which is required to synthesize a particular protein.

During prolonged fasting, protein breakdown makes a significant contribution to the energy supply as the available carbohydrate and fat stores become exhausted. The disadvantage of this is a loss of functional proteins from the blood, cells, and muscles, leading to wasting. No more than 40% of the energy needs of the body can be supplied by protein at any time because of the limited capacity of the liver cells for protein catabolism.

While deficiencies in the quantity of protein in the diet and in its quality (i.e. its amino acid content) can result in malnutrition (see below), too much protein in the diet can also cause problems. In spite of this, a diet based on animal protein seems to produce few ill effects in the Inuit people (Eskimo), who consume a diet largely composed of fish, although this rarely contains more than 40 per cent protein because it is also high in fat. Attempts to survive on lean meat which

---

BOX 2.3 BODY MASS INDEX

Acceptable BMI	20–25 (males)
	19–24 (females)
Obesity	> 30 (men)
	> 28.5 (females)

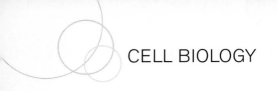

PERSON-CENTRED STUDY: PHENYLKETONURIA

When Lucy was 6 days old, a heel prick sample of blood was taken for the routine Guthrie test. The Guthrie test is a screening test for phenylketonuria (PKU), an inborn error of metabolism resulting from a deficiency of the enzyme phenylalanine hydroxylase. The test gave a positive result, so the child was immediately started on a low phenylalanine feeding plan, since her mother had chosen not to breast feed (human breast milk is lower in phenylalanine than cow's milk).

Lucy's mother was advised that a certain amount of phenylalanine was required for normal growth as it is one of the essential amino acids. However, owing to the enzyme deficiency, Lucy could not adequately metabolize excess amounts of the amino acid, leading to the accumulation of toxic metabolites which damage the nervous system. A dietary restriction was essential, since children with PKU who are given a diet high in phenylalanine suffer irritability, skin rashes, and irreversible brain damage. Nutrition intervention is effective in preventing these symptoms. It was pointed out that problems would arise when Lucy was older and mixed with other children as the PKU diet is rather restrictive.

When a child with PKU has not kept to the special PKU diet, the ultimate results will be mood and behavioural changes and decreased school performance. Some suggest that the PKU diet need not be prescribed for life. However, an elevated raised serum phenylalanine level in older children who are not maintained on a strict PKU diet is thought to be responsible for causing problems such as poor co-ordination, poor memory, and short attention span. Certainly in females it is necessary to recommence the diet in adulthood prior to conception and pregnancy. This is to reduce the risk of toxic metabolites damaging the fetus and causing defects such as congenital heart disease and learning disability.

BOX 2.4 KETOSIS IN DIABETICS AND IN STARVATION

Patients with untreated insulin-dependent diabetes mellitus lacking insulin are unable to use the glucose available in the blood, and show similar symptoms to fasting subjects.
- The fat stores rather than carbohydrate are therefore utilized for energy, which results in weight loss and severe ketoacidosis.
- The ketone bodies are degraded to form acetone, which can be smelt on the breath of ketotic patients. Ketone bodies are acidic, so the pH of the blood may be reduced.

Bizarre slimming programmes based on fat and protein without carbohydrate can also induce ketosis. Any initial dramatic weight loss that results from slimming programmes such as these is largely a result of loss of water, caused by increased urine production accompanying the increased nitrogen excretion.

has a higher proportion of protein may result in severe gut disturbances and a craving for fat. High-protein diets also increase urinary output because of the raised levels of nitrogenous waste (as urea) to be excreted.

Ketone Bodies

The formation of ketone bodies (ketogenesis) arises as a result of excess fatty acid breakdown. Therefore, when cells rely primarily on fats and proteins for energy, ketone bodies accumulate in the blood. This situation occurs during fasting and prolonged endurance exercise. Because fasting occurs during sleep, the levels of ketone bodies in the blood show a diurnal rhythm, with levels peaking after an overnight fast. When levels exceed 70 mg/dl, ketones are excreted in the urine (ketonuria), which provokes an increased urinary output that could lead to dehydration. One of the products of fat catabolism is acetyl CoA, so this molecule occurs in excess when fat is the major energy source. Ketone bodies such as acetoacetate and hydroxybutyrate are formed by the combination of the acetyl CoA molecules; they provide an alternative energy source to glucose (Figure 2.3). They are taken up by the brain, the heart, and skeletal muscles, and they are metabolized for energy. During extended starvation, they may supply up to 60% of the brain's energy needs.

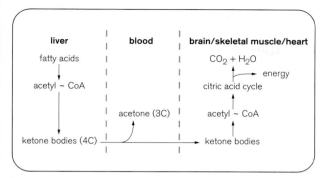

Figure 2.3 The production and utilization of ketone bodies.

However, a blood glucose level of 2–3 mmol/l must still be maintained (Box 2.4).

CONTROL OF ENERGY RESOURCES

The use of stored fuels (fat and glycogen) and protein as energy sources follows a strict pattern to maintain homeostasis. This is well illustrated by the examples of starvation and prolonged endurance exercise, which represent a severe drain on the body's energy supplies.

STARVATION

In starvation, the successive use of energy supplies is controlled in order to optimize survival times. Similar changes occur when patients are on 'nil by mouth' regimens, or when energy intake is insufficient (e.g. in inadequately administered nasogastric or total parenteral feeding). Not all the liver glycogen is released, and even an overnight fast will stimulate gluconeogenesis. As a result, there are increased serum levels of amino acids, fatty acids, and ketone bodies. During the first few days of starvation, the conversion of amino acids (particularly alanine) to glucose can compensate for the dietary shortfall. This loss of protein (together with some minerals, mainly calcium, magnesium and potassium) leads to increased urine production and a rapid initial weight loss through loss of body water. Subsequently, protein loss is minimized, and stored fat becomes the major source of energy.

Some glucose is synthesized from amino acids in the kidney; this organ may be a significant site of glucose production in prolonged starvation. Fat is less dense than carbohydrate and protein, and it has a higher energy content (9 kcal/g compared with 4 kcal/g); hence the loss of body weight in starvation becomes progressively less dramatic with time. Energy resources are conserved by the fall in BMR and the increased feelings of lethargy that reduce energy requirements at

this stage. Circulating levels of free fatty acids and ketone bodies rise, while glucose production by the liver declines dramatically. Survival largely depends on the amount of adipose tissue, so obese subjects have a decided advantage – up to 8 months survival has been recorded if adequate micronutrients and water are provided. Nevertheless, loss of protein from heart muscle resulting in ventricular fibrillation is a significant hazard in prolonged starvation – this is a possible complication of untreated anorexia nervosa (Box 2.5) (see also Chapter 32).

As fat stores are exhausted, functional protein is used to sustain normal energy metabolism. Even at this stage, a succession is evident – the first stage is the mobilization of plasma proteins (to preserve vital organs as long as possible), followed by the loss of protein from metabolically active tissues (particularly the liver, spleen and muscle) even though muscle is the main source of protein in the body. Loss of plasma proteins causes a fall in the osmotic concentration of the blood, so more water moves into the interstitial fluid by osmosis and accumulates between the cells, causing swelling (oedema). Typical examples include the abdominal swelling associated with protein-energy malnutrition, and the ascites found with impaired liver function (e.g. hepatic cirrhosis) – because the liver is the site for synthesis of blood proteins, there are reduced levels of plasma proteins such as albumin.

Tissues accommodate the changing levels of different energy sources to maximize metabolic efficiency. Therefore, they preferentially synthesize the enzymes needed in times of stress. For example, enzymes associated with fatty acid synthesis and glucose utilization decline in starvation, whereas those required for fatty acid utilization and gluconeogenesis increase markedly (because the body draws from its own energy stores).

These adaptive changes associated with fasting are suppressed following trauma or surgery. One reason for this is the over-riding effects on metabolism of the catecholamines (adrenaline and noradrenaline) and glucocorticoid hormones released in response to stress. Consequently a significant loss of muscle mass is observed, with fat stores mobilized and gluconeogenesis increased. The hormones also influence immune function and bone turnover – hence the loss of calcium from the bone matrix (osteoporosis) (see Chapter 39).

The physiological and biochemical adaptations observed in starvation provide invaluable information on strategies for treating cachexia as well as famine victims in developing countries. Protein–energy malnutrition occurs when the body is unable to maintain homeostasis in energy metabolism because of an inadequate and often unbalanced diet with respect to protein and other energy-giving nutrients.

BOX 2.5 DIETARY ASSESSMENT

An assessment of food intake in a day may be acquired by several means.

Dietary history

*   Generally used in clinics, where the person provides information on the amount and types of food eaten and times they are consumed.
*   Very general questions are asked, which may be difficult for the subject to answer accurately, and it supplies details on the patient's life-style.

24 hour dietary recall

The person recalls the previous day's dietary intake.

*   Straightforward technique used by nutritionist, nurse specialists, and in nutrition surveys to gather information about one day only.
*   The information retrieved could be inaccurate, because it relies on a good memory and does not provide details of precise amounts of food taken. Furthermore, the person being studied might 'conveniently forget' foods that were eaten or 'conveniently include' foods that were not eaten.

Food diary

The person weighs or measures all food consumed over several days or weeks, then records this information together with the time and date consumed. It provides information about life-style and dietary habits.

*   This has the advantage of making the subject aware of the food consumed, which is particularly helpful with a weight-reducing programme. However, it relies on the total commitment and honesty of the person.
*   Some of the limitations include distorted data retrieval or modified dietary habits as the person tries to create the impression of a healthy intake.

Which ever method of assessment is used, the nutritional content of dietary intake may be calculated from food tables to evaluate energy, protein, fat, vitamin, and mineral intake. Such information could provide vital evidence for possible excess and inadequate intake of nutrients (e.g. iron, vitamin C).

In developing counties, protein–energy malnutrition exists in two severe clinical disorders:
*   kwashiorkor, a protein deficiency characterized by a distended abdomen caused by fluid retention (oedema); and
*   marasmus, characterized by muscle wasting.

In kwashiorkor, the protein deficiency means that the available energy sources are used inefficiently. Oedema ensues as the osmotic concentration in the blood falls owing to reduced plasma protein levels. Marasmus is largely the result of complete starvation or a totally inadequate diet. The loss of the gastrointestinal activity is significant because it exacerbates the problem by precipitating malabsorption. Thus oral rehydration therapy with a solution of glucose plus electrolytes is particularly useful in contributing towards the restoration of normal gut function (see Chapter 28 for the effects of protein–energy malnutrition on immune function).

Protein–energy malnutrition is not simply confined to the developing countries. It is also associated with diseases of the gut, surgery (particularly surgery involving the gut), cancers, trauma, and sepsis. It may also accompany prolonged and severe illness, or an eating disorder such as anorexia nervosa. In view of the range of possible origins of malnutrition, it is vital to establish the exact cause before treatment (Box 2.6).

EXERCISE AND METABOLISM

Endurance exercise imposes a different problem, for although the body may have enough stored fuel for a run of several hours, the limiting factor is the delivery of sufficient energy to the active muscles. The combined glycogen stores of the liver and muscle will sustain a subject exercising to exhaustion for about 90 minutes. However, the remaining energy must be derived from stored fat mobilized from the adipose stores. The restriction is the blood supply to muscles and its capacity to transport fatty acids. Fat can provide only about half the muscle energy requirements at any time. The rest must come from carbohydrate; hence these two sources of energy have to be used together.

Attempts to conserve glucose levels are provided by a feedback inhibition mechanism operating between fat and glucose metabolism. In essence the net result is that glucose breakdown is kept to a minimum so that carbohydrate stores last as long as possible. As fat stores are utilized to provide ATP via the citric acid cycle, acetyl CoA is provided by fatty acid catabolism rather than by the metabolism of glucose via glycolysis. Eventually, even elite athletes will experience loss of power output as available glycogen stores run out,

---

BOX 2.6 ASSESSMENT OF NUTRITIONAL STATUS

Aims
- detection of under-nutrition and over-nutrition;
- treatment of a disorder;
- evaluation of therapy.

Weight and weight measurement for:
- calculation of Body Mass Index;
- assessment of growth and development in children by comparing these parameters against height–weight percentiles, which can help to identify children 'at risk'.

Skinfold thickness for assessing body fat; limitations include:
- individual variation in fat distribution;
- accuracy of reading – skilled personnel is needed to follow standard protocol;
- reliability of the calipers to give reproducible results;
- oedema and increased muscle mass can affect the result.

Head circumference:
- to assess growth and development in infants and children.

Physical examination of skin, hair nails, mouth, sensory activity

Laboratory investigation of body fluids such as blood and urine:
- to demonstrate a deficiency of specific nutrients by measurement of levels of iron, haemoglobin, vitamin status e.g. serum vitamin B12; serum urea and electrolytes.

Organ function tests (see Chapter 6)
- A comprehensive list of the normal range values for tests performed by pathology laboratories appears in Appendix 2.

---

but the ketone bodies produced make an important contribution to energy needs. During prolonged endurance events such as marathons, gluconeogenesis from amino acids is also evident.

ALCOHOL METABOLISM

Alcohol found in alcoholic drinks is more correctly known as ethanol. Ethanol is a small molecule that is absorbed rapidly from the stomach and small intestine because it has hydrophilic and hydrophobic properties. Although it has a high energy content (7 kcal/g), body cells do not metabolize ethanol efficiently. As a result, this energy is not efficiently harnessed, and the term 'empty calories' is sometimes used to describe this phenomenon. It is possible to double a subject's daily calorific intake by increasing the alcohol intake without a significant increase in body mass. However, it is noteworthy that many alcoholic drinks contain carbohydrates.

Ethanol has some chemical similarities to carbohydrates, but it is not a product of human metabolism, and it cannot be stored in the body. Another important feature is that only liver cells have any significant capacity to metabolize ethanol. Since the affinity of ethanol for water is about 30 times greater than for fat, levels remain low in fatty tissue. As a result, ethanol localizes in highly vascularized areas of the body initially (particularly the brain) and slowly equilibrates with other areas, such as skeletal muscle. In view of these properties, alcohol should certainly be regarded as a drug rather than a nutrient, a view reinforced by its well known effects on the central nervous system and its ability to induce dependence and withdrawal symptoms.

Breakdown of Ethanol

Over 90% of ethanol consumed is metabolized in liver cells (hepatocytes). These cells are packed with smooth and rough endoplasmic reticulum, which is where ethanol and other drugs are metabolized. Two key enzymes are required to detoxify ethanol – alcohol dehydrogenase (ADH) and aldehyde dehydrogenase (ALDH). Both use the coenzyme NAD, which becomes reduced to NADH. A major limiting factor in the liver's capacity to break down ethanol is the rate at which NAD is regenerated:

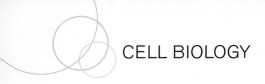

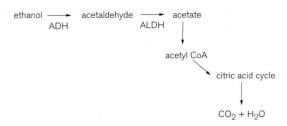

The alcohol metabolizing enzyme, ADH, can act on other alcohols as well, including ethylene glycol (widely used as antifreeze), but unfortunately its metabolites are toxic. Curiously, ethanol is an effective and readily available antidote to ethylene glycol poisoning. It competes with ethylene glycol and allows it to be excreted harmlessly in urine.

There are a number of different forms of ADH and ALDH that metabolize ethanol at different rate; these show some genetic and racial variation. For example, some Chinese people experience unpleasant side-effects, including flushing, choking, and nausea, after consuming alcohol. This is caused by acetaldehyde accumulation because the enzymes of these people work much less efficiently. Drug companies have exploited this phenomenon by designing a drug that evokes unpleasant symptoms when alcohol is consumed; this drug is disulfiram (Antabuse), used for treating chronic alcoholics. The drug works by inhibiting ALDH, which leads to the accumulation of acetaldehyde.

The overall rate of alcohol breakdown is sometimes referred to as the beta-value – the rate at which blood alcohol concentration can be metabolized when no more alcohol is being absorbed from the gut. This is thought to be largely genetically determined, since identical twins show similar beta-values, whereas non-identical twins often differ significantly. Europeans display an average beta-value of 15 mg/100 ml blood per hour, but values between 7 and 26 mg/100 ml blood per hour have been recorded. This indicates that some people metabolize alcohol between three and four times faster than others. Such studies clearly question the validity of the 'safe' alcohol limits for driving.

Liver oxidation of alcohol is also carried out by the microsomal ethanol oxidising system (MEOS), which operates when blood alcohol rises to high levels. This system is inducible, so that people who frequently consume alcohol generally have an increased alcohol metabolizing capacity. Regular drinkers therefore show an increased tolerance towards alcohol because it is removed from the body more quickly. Unlike many other drugs, however, this tolerance is limited by liver function. Chronic alcohol consumption may lead to reverse tolerance and a reduced capacity to metabolize

ethanol because of liver damage. Even short-term ethanol consumption induces dramatic changes in hepatocytes. An alcohol intake of 120 g/day over 18 days has been shown to cause massive proliferation of endoplasmic reticulum, fat accumulation, and enlarged and distorted mitochondria even when no outward signs of intoxication are evident.

Alcohol metabolism generates relatively increased levels of NADH compared to NAD, which has a number of effects notably fatty liver and hypoglycaemia.

Fatty liver

The high levels of NADH generated by alcohol metabolism in turn stimulate fat synthesis (a reductive process) and inhibit fat breakdown. Fats are mobilized from adipocytes and accumulate in the liver, resulting in 'fatty liver'. The liver synthesizes more protein in an effort to export the excess fat as lipoproteins. This results in a further proliferation of the areas where proteins are synthesized for export (i.e. rough endoplasmic reticulum). All this alcohol-induced hyperlipidaemia (too much fat in the blood) can lead to cardiovascular disorders. In addition, heart muscle may already be weakened by the direct toxic effects of acetaldehyde on protein.

Hypoglycaemia

Too much NADH also stimulates the conversion of pyruvate to lactate, causing lactate acidosis and inhibiting gluconeogenesis (the pathways for synthesis of glucose). This can provoke hypoglycaemia in alcoholic people, who are frequently malnourished and have depleted liver glycogen levels. Likewise, consuming alcoholic drinks following prolonged strenuous exercise can have similar effects because of low blood glucose levels. Overall, therefore, the liver is unable to cope with the reducing power of the excess levels of NADH, and cell metabolism becomes distorted and homeostasis is disrupted.

Malnutrition

A number of the symptoms associated with chronic alcohol misuse are caused by micronutrient deficiencies resulting from an inadequate or unbalanced diet. One such condition is Wernicke–Korsakoff syndrome, which is caused by impaired thiamine (vitamin B1) absorption and reduced storage in the liver. It is characterized by ataxia and unco-ordinated eye movements. Thiamine is an essential coenzyme for several enzymes in carbohydrate metabolism, and thiamine triphosphate is required for the biosynthesis of the neurotransmitter acetylcholine.

THE METABOLISM OF VITAMINS AND MINERALS

Micronutrients play a vital role in metabolism. Almost all biochemical processes require the involvement of these compounds at some point, and they are particularly significant in enzyme function. Many vitamins act as coenzymes, and many enzyme cofactors are metal ions.

The presence of micronutrients in the diet does not guarantee that sufficient quantities will be absorbed, however. In the case of iron, for instance, the element needs to be present in the most absorbable form – ferrous iron (Fe^{2+}). This form is most abundant in red meat; the iron that is present in other sources, such as spinach, is poorly absorbed. Vitamin C in the gut will help to ensure that dietary iron is in the most absorbable form, but other dietary components such a phytic acids, found in plant material (dietary fibre), attract metal ions such as calcium and iron, thus reducing absorption.

Vitamins

Vitamins (the word derives from 'vital amines') are essential dietary components that are either not produced in human metabolism or are produced in inadequate amounts. They are classified according to whether they are fat soluble or water soluble, a significant division because their supply is generally related to the fat content of the diet. Thus, diseases that result in fat malabsorption tend to affect the fat-soluble group as a whole. Fat-soluble vitamins are stored in the liver, but (like most dietary fats) they require the presence of bile salts for absorption. Hence, patients with cystic fibrosis, who are deficient in both bile salts and pancreatic lipase, have a malabsorption problem that leads to energy and vitamin deficiencies. This can be alleviated with enzyme preparations encapsulated in microspheres together with vitamin supplementation.

Most water-soluble vitamins are found in meat and cereals, green vegetables, liver, milk, and yeast. They are readily absorbed, and deficiencies are therefore less extensive on a world-wide scale.

Chronic alcoholics suffer from general vitamin deficiencies because of their inadequate and unbalanced diet. Additionally, excess ethanol intake damages the gut mucosa, thereby adversely affecting nutrient uptake – a shortage of B vitamins produces the most dramatic symptoms.

Minerals

The essential dietary minerals may also be classified into two groups: the macrominerals, include calcium, magnesium, potassium, sodium and iron; as well as phosphorus, sulphur, and chlorine, which are present in large amounts in the body fluids and bone.

Trace elements are required in much smaller quantities, mainly for use in proteins and enzymes. They include mainly the metals (chromium, cobalt, copper, manganese, selenium, and zinc), plus fluorine and iodine. Iodine is required for thyroid function. Trace elements are ubiquitous in most foods and water, making it difficult to assess nutritional requirements accurately. However, an excessive intake of any mineral may result in toxicity. (See Appendix 1 for details on the micronutrients.)

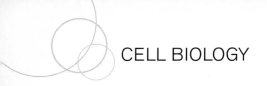

KEY POINTS

- Metabolism refers to all the biochemical processes in the body. The biosynthesis of large and complex molecules from simple molecules is anabolism. The breakdown of complex biomolecules into their basic chemical components is catabolism.
- Energy transfer is an important aspect of metabolic pathways, since all chemical processes lead to energy changes. The chemical energy stored in ATP is used for energy-consuming processes such as muscular contraction.
- Most enzymes are proteins, but many have prosthetic groups chemically bound to them, such as the iron-containing haem group found on cytochrome P_{450}, the drug metabolizing enzyme found in liver cells.
- Enzymes have a highly complex three-dimensional structure that provides one or more active sites, designed to accommodate one specific substrate molecule (absolute specificity) or a range of substrates of similar size and shape (group specificity).
- The energy needed for the body to maintain itself at rest is known as the basal metabolic rate (BMR). BMR declines with age and is normally lower in females than males.
- The formation of ketone bodies (ketogenesis) arises as a result of excess fatty acid breakdown. When cells rely primarily on fats and proteins for energy, ketone bodies accumulate in the blood.
- The use of stored fuels (fat and glycogen) and protein as energy sources follows a strict pattern to maintain homeostasis. This is well illustrated by the examples of starvation and prolonged endurance exercise, which represent a severe drain on the body's energy supplies.
- Ethanol has some chemical similarities to carbohydrates but it is not a product of human metabolism and it cannot it be stored by the body.
- Micronutrients play a vital role in metabolism. Almost all biochemical processes require the involvement of these compounds at some point, particularly in enzyme function. Many vitamins act as coenzymes and many enzyme cofactors are metal ions.

FURTHER READING

Basu TK, Dickerson JWT (1996) Vitamins in Human Health and Disease. CAB International, London.

Eastwood M (1997) Principles of Human Nutrition. Chapman and Hall, London.

Fell D (1997) Understanding the Control of Metabolism. Portland Press, London.

Fidanza F (1991) Nutritional Status Assessment. Chapman and Hall, London.

Halperin ML, Rolleston FS (1993) Clinical Detective Stories: a Problem-Based Approach to Clinical Cases in Energy and Acid–Base Metabolism. Portland Press, London.

Jung RT (1997) Obesity as a disease. Br Med Bull 53:307–21.

Mitchell GA, Kassovska-Bratinova S, Boukaftane Y, et al. (1995) Medical aspects of ketone body metabolism. Clin Invest Med 3:193–216.

Sherwood L Fundamentals of Physiology, 2nd edition. West Publishing Co., New York.

Shikora SA, Blackburn GL (1997) Nutrition Support. Chapman and Hall, London.

Smith I, Cook B, Beasley M (1991) Review of neonatal screening programme for phenylketonuria. BMJ 303:333–5.

Stevens J, Cai J, Pamuk ER, et al. (1998) The effect of age on the association between body mass index and mortality. N Engl J Med 338:1–7.

Suter PM, Russell RM (1987) Vitamin requirements of the elderly. Am J Clin Nutr 45:501–12

Triomphe TJ (1997) Glycogen storage disease: a basic understanding and guide to nursing care. J Pediatr Nurs 12:238–49.

Wilding J (1997) Obesity treatments. BMJ 315:997–1000.

NORMAL AND ABNORMAL CELL GROWTH

3

LEARNING OBJECTIVES

After studying this chapter you will:
- know how normal cell growth and repair is essential to the replacement of certain body tissues and organs
- know the different phases of the cell cycle, including mitosis and the significance of G_0
- be able to list important growth factors, their main effects, and where they can be isolated from
- be able to discuss critically the significance of differentiation in the production of replacement cells
- be able to explain comprehensively atrophy, hypertrophy, hyperplasia, metaplasia, and dysplasia using specific examples

For a clearer understanding of this chapter you would be advised to have read Chapters 1, 7 and 23 and to be familiar with mitosis and meiosis.

INTRODUCTION

Throughout life, cells within the body continue to grow and multiply at varying rates depending on their type. For example, in the basal layer of the skin, mitotic division leads to the production of new cells, keratinocytes, which will, over a period of days, migrate to the surface of the epithelium (the stratum corneum), from where they will be shed. The skin and some other organs in the body, such as the liver, have considerable capacity for regeneration, whereas other cells, such as nerve cells (neurones), have limited capacity in this respect. Indeed, the devastating consequences arising from neuronal damage following events such as oxygen deprivation resulting from a stroke or mechanical damage resulting from spinal injury are well known.

Some tissues in the body are continually being renewed (e.g. non-glandular epithelium, bone marrow and male germ cells), whereas others are conditionally renewed (e.g. the liver, kidney and glandular epithelium). Nervous tissue and the cells of the female germ line, which have little or no capacity for regeneration, are defined as non-replacing.

In addition to normal growth, abnormal growth can also occur. Abnormal cell growth in the body can result in an increase or decrease in the mass of the involved cells. When this type of growth leads to the repair of an organ or tissue, it serves a useful purpose. However it may also be more sinister if it is the mechanism involved in the evolution of a premalignant condition.

NORMAL GROWTH

Any tissue can be separated into:
- parenchymal cells, which are specialized to undertake the functions of the particular tissue that they are in; and
- interstitial cells, which are connective tissue cells that make up the supporting framework of the tissue (see Chapter 1).

The parenchymal cells are mature, differentiated cells, and these cells eventually become senescent and die. Cells have very different life spans depending on their type. Tissues undergoing renewal contain:

- active proliferating cells, which are dividing; and
- potentially proliferative cells, which have the capacity to develop into proliferative cells if required.

MITOSIS AND THE CELL CYCLE

With the exception of the production of gametes, all cell replacement in the body occurs by mitotic cell division. The sequence of events that take place within the life of a cell can be considered in relation to the cell cycle. The cell cycle consists of four main components (Figure 3.1):
- the S (synthetic) phase, in which DNA is synthesized;
- the G_2 (gap) phase, which follows the completion of DNA synthesis during the S phase;
- the M (mitotic) phase, in which the events of mitotic cell division (prophase, metaphase, anaphase, and telophase) take place; and
- the G_1 (gap) phase, which occurs between the S phase and the M phase.

The daughter cells resulting from mitotic cell division may complete an identical cell cycle to the parent cells; this is typical of stem cells, which are required for the replenishment of blood cells. However some cells lose their capacity to divide following mitosis and develop into postmitotic mature cells, which are often well-differentiated cells. Other cells resulting from mitotic cell division may show variability in the length of both the G_1 phase (sometimes referred to as G_{1a}, G_{1b}, and so

on) and the G_2 phase. Finally, some cells may cease progression from the first gap phase and become quiescent; this is known as the G_0 phase, losing any further capacity to divide. They differ from postmitotic mature cells in that they need not have lost the capacity to re-enter the cycle and undergo mitosis, although some may terminally differentiate from the G_0 phase, losing any further capacity to divide. Control and determination of the fate of cells within the cell cycle takes place within the G_1 phase.

Some organs, such as the liver, have a large number of cells in the G_0 phase. These can be returned to the cell cycle if there is a need for tissue replacement (e.g. after a surgical resection). Other organs in which there is continual renewal, such as the skin, have few G_0 cells, and an increase in the proliferation rate is met by reducing the time of the cell cycle or increasing the numbers of cells in the proliferating population.

Genetic control mechanisms have been identified for the cell cycle. Genes that encode for growth factors have been identified; these are expressed during different phases of the cell cycle. For example, in the late phases of G_1 there is transcription of genes that encode for DNA polymerases to be available for use in the DNA synthesis of the S phase.

GROWTH FACTORS

Growth factors are small protein or polypeptide molecules that act as signals to:
- increase proliferation of cells (i.e. growth stimulators);
- decrease proliferation of cells (i.e. growth inhibitors); or
- promote differentiation of cells.

They are important in the regulation of embryogenesis, growth and development, cell survival, haematopoiesis, atherosclerosis, and tissue repair (see Chapters 31 and 32). As discussed in Chapter 5, there is considerable evidence that an imbalance of growth factors may be important in relation to cancer.

Growth factors exert their effects by binding to cell membrane receptors. This leads to the formation of a growth factor–receptor complex that enters the cell by endocytosis. Growth factors can be modulated by extracellular matrix molecules. Extracellular matrix molecules can themselves control cell growth. For example, fibronectin and laminin can stimulate DNA synthesis in some cells, and collagen can result in it being switched off. The mechanism by which the extracellular matrix molecules exert their effects is by binding to special cell surface receptors called integrins. It is likely that one of the ways that growth factors exert their effects is through controlling the expression of integrins (Table 3.1).

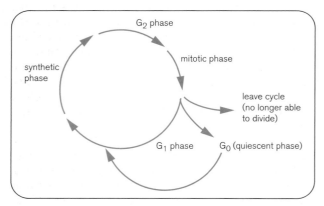

Figure 3.1 Four main components of the cell cycle. After mitosis cell may either leave the cycle (and so become no longer able to divide) or enter into a gap phase (G_1). After this gap phase, cells enter a synthetic phase, after which they enter another gap phase (G_2) before undergoing mitosis again. The length of the G_2 and G_1 phases varies between cell types.

Types of Growth Factors

Growth Factor	Effect
Epidermal Growth Factor (EGF)	stimulates division of many epithelial cells and fibroblasts
Transforming Growth Factors (TGF-alpha and TGF-beta forms)	TGF-alpha appears to be identical to EGF and has similar effects; TGF-beta can be both mitogenic and inhibitory depending on the concentration. Affects smooth muscle cells and fibroblasts
Platelet-Derived Growth Factor (PDGF)	stimulates division of fibroblasts, smooth muscle cells and monocytes
Fibroblast Growth Factor (FGF)	stimulates blood vessel formation (angiogenesis)
Cytokines (e.g. interleukin-1, Tumour Necrosis Factor-alpha (TNF-alpha))	range of effects which include the stimulation of the formation of collagen (see Chapter 25)
Heparin	inhibits fibroblast and smooth muscle proliferation *in vitro*

Table 3.1 Types of growth factors. Some important growth factors are illustrated in this table. EGF is found in body fluids such as saliva and urine. PDGF is, as the name suggests, released by platelets on activation; it is stored in the alpha granules. It can also be produced by macrophages, endothelial cells and smooth muscle cells, as well as by tumour cells. PDGF production can be influenced by the concentration of TGF-beta partly explaining how the latter exerts an effect; in low concentrations of TGF-beta, PDGF synthesis is stimulated but the reverse occurs at high concentrations. Receptors for several of the growth factors have been identified at the cell membrane and receptor binding is important in explaining how some of the effects are brought about.

DIFFERENTIATION

Although mitosis is responsible for the production of new cells, it is the process of differentiation that gives rise to cells with a specific purpose. Differentiation is responsible for the wide varieties of specialized cells present in the body. For example, keratinocytes, neurones, cardiac muscle cells, smooth muscle cells, skeletal muscle cells, and red blood cells are just a few of the highly specialized cells that exist within the body. However, by becoming specialized, some of these cells lose their capacity to reproduce (e.g. neurones and mature red blood cells). All these specialized cells are highly adapted for a specific purpose and are recognizable both by their morphological appearance and biological characteristics. For example, epithelial cells possess desmosomes and produce cytokeratins; nerve cells do not. Mature red blood cells (in humans) have no nucleus and contain haemoglobin, characteristics that make them immediately recognizable.

Differentiation takes place at three different times within the human life cycle. It occurs during embryonic development, when cells are programmed to develop into specific types. There is evidence to suggest that this happens even before the characteristics for the specific cell type become evident. Such cells are referred to as being 'determined'. The mechanisms responsible for this are only partly understood, but growth factors are almost certainly involved. There is also evidence for a reprogramming of cells, which results in a change in gene expression as a result of altering the repressed and activated genes (see Chapter 7). The cell cycle is genetically controlled, and genes that are expressed at different stages of the cycle have been identified. These genes are switched off when cells leave the cell cycle in G_0. Differentiation does not result in a loss of genes, but the balance of expressed and repressed genes varies amongst different cell types.

The second place for differentiation to occur is in the adult, where cells that are already differentiated divide to give rise to new cells. This happens in the case of hepatocytes – mature cells give rise to daughter cells that take on the characteristics of the parent cells. This process is partly under environmental control within the body. Evidence for this comes from cell culture studies. Many human cells can be maintained and grown in *in vitro* cell culture. Although these cells retain many of the characteristics of the mature cells, sometimes certain functions are lost. In some cases, such as with cartilage cells (chondrocytes), the cells actually take on a fibroblast-like form; this is called dedifferentiation.

It is even possible in cell culture to induce trans-differentiation, in which one cell type will differentiate into another. This can be done with epithelial cells grown in culture in conditions will give rise to mesenchymal-like cells. These cells are morphologically identical to mesenchyme but also express similar gene products.

The final type of differentiation is that which occurs from unspecialized stem cells within the body. Stem cells may give rise to daughter cells that either remain as stem cells or will differentiate. During the process, the cells that differentiate may continue to divide. However, they may also develop into cells that are terminally differentiated and that do not have the ability to further divide. In some cases, stem cells give rise only to a single type of cell (e.g. keratinocytes). In other cases, the stem cells give rise to a range of different cell types (e.g. bone marrow stem cells).

Stem cells are found in replacing tissues whose differentiated cells no longer have the capacity to multiply, such as the stratified squamous epithelium of the skin or oral cavity. They also exist within the haematopoietic tissue, where they give rise to the cells that will become differentiated, mature blood cells (see Chapter 31). Stem cells within the bone marrow comprise about 1 per cent of all bone marrow cells. About 5–10 per cent of the cells differentiate every day and give rise to lineages that will in turn become mature blood cells. However, it is not only the stem cells that are responsible for the total numbers of mature cells produced. The daughter cells that are destined to become mature cells will also divide in the process. For example, stem cells destined to become red blood cells will go through between five and eight cycles of division as committed precursors, then a further three to five cycles of division as clearly identified red blood cell precursors. It is these precursors that will give rise to the mature terminally differentiated red blood cells (erythrocytes). This amplification (many cycles of cell division) is important in producing the required numbers of mature specialized cells.

Skin consists of stratified squamous epithelium and the keratinocytes that are organized into a number of different layers (strata) depending on their morphology and function. The horny layer contains the stratum corneum, stratum lucidum, and stratum granulosum. The outer cells are shed from the skin and replaced by cells produced in the germinative layer, which includes the stratum spinosum and the stratum basale. As the cells migrate through the layers, their appearance changes. The dividing stem cells in the stratum basale become spindle shaped as they move into the stratum spinosum. The cells then become granular (stratum granulosum), after which they lose their granules (stratum lucidum) as keratin is formed. The cells finally enter the stratum corneum, from which they are shed in the process of exfoliation.

The stem cells from which keratinocytes are derived are located in the basal lamina. Only about one-tenth of the basal cells are stem cells with proliferative capacity. The replicating capacity of the skin is considerable – mouse epidermis produces 10^7 cells per day. It is likely that it is not just stem cell division that gives rise to skin cells, but that there are further divisions of the cells in transit as they migrate towards the horny layer. Cell kinetic studies suggest up to three divisions of the transit cell population may take place.

Within the small intestine, cell proliferation takes place at the base of the crypts. The daughter cells migrate towards the villus tip at the rate of about one or two cell positions per hour. The cells are shed from the villus at the apical extrusion zone and, in humans, about 10^{11} cells are shed from the small intestine each day. It is thought that a relatively small number of cells within a crypt act as stem cells. A ring of cells around the circumference of the crypt contains approximately 16 cells. It has been suggested that there may be two rings of stem cells for each crypt, although only one of them might be active. The daughter cells almost certainly continue to divide as they migrate upwards, giving up to six transit cell generations.

Control of the division of stem cells and the differentiation of the daughter cells is only partly understood. Environmental modulation through contact with other cells and the extracellular matrix is important, as are growth factors. It is significant that many growth factors have an effect on the production of extracellular matrix components.

ADAPTATIONS OF CELL GROWTH AND DIFFERENTIATION

If the external environment of cells remains unchanged, then the cells will exist in what is known as a steady state. This is a situation that occurs in health where the cells have an adequate supply of nutrients and, in the case of proliferating tissues, where the rate of cell turnover is normal. Even in health, however, there may be changes in the demands of cells. A person who undertakes healthy exercise or participates in sport or weight training places additional demands on cells within the body. Individual cells have considerable capacity to adapt to new demands placed on them, either in health or as a result of disease.

The following is an account of some of the adaptive changes that may take place as a result of different demands being placed on cells. If the stress on cells exceeds their capacity for adaptation, cell death will occur.

ATROPHY

Atrophy is defined as the shrinkage in the size of a cell, tissue, or organ. It occurs through the loss of cell substance or, in the case of tissues and organs, through reduction in the size or number of cells. Atrophied cells are in a new equilibrium (adapted state) that allows them to survive in an altered environment through reducing cell volume and metabolism.

Atrophy can be considered to be either physiological or pathological. Physiological atrophy includes the changes of ageing, such as the shrinkage of the endometrium following the menopause; this atrophy results from diminished hormonal stimulation. From another perspective, any reduction in the workload on a tissue or organ can result in disuse atrophy. For instance, a limb that has been encased for weeks in plaster will have a decreased muscle mass because the cells have not being used (see Person-Centred Study: Paralysis Following a Car Accident).

Other forms of atrophy are pathologically induced. For example, muscular dystrophies are caused by defects in the dystrophin gene (deletions of long stretches of genetic sequence; see also Chapter 7). This results in atrophy of muscle fibres and leads to muscle weakness. Interference with the nervous supply to a tissue or organ can result in a decrease in its size. This is not just due to disuse but seems to be a result of degenerative changes – this is called neuropathic atrophy. Following infection with polio viruses, the anterior horn cells in the spinal cord are destroyed, which in turn leads to muscle wasting. In addition, fever results in the increased protein catabolism, and this may cause atrophy. Polio is just one example of atrophy that has more than one causal factor (i.e. the infection causes neurodegenerative and metabolic changes).

Starvation causes a loss of body weight as a result of the utilization of fat stores as a source of energy; this loss of body weight is not atrophy. However, prolonged starvation causes true atrophy of tissues and organs when there is a reduction in the weight of the liver, spleen, kidneys, and heart (Box 3.1).

Diminished blood supply to an organ can also cause atrophy. For example, it is known that atrophy of the brain occurs in late life; this is almost certainly due to inadequate blood circulation and may be the result of atherosclerosis (see Chapter 32). In old age, there is often a loss of structural components of the cells making up a tissue or organ. Within cells, there is increased evidence of autophagy in that there exist more autolysosomes (see Chapter 4). Some of the changes occurring in tissues and organs characteristic of old age are referred to as senile atrophy. This includes the accumulation of the pigment lipofuscin, which is most frequently detected in tissues such as the liver, the heart, and nerves; it is sometimes called 'brown atrophy'. However, it should be noted that lipofuscin does not radically affect the cellular structure and function.

Regardless of the cause of atrophy, it is, by definition, reversible. If the factors responsible are revoked, then the cells will return to normal functioning and size. For instance, patients with hypothyroidism (thyroid deficiency) have atrophy of the skin, which can be reversed by the administration of thyroid hormone.

HYPERTROPHY

Hypertrophy and hyperplasia (see below) can and do frequently exist together. The expansion of the pregnant uterus in response to oestrogen and progesterone stimulation is a classic example of this.

Hypertrophy is the increase in the size of cells. It results in the increase in the size of a tissue or organ and is an adaptive response to a changed environment. Both physiological and pathological factors are recognized. An example of physiological hypertrophy is that seen in cardiac or skeletal muscle as a result of increased workload. These tissues have great capacity for hypertrophy, which compensates for their inability to increase the number of cells (hyperplasia). The large muscles of the bodybuilder or athlete are due to the cells undergoing expansion as an adaptive change to an increased workload (Figure 3.2).

PERSON-CENTRED STUDY: PARALYSIS FOLLOWING A CAR ACCIDENT

Asif, aged 35, was in a car accident that resulted in a broken neck and extensive paralysis – because of the damage to the nerves, he lost the use of both legs and most of his left arm. Over a period of time, the reduced use of the muscles in his legs and in his left arm led to atrophy of the muscles and a decrease in their size, which is characteristic of this sort of injury. He remained able to use his right arm, however, and this arm became very well toned with some hypertrophy of the muscles. This is because it received greater use than previously when both his arms had been functional.

BOX 3.1 MALNUTRITION

Malnutrition is not present only in developing countries; it is also seen in Western countries; examples include:

- HIV wasting syndrome;
- cachexia in patients with malignancy;
- patients prescribed nasogastric and intravenous feeding where the full diet is not administered;
- children given high-fibre, low-energy diets (because the parents perceive this type of diet as 'healthy');
- anorexia nervosa.

Adaptive features exhibited in malnutrition include changes in body composition and a decrease in subcutaneous adipose tissue and muscle mass. Initially the function and mass of the vital organs are conserved at the expense of the adipose and muscle tissues. However, if a person remains undernourished and is not treated, ultimately the viscera and central nervous system will be affected.

Physical and metabolic changes also occur; these include decreased mechanical and spontaneous activities and a fall in the basal metabolic rate to conserve energy; decreased ability to maintain normal body temperature (resulting in an increased risk of hypothermia); reduced sodium–potassium pump activities within cell membranes; compromised immune function; and an increased susceptibility to infection. The function of the liver, kidney, heart, gastrointestinal tract, and central nervous system is also reduced in malnourishment.

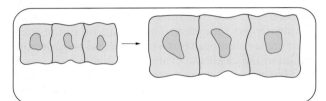

Figure 3.2 Hypertrophy. Cells that increase in size are said to undergo hypertrophy, which is an adaptive response to a changed environment.

A further example of physiological hypertrophy occurs in the thyroid. If there is overproduction of thyroid stimulating hormone (TSH) (e.g. because of iodine deficiency), then hypertrophy (and also hyperplasia) of the thyroid follicle cells occurs (see Chapter 35).

Pathological hypertrophy is seen in the heart after long periods of raised blood pressure (hypertension) or aortic stenosis. Hypertension places greater demands on the heart as it attempts to pump blood around the body. The cardiac muscle responds by becoming hypertrophied, and this is particularly evident in the region of the left ventricle. It is possible for the weight of the heart to double from its original value. This left ventricular hypertrophy cannot continue indefinitely and eventually leads to a point where the heart can no longer adapt and degenerative changes take place, resulting in cardiac failure (see Chapter 32).

HYPERPLASIA

Hyperplasia is characterized by an increase in the number of cells in a tissue or organ, which leads to a rise in the volume of the tissue or organ. Hyperplasia can, like hypertrophy, be separated into both physiological and pathological responses.

Examples of physiological hyperplasia include:
- the hormonal hyperplasia that results in an increase in the glandular epithelium of the human female breast following hormonal stimulation at puberty;
- the compensatory hyperplasia that is seen in the regeneration of hepatocytes that can occur following partial hepatectomy.

Compensatory hyperplasia also occurs as a physiological response in wound healing. When skin is removed, the cells at the edge of the wound divide and increase in number until the wound is repaired and the stimulus for the hyperplasia is removed. It is likely that growth factors are associated both with stimulating cell proliferation while the restoration is taking place and with inhibiting cell division once the tissue is regenerated (Figure 3.3).

An example of pathological hyperplasia is endometrial hyperplasia that results in abnormal menstrual bleeding. This occurs when the response to the ovarian steroids (oestrogen and progesterone) exceeds that needed in the physiological process of proliferation to replace the shed endometrial cells. However, even pathological hyperplasia is under some controlling influence, and the process

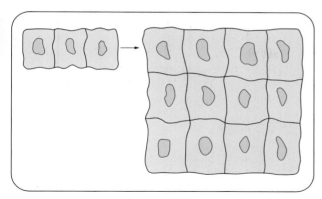

Figure 3.3 Hyperplasia. When there is an increase in the number of cells in a tissue or organ, hyperplasia is said to occur.

will stop when the stimulus is removed. Hyperplasia of the endometrium is a potentially serious condition in that it can progress to cancer. Oestrogen-secreting tumours of the ovary can induce endometrial hyperplasia, and hormone replacement therapy also results in some endometrial hyperplasia (see Chapters 5 and 37).

Enlargement of the prostate can produce urinary problems through the increase in size of the prostate gland. This is a very common condition in older men; it results from hyperplasia of the epithelium, stroma, and smooth muscle within the prostate gland.

Pathological hyperplasia can also occur as a result of infection. Certain viruses can cause hyperplasia. They seem to exert their effects through growth factors. The effects of the human papilloma virus infection are seen in skin warts, which are a consequence of hyperplasia of the epithelium. Human papilloma virus has also been implicated as a causative factor in squamous cell carcinoma of the cervix.

An increase in the requirement for blood cells, such as occurs following blood loss or lung disease or cyanotic heart disease, results in bone marrow hyperplasia. After haemorrhage there is, typically, erythroid hyperplasia with the red marrow extending into the shafts of the long bones.

METAPLASIA

Metaplasia results when an adult epithelial or mesenchymal cell type is replaced by another cell type. It results in the appearance of cells that are abnormal for the particular histological location. Metaplasia is considered to be an adaptive response to stressful stimuli on cells. The word 'metaplasia' is essentially the Greek word that means 'a moulding afresh'.

The epithelial lining of the bronchus and bronchioles of the respiratory tract is composed of pseudostratified ciliated columnar epithelium. During habitual cigarette smoking, these cells are exposed to toxic chemicals contained within the smoke. The response is seen in the squamous metaplasia that occurs – the sensitive respiratory epithelium is replaced following repeated injury by stratified squamous epithelium, which is abnormal for this location. The replacement can be over wide areas or in specific foci. The stratified squamous epithelium is more resistant and better able to survive than the original pseudostratified columnar epithelium, but it is non-functional and cannot produce mucus or aid in the ciliary movement of inhaled particles from the respiratory tract. Chronic infections within the respiratory tract can also result in squamous metaplasia, as can a deficiency in vitamin A.

In the urinary bladder, squamous metaplasia can occur as a result of calculi or schistosomiasis infection. A different type of metaplasia, glandular metaplasia, may result from chronic cystitis or pyelonephritis (see Chapter 36). In this type of metaplasia, the urothelium (bladder epithelial cells) is replaced with glandular epithelium.

Stones in the bile ducts, salivary gland ducts, or pancreatic ducts can cause irritation and result in replacement of the columnar epithelium of these ducts by stratified squamous epithelium.

Intestinal metaplasia can occur in the stomach, resulting in the replacement of the gastric glands with crypts identical to those found in the small intestine. In Crohn's disease, the opposite may occur, with the formation of gastric epithelium in the small intestine.

Within the ovary, as a result of the repeated trauma of ovulation, the germinal epithelium can undergo hyperplasia. This leads to the formation of cysts lined with metastatic epithelium of a range of different types.

Metaplasia occurs in mesenchymal cells, but less so as an adaptive response. Fibroblasts can develop into functioning chondroblasts (cartilage cells) or osteoblasts (bone cells) which can form cartilage or bone respectively. This can result in the production of bone, for example, in soft tissues. Such changes may arise after mechanical trauma to muscles, in surgical scars, in lungs following mitral stenosis, in the walls of sclerotic calcified arteries (Figure 3.4), or in calcified heart valves.

THE RELATIONSHIP BETWEEN METAPLASIA AND MALIGNANT CHANGE

Although metaplasia is an adaptive response, it invariably represents undesirable change. The squamous metaplasia associated with cigarette smoking, for instance, is a change that may be a forerunner of malignant change. Squamous cell carcinoma is the most common

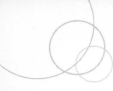

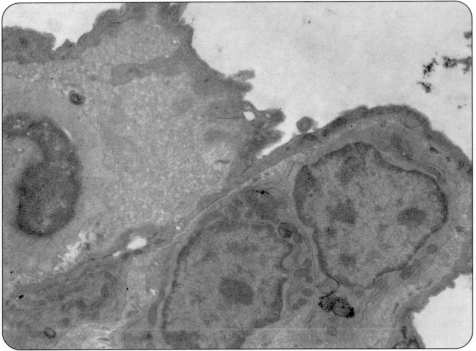

Figure 3.4 Abnormal changes in the intima of an artery. This electron micrograph shows part of the intima from an artery in which there is evidence of abnormal changes. The intima is thickened and white cells can be observed below the endothelium. The internal elastic lamina is apparent at the bottom edge of the micrograph. Normally the intima is a uniform thickness, but there is evidence of disruption. This sort of change can result from the injurious agents that result from smoking or hyperlipidaemia (× 5000).

cancer in the respiratory tract. It is of note that the cancerous cells are similar to the new tissue rather than the parent tissue, which, in health, has a completely different epithelium (Figure 3.5).

In the bladder, squamous metaplasia may also give rise to squamous cell carcinoma. If the factors that lead to metaplastic change continue, malignant change may occur. Metaplasia is associated with chronic tissue irritation and damage, and this is true for many cancers. It is also noteworthy that many cancers occur at the border between two tissue types, and metaplastic change results in the creation of new and probably unstable borders.

DYSPLASIA

The term 'dysplasia' means 'deranged development'. It is usually restricted to epithelial or mesenchymal cells that have undergone hyperplasia, leading to the formation of daughter cells with abnormal characteristics.

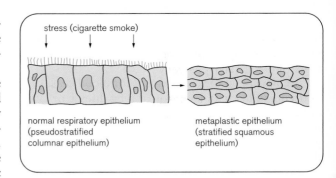

Figure 3.5 Metaplasia. Metaplasia is an adaptive response but it represents an undesirable change. For instance, this occurs in squamous metaplasia when respiratory epithelium changes from normal pseudostratified columnar epithelium to a more resistant type, stratified squamous epithelium. It may arise as a result of exposure to the toxic components within cigarette smoke. Metaplasia is a change from one adult epithelial or mesenchymal cell type to another.

These abnormal characteristics include both altered and variable shape and size.

Dysplasia involving epithelium results not only in alterations to the cells, but also in changes in the architecture of the tissues and in the relations of the cells to each other. It is the alteration to the cellular or tissue architecture that allows the term 'dysplasia' to be used. Typically, lining epithelia are affected and there is hyperplasia of the basal cells with deranged ordering of the cells as they migrate to the surface. Dividing cells, as evidenced by mitotic figures, are observed in the basal layer. Dysplasia is common following squamous metaplasia in the respiratory tract. It is also seen in the cervix. In the respiratory tract the evidence is that epithelial dysplasia is a forerunner to malignant change, although it is possible that removal of the noxious stimulus (e.g. cigarette smoke) may allow the epithelium to become normal again (i.e. the dysplasia is an adaptive change that is potentially reversible if the noxious stimulus is removed.

KEY POINTS

- Cells grow and multiply at varying rates, depending on their type. Some tissues exhibit a considerable capacity for regeneration (e.g. liver and skin); this is normal growth. Abnormal cell growth can result in an increase or decrease in cell numbers or cell mass.
- The sequence of events in the life of a cell i.e. the cell cycle, is genetically controlled, and may be divided into four phases: S phase (DNA synthesis), G_1 phase, M phase (mitotic division), and G_2 phase.
- Mitosis is responsible for the production of new cells.
- The process of differentiation gives rise to cells with a specialized function. In the embryo, cells are programmed to develop into specific cell types. In adults, differentiation gives rise to new cells in regeneration processes (e.g. the range of blood cell types derive from bone marrow stem cells).
- Atrophy is a shrinkage in the size of a tissue, cell, or organ, and is an adaptive change to help the cells to survive in an altered environment.
- Hypertrophy is an increase in the size of cells, which may be induced by pathological or physiological factors.
- Hyperplasia is an increase in the number of cells of a tissue or organ (e.g. regeneration of skin in wound healing).
- Metaplasia occurs when adult epithelial or mesenchymal cells are replaced by another cell type as an adaptive response to a stressful stimulus, and invariably represents undesirable change.
- Dysplasia is a deranged development of cells that leads to abnormal characteristics in their shape and size, often with changes in the architecture of the tissues which they form. Dysplasia is a forerunner of malignancy, but it is potentially reversible if the noxious stimulus is removed.

FURTHER READING

Chandrasoma P, Taylor CR (1997) Concise Pathology, 3rd edition. Prentice Hall International (UK), London.

Cotran RS., Kumar V, Robbins SL (1994) Robbins' Pathologic Basis of Disease, 5th edition. WB Saunders, Philadelphia.

Lakhani SR, Dilly SA, Finlayson CJ (1998) Basic Pathology: an Introduction to the Mechanisms of Disease, 2nd edition. Edward Arnold, London.

McGee JO, Issacson PG, Wright, NA (eds) (1992) Oxford Textbook of Pathology, volume 1. Principles of Pathology. Oxford University Press, Oxford.

Anderson JR ed (1992) Muir's Textbook of Pathology, 13th edition. Edward Arnold, London.

Rubin E, Farber JL (eds) (1995) Essential Pathology, 2nd edition. JB Lippincott, Philadelphia.

Tausigg MJ (1998) Processes in Pathology and Microbiology, 3rd edition. Blackwell Scientific, Oxford.

Woolf N (1998) Pathology: basic and systemic. WB Saunders, Philadelphia.

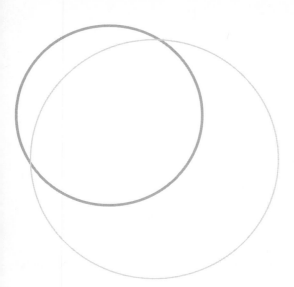

CELL INJURY

For a clearer understanding of this chapter you are advised to have read Chapters 1, 2, and 3.

INTRODUCTION

In the body of a healthy person, individual cells perform specific functions essential to the well-being of the person. They have a limited capacity to adapt to change, and they can do so only within defined limits. For example, hypertrophy of skeletal muscle cells takes place during weight training as an adaptive response to an increased workload and the associated rise in metabolic activity (see Chapter 3). However, if the stresses placed on a cell exceed its capacity to adapt, then the cell will be injured. Depending on the extent of these stresses, this injury will either be sublethal or lethal; in the latter case the injury precedes death of the cell. This chapter is concerned with the causes of cell injury, the changes that take place in cells during sublethal and lethal injury, and the characteristics and consequences of cell death.

CAUSES OF CELL INJURY

Cells can be injured by :
• microbial agents;
• physical agents;
• chemical agents;
• immune injury;
• lack of nutrients and oxygen;
• metabolic changes.

MICROBIAL AGENTS

The effects of micro-organisms on cells are discussed in the section on Microbiology (see Chapters 15–21). In this context, it is sufficient to note that the invasion of cells by micro-organisms can result in cell death. Bacteria, viruses, fungi, protozoa, and helminths can all bring about destruction of cells, with serious consequences for the host (Figure 4.1).

For example, invasion of cells by the human immun-odeficiency virus (HIV) and the eventual replication of the virus in these cells is responsible for the effects of the acquired immunodeficiency syndrome (AIDS) (see Chapter 28). In this condition, it is destruction of the T helper lymphocytes during viral replication that renders the host susceptible to malignancies and infection.

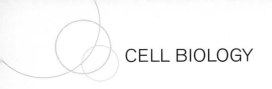
As another example, parasites belonging to the genus *Plasmodium* are responsible for malaria; after invading and multiplying in red blood cells, the parasites are eventually released into the blood stream with consequent rupturing of the red blood cells. It is the destruction of the red blood cells that results in the clinical features of malaria and the characteristic fever.

PHYSICAL AGENTS

Physical Force

A range of physical agents can result in cell injury and cell death. Physical force can disrupt cells; obvious examples of this are bullet wounds, knife wounds, and the forces resulting from a road traffic accident. If sufficient cells are damaged, then tissues and organs may no longer function effectively, with disastrous consequences.

Extremes of Temperature

The effects of extremes of temperature can have serious effects on cells. The range of body temperatures that is conducive to survival is from 31°C to 41°C (see Chapter 2).

The effects of cold on cells include degenerative changes and metabolic dysfunction. Individual cells may be able to tolerate cold temperatures and can even be stored at very low temperatures, a technique that is utilized when storing certain blood products or sperm. However, the consequences of hypothermia on the body as a whole are potentially fatal.

A patient is diagnosed with hypothermia when the core body temperature is less than 35°C:
- mild hypothermia occurs when the core body temperature is 34–35°C;
- moderate hypothermia occurs when the core body temperature is 30–34°C;
- severe hypothermia occurs when the core body temperature is less than 30°C.

The symptoms of mild hypothermia include:
- shivering;
- increased heart rate;
- vasoconstriction with a possible rise in blood pressure;
- hyperventilation;
- increased urinary output with the subsequent risk of dehydration.

As body temperature falls below 34°C, there is a decline in the shivering response and muscle rigidity occurs. Heart rate and blood pressure decrease, respiratory difficulties occur, and the coughing reflex is affected. Other features included a fall in metabolic rate and the subsequent reduction in oxygen utilization and carbon dioxide output (see Chapter 2).

Examples of patient groups most at risk of hypothermia include neonates and the elderly, in whom the homeostatic ability to maintain body temperature is diminished – this is compounded by illness and social deprivation; those suffering from malnutrition or hypothyroidism , in which there is a decline in metabolic rate; alcoholics; and those with cardiovascular disease.

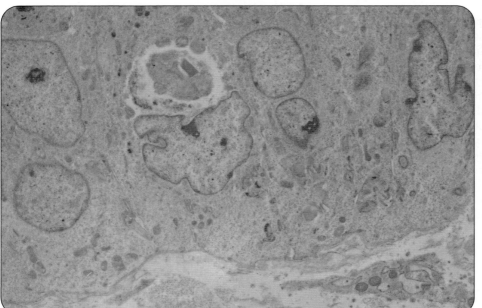

Figure 4.1 The boundary between intestinal epithelium and the underlying connective tissue. In this electron micrograph, epithelial cells are resting on the basal lamina and within one of the cells a protozoon parasite can be seen (× 3000).

High temperature is also damaging to cells, and high temperatures cause denaturation of the protein within the cells (see Person-Centred Study: Hyperaemia). The outcome of this depends on how much of the body has been damaged as a result of exposure to high temperatures. In general, burns exceeding 70% of the body surface prove fatal.

In the skin, partial thickness burns can result from exposure to temperatures that cause reversible cell injury but do not irreversibly damage the dermis. Exposure to higher temperatures will result in full thickness burns which differ from the former in that there is complete destruction of the skin affected. Epithelial regeneration often has to be supported through skin grafting.

Ionizing Radiation

Ionizing radiation is an important cause of cell injury and cell death. Ionization is produced by the displacement of electrons from the atoms within the cells that the radiation passes through. The ionized molecules are highly unstable and are converted into highly reactive species known as free radicals (see below). It is these free radicals that result in damage to the affected cells. However, X-rays cause ionizing radiation, and these are used for diagnostic purposes and also as cancer therapy. Gamma-rays and radiation that consists of electrons (beta-particles), protons, neutrons, and alpha-particles (two neutrons and two protons) are also used.

Ionizing radiation is more damaging to dividing cells than to cells that are non-dividing. The reason for this is that the DNA is affected, and this only becomes apparent during cell division. In radiotherapy, where ionizing radiation is used to destroy cancer cells selectively, differentiated non-dividing cells exposed to the radiation are less damaged than cells that are dividing rapidly (e.g. cells within the bone marrow, intestine, and skin are easily damaged).

Ionizing radiation can be a cause of cancer, and the relationship between ionizing radiation and a number of cancers is well established (see Chapter 5). Depending on the dose, the effects of ionizing radiation will either be sublethal or lethal. At higher doses it is particularly harmful to cells and will produce considerable damage.

Ultraviolet Radiation

Ultraviolet radiation does not result in ionization, but nevertheless it is very damaging to cells. DNA can absorb photons of energy from ultraviolet light, which leads in alterations in the genetic bases (i.e. adenine, guanine, thymine, and cytosine) and can result in dimerization, that is linking of adjacent bases. Pyrimidines are important in this respect. Accordingly, when thymine dimers are formed, they can prevent the normal replication of DNA (see also Chapter 7).

CHEMICAL AGENTS

Cells can be injured by the effects of poisons. Almost all chemicals will act as poison if the concentration is sufficiently high, but a number of chemicals are poisonous at very low concentrations. Cyanide, for example, injures cells by affecting cytochrome oxidase, an enzyme that is found in the mitochondria and that is part of the oxidative phosphorylation pathway (this metabolic pathway is also referred to as the electron transport chain; see Chapter 2). Other chemicals, such as lead, are only poisonous when accumulated following continual exposure. Oxygen, which is essential for aerobic respiration, can be severely toxic under high concentrations.

In the modern world, people are exposed to high levels of toxic and potentially toxic chemicals. These include environmental and air pollutants, pesticides, and carbon monoxide. Carbon monoxide can indirectly damage cells by binding to haemoglobin to form carboxyhaemoglobin; this restricts the supply of oxygen

PERSON-CENTRED STUDY: HYPERAEMIA

Marc, aged 4 years, wandered into the kitchen without his mother noticing. He was just able reach up and pull a white flex that led to a kettle containing water that was close to boiling. He pulled this flex and the kettle fell on top of him, spilling some hot water on his arm. His arm was badly scalded, and soon the skin started to go red because of hyperaemia (increased blood flow to the area). This was then followed by blistering despite the attempts of his mother to administer first aid by pouring cold water on the wound. Fortunately, the scald was superficial and did not result in damage to the dermal structures. Eventually the blisters resolved and the affected tissues returned to normal with almost no scarring.

to cells in the body. Drugs used for therapeutic purposes are invariably poisonous and the toxic effects have to be balanced against the benefits associated with use. In an ideal therapeutic drug, the dose required for therapeutic benefit should be significantly less than the dose that has a lethal effect (see the section on Pharmacology, Chapters 8–14).

IMMUNE INJURY

Although the immune system is extremely important to a person's well-being and in defence against disease, it can also be involved in cell injury. Immunological mechanisms are known to contribute to a number of diseases. Autoimmune injury is the consequence of immunological attacks on the body's own tissues and cells by the action of antibodies or T-lymphocyte-mediated reactions (see Chapter 27).

It appears that opsonization and phagocytosis of red blood cells is the main factor responsible for destruction of the cells in autoimmune haemolytic anaemia. In systemic lupus erythematosus, autoantibodies (and in particular antinuclear antibodies) arise from a probable defect in the regulatory mechanisms that maintain self tolerance. The patient's skin, joints, kidney, and sclerosal membranes are often damaged as a result. (The immune system is discussed in Chapters 22–30).

LACK OF NUTRIENTS AND OXYGEN

Poor diet and nutritional imbalances can result in cell injury. Insufficient oxygen results in a reduction in oxidative phosphorylation within cells, which can lead to cell injury (see below). Similarly, if there is insufficient glucose, cells have to obtain their energy from alternative macronutrients. Likewise, insufficient protein in the diet leads to a deficit of basic materials to support cell repair mechanisms, and injury could result.

Diseases associated with nutritional deficiencies are well known, as are the effects of malnutrition. It is also worth noting that there are diseases that are associated with dietary excess, and there is good evidence that vascular endothelium can be injured through a lipid-rich diet (see Chapter 2).

METABOLIC CHANGES

Metabolic changes, such as an excess or deficiency of hormones, acid–base and electrolyte imbalances, and an excess of growth factors, can result in cell injury (see Box 4.1).

After cell injury, it may be some time before morphological effects are apparent at both the ultrastructural and light microscope levels. For example, cell

---

BOX 4.1 MECHANISMS OF CELL INJURY

Injurious agents can affect the cell at a number of levels, by damaging:
- the plasma membranes, rendering them ineffective as selective barriers between the internal environment of the cell and the extracellular fluid
- aerobic respiration and the production of adenosine triphosphate (ATP)
- the synthesis of proteins (i.e. those important as enzymes and structural proteins)
- the genetic machinery of the cell

---

swelling can occur in minutes and is frequently reversible, whereas the changes seen in cardiac muscle cell death resulting from anoxia do not appear until some 10–12 hours after the tissue has become anoxic. Typically, a series of events will occur after a harmful effect. Some cells, such as skeletal muscle cells, can survive extended periods without oxygen; nerve cells, on the other hand, are extremely sensitive and will be lethally injured follow ischaemia of about 4 minutes.

EFFECTS OF HYPOXIA

Cells that rely on aerobic respiration undergo change if their oxygen supply is affected. The first system to be influenced is the mitochondrion, within which oxidative phosphorylation takes place, so the production of ATP will be reduced.

The decrease in cellular ATP results in a rise in adenosine monophosphate (AMP). In turn, this stimulates enzymes resulting in an increased rate of glycolysis, which is not dependent on oxygen. As was noted in Chapter 2, glycolysis is less effective in producing ATP than oxidative phosphorylation. Within certain cells, ATP can be produced anaerobically from creatine phosphates following the action of creatine phosphatase. An increase in glycolysis within a cell will result in a depletion of glycogen, and this is apparent morphologically. Lactic acid accumulates, leading to a reduction in the intracellular pH; this can result in the clumping of chromatin within the nucleus.

At the cell membrane, a reduction in ATP affects the sodium–potassium pump mechanism, which in health is responsible for removing sodium ions from the cell and transferring potassium ions from the extracellular fluid into the cell. The consequence of this is that these ions move freely across the selectively permeable cell membrane, as would be expected (owing to the concentration differences in sodium and potassium between the intracellular and extracellular fluids) Thus, potassium diffuses from the cytoplasm into the extracellular fluid and sodium moves in the opposite direction. Because sodium has a larger hydration shell than potassium, water moves into the cell, and the cell swells as a result of this water.

Other effects seen include a dilation of the endoplasmic reticulum, detachment of ribosomes from the granular endoplasmic reticulum, and disassociation of the polysomes ('strings' of ribosomes). Further hypoxic injury can result in mitochondrial damage, blebbing of the cell membrane, and the loss of microvilli if these were a normal feature of the cell. Parts of the outer cell membrane as well as membranes of intracellular organelles may be found in whorls that look like the sheath of nerves and are therefore called myelin figures. Typically, the damaged mitochondria are swollen (Figure 4.2, Box 4.2).

Most of the features of hypoxia are reversible in many cells providing that the reduced supply of oxygen does not continue indefinitely. If it persists, however, severe vacuolization of the mitochondria, further damage to the plasma membranes, and the movement of calcium into the cells represent the next stages. The damaged cell membranes allow the flow of essential

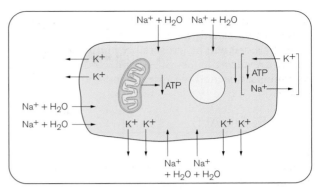

Figure 4.2 Effects of reduced oxygen supply on cells. Inhibition of ATP production leads to a reduction in the sodium–potassium pump mechanism, and extracellular sodium therefore enters the cell and potassium leaves it. This results in cloudy swelling, dilatation of the endoplasmic reticulum, dissociation of the ribosomes, mitchondrial damage, and cell blebbing.

proteins from the cells. If the lysosomal membranes are disrupted, then potent enzymes are released into the cell cytoplasm, and when this occurs cell death is inevitable. The leakage of intracellular enzymes from irreversibly injured cells are important clinical measures of cell death. For example, the measurement of aspartate aminotransferase, lactic dehydrogenase and creatine kinase are important clinical indicators of myocardial death (see Chapter 6).

BOX 4.2 PRESSURE SORES

An example of hypoxic injury is the development of pressure sores.

- Immobile patients are particularly vulnerable to developing pressure sores.
- Pressure sores are localized areas of tissue necrosis and are a consequence of a time–pressure relationship, i.e. the risk of developing a pressure sore is increased with (i) greater pressure and (ii) a longer duration of remaining in one position.
- When pressure is constantly applied to the skin surface it causes a decrease in blood flow leading to tissue hypoxia. This is accompanied by changes in the cellular metabolism to compensate for the lack of oxygen, and cellular damage (Figure 4.3).

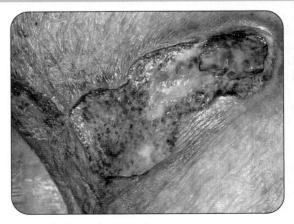

Figure 4.3 Sacral pressure sore. Cellular damage due to lack of oxygen. By kind permission of Dr. Mark Cottee, St. George's Hospital Healthcare Trust, London.

It is clear that the ability of the plasma membrane to function normally is a critical factor in determining whether a cell will be irreversibly injured. Membrane damage resulting in loss of essential components from the cell is associated with irreversible injury.

FREE RADICALS

In recent years there has been considerable investigation of the role of free radicals and their generation of membrane damage. Free radicals are extremely energetic and reactive chemical species that have single unpaired electrons in their outer orbitals. Furthermore, they are extremely unstable and can interact with a wide range of biological molecules, including nucleic acids, membrane proteins, and lipids. Free radicals are produced by the absorption of ionizing or non-ionizing radiation (see above), by oxidative reactions that occur during metabolism, or through the enzymatic breakdown of chemicals or drugs.

The most important free radicals in the body include the oxygen-derived radicals. These radicals can be produced as a result of the activity of a variety of oxidative enzymes in different parts of the cell. They include:
- superoxide (O_2^-);
- hydrogen peroxide (H_2O_2); and
- hydroxyl radicals ($OH^\bullet$).

Superoxide is generated during oxidation in mitochondria or by cytoplasmic enzymes such as xanthine oxidase, cytochrome P_{450}, and other oxidase enzymes. Superoxide inactivates spontaneously, though it is inactivated more quickly in the presence of the enzyme superoxide dismutase. It forms hydrogen peroxide (Figure 4.4) regardless of the route of inactivation.

Hydrogen peroxide can also be produced in cells by the oxidases that are present in peroxisomes, which also contain the enzyme catalase. Catalase can remove hydrogen peroxide:

$$2H_2O_2 \longrightarrow O_2 + 2H_2O$$
$$\text{catalase}$$

The effective activity of certain immune cell types relies on the release of hydrogen peroxide to aid the phagocytic process (see Chapter 22).

Hydroxyl radicals are oxygen-derived radicals that are also generated by the hydrolysis of water by ionizing radiation. They can be produced by the interaction of hydrogen peroxide with transitional metals such as iron and copper or by the interaction between hydrogen peroxide and superoxide, which is known as the Haber–Weiss reaction. Lipid peroxidation is typically initiated by hydroxyl radicals, which generate organic acid-free radicals that react with oxygen to form peroxides. The peroxides then act as free radicals, initiating a chain reaction that results in extensive membrane damage. The oxygen-derived radicals can also damage proteins and DNA.

Antioxidants (sometimes known as scavengers) are important in terminating free radical reactions. Vitamin E and glutathione and some serum proteins (e.g. caeruloplasmin, a copper-transport protein) block the initiation of free radical formation and inactivate free radicals.

Superoxide dismutase converts superoxide to hydrogen peroxide (Figure 4.4). Glutathione peroxidase catalyses the release of hydrogen from reduced glutathione (GSH) to a hydroxy radical or to hydrogen peroxide:

$$2OH^\bullet + 2GSH \longrightarrow 2H_2O + GSSG$$
$$\text{glutathione peroxidase}$$

$$H_2O_2 + 2GSH \longrightarrow 2H_2O + GSSG$$
$$\text{glutathione peroxidase}$$

All the main categories of biological molecules can be attacked by free radicals and lipids are very susceptible. Cell membranes contain large quantities of polyunsaturated fatty acids (PUFAs) which are readily attacked by free radicals in a process known as lipid peroxidation.

Figure 4.5 shows how lipid peroxidation takes place. It is very damaging because it proceeds as a self-perpetuating chain reaction which can lead to widespread membrane damage within the formation of visible injury such as blebbing.

FATTY CHANGE

It has been noted above that hypoxia can result in the accumulation of water within cells. Similarly, cell injury can result in the intracellular accumulation of lipids, which is known as fatty change. The excess lipid can be seen as small droplets or as a large drop within the cell. During conventional preparation for light microscopy, lipid tends to be removed from the cell; however, special techniques, such as frozen sections followed by staining with lipid soluble dyes such as oil red O, can demonstrate the fat within affected cells.

Fatty change can be seen within the supportive or parenchymal cells of the liver, heart, and kidney, and affected organs have a greasy feel. A range of mechanisms may be responsible for the accumulation of fat within liver cells (hepatocytes). The liver receives fat from non-esterified free fatty acids derived from adipose tissue stores during lipolysis (see Chapter 2). It also

superoxide generation

$$O_2 \xrightarrow{\text{oxidase}} O_2^-$$

superoxide inactivation and formation
of hydrogen peroxide

$$O_2^- + O_2^- + 2H^+ \xrightarrow[\text{dismutase}]{\text{superoxide}} H_2O_2 + O_2$$
$$\text{(SOD)}$$

hydroxyl radical generation

$$H_2O \xrightarrow[\text{radiation}]{\text{ionizing}} H^\bullet + OH^\bullet$$

$$Fe^{2+} + H_2O_2 \longrightarrow Fe^{3+} + OH^\bullet + OH^-$$

$$H_2O_2 + O_2^- \longrightarrow OH^\bullet + OH^- + O_2$$

Figure 4.4 Production of free radicals. Superoxide can be produced within the mitochondria and in the cytoplasm. In the cytoplasm it occurs by enzyme such as cytochrome P_{450} or xanthine oxidase. In the mitochondria it normally occur through auto-oxidation.

$$LH + R^\bullet \longrightarrow L^\bullet + RH$$
$$L^\bullet + O_2 \longrightarrow LOO^\bullet$$
$$LOO + L^1H \longrightarrow LOH + L^{1\bullet}$$
$$LOOH \longrightarrow LO^\bullet, LOO^\bullet, \text{aldehydes}$$

Figure 4.5 Lipid peroxidation. Oxidation of the PUFA (LH) by a free radical (R•) generates a fatty acid radical (L•) that combines with oxygen to form a fatty acid peroxyl radical (LOO•). The peroxyl radicals can oxidise new PUFA molecules and initiate new change producing lipid hydroperoxides (LOOH) which can in turn break down to give new radical species and a wide range of other compounds including aldehydes which are always formed when lipid hydroperoxides breakdown.

receives fat in the form of chylomicrons, which are large molecules synthesized within the epithelium of the small intestine. Chylomicrons consist of triglyceride, phospholipid, and apoprotein B. In hepatocytes, hydrolysis of chylomicrons occurs, releasing free fatty acids and glycerol. Free fatty acids arriving at the liver are esterified to form triglycerides, some of which are incorporated into phospholipid and others into cholesterol. Triglyceride within the liver is coupled to apoprotein (a lipid acceptor protein) and secreted from the liver in the form of very low density lipoprotein. An injured hepatocyte may not be able to produce sufficient apoprotein, and the accumulation of lipid can occur. Alternatively, fatty change can result from an increase in the amount of triglyceride being brought to the liver.

During starvation or in some diseases (e.g. diabetes mellitus), increased fat metabolism takes place to make up for energy shortfalls. This leads to the breakdown of fat in adipose tissue stores and results in an increase in the plasma concentration of free fatty acids.

If the cells are damaged as a result of hypoxia caused by congestive cardiac failure or through malnutrition, which prevents the production of apoproteins, then triglyceride accumulation can occur. People who misuse alcohol often have significant liver cell injury, which is manifested through fatty change. It may well be that this is due to interference with the oxidation of fatty acids.

Poisons such as carbon tetrachloride (as found in dry cleaning fluid) can reduce the production of protein by liver cells; again this can result in fatty change.

MORPHOLOGICAL INDICATORS OF CELL INJURY

Some of the morphological changes that occur have already been discussed. Our ability to recognize these depends on whether the cells are being examined by light microscopy or at the electron microscopic level. These visible modifications frequently represent the after-effects of injurious agents on some vital function or structural component of the cell. The changes seen include alteration to the plasma membrane (e.g. blebbing), changes to microvilli, and disruption of the membrane. Blebbing and disruption of microvilli can occur quickly but they may be reversible, whereas the effects on the plasma membrane may be irreversible.

Swelling of the mitochondria is a further characteristic of irreversible change. Typically, there may be initial condensation of the mitochondria after an injury such as that produced by poison. This condensation is reversible, but by the time swelling has taken place, a later stage has been reached and the process has usually become irretrievable.

Dilatation of the endoplasmic reticulum, detachment of ribosomes, and the break-up of polysomes has previously been mentioned. Lysosomes may swell following injury, and, although this is reversible, damage to the lysosomal membrane and the loss of the lysosomal content of the cell is associated with irreversible change.

CELL DEATH

If a cell is irreparably damaged, cell death will occur. Different morphological changes are observed after cell death or necrosis.

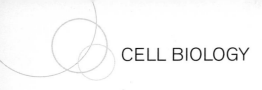

CELL BIOLOGY

Coagulative Necrosis

Coagulative necrosis results in a cell retaining its outline, often for periods extending into several days. The nucleus from the cell is lost and the cell appears as a mass of pink-staining homogeneous material when examined in a routine histological section. A key feature of this type of necrosis appears to be the denaturation of cytoplasmic proteins through the release of lysosomal enzymes. It characteristically occurs in organs such as the kidney and the heart, where cell injury usually results from anoxia. It is also seen in the skin following burns.

Liquefactive Necrosis

Liquefactive necrosis occurs when lysosomal enzymes cause rapid liquefaction, which happens when the action of these enzymes on a cell results in autolysis. It is typically seen in the brain following an ischaemic injury. Liquefactive necrosis is also responsible for pus formation after the action of neutrophil enzymes (see Chapter 22).

Fat Necrosis

Fat necrosis can be separated into enzymatic and non-enzymatic types. In enzymatic fat necrosis, the enzymes from an organ such as the pancreas are liberated from the duct into surrounding tissues. The lipases act on the triglycerides and fat cells and break them down into glycerol and fatty acids, which then form complexes with calcium ions to form soaps. If the lipids enter into the blood stream, widespread fat necrosis throughout the body can occur.

In non-enzymatic fat necrosis, trauma is often suspected as causing an inflammatory response. It is characterized by the appearance of foam cells, neutrophils, and lymphocytes; this is followed by fibrosis, which results in the production of a mass. It is sometimes known as traumatic fat necrosis.

Caseous and Gummatous Necrosis

Caseous ('cheese-like) and gummatous ('gum-like' or 'rubber-like') necrosis occurs in infectious granulosis and is frequently associated with infections such as tuberculosis (see Chapter 26).

Fibrinous Necrosis

Fibrinous necrosis is seen in autoimmune diseases such as rheumatic fever and systemic lupus erythematosus (see Chapter 27). It is characterized by the loss of the normal structure and the replacement of cells by homogeneous, bright pink staining material that looks like fibrin microscopically in histological sections. Typically, these areas of necrosis contain immunoglobulins and complement, breakdown products of collagen, and fibrins (see Chapters 24 and 25).

Gangrene

Gangrene is a term used to denote a condition in which extensive tissue necrosis is complicated by secondary bacterial infection and may be classified as dry or wet gangrene.

In dry gangrene there is coagulative necrosis of tissues resulting from ischaemia that is secondary to arterial obstruction. The necrotic area has a black, dry, and shrivelled appearance, and it is separated from adjacent tissue. There is usually insignificant secondary bacterial infection and the gangrene can be removed surgically.

Wet gangrene occurs when there is severe bacterial infection amongst necrotic tissue. It can occur in the extremities as well as the internal organs, including the intestine. Acute inflammation and the growth of invading bacteria result in the necrotic area becoming swollen and reddish-black, with liquefaction of the dead tissue owing to poor venous return. Unlike dry gangrene, wet gangrene is not separated clearly from the adjacent tissue and it is difficult to treat surgically. The bacteria can cause fermentation with a characteristic foul smell.

Gas gangrene results from wounds infected by *Clostridium perfringens* as well as other *Clostridium* species. There is extensive necrosis of the tissue and production of gas by bacteria. It looks like wet gangrene except that there are bubbles of gas in the tissues. Both wet gangrene and gas gangrene are associated with high mortality (see Chapter 16).

LYSOSOMES AND CELL INJURY

Lysosomes are extremely important in relation to cell injury. Release of their contents can result in irreversible cell injury following exposure to a damaging agent – lysosomes are membrane-bound vesicles that contain a potent mix of hydrolytic enzymes. They are produced within the rough endoplasmic reticulum, from where vesicles transfer to the Golgi apparatus, which gives rise to mature lysosomes (see Chapter 1). Lysosomes that have not undergone any reactions are known as primary lysosomes or virgin lysosomes. These primary lysosomes contain a full range of enzymes, which, if they were to leak into the cell, would cause irreversible damage. Lysosomal membranes have specific properties that prevent the contents being released.

In health, lysosomes undertake a number of functions, including heterophagy and autophagy. In heterophagy, lysosomes fuse with phagosomes, vesicles that contain particles of phagocytosis, thereby forming a secondary lysosome sometimes referred to as a heterophagic phagolysosome. The release of the lysosomal enzymes into the heterophagosome results in the digestion of the ingested particle. The particle that is left is referred to as a residual body, which contains the indigestible remains of the heterophagic phagolysosome.

In autophagy, autophagic vacuoles are formed by surrounding worn-out cell organelles with a membrane. Primary lysosomes fuse with this autophagic vacuole to create a secondary lysosome, within which the worn-out organelle can be digested. This again leads to the formation of a residual body. Autophagy is particularly common in cells undergoing atrophy (see Chapter 3).

Occasionally the process of heterophagy can result in cell injury. For instance, it will happen if the cell tries to ingest a particle such as asbestos. This leads to the production of an unstable secondary lysosome, and there can be leakage of the lysosomal contents into the cell, with disastrous consequences. Heterophagy is a common process undertaken by phagocytic cells.

KEY POINTS

- Cells have a limited capacity to adapt to change, and do so only within defined limits. Therefore, if the stress placed on a cell exceed its ability to adapt, it will be injured.
- Physical forces and extremes of temperature can result in degenerative changes and metabolic dysfunction. Ionizing radiation used in diagnosis and therapy may damage DNA, and thus affect cell division if given in high enough doses.
- Certain chemical agents are metabolic poisons that can inhibit enzymes (e.g. cyanide). Some drugs may also be lethal if given at an inappropriate dose.
- Cellular injury may be sustained after changes in oxygen supply; respiration is thus affected and other metabolic changes ensue. The consequences of hypoxia on cell structures include increased permeability of the outer membrane, which encourages the influx of water, and disruption of cellular organelles.
- Free radicals are extremely energetic chemical species that can interact with a range of biological molecules, but can be inactivated by enzymes (e.g. superoxide dismutase) and by antioxidants (e.g. vitamin E).
- The accumulation of lipid is known as 'fatty change', which can be seen on light microscopy. Fatty changes occur after metabolic disturbances (e.g. diabetes mellitus and long-term misuse of alcohol).
- If a cell is irreversibly damaged, cell death will occur, and different morphological changes can be observed. Necrotic changes differ in their presentation, depending on the type of injury sustained.
- Gangrene denotes a condition in which extensive tissue necrosis is complicated by a secondary bacterial infection.

FURTHER READING

Ardire L (1997) Necrotizing fasciitis: case study of a nursing dilemma. Ostomy Wound Management 43:30–4.

Burkitt HG, Stevens A, Lowe JS , Young B (1996) Wheater's Basic Histopathology: a Colour Atlas and Text, 3rd edition. Churchill Livingstone, Edinburgh.

Castledine G (1994) Nurse-aid management of hypothermia. Br J Nurs 3:185–7.

Chandrasoma P, Taylor CR (1997) Concise Pathology, 3rd edition. Prentice Hall International (UK), London.

Eastwood M (1997) Principles of Human Nutrition. Chapman and Hall, London.

Fell D (1997) Understanding the Control of Metabolism. Portland Press, London.

Jordan BS, Harrington DT (1997) Management of the burn wound. Nurs Clin North Am 32:251–73.

Laing HJ (1997) Perioperative burn nursing. Semin Perioper Nurs 6:210–22.

Lewis RT (1998) Soft tissue infections. World J Surg 22:146–51.

Majno G, Joris I (1996) Cells, Tissues and Disease. Principles of General Pathology. Blackwell Scientific, Oxford. <19>

Sedlak SK (1995) Hypothermia in trauma: the nurse's role in recognition, prevention, and management. Int J Trauma Nurs 1:19–26.

Shikora SA, Blackburn GL (1997) Nutrition Support. Chapman and Hall, London.

Smith GL, Bunker CB, Dinneen MD (1998) Fournier's gangrene. Br J Urol 81:347–55.

Stewart-Amidei C (1995) Delayed effects of therapeutic brain irradiation. Crit Care Nurs Clin North Am 7:125–33.

Tausigg MJ (1998) Processes in Pathology and Microbiology, 3rd edition. Blackwell Science, Oxford.

Woolf N (1998) Pathology: basic and systemic, WB Saunders, Philadelphia.

NEOPLASIA

5

LEARNING OBJECTIVES

After studying this chapter you will:
- understand the different terminologies used to describe benign and malignant neoplasms
- know the difference between benign neoplasms and malignant neoplasms (cancer)
- be able to consider the routes of invasion that exist for different types of neoplasms
- understand the mechanisms by which metastases are established
- be able to evaluate critically the influence of key carcinogens in the establishment of cancer
- understand how a study of epidemiology can provide information on possible causes of cancer
- be able to discuss the role of oncogenes in the development of malignant neoplasms

Before reading this chapter, you should be familiar with the information in Chapters 1, 3, and 7.

INTRODUCTION

This chapter is about neoplasia and, in particular, about malignant neoplasms or cancer. It explores the causes of cancer and the biological effects of cancer on the body.

DEFINITIONS

The word neoplasm is derived from the Greek and simply means 'new growth'. It has been defined as being an abnormal mass of tissue where the growth both exceeds that of the normal tissues and is unco-ordinated with that of the normal tissues. The growth persists in the same excessive manner even after the stimulus that evoked the change has been removed. Conversely, in hyperplasia, such as occurs following injury to the skin (see Chapter 3), the rapid growth ceases once the stimulus has been removed (in this case, once the wound has been repaired). However, neoplasms continue to grow in the absence of any stimuli. They are autonomous and their growth is to the detriment of the host.

A tumour is simply a swelling. The term is used to describe one of the cardinal signs of inflammation, but in the context of neoplasia it means a growth or swelling. Not all neoplasms result in tumours. The word cancer is derived from the Latin for 'crab', for reasons that are explained later in this chapter. It is the common name used for malignant neoplasms. The behaviour of neoplasms determines whether or not they are benign or malignant (cancer).

Oncology, a term derived from the Greek *oncos*, which means tumour, is the study of tumours or neoplasms, and oncologists are medically qualified staff working in the field of oncology.

TERMINOLOGY USED TO DESCRIBE DIFFERENT TYPES OF NEOPLASMS

There are two components to both benign and malignant neoplasms:
- the parenchyma, which is composed of proliferating neoplastic cells;
- the stroma, which is the connective tissue and blood vessels that support the parenchymal cells.

CELL BIOLOGY

The terminology applied to tumours is based on the parenchymal component. The following describes the cells originating from mature specialized cells. Benign neoplasms derived from epithelium are adenomas if they arise from glandular epithelium, and papillomas if they have a papillary shape. The term adenoma is used with the tissue of origin, for example, a liver cell adenoma or a parathyroid adenoma. Similarly, the term papilloma is also used with the cell of origin, such as a urothelial papilloma or a squamous papilloma.

Malignant neoplasms arising from epithelium are called carcinomas. If they are derived from glandular epithelium, they are adenocarcinomas. The term carcinoma is also used with the tissue of origin, such as transitional cell carcinoma, squamous cell carcinoma (see Person-Centred Study: Squamous Cell Carcinoma), and basal cell carcinoma.

Benign neoplasms arising from mesenchymal tissue are named after the cell of origin with the suffix -*oma* added. Examples include fibroma, chondroma, schwannoma, lipoma. Malignant mesenchymal neoplasms have the suffix -*sarcoma*. Examples include fibrosarcoma, chondrosarcoma, osteosarcoma, liposarcoma, and haemangiosarcoma.

In addition to the neoplasms that are derived from mature cells, neoplasms can also be derived from totipotent cells (i.e. cells that are capable of maturing into any cell in the body). After birth, the only such cells in the body are the germ cells. Neoplasms that are derived from germ cells include teratomas, which may be benign or malignant. They can form a range of fetal tissues, and mixtures of these tissues typically exist within a single teratoma. Teratomas that are mature are those that are well differentiated and composed of adult tissue types. Immature teratomas contain fetal-type tissues and are malignant.

Neoplasms can also arise from pluripotent cell types. Pluripotent cells are those cells that can develop into several different cell types. They mainly exist in the fetus and during the first few years of childhood. For this reason, these neoplasms are characteristic of childhood; examples are malignancies such as retinoblastoma, nephroblastoma, neuroblastoma, and medulloblastoma.

As with all classification systems, there are exceptions. There are a number of malignant neoplasms whose names sound benign, including melanomas, lymphomas, gliomas, plasmacytomas, and astrocytomas. The cell of origin is obvious, that these neoplasms are malignant is indicated by prefixing them with the word 'malignant'. In practice, there is little ground for confusion because none of these neoplasms is ever benign. Therefore, both melanoma and malignant melanoma are used interchangeably to describe the same malignancy. There are no benign neoplasms that derive from melanocytes.

Mixed tumours are neoplasms that contain more than one neoplastic cell type, and so they have two parenchymal cell types. These may both be derived from epithelial components or mesenchymal components or there may be a mixture of both. For example, the adenosquamous carcinoma consists of both glandular and squamous epithelial tissue; the malignant fibrous histiocytoma consists both of malignant cells derived from fibroblasts and from histiocytes; and the carcinoma sarcoma of the lung consists of both epithelial and mesenchymal cells.

Neoplasms arising from blood-forming tissues are all malignant and are called leukaemias. Neoplasms derived from red blood cells are called erythroblastic leukaemias; neoplasms derived from myeloblasts are called myeloid leukaemia; and neoplasms derived from

PERSON-CENTRED STUDY: SQUAMOUS CELL CARCINOMA

Patrick, aged 56, had been a heavy cigarette smoker since he was 14 years old. He was used to coughs and sore throats, but he had always felt that he would be one of the lucky ones. After all, his grandfather had smoked until dying from a road accident in his mid-80s.

One winter, Patrick had a cough that would just not go away. He put it down to a long-standing cold, but it continued to persist right through until the spring. He was also starting to feel very tired and described himself as 'chesty'. He decided to seek help from his general practitioner, who referred him for a chest X-ray.

On the X-ray there was evidence of a mass in his right lung, and he was referred for bronchoscopy. Examination of the cells from the lesion showed a squamous cell carcinoma. Pneumonectomy was considered but it proved not to be possible. He has had both chemotherapy and radiotherapy and remains well some 6 months later.

monoblasts are called monocytic leukaemia (see Chapter 31). Within the lymphoid tissue, lymphoblasts and lymphocytes can rise to malignant lymphomas, lymphocytic leukaemias, and myeloma; histiocytes give rise to malignant histiocytosis. It was noted above that not all malignant neoplasms give rise to tumours. Leukaemias are an example of this in that they rarely produce tumours and are characterized by the proliferation of malignant cells in the peripheral blood and the bone marrow.

CHARACTERISTICS OF BENIGN AND MALIGNANT NEOPLASMS

In the majority of cases, morphology is used to distinguish between benign and malignant neoplasms. However, there are problems associated with this because morphology is subjective. A diagnosis based on morphological features is in effect a prediction of the future course and behaviour of the neoplasm. There can frequently be a marked discrepancy between the morphological appearance of a neoplasm and its behaviour.

DIFFERENTIATION AND ANAPLASIA

The term differentiation refers to the extent to which the parenchymal cells within a tumour resemble comparable normal cells, both morphologically and functionally. Well differentiated tumours are composed of cells that resemble the mature normal cells of the tissue of origin. Poorly differentiated and undifferentiated tumours have primitive or unspecialized cells. In comparison, all benign tumours are well differentiated.

Malignant neoplasms range from well differentiated to undifferentiated, and those that are composed of undifferentiated cells are called anaplastic. The word 'anaplasia' means 'to form backwards' and refers to a lack of differentiation. The term 'poorly differentiated' often appears on histopathological reports (Table 5.1).

RATE OF TUMOUR GROWTH

The growth rate of tumours correlates with their level of differentiation. Most malignant tumours grow more rapidly than benign tumours. Poorly differentiated tumours tend to grow more rapidly than well-differentiated tumours. Rapidly growing tumours often contain central areas of ischaemic necrosis. The reason for this is that they have outgrown their blood supply. Hormone dependency as well as the blood supply can also influence growth.

Characteristic Features of Anaplastic Cells

- The cells and nuclei display pleomorphism (i.e. both the cells and nuclei show variations in size and shape in comparison with their neighbours)
- The nuclei are hyperchromatic or dark-straining
- The nuclei are disproportionately large for the cell, and the nuclear–cytoplasmic ratio may reach 1:1 (normally this ratio is 1:4 or 1:6 in healthy non-malignant cells)
- The chromatin is clumped and distributed at the nuclear membrane
- Large nucleoli are present
- There are large numbers of mitoses
- Atypical mitoses are present
- Tumour giant cells are formed
- The cell orientation is disorganized
- Within the connective tissue supporting the tumour, the vascular stroma is often minimal and this leads to necrosis

Table 5.1 Characteristic features of anaplastic cells.

LOCAL INVASION
Benign Tumours
These grow as masses that remain localized to their site of origin. They do not have the capacity to infiltrate, invade, or metastasize (see below) to distant sites as malignant neoplasms do. Benign tumours usually possess a fibrous capsule. They exist as palpable and easily movable masses, and they can often be surgically enucleated.

Malignant Tumours
Malignant tumours are cancers that grow and progressively infiltrate, invade, and destroy the surrounding tissue. They are poorly demarcated from the surrounding tissue. Typically, cords of tumour cells extend into the surrounding tissue and on histological section these cords resemble crab-like feet emerging from the main tumour mass (see Chapter 6). It is this feature that has resulted in the name 'cancer' (Latin for 'the crab') being used for malignant neoplasms. Cells from malignant neoplasms can enter lymphatic vessels, blood vessels, and body cavities (see below). Unlike benign neoplasms, malignant neoplasms are often extremely difficult to resect satisfactorily. There are differences in the vulnerability of tissues to the spread of malignant neoplasms. For instance, connective tissue stroma presents the least resistance to malignant spread, whereas cartilage is strongly resistant to invasion.

A carcinoma *in situ* may be found within a range of tissues, including the bladder, breast, cervix, and skin. This type of cancer is considered to be a pre-invasive stage that will eventually result in a malignant tumour. The cells of a carcinoma *in situ* have the characteristics

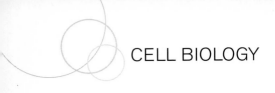
of a malignant neoplasm but there is no evidence of invasion of the tumour and the cells have not crossed the basement membrane. (The basement membrane is the term given to the connective tissue layer observed between all epithelia and the underlying tissue when observed under the light microscope.)

METASTASIS

In the context of neoplasia, metastases are tumour implants that are discontinuous with the primary tumour. It is the presence of metastases that marks a tumour as being malignant. Benign neoplasms do not metastasize, whereas, with very few exceptions, all malignant tumours have the capacity to metastasize (see Box 5.1).

Metastasis can take place via three main routes. These are:

- spread into body cavities;
- invasion of lymphatic vessels;
- haematogenous spread.

Spread into Body Cavities

This occurs when the tumour cells spread via the body cavities, which include the peritoneal cavity, the pleural cavity, the pericardium, and the subarachnoid spaces. An example of this is carcinoma of the ovary, which spreads transperitoneally from the ovary to the liver or to other abdominal viscera.

Invasion of Lymphatic Vessels

Some tumour cells gain access to lymphatic vessels, from where they are transported in the lymph to nodes. This method of invasion is particularly common for carcinomas. For example, breast cancer frequently spreads to the axillary or internal mammary lymph nodes. Involved lymph nodes become enlarged, and although this may be due to the growth of tumour cells within the lymph node, it may also on occasions be due to a reactive hyperplasia of the immune cells within the lymph nodes (see Chapter 30).

Haematogenous Spread

This occurs when tumour cells gain access to blood vessels. It is typical for sarcomas but it is also an important route of spread for certain carcinomas. Veins are more often invaded than arteries. The lungs and the liver are common sites for the establishment of metastases that have been spread via the blood vessels, but the brain and the bones are also frequently involved.

ESSENTIAL STEPS IN THE METASTATIC PROCESS

A number of different stages in the metastatic process can be identified. These are, in reality, part of a continuous process, but the stages described below are useful in defining some of the key mechanisms that must take place to establish successful metastasis (see

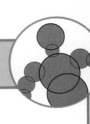

PERSON-CENTRED STUDY: MALIGNANT MELANOMA WITH METASTATIC SPREAD

Moira, a city lawyer, had fair skin and a tendency to develop freckles on exposure to the sun. With a good source of income, she was accustomed to taking frequent holidays in the sun. She loved sunbathing, and between holidays she would top-up her tan at the local health club. Although she tended to go red very quickly, she did not find sunburn particularly uncomfortable and was prepared to put up with it for the sake of a good tan.

One morning, she noticed a lesion on her shoulder that was starting to bleed. It was quite small and she knew that, if caught early, skin cancer was treatable. When the lesion continued to bleed and ooze over a period of days, she sought advice from her general practitioner, who immediately referred her to a consultant dermatologist.

The dermatologist arranged an immediate admission into hospital for her to have the lesion removed. On histological section, it was found to be a malignant melanoma and, although there was no evidence of metastasis, it was a worrying biopsy because there was evidence of the cells having entered into the dermis. Nine months later, she developed jaundice, and a scan suggested that there were secondary deposits (metastases) of the malignant melanoma which had lodged in the liver. Her disease was now widespread with secondary metastases present both in liver and in brain. She died shortly afterwards.

Figure 5.1 and Person-Centred Study: Malignant Melanoma with Metastatic Spread).

Local Invasion

For cancer to establish metastases, there has to be penetration of the host tissue immediately adjacent to the primary tumour. Penetration of the host tissue results from a number of factors.

Growth of the tumour cells results in an increase in pressure within the neoplasm. However, the importance of pressure in facilitating local invasion may not be a major factor. Evidence for this comes from the fact that the speed of growth does not correlate with the invasiveness of a tumour.

Motility of tumour cells does not seem to be related to their invasive potential. Local spread tends to follow the line of least resistance.

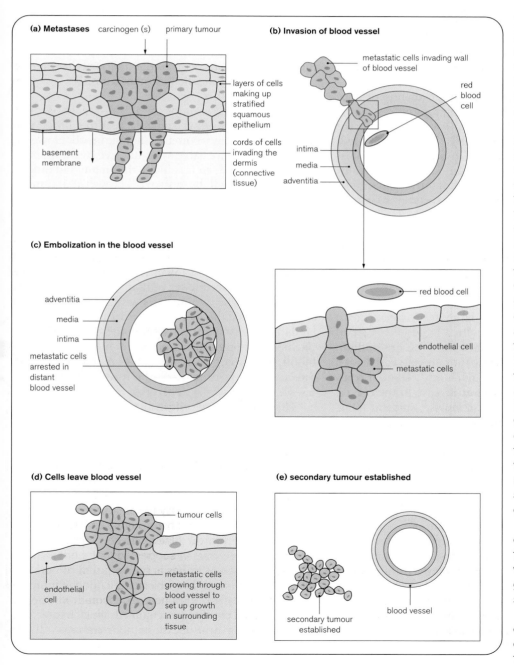

Figure 5.1 Metastases. The stages in the spread of (a) malignant neoplasm, if a tumour arises within the epithelium. a. Local invasion leads to the cells crossing the basement membrane of the epithelium. The cords of cells leaving the epithelium from which the tumour originated appear on histological section like a crab – hence the term 'cancer'.
(b) Malignant cells gain access to a fluid compartment such as a blood vessel; this is typical for carcinomas. Metastatic cells cross the basement membrane of the blood vessel.
(c) The metastatic cells are embolized in the lumen, where they will either be arrested mechanically or by adhesion to the endothelial cells.
(d) The metastatic cells then grow through the blood vessel and set up growth in the surrounding tissue.
(e) Secondary tumour established at site distant from primary tumour.

Tissue destruction results from invasion of the tumour cells. The tumour may obstruct the blood vessels supplying the tissue, which can lead to ischaemia and eventually to ischaemic necrosis (see Chapter 4).

Tissue destruction can also result in the release of cytolytic products from the tumour cells (e.g. collagenase, which digests the collagen in connective tissues). Some malignant cells are able to secrete lytic enzymes. Others can act on the host cells and stimulate secretory mechanisms within these. For example, the invasion of bone appears to be mediated by the enzymatic activity of osteoclasts, which are normally involved in the shaping of bones during development and repair (see Chapters 1 and 39). Fibroblasts can also secrete high levels of collagenase when they are cultured together with tumour cells.

Tissue destruction can also result from host defence actions in response to the growing tumour.

A further important factor in local invasion is the level of differentiation of the cells. Tumour cells dedifferentiate and this can result in increased mobilization of the cells from the main tumour bulk. Typically, dedifferentiation involves the loss of intracellular junctions and a decrease in tumour associated basement membrane.

Detachment from Primary Tumour

This is a second stage that must take place for metastases to be established. Detachment from the primary tumour may occur before or after blood vessel invasion. The number of tumour cells released from the primary tumour can be very large. It has been shown that mammary carcinomas with a mass of 2–4 g can release cells at a rate of around 3 million or 4 million cells/g of tumour per day. The tumour cells can detach either as single cells or as small clumps. Tumour trauma or massage can lead to an increase in the release in tumour cells and clumps. Likewise, surgical intervention can also lead to the spread of tumour cells. This is why a suspected testicular tumour is never biopsied; instead an orchidectomy (removal of the testicle) is performed. Spread of a tumour caused by surgical intervention is known as iatrogenic dissemination.

Blood Vessel Invasion

The invasion of blood vessels by tumour cells represents an important stage in the establishment of metastases. The cells may invade a blood vessel singly or with other tumour cells. The structure of blood vessels does not make invasion straightforward. The tumour cells have to cross a number of cellular layers before they gain access to the lumen (i.e. connective tissue of the adventitia, the media, the intima, including the vascular endothelial cell).

The degree of development of the layers of blood vessels differs from the small capillaries to large arteries. Because veins have thinner walls than arteries, it is easier for tumour cells to gain access to veins than to arteries. Some tumour cells are able to release angiogenic factors that promote the growth of blood vessels towards the tumour cells, and these young vessels have delicate walls that can be easily penetrated.

It is well known that tumours frequently outgrow their blood supply, and where this occurs it results in areas of necrosis. These necrotic areas can release toxic products, which can diffuse into surrounding blood vessels and exert damaging effects. Accordingly it can render the blood vessels more easily penetrable by tumour cells. The process of the tumour cells entering the blood vessels is called intravasation.

Transport

Once tumour cells have gained access to a blood vessel, they may be transported within the blood. However, the tumour cells are liable to be attacked by the immune cells in the blood, so it is likely that many potentially metastatic cells will be destroyed. However, if tumour cell emboli form, blood vessels can be blocked by the tumour cells (Box 5.1).

Lodgement

Most tumour cells are arrested in the first capillary bed that they encounter. However, this does not guarantee the growth of a secondary tumour. It seems likely that interaction of the tumour cells with platelets or fibrin could influence the metastatic process. Where vascular damage exists, this can expose the subendothelium (including the endothelial basement membrane) to the blood, and it is possible that this may have a more direct effect on influencing the formation of metastases.

The movement of cells from the blood vessel to the surrounding tissue is called extravasation. For this to happen, the tumour cells must first become lodged within the blood vessel. This can occur as a result of mechanical entrapment, specific adhesion between the tumour cells and the cells of the blood vessel, or selective adhesion. In some instances, the tumour cells will immediately leave the blood vessel and set up active metastases. At other times the cells may become dormant either within the blood vessel or after extravasation and give rise to metastases at a later stage. Alternatively, the cells may lodge within the blood vessel and not survive. The various cells of the immune system can destroy tumour cells through antibody-dependent and cytolytic mechanisms (see Chapter 30).

Before extravasation, the tumour cells may divide and accumulate within the lumen of the blood vessel and then invade outward *en masse*, with possible destruction of the affected blood vessel. Alternatively, the tumour cells may migrate singly between the endothelial cells, and there is some evidence that the tumour cells may follow leukocytes as they emerge naturally from blood vessels (see Chapter 22). Finally, the cells could also pass directly through the endothelial cells themselves, resulting in damage to the endothelium. Once the tumour cells have passed through the endothelium they also have to cross the basement membrane of the vessel.

Growth

It is estimated that less than 1 per cent of cells that successfully complete these processes will establish a metastasis. The ability of the malignant cells to resist the host immune defence mechanisms is an important criteria for survival. Similarly, their availability and responsiveness to growth factors are also significant, for growth of the tumour cells is important for the successful establishment of the metastatic deposit.

Invasion

Two types of invasion are recognized. Type I invasion occurs when there is invasive growth and the malignant cells invade the tissue *en masse*. When this occurs there is a general pattern of lytic activity – this sort of invasion is characteristic of carcinomas. In type I invasion, proliferation rather than locomotion is important. After mitosis, two cells have to occupy the site where a single cell used to be, and the ensuing pressure leads to invasion.

In type II invasion, it is the migration of individual cells or cell islands that is significant. Lytic activity is restricted to the environment of the invasive cells and both locomotion and proliferation take place. Cellular dedifferentiation is important in mobilizing the tumour cells from the main mass. This seems to be common in sarcomas and malignant melanomas.

Resistance to Invasion

Some tissues are highly resistant to invasion. These include uncalcified cartilage, heart valves, the cornea, and the lenses. Uncalcified cartilage is resistant to blood vessels invasion, and, inevitably, tissues that lack a blood supply are resistant to invasion by tumours transported in the blood vessels.

There are a number of different types of collagen (Types I, II, III, IV); type II collagen is more resistant to destruction than types I and III are. Proteoglycans are known to have an anti-invasive effect. Two major classes of inhibitory substances are known to be present in cartilage. These include proteinase inhibitors and endothelial growth inhibitor.

SPREAD OF CARCINOMAS AND SARCOMAS

The previous section has dealt primarily with spread of cancers via the blood but, as already stated, tumours can spread via the lymphatic system and through body cavities. Carcinomas typically spread through the lymphatics, and it may well be that the environment within lymph

---

BOX 5.1 THE MECHANISM OF INVASION AND METASTASIS – BLOOD VESSEL SPREAD

- Transformation of a cell has to take place in order for a primary tumour to form.
- There has to be clonal expansion of this transformed cell, leading to growth and diversification.
- Typically, a metastatic subclone will form. Tumour cells are not heterogenous, and it is likely within any primary tumour that there is a subset of cells that have the potential to metastasize successfully.
- The cells have to pass through the extracellular matrix, assisted by various

  factors including the release of potent enzymes, and gain access to blood (or lymphatic vessels).
- Interaction within the blood or lymphatic vessels with the host lymphoid cells will take place and may result in a tumour cell embolus.
- Eventually the tumour cell embolus will be arrested, either mechanically or by selective adhesion to the wall of a blood vessel.
- Extravasation of tumour cells into the tissue will take place.

nodes is more suitable than blood vessels for carcinomas. However, it could also be that some tumours find it easier to invade blood vessels. Epithelial tissue does not contain lymphatic vessels or blood vessels, and therefore the spread has to involve prior detachment of the cells from the tumour mass.

GRADING AND STAGING OF CARCINOMAS

The grading and staging of carcinomas is important in indicating the prognosis of the disease, which in turn may influence the treatment options for the patient.

Grading

Grading is based on the degree of differentiation and the number of mitoses seen within a tumour. Typically grading runs from grade I to grade IV, with the higher values being given to tumours with an increased level of anaplasia. Higher-grade tumours tend to be more aggressive than lower-grade tumours. However, the grading of a tumour is an imperfect definition, because different parts of the same tumour may display different degrees of differentiation, and because the grade of the tumour may change as the tumour grows.

Staging

Staging is based on the anatomic extent of the tumour, the size of the primary tumour, and the degree of the local and distant spread. The TNM system is often used:

- T refers to the size of primary tumour;
- N refers to regional lymph nodes;
- M refers to metastasis.

The T value ranges from T1 to T4 with increasing size, and T0 refers to a carcinoma *in situ*. N1 increases to N3 with increased node involvement. M0 means no metastases, increasing to M2 when metastases are widespread (Box 5.2).

EPIDEMIOLOGY OF CANCER

The study of epidemiology provides information on the causes of cancer. Important information is gained from mortality studies (annual rate of death), as well as studies on the incidence (frequency of new cases arising in a population) in relation to malignant disease. Epidemiological studies only provide details on possible causes, and epidemiological data does not provide information on the mechanism(s) by which a causative agent may result in the development of cancer. All too often, the popular press publicizes a 'new link' between some suspected cause of cancer and the disease. These 'links' are often drawn from epidemiological studies, where a link may indeed be demonstrated, but this does not definitely mean that a cause-and-effect relationship can be established, or that the mechanisms for such a relationship can be determined.

Cancer is a significant cause of mortality and morbidity in the Western world. The incidence of cancer is increasing and this may be related to the fact that people now live longer than they used to, and furthermore, are exposed to higher levels of carcinogenic agents (see below). The following provides some information to demonstrate the role of epidemiology in drawing links between a range of variables and the development of malignant disease.

AGE

There is an increasing incidence of cancer with an increase in age. As always, there are exceptions to this general rule, and these exceptions include the leukaemias, lymphomas, neuroblastomas, retinoblastomas, Wilms' tumours, and sarcomas of bone and skeletal muscle. Within the younger age group, the overall incidence of cancer is higher in children from birth up to 5 years of age than it is in the age range 5–15 years. It is suspected that if men live long enough they have a 100 per cent chance of developing cancer of the

---

BOX 5.2 CHARACTERISTICS OF MALIGNANT CELLS IN IN-VITRO CELL CULTURE

- Cells derived from malignant neoplasms have a characteristic behaviour. They tend to show a loss of growth control, and reduced amounts of serum is required as a supplement in the growth medium compared with normal cells in order for growth to take place. Frequently, they are 'anchorage-independent', in that they do not require a base on which to grow.
- They are immortal in that they are not restricted to a finite number of cell doublings as are other cells.
- They show a reduced cohesiveness and, when transplanted into animals, they result in the production of tumours.

prostate. This is based on autopsy studies in which elderly men who have died from causes other than cancer of the prostate have been shown to have small foci of prostatic cancer that have been undetected.

SEX

In childhood there is a higher incidence of cancer in males than in females. In later life, that is over the age of 60, again the incidence of cancer in males is higher than in females. Between the ages of 30–60, however, there is a higher incidence of cancer in females, and this is mainly due to breast, ovarian, and cervical cancer. However, overall, there tends to be a higher incidence of cancer in males than in females.

ENVIRONMENTAL FACTORS

A number of environmental factors seem to be important in determining the incidence of malignant disease. Some of these are the result of personal habits. Cigarette smoking is associated with a large range of cancers, and lung cancer in particular. Before cigarette smoking becoming popular in the UK at the end of the 19th century, lung cancer was almost unknown. There has been an unparalleled increase in this disease as cigarette smoking became popular, first among the male population, and women are now also seriously affected. Lung cancer is still rare in non-smokers, although the effects of passive smoking are thought likely to be responsible for some of the cancers that are seen in non-smokers. It was Professor Sir Richard Doll and his colleague, Professor Austin Bradford-Hill, who first demonstrated the link between cigarette smoking and lung cancer in the 1950s. Even today, although we know of the many carcinogens that exist within cigarette smoke, we do not know precisely the mechanisms by which these carcinogens result in lung cancer.

Other lifestyle factors are important. Cervical cancer is very rare in nuns, virgins, and Jewish women. In the last-named group this is thought to be due to male circumcision. Breast cancer is more common in women who have not had children (i.e. nulliparous women).

Diet has been implicated in the development of malignant disease. High salt levels, a diet rich in smoked foods, and high alcohol consumption are all linked to different types of malignant disease. High consumption of alcoholic beverages, in particular spirits, is associated with an increased incidence of cancer of the oesophagus.

Certain occupations are associated with a range of cancers. A link between an occupation and the development of malignant disease was first noticed by the physician, Percival Pott. He noted that the boys who were used to clean chimneys had a much higher incidence of cancer of the scrotum. This is a good example of how epidemiology can demonstrate a possible link. At the time of Percival Pott's observation, the causal effect was not known, and the substances that the children were being exposed to had not been identified as possible risk factors. It was many years later (see below) that the causative agents were identified. Another occupational hazard is the chemicals used in the dye industry (see below), which are associated with bladder cancer. Exposure to asbestos is associated with an increased incidence of lung cancer (particularly if the exposed person is a smoker) and with mesothelioma, a tumour derived from mesotheial cells which line the visceral and parietal surfaces of, in this case, the pleura.

GEOGRAPHICAL LOCATION

There are remarkable variations in the incidence of various cancers in different parts of the world. Stomach cancer is very much more common in Japan that it is in the USA. Cancer of the colon is common in western Europe, North America, and New Zealand, but rare in Africa and Japan. Liver cancer is common in parts of Africa and at one time this was thought to be due to the presence of aflatoxins in the diet. However, it now seems more likely that the high incidence of hepatitis B is the real cause. Again, this shows how epidemiological data has to be considered cautiously.

CARCINOGENESIS

A carcinogen is a substance that is responsible for causing cancer. Carcinogens can be chemicals, physical agents, or viruses.

CHEMICAL AGENTS AS CARCINOGENS

In 1775, Percival Pott first noted that chimney sweep boys were likely to develop cancer of the scrotum. At that stage, the occupational hazard had been identified but the components responsible were not known. Identifying chemical carcinogens is frequently very difficult because they often exist within complex mixtures. For example, tobacco smoke contains many thousands of chemicals and only a few of these are carcinogens. The identification of chemical carcinogens involves animal experimentation, in which the activities of chemically purified substances are investigated. The following are examples of known chemical carcinogens.

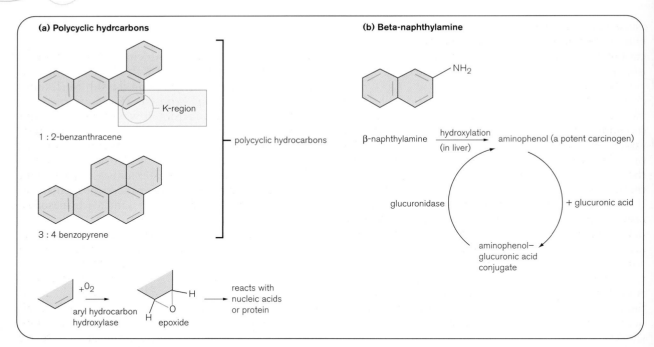

Figure 5.2. Chemical carcinogens. (a)1:2-benzanthracene and 3:3-benzpyrene combine with oxygen to form an epoxide. Epoxide can react directly with nucleic acids or proteins. (b) Beta-naphthylamine is metabolized in the liver to form an aminophenol that is then conjugated with glucuronic acid. Glucuronidase in the bladder metabolizes this conjugate back to aminophenol which is then involved in development of bladder cancer.

Polycyclic Hydrocarbons

Polycyclic hydrocarbons were the first carcinogenic chemicals to be recognized. They are widespread in the environment, in cigarette smoke, in polluted city air, and in some smoked foods. They are produced by the combustion of carbon-containing materials. In 1915 it was shown that coal tar could induce skin tumours. It was later shown that the active component of the coal tar that was responsible for this was a benzanthracene-like structure. 1:2,5:6-dibenzanthracene was the first pure carcinogen to be discovered, but it is not actually present in coal tar (it was chemically synthesised). 3:4-benzopyrene was, however, isolated from coal tar. In those early days, analytical techniques and isolation techniques were not well refined and it took 2 tons of coal pitch to isolate just 50 g of 3:4-benzopyrene. This chemical compound is common and can induce a wide variety of tumours depending on the route of administration.

In the case of the polycyclic hydrocarbons, close structural relationships do not imply similar carcinogenic properties. The critical chemical bonds determine the carcinogenicity, and the addition of oxygen to kappa-region double bonds occurs to form an epoxide, which can react with the cellular DNA. Polycyclic hydrocarbons induce the production of microsomal enzymes in the cell, and these enzymes catalyse the reaction between the oxygen and the kappa-region double bond (Figure 5.2). Polycyclic hydrocarbons are very important in the development of lung cancer.

Aromatic Amines, Azo-Dyes, and Aminofluorenes

At the end of the 19th century it was noted that aromatic amines had carcinogenic properties. It had been noticed that there was a very high incidence of bladder cancer amongst workers who were exposed to aniline dyes. It was not the aniline dyes themselves that were responsible for these cancers, but rather aromatic amines, such as beta-naphthylamine and benzidine, that were used in the industry. Aromatic amines cause production of tumours at distant sites, unlike the polycyclic hydrocarbons, whose effect is at the site of contact. The term given to the production of tumours distant to the site of contact is remote carcinogenesis.

Among the aromatic amines and the azo-dyes, molecules with minor structural differences may have very marked differences in carcinogenic properties. It is not the actual molecules of the aromatic amines and azo-dyes that are carcinogenic; rather, they are metabolized into carcinogenic derivatives. These derivatives are called ultimate carcinogens. A good example of this occurs with beta-naphthylamine.

Beta-naphthylamine is converted to an aminophenyl in the liver; the aminophenyl is then conjugated to glucuronic acid. Aminophenyl is toxic, but the glucuronic acid–aminophenyl conjugate is not toxic, and this conjugation is part of the detoxification process. In humans, the bladder contains the enzyme glucuronidase, and this has the effect of acting on the glucuronic acid–aminophenyl conjugate to release the strongly carcinogenic aminophenyl. This results in the development of tumours in the bladder (see Chapter 36). Dogs as well as humans have bladder glucuronidase, but it is not present in all species; species that do not possess bladder glucuronidase are not susceptible to this carcinogenic effect of aminophenyl.

It should be noted that as well as people in the dye industry, people working in the rubber and cable manufacturing industries, the printing industry, and the gas industry are also exposed to aromatic amines and have a high risk of developing bladder cancer. Absorption of these substances is primarily by inhalation. There is an induction period of between 15 and 20 years, and these neoplasms typically occur in middle life. Cancer of the bladder is also strongly associated with cigarette smoking.

Nitrosamines

Nitrosamines are formed in the stomach from the nitrates used as preservatives in certain foods (e.g. smoked meats). Their formation can be inhibited by vitamin C. Although nitrosamines have not been shown to be directly responsible for human cancers, many are carcinogenic in animal studies. Some nitrosamines, such as dimethylnitrosamine, have been withdrawn as solvents in the chemical industry because they caused liver cancer in animals. Nitrosamines, including *N*-nitrosopiperidine, are present in tobacco smoke.

Alkylating Agents

Alkylating agents are a group of chemical carcinogens that do not require any conversion to produce ultimate carcinogens. They include a number of very reactive molecules that combine directly with DNA. Mustard gas, beta-propiolactone, methyl nitrosourea, and cyclophosphamide are all examples of potent alkylating agents.

Aflatoxin

Aflatoxins are produced by the fungus, *Aspergillus flavus*, and are associated with human liver cancer. Previously it was thought that exposure to aflatoxin was the sole important cause of liver cancer, but it now seems that areas of the world where contamination of food stuffs with aflatoxin occurs are also areas where hepatitis B is common. It is likely that hepatitis B virus is the major cause of the liver cancer, although the situation is probably exacerbated by the presence of aflatoxins.

PHYSICAL AGENTS AS CARCINOGENS

Ultraviolet Radiation

The sun's energy contains ultraviolet (UV) radiation. Ultraviolet radiation consists of UVA waves (with a wavelength of 315–400 nm), UVB waves (280–315 nm), and UVC waves (210–280 nm). UVC cannot penetrate the ozone layers of the atmosphere but both UVA and UVB do. UVB can penetrate the skin to the depth of the superficial dermis, and it produces damage, including erythema and sunburn with blistering. However, UVB is unable to penetrate window glass, and sunscreens are effective in blocking it. The longest wavelength of ultraviolet light is UVA, which is responsible for ageing of the skin and tanning.

Ultraviolet can cause damage to DNA by the formation of pyrimidine dimers. This damage may be responsible for skin cancer as a result of UV exposure. Fair-skinned people and those who have had frequent sun damage to the skin are most at risk. Skin carcinomas and melanomas are both associated with high exposure to UV. People with xeroderma pigmentosum, a condition in which there is impairment of DNA repair mechanisms, are very susceptible to skin cancer as a result of UV exposure.

Ionizing Radiation

As already noted in Chapter 4, ionizing radiation can result in the hydrolysis of water to produce free radicals. These free radicals can interact with the nucleic acids and give rise to a range of malignancies. There is plenty of evidence to demonstrate that exposure to ionizing radiation is associated with the development of cancers. The incidence of leukaemia was greatly increased in survivors of the Hiroshima atomic bomb. Malignancies were also noted in the early workers with radiation as it was being developed for use as a diagnostic tool. The therapeutic use of radiation to treat malignancies in the head and neck of children is associated with a higher risk of developing thyroid cancer later in life.

Indeed, the most frequently observed cancers following exposure to ionizing radiation are myeloid leukaemias and thyroid cancers in children. Cancers of the breast and lung occur less frequently, and occurring even more infrequently are cancers of the skin, bone, and intestinal tract

Although these cancers may result from the production of free radicals, it is possible that radiation energy can also have a direct effect, especially with the particulate radiations such as alpha-particles and neutrons, but also with electromagnetic radiation such as gamma-rays and X-rays.

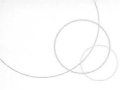

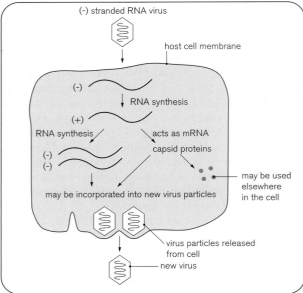

Figure 5.3 RNA viruses and the host cell. When negative-stranded RNA viruses enter a cell, viral nucleic acid is released into the cytoplasm. A copy of the RNA is made (the positive strand), which can then be used either to synthesize further negative-stranded RNA for making new virus particles, or to act directly as messenger RNA (mRNA) to synthesize proteins. These proteins are then used within the cell or incorporated into virus particles that are then shed from the cell.

VIRUSES AND CANCER

Viruses can be described as intracellular parasites; and are obligate 'parasites' in that they can multiply only inside cells. Viruses contain either DNA or RNA and may be double-stranded or single-stranded. Large viruses have coding potential within their nucleic acid for up to 200 proteins; at the other extreme, small viruses code for as few as five proteins.

The virus nucleic acid is referred to as the genome and is enclosed in a capsid, which is a protein coat. The nucleic acid and protein are together known as the nucleocapsid. Some nucleocapsids are surrounded by a phospholipid bilayer. This is typically formed from the plasma membrane of the cell during the shedding of virus particles. Viruses with a phospholipid coat are termed enveloped viruses.

The entry of a virus into a host cell is a complex process. Viruses first attach to the plasma membrane of the host cell, and this involves surface molecules on the membrane of the host cell acting as a receptor for molecules on the surface of the virus. Following this,

the virus has to penetrate the cell, and this typically occurs through endocytosis. The production of viral proteins and the assembly of new virus particles depends on the type of virus. In the case of double-stranded DNA viruses, the nucleic acid enters the nucleus of the cell where it can be replicated to form new DNA for incorporation into new virus particles.

RNA viruses do not enter the nucleus of the cell. Instead, the positive-stranded RNA from the virus acts as messenger RNA, which is translated into fresh capsid proteins. Additional parts of the nucleic acid will be translated to manufacture an enzyme that will catalyse the replication of the RNA molecule to make the new virus particles. With negative-stranded RNA, the nucleic acid has first to be copied in order to generate the complementary strand of nucleic acid to be translated (i.e. a positive-stranded RNA is made). After this has occurred, the newly made positive-stranded RNA can be used to provide new virus proteins and more nucleic acid for incorporation in the new virus particles (Figure 5.3).

Retroviruses are an important group of viruses. They contain single-stranded RNA but they replicate by way of a DNA intermediate. These viruses contain an enzyme called reverse transcriptase, which enables a unique biological event to occur. Reverse transcriptase results in the transcription of DNA from the viral RNA, and this acts as the template. All this takes place within the nucleus of the host cell, and the DNA that has been copied becomes incorporated into the DNA of the host cell. The segment of DNA derived from the virus within the host cell chromosome is known as a provirus. The provirus gene can be transcribed into RNA and acts either as messenger RNA for the production of new proteins, or as RNA for packaging into new viruses.

A number of viruses are associated with malignancies. Of the double-stranded DNA viruses, the *Papovaviridae*, which include polyomavirus and simian virus 40 are known to be able to induce tumours in animals. Also belonging to this group are the papillomaviruses, which result in human warts. The human papillomaviruses (HPV) used to be considered as just a nuisance, but they are now of significant interest because they are one of the very few infectious causes of cancer.

In the 1930s it was known that papillomas on the skin of cottontail rabbits often became malignant. A similar phenomenon was observed in dogs and cattle. In humans, an association between infection with HPV and cervical cancer is well established. Cervical cancer is very common, particularly in women in Africa, Asia, and Latin America. As has been noted elsewhere, cervical cancer is virtually unknown in virgins.

Molecular techniques have established that in almost all cases of cervical cancer there is evidence of HPV infection, and in particular HPV16 infection. (HPV16 is one of the many subgroups of this virus.) This particular subgroup is found in almost two-thirds of cases of cervical cancer in the UK. Clearly, people who have had multiple sexual partners are more likely than other people to come into contact with partners who have been infected with HPV. In addition to the risk of developing genital warts, there is also a very real risk associated with developing cervical cancer.

Before HPV was identified as being associated with cervical carcinoma, it had been thought that herpes simplex virus, which causes cold sores and genital herpes, might have been responsible. However, this is now not believed to be the case at all.

Infection with human immunodeficiency virus (HIV) is associated with the development of Kaposi's sarcoma. This type of malignancy used to be rarely seen, but is now more widespread as a result of infection with HIV. It is likely that it is not an oncogenic effect of HIV that is responsible for this relationship, rather a side-effect of the influence that HIV has on the immune system (see Chapter 28).

Within the animal kingdom, the Rous sarcoma virus can cause sarcomas in poultry. This was first identified in 1911. The Rous sarcoma virus is a retrovirus that is similar to HIV. Feline leukaemia virus is another retrovirus; it can cause leukaemia in cats. Other *Papovaviridae* that can cause cancer include polyomavirus, which can cause tumours in rodents, and simian virus 40, which can cause tumours in monkeys. Marek's disease virus causes lymphoma in poultry. It is a herpesvirus in the same family as herpes simplex virus and Epstein–Barr virus (EBV), the causative virus of glandular fever and, in parts of Africa, Burkitt's lymphoma. EBV is associated with nasopharyngeal carcinoma and EBV DNA can be identified in tumours. The human T-lymphatrophic viruses 1 and 2 are also associated with malignancies in humans.

Evidence that Viruses Can Cause Cancer in Humans

Evidence for the oncogenic effect of viruses has been obtained both directly and circumstantially. In the case of HPV and cervical cancer, there is direct evidence of the presence of viral nucleic acid sequences in the transformed cells that make up the tumour. This is also the case with Epstein–Barr virus – nasopharyngeal cancer cells consistently show the presence of this virus. In the case of hepatitis B virus and its association with the development of primary liver cell cancer (see above), there is no direct evidence but the association is nevertheless very strong. The current thinking is that viruses are important in only a very small number of human and animal cancers, but a study of how they exert their effects has yielded considerable information about the molecular basis of cancer.

Molecular techniques have provided evidence that gene alteration takes place in cancers. Using molecular biological techniques, altered DNA sequences can be removed from cancer cells and copied (see also Chapter 7). These isolated, altered genes can then be placed in normal cells in culture, where their effect is to transform the cells and make them behave as if they were malignant. Cells prepared in this way in culture will result in tumours when introduced to animals, although these tumours are often small and do not result in significant disease. A number of oncogenes have been identified (Table 5.2).

It is clear that several mutations are necessary to cause a normal cell to develop into a cancerous cell, and it may well be that additional mutations are required beyond that of producing a benign neoplasm to give rise to cancer. Current thinking is that five critical genes have to be altered within a cell before it becomes transformed. We have already seen that a

Some Oncogenes, Associated Retroviruses and Tumours, and the Proteins for which they Code

Oncogenes	Associated Retroviruses	Tumour	Protein for which the Gene Codes
H-ras	Harvey murine sarcoma virus	various human cancers (bladder, colon, lung, leukaemia, neuroblastomas)	GTP-binding proteins with GTPase activity
src	Rous sarcoma virus	no human tumours	tyrosine-specific cancers
myc	Avian myelocytomatosis virus	Burkitt's lymphoma, small cell lung cancer, neuroblastoma	nuclear-binding protein

Table 5.2 Some oncogenes in terms of associated retroviruses, tumours they are thought to cause and the proteins they code for.

spectrum of change is apparent in a range of malignant diseases. For example, the changes resulting from cigarette smoke exposure to the bronchial epithelium range from squamous metaplasia followed by dysplasia to cancer if the irritation is not removed. Similarly, carcinoma *in situ* in the uterine cervix exists, in which all the signs of malignancy are present but the cells have not crossed the basement membrane.

The critical mutations that have to take place to change a cell into a cancer cell occur over time. The cells are being continually damaged but it is only when critical mutations have taken place that tumour cells result. One of the most surprising observations that a study of tumour viruses demonstrated was that the segments of nucleic acid responsible for transformation were, in many cases, not special cancer genes but homologous with genes present in normal cells. The name given to these genes in oncogenic viruses was viral oncogenes (v-onc) (Table 5.3). The sequences found in normal healthy cells that were homologous were termed proto-oncogenes. *Why is it that cells could contain 'cancer' genes and be normal, yet the possession of these genes was also associated with transformation of cells in culture?* Although, the following is very much an oversimplification, it has been an investigation of this question that has helped explain at the molecular level what changes normal cells into cancer cells.

Proto-oncogenes are normal genes that code for proteins that are essential for a cell's survival. What immediately became apparent was that an overproduction of normal proteins may be responsible for the transformation of a cell. This could occur in different ways.

If a viral oncogene was inserted into the nucleic acid of a cell, this could result in it producing an excess of 'normal' protein. This overproduction of protein could result in a cell becoming altered. Furthermore, viral genes are often rapidly expressed, so the insertion of viral nucleic acid close to a proto-oncogene could cause overexpression of the proto-oncogene, resulting in it producing an excess of the 'normal' protein, which again could lead to the cell becoming malignant.

To distinguish the normal proto-oncogene from the proto-oncogenes produced in a cell in which it has been altered to overexpress, the term 'cellular oncogene' is used. Cellular oncogenes are altered proto-oncogenes, which, when expressed, result in the cell becoming transformed. A final twist is that proto-oncogenes can become cellular oncogenes if their gene product is altered in some way. This therefore helps explain how chemical or physical agents might bring about cancer. The effects of chemical carcinogens or physical carcinogens on a proto-oncogene may be to alter it slightly so that an altered gene product accumulates in the cell, which may be responsible for malignant change. Some examples of known oncogenes and their gene products are provided in Table 5.2.

ONCOGENES AND THEIR GENE PRODUCTS

Changes in the gene expression of a proto-oncogene result from:

- amplification of a proto-oncogene;
- mutation within a proto-oncogene, leading to an altered gene product; or
- chromosomal transformation.

The transfer of part of one chromosome to another (as happens in chromosome translocation) occurs in a number of neoplasms, including Burkitt's lymphoma. In this case, there is an exchange of chromosomal material between chromosomes 8 and 14. The effect is to alter the expression of an oncogene, which results in a protein product that results in cell proliferation.

The genetic changes in tumour cells may affect one or both copies of a gene. During fertilization, the zygote contains one set of chromosomes from the male and the one from the female, each carrying a separate set of homologous genes. Some tumour mutations can exert their effects by damaging only one gene. Such mutations are known as oncogenic mutations. In other cases, both copies of a gene have to be altered to make the cell behave differently. These are sometimes referred to as 'recessive' mutations. These types of mutations where both copies have to be affected are known as tumour suppressor gene mutations. The reason for this is that if only a single copy of the gene is activated, the other copy can make the protein and this is able to prevent any effects on the behaviour of the cell (Figure 5.4).

Oncogenes	
Oncogene	Effect
proto-oncogene	normal cellular gene producing protein important for growth and differentiation
viral-oncogene (v-onc)	gene present within an oncogenic virus that can, following infection of the cell, result in malignant transformation
cellular-oncogene (c-onc)	the name given to a proto-oncogene that has been altered or is being inappropriately expressed resulting in malignant transformation

Table 5.3 Oncogenes.

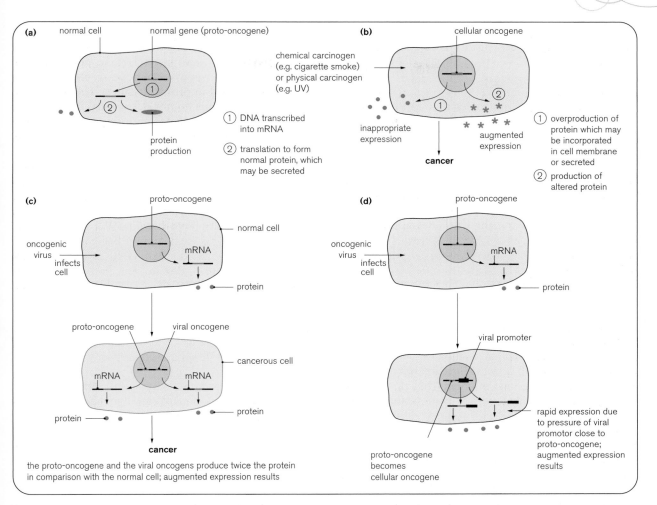

Figure 5.4 How oncogenes exert their effect on cells. (a) A normal gene (in this case a proto-oncogene) codes for normal proteins. DNA is transcribed to messenger RNA (mRNA) for protein synthesis. (b) The proto-oncogene may be altered to a cellular onogene by exposure to a chemical carcinogen (e.g. cigarette smoke) or a physical carcinogen (e.g. ultraviolet light). The cellular oncogene can have one of two effects: it can either cause excess production of the normal protein, or it can cause production of slightly altered protein. This inappropriate expression of the protein can result in the cell becoming a tumour cell. An oncogenic virus can affect a normal cell by: (c) causing two copies of the gene being made: the original proto-oncogene, and a viral oncogene derived from the oncogenic virus. This can lead to overproduction of the normal cellular protein, which in turn can lead to cancer; or (d) placing a rapid replicating gene close to a proto-oncogene. This can result in the proto-oncogene becoming a cellular oncogene.

The *ras* proto-oncogenes are activated by point mutations, which can result from exposure to chemical carcinogens or physical agents. Chromosomal translocations activate proto-oncogenes by placing the genes next to a strong promoter, such as occurs in Burkitt's lymphoma, in which the small *c-myc* gene on chromosome 8 is placed in close proximity to the actively expressed gene for the immunoglobulin heavy gene on chromosome 14. A second effect of translocation may be the fusion of a gene with other genes to produce an altered protein. Gene amplification through reduplication of a proto-oncogene can also lead to increased expression or activity and *N-myc* amplification occurs in neuroblastomas and *c-neu* gene amplification can also occur in breast cancers.

It is the overexpression of these normal or extenuated proteins that can result in a cell becoming malignant. In conclusion, an understanding of oncogenes has helped in the understanding of the molecular basis of cancer and the interaction between the known observations on the effects of oncogenes, chemical carcinogenesis, and physical agents as causes of cancer.

TUMOUR MARKERS

Tumour markers are molecules that can be detected both in the blood and in other body fluids. They can aid the diagnosis of certain tumours. Alpha-fetoprotein (AFP) is normally produced by the fetal yolk sac and liver cells. In certain types of cancer (e.g. carcinoma of the liver, testicular germ cell tumours), there are elevated levels of this protein detectable in the patient's blood. Cirrhosis of the liver and hepatitis also result in an increase but the levels are not usually as elevated as they are with carcinoma. Measurement of the serum AFP level is therefore useful in detecting the presence of these tumours. Similarly, prostatic acid phosphatase is an enzyme whose serum levels are markedly elevated in prostatic cancer. Unfortunately, detectable elevations do not occur until the disease is at an advanced stage. Human chorionic gonadotrophin (hCG) can also be detected in germ cells and tumours. Carcino-embryonic antigen (CEA) is normally produced by fetal, liver, gut, and pancreatic cells, but significant increases occur in cancers of the pancreas, colon, and breast. Detection of CEA is used to estimate the size of colorectal cancer and to detect recurrences after surgery (see Chapter 30).

KEY POINTS

- A neoplasm is an abnormal mass of tissue whose growth exceeds and is uncoordinated with that of the normal tissues.
- Benign tumours grow as masses that remain localized to their site of origin. They do not have the capacity to invade or metastasize to distant sites.
- Malignant tumours are cancers that grow and progressively invade and destroy the surrounding tissue. They are poorly demarcated, and cords of tumour cells extend into the surrounding tissue.
- Metastases are tumour implants that are discontinuous with the primary tumour and take place via three routes: spread into body cavities, invasion of lymphatics, and haematogenous spread.
- The grading and staging of carcinomas is important in indicating the prognosis of the disease, which in turn influences the treatment options for the patient.
- Grading is based on the degree of differentiation and the number of mitoses within a tumour. Staging is based on the anatomic extent of the tumour, size of the primary tumour, and degree of local and distant spread.
- Epidemiology data provide evidence for the causes of cancer (e.g. age, sex, and environmental agents such as diet, pollutants, geographical location). Such data do not provide information on the mechanisms by which a causative agent may result in cancer development.
- A carcinogen is a substance responsible for causing cancer e.g. chemical agents, physical agents, or viruses.

FURTHER READING

Bingham SA (1997) Epidemiology and mechanisms relating to diet to risk of colorectal cancer. Nutr Res Rev 9:197–239.

Bryla CM (1996) The relationship between stress and the development of breast cancer: a literature review [Review]. Oncol Nurs Forum 23:441–8.

Clavel J, Conso F, Limasset JC, et al. (1996) Hairy cell leukaemia and occupational exposure to benzene. Occup Environ Med 53:533–9.

Department of Health Committee on Medical Aspects of Food Policy Working Group (1997) Nutritional Aspects of the Development of Cancer. Her Majesty's Stationery Office, London.

Doll R (1996) Cancers weakly related to smoking [Review]. Br Med Bull 52:35–49.

Hansson LE, Nyren O, Hsing AW, et al. (1996) The risk of stomach cancer in patients with gastric or duodenal ulcer disease. N Engl J Med 335:242–9.

Li CY, Theriault G, Lin RS (1996) Epidemiological appraisal of studies of residential exposure to power frequency magnetic fields and adult cancers [Review]. Occup Environ Med 53:505–10.

Liede A, Tonin PN, Sun CC, et al. (1998) Is hereditary site-specific ovarian cancer a distinct genetic condition? Am J Med Genet 75:55–8.

Tawn EJ (1995) Leukaemia and Sellafield: is there a heritable link? J Med Gen 32:251–6.

THE ROLE OF THE LABORATORY IN THE INVESTIGATION OF DISEASE

LEARNING OBJECTIVES

After studying this chapter you will have a clearer understanding of:
- the help that laboratory tests can give in clinical problem solving at the bedside
- the investigative tests used and their basis in the pathophysiology of disease
- the way in which investigations can be used to assess the severity of a disease or its complications
- the way in which investigations can determine a predisposition to a disease in an asymptomatic person

INTRODUCTION

Clinical problem-solving can be divided into two stages. The first stage, which occurs usually in a hospital ward or a clinic, is the taking of the patient's medical history and the examination of the patient for abnormal signs in a particular body system or organ. After gathering this information, possible links may be constructed to find a reason behind the symptoms and possible diagnoses can be considered (i.e. a differential diagnosis). The second stage concerns management of the patient, in which the possible diagnoses are investigated, and disease and symptoms are treated (Figure 6.1).

Investigations can therefore be divided into initial (general) tests, which screen for a differential diagnosis, and specialized (specific) tests, which focus on a particular disorder, body system, or organ. In this way, pathology laboratories play an important role in helping to make a clinical decision regarding the nature of a health-related disorder, monitoring the progress of a disease and its response to treatment. Clinical investigation may be requested under one of the following categories:
- to confirm a diagnosis suspected from the clinical information;
- to assess the severity of the disease and its complications;
- to follow the course of a disease, its response to treatment, and its complications, and to give information on its likely outcome (prognosis); and

- to look for a disease or a predisposition to a disease in asymptomatic and healthy people (e.g. the Guthrie test is performed on all new-born infants to screen for phenylketonuria – see Chapters 2 and 7 – and measurement of total serum cholesterol can be used to indicate an early predisposition to cardiovascular disease).

There are many types of pathology laboratories involved in the care of patients, including haematology, immunology, clinical biochemistry, microbiology, and histopathology laboratories. Laboratory tests are often performed in conjunction with other appropriate, more intensive and specialized investigations. Some procedures 'visualize' organs (e.g. X-rays, catheter studies), whereas others are physiological studies that evaluate more functional aspects of the organ being examined [e.g. electrocardiograms (ECG), electroencephalograms (EEG)).

WHY PERFORM LABORATORY TESTS?

The results of any laboratory test can be interpreted only in the context of the clinical history, symptoms, and signs of the patient. In general, there is no such entity as a 'specific' test for a disease; instead a series of different investigations are performed to confirm or refute a particular clinical diagnosis. There should always be a reason to request an investigation, because they are costly in terms of both laboratory time and money, and also because

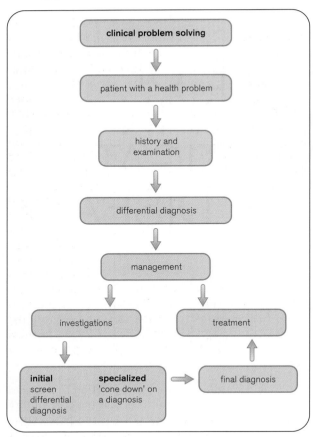

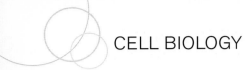

Figure 6.1 Stages in the diagnosis of a health-related disorder.

Inside the figure:

clinical problem solving

patient with a health problem

history and examination

differential diagnosis

management

investigations

treatment

initial
screen
differential
diagnosis

specialized
'cone down' on
a diagnosis

final diagnosis

they may be dangerous to the patient. For many tests, the results obtained from normal subjects show a distribution around an average value (i.e. within a normal range) (see below). But no two results of the same test are necessarily going to be identical, even in the same person, and serial laboratory tests are therefore often important in diagnosing an abnormality. The position may be clearer when tissues are available for histology and histochemical studies, in which case the anomaly in tissue morphology can be seen under the microscope.

COLLECTION OF SAMPLES

Most laboratory investigations are carried out on whole blood (plasma or serum, and cells), urine, faeces, calculi (e.g. renal stones), sweat, saliva, amniotic fluid, pleural fluid, peritoneal fluid, or joint fluid (see Chapter 39); less frequently, cerebrospinal fluid (CSF) is examined. Samples of body tissues or fluids must be collected and transported with care, and they must be correctly labelled with details of the patient (i.e. name, hospital

number, ward or clinic, and the name of the patient's clinician). All samples should be regarded as potentially infectious, and care taken in handling them; each sample should be treated as though it were a high-risk sample (e.g. as though it were infected with hepatitis B or human immunodeficiency virus (HIV)). Vigilance is also required by the health care professional to ensure that the sample of body tissue or fluid is put into the appropriate bottle or container for the particular laboratory test requested (e.g. a tube containing sodium citrate is needed for clotting studies).

Blood

Care must be taken when venesecting the patient so that the blood does not become haemolysed. This can easily happen if the size (gauge) of hypodermic needle is too small, for then the cells may be broken up while the blood is being drawn into the syringe. The plasma is then contaminated with the intracellular contents of red blood cells, and this could lead to inaccuracy of the laboratory results. Similarly, when the patient is receiving an intravenous infusion, blood must always be taken from the opposite arm, so the specimen does not contain a disproportionate amount of the fluids being administered.

When the sample is taken may also be important in relation to diet or time of day. For instance, serum lipid estimations need to be performed on blood taken following an overnight fast. Similarly, the circulating level of certain hormones fluctuate throughout the day (i.e. they exhibit diurnal variation), and therefore blood samples for analysis of these parameters must be taken at a specific time (see Appendix 2).

Many laboratory investigations are performed on clotted blood, and occasionally a preservative may be required in a collection tube. The type of preservative is identified by the specific colour-coding of the bottle. For example, a sample for blood glucose analysis must be taken into a tube containing fluoride. In this case the fluoride is necessary to prevent the blood cells (which are still 'alive' in the tube) from metabolizing the glucose in the plasma. If the cells were able to use the glucose for energy, then a falsely low result would be estimated by the laboratory.

Whole blood specimens must be separated into cells and supernatant fluid before storage. The fluid is usually serum, but it may be plasma if the sample was collected into a tube containing an anticoagulant, such as heparin, EDTA, or sodium citrate. Although the concentration of most blood components is the same in these different fluids, the obvious difference between serum and plasma is the absence or presence of the different clotting factors. These factors are present in plasma but are removed from serum when they are used up in the clotting process. Plasma and serum samples can be stored in a refrigerator (at 4°C) or in a freezer (at –20°C or –80°C) depending on the stability of the plasma or serum component (also referred to as an 'analyte') being measured. Some analytes are unstable at 4°C. It is particularly noteworthy that samples of whole blood should never be frozen. This is because the blood cells are broken up (lysed) in the thawing process, thereby causing inaccuracies in the laboratory analyses of the plasma and cells.

Urine

Although some analyses can be carried out on random (untimed) specimens of urine, most investigations require a sample from a carefully timed urine collection (over 24 hours). Often the urine bottle needs to contain specific additives and to be refrigerated in order to prevent alteration in the levels of the analytes by the bacteria that are inevitably present in urine samples.

Collection over 24 hours requires specific instructions to be given to the patient. To obtain a complete collection, the first urine sample immediately before starting the test must be discarded and the time recorded. Thereafter, from the beginning of the test (e.g. at 9.00 am) until its completion (24 hours later at 9.00 am the next day), all samples should be added to this container. At the end of the test, the patient should empty the bladder, and this urine sample should be included in the collection.

Faeces

Collection of faecal specimens are generally made for microbiological investigation (see Chapter 17). Faecal specimens are less frequently required for analysis by the clinical biochemistry laboratory, but it may be important to detect fat globules by microscopy or a specific measurement of fat. Again, for a precise analysis, specific instructions need to be adhered to by trained staff, so a complete collection is achieved (see below).

ANALYSIS OF BODY FLUIDS BY PATHOLOGY LABORATORIES

GENERAL PRINCIPLES OF LABORATORY INVESTIGATIONS

Bedside Biochemical Tests

Certain laboratory investigations may be carried out at the bedside, at home, or in the clinic. Dipsticks, which are commercially prepared 'sticks', may be used to measure analytes in blood or urine. For instance, measurements of glucose, albumin, and ketones in urine are very useful in screening for and monitoring diabetes

mellitus. Similarly, a dipstick may be used for a rapid measurement of the bilirubin level in blood when a patient is suspected of having liver disease. Some hospitals have 'minilabs' or 'near-patient' testing equipment (e.g. blood gas analyses in intensive care units, and bilirubinometers in neonatal intensive care units).

Although at first sight these may appear attractive and useful to the clinician, there are pitfalls in using such equipment. If such instruments are not well maintained, or if they are used by untrained staff, then the results obtained may be inaccurate and dangerous to the patient. The worst scenario is if the clinician's management of the patient is changed as a consequence of a wrong result, and it leads to deterioration instead of improvement in the patient's health. With improved mechanical systems for transportation of the samples to the laboratory (in hospital), and by courier from general practitioner surgeries, there is probably less need for any near-patient testing equipment. This also leaves the clinician free to concentrate on the clinical aspects of the patient, rather than having to carry out biochemical analyses. The exception to this rule is the glucometer (see below).

Precision of Results Obtained from Analysis of Body Fluids

When a specimen has been taken to the laboratory for analysis, the result of the analyte measurement should be accurate (i.e. repeatable and precise). As far as possible, the laboratory technician must ensure that the results are sufficiently reliable; hence the analytical methods used are subject to rigorous control. Internal and external audit of quality of the methods has been practice in hospital laboratories for many years (e.g. the National External Quality Assurance Schemes). After these quality-controls checks, the results are reported, mainly by computers linked to the analytical instruments, for them to be relayed to the ward or clinic. This allows storage of the pathology reports and the ability to retrieve and review the data.

The Normal Range of a Laboratory Test

The 'normal range' for a particular analyte identified and measured in a body tissue or fluid (e.g. serum albumin level) is a difficult concept. In effect, analysis is made on a population of healthy subjects, and then the results are plotted on a graph and subjected to statistical analysis. When the results have been plotted, their distribution on the graph gives a 'bell-shaped' curve (Gaussian distribution). The range of values that encompasses around 95 per cent of the total number of tests (i.e. the mean and two standard deviations) is used as the normal range. When the laboratory is establishing a normal range for certain investigations, a number of different variables need to be considered (e.g. age, sex, body size, and race of the subjects; the timing in the menstrual cycle when the samples were collected). (See Appendix 2 for a comprehensive list of normal ranges for laboratory tests performed in haematology, clinical biochemistry, and immunology laboratories.)

Although the normal range defines a range of values expected to occur in most people, it is noteworthy that certain anomalies may be found. For instance, around 5 per cent of people fall outside the normal range. Furthermore, a person's result might be within the normal range for the population of people who have been studied, but the value obtained might still be an abnormality for that individual person. Thus, any laboratory result must be interpreted in conjunction with the findings of other clinical investigations, and an explanation sought for any discrepancy that occurs.

Measurement of Plasma Enzymes for the Diagnosis of Disease

Determination of the levels of a particular enzyme for diagnostic purposes can be made on samples of blood, serum, or other body fluids. Most enzymes are present in much higher concentrations inside cells rather than in blood, because it is inside cells that they are required for metabolic processes (see Chapters 1 and 2). The assumption is that the enzyme is released by damage to the cell or intracellular component (organelle). Cell division and cell death are continuous parts of the normal growth and repair mechanism within the body, so a certain presence of intracellular enzymes in body fluids is acceptable. Normal plasma or serum enzyme levels (or concentrations) reflect the balance between:

- the rate at which the enzyme is produced by a cell;
- the rate at which it is released into the plasma during cell turnover (i.e. it is increased during cell damage by disease); and
- the rate of clearance from the circulation.

Depending on which organ is affected by a disease, an increase in plasma concentration of an enzyme being measured might indicate that there is either:

- an increase in the amount of enzyme being produced or released from the cells; or
- a decrease in the clearance of the enzyme from the blood (see also Chapter 4).

Enzymes used in the diagnosis of disease are not measured only in body fluids; they can also be detected by specific measurement in tissue biopsy samples or by histochemical stains. However, knowledge of plasma levels of an organ-specific enzyme can often obviate the need for obtaining a tissue sample.

Certain drugs may affect the enzyme activity by inducing their synthesis; for instance phenobarbitone enhances the synthesis of drug-metabolizing enzymes in the liver. Thus an increase in plasma and tissue enzyme concentrations may occur in the absence of a specific disease. Similarly, a lower than normal plasma enzyme activity may be found. This could be due to either a reduction in enzyme synthesis or to a genetic defect that leads to a deficiency in the levels of the enzyme. Some people possess enzymes that do not work as effectively as they do in most people (e.g. the presence of inherited variants which have a lower than normal biological activity) (see Chapter 9).

SPECIFIC INVESTIGATIONS

INVESTIGATION OF CARDIAC DISEASE

The viability of heart muscle depends critically on its blood supply (see Chapter 4). If the blood supply to the myocardium is reduced, there is tissue ischaemia, the cells die, and infarction occurs (i.e. there is an area of tissue death). Ischaemic heart disease (IHD) can be divided into chronic IHD and acute IHD. In chronic IHD, the patient experiences chest pain (i.e. stable or unstable angina). However, in acute IHD, there are varying forms of myocardial damage (called myocardial infarction) and sudden death. The major cause of ischaemia is narrowing of the coronary arteries due to atheroma. Atheroma is increased by abnormal levels of circulating lipids (e.g. cholesterol and triglyceride) (see Table 6.1).

Measurement of Plasma Enzymes in Myocardial Infarction and Ischaemic Heart Disease

Diagnosis of myocardial infarction (MI) and assessment of the degree of damage to the myocardium can be confirmed by performing an ECG and by measuring specific enzymes (originating from the cardiac muscle) in serum. Treatment is also given to dissolve any blood clots (thrombolysis with streptokinase) and the patient may require other confirmatory tests involving other investigative specialities during the recovery period; for example, exercise ECG or coronary angiography to demonstrate narrowing or occluded blood vessels (see Chapter 32).

Diagnosis of acute MI is a good example of enzymes acting as markers for cellular components that change as a result of disease. The three enzymes commonly measured are creatine kinase, lactate dehydrogenase, and aspartate aminotranferase. In a patient who has been admitted to hospital with a suspected MI, these enzymes are measured daily on admission for the first 3 days (see Person-Centred Study: Myocardial

Infarction), in conjunction with regular clinical and ECG monitoring of the heart (Figure 6.2).

Creatine kinase

Creatine kinase specific to cardiac muscle (CKmb) is released by the damaged myocardium and an increased serum level is a good clinical indicator of the early stages of cardiac muscle damage in an MI. Following an MI, blood levels peak within 24 hours and often return to a normal level by 48 hours.

Plasma creatine kinase levels may also be elevated in patients with myocarditis or cardiomyopathy, and after cardiac surgery or cardiac arrest with resuscitation. A common cause of a non-specific rise in creatine kinase is damage to skeletal muscle such as might occur after an intramuscular injection. Creatine kinase is an enzyme that is not only produced by the myocardium but also by the brain and skeletal muscle. The laboratory tests can distinguish between the enzymes derived from the three different sources of creatine kinase. They may be referred to on the laboratory report as:
- CKmb, which is creatine kinase from the myocardium;
- CKmm, which is creatine kinase from skeletal muscle; and
- CKbb, which is creatine kinase from the brain.

Lactate dehydrogenase

Lactate dehydrogenase (LDH) is released from damaged myocardium. The serum level peaks within 3–4 days of an MI and remains elevated for up to 10–14 days. Like creatine kinase, the enzyme may originate from a number of different sources (skeletal muscle, red blood cells, and the liver). Thus a raised serum LDH levels on its own is not a good marker for MI. Raised levels of serum LDH also occur where there is tissue damage such as metastatic carcinoma of the liver, in blood disorders such as leukaemia and haemolysis, and in muscular dystrophy.

Aspartate aminotransferase

Aspartate aminotransferase (AST) levels in serum peak about 24–48 hours after an MI and return to normal within about 72 hours. This enzyme is also found and released from red blood cells, liver, kidney, and lungs, and again increased levels may be detected in liver and heart failure.

Alanine aminotransferase

Alanine aminotransferase (ALT) levels may be normal or slightly elevated after an MI. This enzyme is also detectable in the liver, kidney, and skeletal muscle, and a raised serum level is also indicative of hepatocellular damage.

PERSON-CENTRED STUDY: MYOCARDIAL INFARCTION

Sebastian, a 45-year-old business director, suddenly developed a crushing central chest pain that radiated to his left arm. The pain was associated with nausea and sweating. On admission to Accident and Emergency, he was given an intramuscular injection of diamorphine. The significant points in his clinical history were that he had a family history of heart disease under the age of 55 years, he smoked 60 cigarettes a day, he did not exercise, and he ate a diet of junk food.

In the Accident and Emergency department, the **differential diagnosis** was between a myocardial infarction, angina, and hypertension.

General investigations showed an abnormal ECG and serum creatine kinase levels of > 2000 U/L. Specific investigations included a cardiac muscle specific enzyme measurement (CKmb), since he had had an intramuscular injection of diamorphine; the CKmb was > 6 per cent, confirming a myocardial infarction. He was treated with oxygen, thrombolysis, and later aspirin.

Further specific investigations revealed an increase in the serum levels of lactate dehydrogenase (LDH) and alanine aminotransferase (ALT) and an increase in circulating cholesterol and low-density lipoprotein (LDL) cholesterol, which were treated with simvastatin and a diet low in saturated fat.

At follow-up in the outpatient clinic, his serum enzymes levels (CK, ALT and LDH) were normal, and his total and LDL cholesterol were normalizing. He had taken advice and stopped smoking.

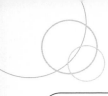

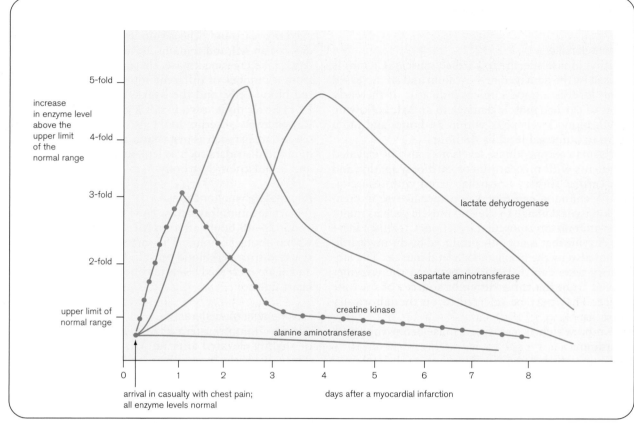

Figure 6.2 Enzyme levels following a myocardial infarction. Serum enzyme levels used for the diagnosis of myocardial infarction and in post-infarction monitoring.

Troponin

Recently, a more cardiospecific muscle protein troponin has been used as an indicator of an MI. Troponin concentration increases in the blood about 4–8 hours after the onset of anginal symptoms, peaks within 48 hours, and again at 4 days. The important distinction in this test is that the troponin level may remain increased in the circulation for up to 14 days. Therefore it is useful to confirm an MI that occurred a number of days ago.

Measurement of Blood Lipids

Lipids are not soluble in water, so they are converted to a more transportable form in the liver in order that they may be easily transported in the blood. In effect, protein is attached to the lipids to produce a lipoprotein particle which enables them to be transported and metabolized in the body. Within an hour of consuming a meal, chylomicrons can be detected in blood; chylomicrons are particles that are mainly triglyceride lipid with very little protein attached. (If blood is taken from a patient soon after a meal, and the sample is allowed to separate into cells and supernatant, the plasma or serum is liable to look very creamy owing to the presence of chylomicrons. This may interfere with the analysis of other lipoproteins.)

After being acted on in the liver, the chylomicrons are converted to one of the three main types of lipoprotein, which can be measured by the clinical biochemistry laboratory. Serum lipoprotein profiles are performed on blood taken following an overnight fast, as the presence of the chylomicrons would invalidate the results obtained (see Table 6.1)

Measurement of lipids is essential in any patient with a family history of IHD, since an increase in the level of low-density lipoprotein or very low-density lipoprotein cholesterol exacerbates atheroma. This will predispose the patient to coronary (and cerebral) arterial narrowing, blood clots, and consequent ischaemia or infarction (see Chapter 4).

Classification of Serum Lipoproteins

Lipoprotein	Lipid composition				Functions
	Cholesterol (%)	Tryglyceride (%)	Phospholipid (%)	Protein (%)	
Chylomicrons	5	90	4	1	transport of triglyceride from the gut to the liver
Very low-density lipoprotein (VLDL)	20	65	10	5	transport of triglyceride from the liver to other body organs and tissues
Low-density lipoprotein (LDL) – 'bad'	50	10	20	20	transport of cholesterol from the liver to other body organs and tisues
High-density lipoprotein (HDL) – 'good'	35	5	35	25	transport of cholesterol from extrahepatic tissues to the liver

Table 6.1 Classification of serum lipoproteins. Normal ranges: serum cholesterol: <5.2 mmol/l; serum triglyceride: 0.8–2.0 mmol/l. The class of circulating lipoproteins may be affected by life-style (e.g. diet, exercise, obesity, smoking, alcohol) and some drugs. The class of circulating lipoproteins may be changed by (and also may predispose to) diseases such as ischaemic heart disease and diabetes (see Chapter 32). Levels of circulating lipids are estimated to evaluate the effectiveness of and compliance with lipid-lowering therapies (i.e. dietary and other life-style changes, and lipid-lowering drugs).

INVESTIGATION OF LIVER DISEASE

The liver is an organ with multiple functions. It plays an essential role in the body's metabolic processes. An abnormal liver function test may be the result of a primary disease (e.g. caused by a genetic defect or an infection in the liver) (see Chapter 34); however, more frequently abnormal liver function tests reflect a disease state in another body system (e.g. heart failure). Therefore, they may provide vital information in the detective work involved in trying to make a diagnosis.

Investigations of the liver may be used to indicate specific abnormalities of the hepatocytes (liver cells) or biliary tract. The functional mass of liver cells or biliary tract cells are evaluated. New imaging techniques (e.g. ultrasound, magnetic resonance imaging, and endoscopic examination) enable parts of the liver and biliary tree to be visualized with precision, and this often obviates the need for more invasive procedures, such as laparoscopy or biopsy. However, liver biopsy may be important in determining the precise cause or extent (staging) of certain liver diseases.

Liver Function Tests

Assessment of liver function includes measurements of bilirubin, albumin, and prothrombin (which are all made by the liver), and a measurement of glucose (which is utilized by the liver to make glycogen). The levels of these components in blood will be abnormally *increased* if the excretory, detoxification, or storage functions of the liver are disturbed. However, if the ability of the liver to synthesize is impaired, then inevitably blood levels will be *reduced*. Impaired excretory function of the liver (cholestasis), may occur where there is partial or total obstruction of the biliary tract affecting excretion from the liver into the intestine (e.g. in gallstones, cancer of the pancreas, or primary biliary cirrhosis).

Liver Enzyme Tests

Enzymes can be used as markers of the outer membrane of the hepatocyte, the intracellular component, or the biliary tract. The three enzymes whose concentrations in blood are commonly measured to assess whether the patient has a disease of the liver are:

- alanine aminotransferase (for the hepatocyte);
- alkaline phosphatase (for the biliary tract); and
- gamma-glutamyl transpeptidase (for the biliary tract).

These enzymes are found in the hepatocytes and the cells in the biliary tree, and they are therefore indicators of the viability of these cells. An abnormality in these enzymes can indicate the predominant area of damage in a particular disease process (e.g. virus-

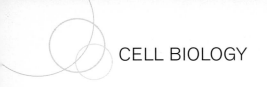

Serum Enzyme Levels for Assessment of Liver Damage

Enzyme	Normal range in serum	Comments
alanine aminotransferase	5–40 U/l	raised level is a likely indicator of hepatocellular damage
alkaline phosphatase	30–100 U/l	raised level associated with damage to the liver and biliary tract
gamma-glutamyl transpeptidase*	<60 U/l (females), <30 U/l (males)	sensitive indicator of liver disease; raised level indicates damage to the biliary tract

Table 6.2 **Serum enzyme levels for assessment of liver damage.** *Also known as gamma-glutamyl transferase.

induced hepatitis, liver problems caused by alcoholic, or genetic disease) (Table 6.2). Thus, measuring the serum levels can be helpful in revealing the major categories of liver disease (see Person-Centred Study: Alcoholic Hepatitis).

Investigations for the presence of rare genetic diseases such as haemochromatosis (a genetic disorder of iron storage) and Wilson's disease (a genetic disorder of copper storage) require more specific protein measurements. For instance, in Wilson's disease, serum levels of copper and caeruloplasmin (a copper-binding protein in plasma) are measured.

INVESTIGATION OF GASTROINTESTINAL DISEASE

Laboratory tests play a lesser role in the diagnosis of diseases of the gastrointestinal system. Such tests are always likely to be carried out in conjunction with radiological investigations (e.g. barium meal, barium enema, nuclear medicine scans, and endoscopic and colonoscopic procedures) (see Chapter 34). However, these procedures can be a means of obtaining gastrointestinal fluids and samples of tissue by biopsy for biochemical and histological analysis. Tests of gastrointestinal function largely determine the response of the gut (following an overnight fast) to the administration of a meal with a known content of nutrients (e.g. glucose, fat, protein) or the administration of a hormone. They are known as dynamic tests.

Stomach

Gastric fluid found in the stomach may easily be obtained via a nasogastric tube or at the time of endoscopy. Measurement of acid, microscopic analysis for the presence of the micro-organisms, such as *Helicobacter pylori* (see Chapter 17), and biopsy of the gastric mucosa will aid the diagnosis of gastritis, gastric or duodenal ulcers, gastric atrophy, or carcinoma.

PERSON-CENTRED STUDY: ALCOHOLIC HEPATITIS

Clive, aged 50 years, is a publican who had drunk 50 units of barley wine (1 unit of alcohol is 8 g) each week for many years. He was admitted with abdominal discomfort and swelling.

On admission, he was noted to have the cutaneous stigmata of chronic liver disease, hepatomegaly, and jaundice. The differential diagnosis included acute alcoholic hepatitis, cirrhosis, portal hypertension, or hepatocellular carcinoma.

Biochemical tests confirmed abnormal levels of serum liver enzymes (with raised aminotransferases and gamma-glutamyl transpeptidase) and alterations in the liver function tests (prolonged prothrombin time and low albumin).

Liver biopsy showed fatty change with features of early cirrhosis.

At discharge he was advised to stop drinking alcohol, which he did, and over the next few months his liver enzymes fell to within the normal range and liver function returned to normal. On one occasion after a drinking 'binge', his serum gamma-glutamyl transpeptidase level again became abnormal.

Previously, gastric function tests were generally used to assess the success of a vagotomy (surgery performed to decrease acid production by the stomach). However these tests may also be performed on patients where there is suspected decreased acid production, as occurs in achlorhydria, which may be found in older adults and those with pernicious anaemia (see Chapter 27).

Specific measurement of hormones (e.g. gastrin, calcitonin, somatostatin) are reserved for the investigation of much rarer conditions. For example, the plasma gastrin level (normal level < 40 pmol/l) may be estimated in patients being investigated for Zollinger–Ellison syndrome, a gastrin-producing tumour.

Small Intestine
The small intestine extends from the duodenum to the terminal ileum inclusively. It has a large surface area for absorption, formed by the mucosal folds and villi. The main function of the small intestine is to transfer digested nutrients, salts, and water across the intestinal epithelial cells; in order to achieve this, it produces many enzymes and hormones. Most constituents of the gut lumen can be absorbed through the epithelium, with the exception of vitamin B12-intrinsic factor complex and bile, which both have a specific receptor in the terminal ileum for their transport.

General tests to screen for malabsorption
Diseases of the small intestine are included in the differential diagnosis of abdominal pain, weight loss, diarrhoea, steatorrhoea (fatty, frothy stools), and nutritional deficiencies. The preliminary tests to investigate these possibilities include a full blood count, an estimation of the levels of serum vitamin B12 and folate, and measurement of serum albumin, serum calcium, and alkaline phosphatase (which might indicate osteomalacia or adult vitamin D deficiency; see Chapter 39).

Fat malabsorption
Fat malabsorption can be detected by collecting a faecal specimen and looking for the presence of fat globules under the microscope. The presence of fat in the stool is called steatorrhoea, and it may be apparent from the clinical appearance of the voluminous and smelly pale stools (e.g. in patients with coeliac disease, cystic fibrosis, or pancreatic disease). Normal fat excretion is less than 6 g per day. To measure fat excretion, the total faecal output is collected over 3 days while the patient takes a regulated diet containing a known amount of fat. Thus, by knowing the fat consumed, the proportion of fat excreted in the stools can be measured.

To avoid faecal collection, which can be unpleasant for patient, fat absorption can also be measured by breath analysis following the oral administration of a radioactive-labelled fat load. The lipases in the intestine split (hydrolyse) the fat, which is then absorbed, and a detectable radioactive form of carbon dioxide is produced from fat metabolism in the body (see Chapter 2). This can be measured in the air that is expired from the lungs. Thus, an indication of the extent to which fat is or is not being absorbed can be calculated from the level of radioactive carbon dioxide in the expired breath.

Steatorrhoea can be confirmed by measuring the wet weight of stool (normally < 100 g per day, but is substantially increased in steatorrhoea).

INVESTIGATION OF ENDOCRINE DISEASE
Laboratory investigations for endocrine disease cover a wide range of organs and can largely be divided into simple measurement of the levels of the target hormone produced by the endocrine gland (e.g. measurement of the levels of thyroxine and tri-iodothyronine, released from the thyroid gland). Alternatively measurement of the plasma levels of the substance that the hormone 'works on' or regulates may be more appropriate. A classic example is measurement of blood and urine glucose concentrations in patients suspected of, or suffering from, diabetes mellitus.

Feedback mechanisms operate between the hypothalamus, the pituitary, and other endocrine glands in a healthy person, in order to ensure equilibrium in hormone secretion (see Chapter 35). However, because the functions of the endocrine system are very much inter-related, a defect in one gland can influence the activities of another.

One of the golden rules in the investigation of these disorders, is that if a deficiency disorder is suspected, a stimulatory test should be performed, whereas if excess hormone secretion is suspected, then a suppression test should be performed.

Diabetes Mellitus
Diabetes mellitus is a common disorder of carbohydrate metabolism. It usually presents either in childhood or in middle life (see Chapter 35). It may also occur during pregnancy (gestational diabetes) or as a consequence of disease in another system (e.g. in chronic pancreatitis or haemochromatosis, in which the pancreas is damaged, or in Cushing's syndrome or acromegaly, in which increased hormone production affects the metabolism of glucose).

General tests for diabetes mellitus
Initially, the presence of glucose in the urine may indicate diabetes, but it may also be associated with a low

renal threshold for glucose. Diagnosis depends on finding a fasting venous glucose level > 7.8 mmol/l or a random glucose level > 11.1 mmol/l. If diabetes is suspected from a raised fasting blood glucose level, a blood glucose level in a 2-hour post-prandial sample (after a meal) is measured; if elevated (> 11.1 mmol/l), it indicates that the person has diabetes mellitus.

The traditional glucose tolerance test (GTT) should only be used rarely, since it requires giving an oral glucose load, which could produce dangerously high glucose levels in a person with diabetes. Thus, the GTT is largely reserved for detection of pregnancy-associated diabetes and for investigating people with impaired glucose tolerance (glucose handling). The procedure is as follows: the patient is asked to fast overnight and blood is taken for estimating the glucose level, then the person is given an oral glucose load of 75 g glucose in water. Serial blood samples are then taken at 60 and 120 minutes. An impaired GTT is indicated by a glucose level in venous blood of 6.7–10 mmol/l and in capillary and whole plasma of 7.8–11.1 mmol/l at 2 hours (Figure 6.3).

Monitoring diabetic control

The response of a person with diabetes to treatment may be monitored by regularly testing the urine by using reagent tablets or dipsticks. Another procedure is the measurement of blood glucose. There are dipsticks available for this purpose which can be read by eye, or by an apparatus called a glucometer, which the patient can be trained to use at home. Such tests are performed on a day-to-day basis. Glycated haemoglobin, another blood component, can be measured as an indicator of adequate control of blood glucose over the past month. This test measures how much of the excess glucose becomes bound to haemoglobin to produce the glycated form of the protein. The proportion of glycated haemoglobin indicates the control of diabetes over the previous few weeks. Good control is indicated by levels of <6 per cent; levels of >20 per cent indicate poorly controlled diabetes. (Some laboratories use other glycated proteins, such as serum fructosamine, which is a measure of the glycation of plasma proteins, notably albumin.)

In the sick diabetic patient, the ketoacidosis state frequently involves hospital admission, with measurement of blood gases to detect the level of acidosis, as well as measurement of renal function and serum lactate. Diabetic patients may also have lipid abnormalities – hypertriglyceridaemia may be present in insulin-dependent diabetes, with raised serum levels of very low-density lipoprotein, whereas in non-insulin-

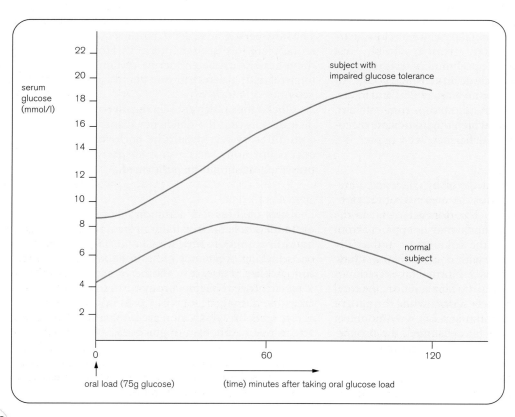

Figure 6.3 Glucose tolerance test. The serum glucose levels after an oral load of 75 g of glucose in a healthy person with normal glucose tolerance and in a person with impaired glucose tolerance.

dependent diabetes, raised serum levels of very low-density lipoprotein and low-density lipoprotein (i.e. a mixed pattern) is more common (see Table 6.1). Normalisation of aberrant serum lipid profiles is likely to occur with good diabetic control.

Investigation of the Thyroid Gland

Tests may be performed to establish the presence of an abnormality in the function of the thyroid gland. The general tests are usually concerned with measurement of the levels of total and free thyroid hormones (thyroxine and tri-iodothyronine) and of the thyroid-binding protein (the transport protein for the thyroid hormones in blood). The levels of these components in blood not only vary in thyroid disorders, but also during pregnancy and in women taking the oral contraceptive pill. In addition, thyroid antibodies may be measured in patients suspected of having an autoimmune thyroid disorder (see Chapter 27).

Thyroid stimulation test

This test involves giving a known amount (usually 200 μg, administered intravenously) of thyroid-releasing hormone (TRH), a hormone normally produced by the hypothalamus. Serial blood samples are taken just before administration, and at 20 and 60 minutes after the injection in order to measure the level of serum thyroid-stimulating hormone (TSH). This is to assess the extent to which the pituitary gland has been stimulated in response to the injected hormone. The serum level of thyroid hormones produced by the thyroid gland are also estimated.

This test is performed in patients suspected of having thyroid disease in order to ascertain whether the problem is in the thyroid gland itself or in one of the other glands involved in controlling its hormonal output (i.e. the hypothalamus and pituitary) (Figure 6.4).

Radioactive iodine uptake test

Radioactive iodine (^{131}I) may be given orally as a capsule or intravenously to investigate an overactive thyroid gland. The test is generally performed in the fasting state and the patient is not allowed to eat for about 1 hour after the oral dose of radioactive iodine has been given, since food can affect its uptake. The amount of radioactivity in the thyroid gland is measured just before administration (i.e. a baseline measurement), and 2, 6, and 24 hours later. By administering a radioactive source of iodine, the amount taken up by the gland can be effectively and accurately detected on thyroid scans. Thus, the metabolic activity of the thyroid can be assessed.

Use of a technetium (Tc) scan can detect:
- carcinoma, in which thyroxine production is normal;

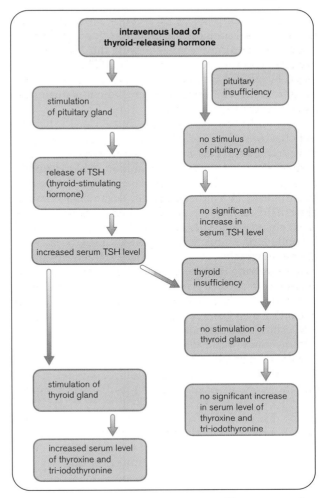

Figure 6.4 Thyroid stimulating test. This test can be used in the invesigation of thyroid disease.

- an underactive thyroid gland; and
- the presence of a goitre (thyroid swelling).

Investigation of the Adrenal Gland

Although disorders of the adrenal gland are very rare, tests of adrenal function need to be performed to exclude them as a possible diagnosis when investigating common symptoms and disorders. A general test is the measurement of serum and urine cortisol to confirm adrenal hypofunction (Addison's disease) or adrenal hyperfunction (Cushing's disease or Cushing's syndrome). Serum cortisol levels exhibit diurnal variation and must therefore be collected at standard times. A 24-hour collection of urine for cortisol measurement may also be helpful, because the level is increased in Cushing's disease (see Chapter 35).

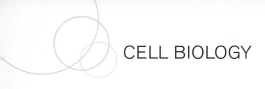

Adrenal hypofunction

Although Addison's disease (underactive adrenal gland) is rare, diagnosis is essential because the disease is life-threatening. The presence of the disease might be indicated by a low serum sodium level (<120 mmol/l); the specific test is the synacthen test, which is a stimulatory test (see Chapter 35).

Adrenal hyperfunction

An adrenal suppression test is used when Cushing's disease is suspected. In this investigation, a blood sample is taken before the test to measure the baseline serum cortisol level. A synthetic steroid, dexamethasone (at a dose of 0.5 mg) is given at regular 6-hourly intervals over 48 hours to reduce the activity of the adrenal gland. A second blood sample is taken 6 hours after the last dose to assess whether cortisol output was decreased as a result of giving dexamethasone. A lack of suppression (high serum cortisol level) indicates an adrenal tumour (Cushing's syndrome). However, suppression of adrenal gland activity (i.e. a reduced serum cortisol level) occurs in Cushing's disease but not in an adrenal tumour. This suppression test can therefore be used to distinguished between the two 'Cushing' conditions.

INVESTIGATION OF RENAL DISEASE

Many diseases affect renal function as well as diseases which originate in the kidney. Therefore, the biochemical tests for renal function are important in determining and confirming renal dysfunction, but they may not diagnose the cause of the impaired renal function.

General Tests of Renal Function

Measurement of the levels of serum urea, electrolytes (sodium and potassium), and creatinine will give information about the function of glomeruli and tubules. Plasma creatinine (normal range 60–110 mmol/l) is filtered freely at the glomerulus with only small amounts reabsorbed by the tubules, and is a good marker of glomerular function. However, slight individual variation in creatinine levels may be found because it is affected by body mass and muscle bulk (see Chapter 2).

A further assessment of renal function includes the creatinine clearance test. This is performed on a complete 24-hour urine collection to measure total creatinine output. Blood is also taken at the end of the 24 hours to estimate the plasma creatinine level. Knowing the level of creatinine in both the urine and the plasma enables the amount of creatinine being cleared by the kidneys to be determined.

Renal tubular damage is signalled by the loss of concentrating ability, indicated by a low urine osmolality. In patients with renal failure, this needs to be assessed and compared in relation to plasma osmolality. When the kidney fails to maintain adequate homeostatic control of electrolytes, notably sodium and potassium, a restricted diet with respect to salty foods and fluid intake may be indicated (Box 6.1 and Table 6.3).

INVESTIGATION OF BONE AND CALCIUM DISORDERS

Circulating calcium levels are controlled by parathyroid hormone and activated vitamin D (1,25 dihydroxycholecalciferol), both of which act to increase calcium concentration in the blood. In addition, calcium homeostasis is regulated between the plasma and a number of organs (the kidney, the liver, bone, and the intestines) and other hormones (oestrogen, glucocorticoids, thyroxine, testosterone, and growth hormone) (see Chapter 39).

The levels of serum calcium, phosphate, and alkaline phosphatase are good markers of calcium metabolism. Plasma calcium concentration may need to be 'corrected' for changes in albumin concentration, which affect total calcium concentration. The most usual formula is that for every gram of albumin over 40 g/l,

---

BOX 6.1 TYPICAL SIGNS OF ACUTE AND CHRONIC RENAL FAILURE

Acute renal failure

Oliguric phase
  low urine output
  decreased serum sodium
  increased serum urea, creatinine, potassium, and hydrogen

Diuretic phase (which follows the oliguric phase)
  decreased serum potassium
  elevated serum urea and creatinine (if adequate renal function has not yet been re-established)

Chronic renal failure
  reduced glomerular filtration rate
  increased serum urea and creatinine
  retention of sodium and water retention, leading to weight gain and rise in blood pressure

Clinical signs associated with changes in levels of serum potassium and sodium

Condition	Serum level	Causes	Symptoms	Signs
Hypokalaemia	potassium <2.5 mmol/l	gastrointestinal disturbances (diarrhoea, vomiting); drugs (e.g. diuretics); renal disease; endocrine disease	muscle weakness; muscle cramps	gastric stasis and ileus; confusion; depression
Hyperkalaemia	potassium >5.6 mmol/l	renal disease; excess potassium intake	confusion	cardiac dysrhythmias; cardiac arrest; convulsions
Hyponatraemia	sodium <120 mmol/l	excess intravenous infusions; water intoxication (rare); inappropriate ADH secretion (e.g. in bronchial carcinoma)	confusion; central nervous system irritability	confusion; oedema
Hypernatraemia	sodium >160 mmol/l	water depletion; dehydration; excess sodium intake (usually intravenous); diabetes insipidus	swelling	oedema; weight gain; congestive cardiac failure

Table 6.3 Clinical signs associated with changes in levels of plasma potassium and sodium. Normal ranges: serum potassium: 3.5–4.7 mmol/l; serum sodium: 135–145 mmol/l.

0.02 mmol/l should be subtracted from the total calcium level as measured, and for every gram of albumin under 40 g/l, 0.02 mmol/l should be added to the total measured calcium level. Measurement of ionized calcium in serum can be performed in cases of suspected serious hypocalcaemia or hypercalcaemia. Serum calcium, phosphate, and alkaline phosphatase levels are measured when hypercalcaemia is being investigated, and they will indicate causes such as hyperparathyroidism, malignancy, and rarer conditions, such as vitamin D intoxication and sarcoidosis (Box 6.2).

ANALYSIS OF RESPIRATORY GASES

The main indications for estimating blood gases are the investigation and management of patients with respiratory diseases, the management of critically ill patients in the Intensive Therapy Unit who require assisted ventilation, and the investigation and management of certain metabolic disorders (e.g. metabolic acidosis and alkalosis). The levels of carbon dioxide ($paCO_2$) and oxygen (paO_2) in arterial blood can in turn have an effect on hydrogen ion concentration and thus the acid–base balance of the body (i.e. the pH) (see Chapter 33).

Estimation of blood gases are performed on an arterial blood specimen collected into a tube that contains heparin. Care should be taken when drawing the blood in order to avoid haemolysis, which could affect the result. The sample should be kept on ice before blood gases are estimated, and air should be excluded

---

BOX 6.2 HYPOCALCAEMIA AND HYPERCALCAEMIA

Serum calcium level normal range – 2.15–2.55 mmol/l

Hypocalcaemia

Signs
muscle and abdominal cramps, paraesthesia, tetany, hypotension

Causes
vitamin D deficiency, renal insufficiency, hypoparathyroidism

Hypercalcaemia

Signs
thirst, polyuria, epilepsy

Causes
hyperparathyroidism secondary to malignancy, certain drug treatments (e.g. thiazide diuretics), renal transplantation

from the syringe once the blood has been collected because air subsequently dissolved in the sample could influence the final result. The measurements are performed at 30°C, even if the patient's own body temperature is elevated. The test should ideally be done immediately after the blood has been taken. Thus, to avoid delays equipment for estimating arterial blood gas is often available in the Intensive Therapy Unit or the Accident and Emergency department.

ANALYSIS OF BODY TISSUES BY PATHOLOGY LABORATORIES

PREPARATION AND EXAMINATION OF SOLID TISSUES

Tissues removed surgically for histopathological examination must first be stabilized (fixed) to prevent decay, otherwise the tissue will undergo autolysis and be subject to attack from micro-organisms. Normally the tissue is stabilized by the use of chemical fixatives, in particular formaldehyde. This arrests decomposition and maintains the tissue in a state suitable for further examination. Other chemical fixatives, such as glutaraldehyde, are sometimes used, especially when examinations are likely to be required beyond the light microscope level. For example, if an electron microscope is to be used, then better subcellular preservation is obtained using glutaraldehyde rather than other fixatives, such as formaldehyde.

Fixation

Fixatives are agents which preserve the morphology and the chemical constituents of tissues and cells. Typically, the fixatives act on the protein components of biological tissues to achieve structural stabilization. The degree of fixation should be such that the tissue retains as closely as possible its structural relationships in life. Good fixatives kill cells, tissues, and organs quickly, thus minimizing shrinking and swelling artefacts. They penetrate the tissues rapidly and evenly, and inhibit bacterial decay and autodigestion. They should also prepare the tissue for further examination, and, ideally, the natural colours of the tissues should remain. The fixative used should be economical. No ideal fixative exists, and compromises frequently have to be made between preserving cellular components for immunological staining on the one hand and preserving good tissue architecture following cell death on the other.

Formaldehyde, one of the most widely used fixatives, is a gas produced by the oxidization of methanol. It is soluble in water to a level of 40 per cent by weight, and in this state it is known as formalin. For many specimens, a solution is used which consists of one part of 40 per cent formaldehyde with nine parts of distilled water, within which 8.5 g/l of sodium chloride is dissolved. This is an excellent fixative for post-mortem material, but the process is slow – the period of fixation required is 24 hours or more. A solution of 10 per cent neutral-buffered formalin is also frequently used for the preservation of surgical, post-mortem, and research specimens; this also requires 24 hours of fixation. The period of fixation is partly dependent on the size of the specimens. Tissues smears can be fixed very rapidly typically using alcohol–ether.

Calcium is present in bone and some other tissues, and this has to be removed. Acids are used to decalcify these tissues, and the extent of decalcification can be satisfactory determined by X-ray examination. It is important that decalcification is completed before the tissue is subjected to sectioning.

In addition to chemical fixatives, it is possible to freeze tissue and to cut sections of the frozen tissue, which can be stained and examined using the light microscope. This can be extremely important when a very rapid diagnosis is required. For example, this used to be the standard procedure for examining the biopsy of a breast lump suspected of being malignant, because the results of the examination could determine the future course of the operation. There were also advantages in obviating the need for a patient to have a general anaesthetic for a biopsy which might have to be followed by a later operation based on the histopathological result. Changes in breast cancer surgery have meant that the examination of the frozen sections from the biopsy is less frequently used, but it retains a use in many other types of surgery including parathyroid surgery.

Although the frozen section is quick to prepare, the quality of preservation is less satisfactory than that obtained with chemical fixation. Chemical fixation does, however, take some time.

PREPARATION OF FIXED TISSUE SAMPLES FOR MICROSCOPY

Once they are fixed, tissues have to be dehydrated by solutions such as alcohol or acetone, after which they are cleared to remove the alcohol from the blocks and sections. Clearing solutions, such as xylene, cause the tissues to appear transparent (hence the term 'clearing'). The tissues are then impregnated with paraffin wax, normally using an automatic tissue presser; this is usually done overnight. After this procedure, the tissues are embedded using wax moulds, and sections are cut for histological examination using a microtome.

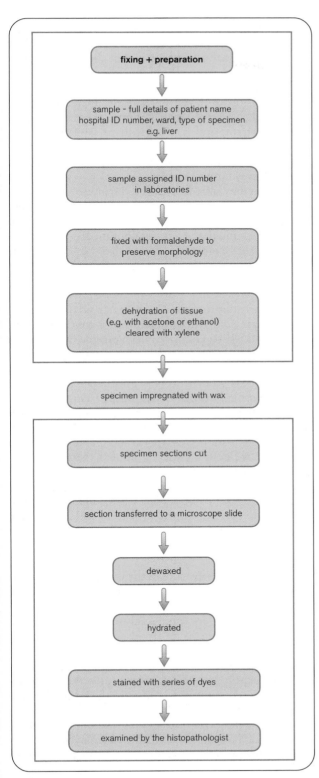

Figure 6.5 Stages in the preparation of a tissue specimen for examination by the histolopathologist.

Tissue Sections

Section cutting is a skilled job; to produce sections of consistently good quality takes considerable patience. Once cut, the sections are dewaxed, hydrated, and then stained using natural dyes that confer contrast to the tissues. The stains most typically used are haematoxylin and eosin. A wide range of so-called special stains are also used to demonstrate specific cellular components. After staining, the slides containing the tissue are washed and then covers mounted on to them; they are then forwarded for examination by the histopathologist (Figure 6.5).

Histopathological diagnosis depends on scrupulous labelling and recording of sample data. Any mix-up in specimens could have disastrous consequences for patients. Another investigation sometimes used is the technique of fine-needle aspiration. This involves the removal of cells, connective tissue, and tissue fluids from tumours or other lesions that are easily palpable and accessible through the skin. The aspirated cells are smeared and stained in a similar way to that of the staining of tissue sections.

In some tissues and tumours, cells are gradually shed. Cells are shed from epithelial surfaces, including the oral cavity, skin, stomach, bladder, and cervix. Shed cells from areas suspected of being malignant can be examined microscopically and an assessment made on the nature of the tumour. Although false-positive results are very rare, sampling error makes the false-negative result less infrequent.

Information Obtained from Histological Sections

Using the light microscope, the histopathologist is able to identify tissue changes that result in disease processes. Quite often, it is possible to identify the features associated with neoplasia, (see Chapter 5). However, histopathological diagnosis is subjective and there are a number of occasions when it is not possible to be absolutely certain whether a tumour is benign or malignant.

At the histopathologist's disposal are a range of special stains and antibodies linked to markers that are specific for cellular components. These markers can greatly assist the histopathologist in determining the origin of tumour tissue as well as indicating whether or not the tissue is benign or malignant. Furthermore, the electron microscope, although not used as a routine diagnostic tool, can provide additional information at the ultrastructural level. It is particularly useful in the examination of renal biopsies.

Sampling Errors

One of the major difficulties in the evaluation of tissue histopathologically is that only a relatively small sample of tissue is being examined. For this reason, the description of the tissue as it arrives in the laboratory from the operating theatre is very important. At this stage, the histopathologist has to be very sure that the tissue received by the laboratory is representative of the areas of tissue being sampled. Where a small tumour exists, it is likely to be surrounded by biologically normal tissue, so there is a danger that a false-negative result could be recorded.

Histopathological Reports

The histopathological report is prepared by a qualified pathologist and is sent to the attending physician, who will use it to inform further treatment options for the patient. For example, it may be acceptable to consider certain types of chemotherapy for an aggressively malignant tumour; the same chemotherapy may be less acceptable for a slowly growing, well-differentiated cancer.

Autopsy Examinations

Autopsy examinations are conducted for a number of purposes. These include determining the cause of death, learning more about disease processes, and instructing junior medical staff. During an autopsy, the histopathologist carefully records the condition of the body and the external organs. It is often possible to determine the cause of death and, because of this, autopsy examinations are sometimes mandatory for medical or legal reasons. For example, any sudden death in the UK necessitates a post-mortem examination. Similarly, death that occurs within a period of 24 hours from surgery also requires a post-mortem examination.

Sometimes, particularly when there are forensic considerations, a post-mortem examination may involve staff other than a histopathologist; for instance, toxicologists may need to be there to undertake chemical analysis on tissue fragments.

Preparation and Examination of Blood

The haematology laboratory is concerned with investigating disorders of the blood, including:
- anaemia, and diagnosis of the underlying pathology;
- disorders associated with abnormal proliferation of blood cells, such as leukaemia; and
- inherited blood clotting disorders, such as haemophilia.

Disorders of blood that are commonly seen in clinical practice are discussed in Chapter 31.

Collection of blood

For haematological investigation, both capillary and venous blood can be used. There must be good mixing of the blood with an anticoagulant, and typically a rotating mixer is used. Capillary blood samples can be used, but they present a number of problems in the laboratory. Their advantage is that they can used for young children, from whom it is often difficult to collect venous blood, and for adults with veins that make the collection of a venous sample difficult. Unfortunately, because of small volumes there is a risk of sampling error, and it is difficult to repeat tests in a laboratory because usually the whole sample has to be used. Larger volumes of blood are most easily obtained using venous blood samples.

Plasma may only be separated from the blood cells if the specimen has been maintained in an anticoagulated state. If serum is required, the blood is allowed to clot in a tube that does not contain any anticoagulant, and the serum and cells can then be separated by centrifugation.

Typically, blood is examined by making a blood film (i.e. by pressing a drop of blood on a slide and using a spreader to draw the drop across the slide). In this way an evenly distributed film is made, and this can be stained to examine the blood cells. Different sorts of stains may be used, such as the Leishmann stain and the Giemsa stain. With the Leishmann stain, the nuclei of leukocytes appear purple, the eosinophilic granules appear orange–red, and the basophilic granules appear dark blue. Lymphocytes have dark purple nuclei with pale blue cytoplasm and the red blood cells have a slight salmon-pink appearance. With the Giemsa stain, the nuclei of leukocytes appear reddish purple, the eosinophilic granules appear red to orange, and the basophilic granules appear blue. Lymphocytes appear as dark purple nuclei with a light blue cytoplasm. The platelets again appear as violet to purple granules.

Automation in Haematology

One of the major advances in the haematology laboratory has been the introduction of automation. There are now a variety of machines that enable the laboratory to provide a very rapid analysis of the blood cells. Although automation in blood cell counting is very widely used, it needs to be subject to stringent quality control procedures.

Haemoglobin concentration is also measured by the automated counter to estimate the oxygen-carrying capacity of the blood. This is important in the detection and diagnosis of diseases that result in a deficiency or excess of haemoglobin. Further haematological tests include the packed cell volume (PCV) or the haematocrit. This is a measure of the relative mass of red blood cells present in a sample of whole blood. Normal values for the PCV are known, and these may differ in males and females (see Appendix 2).

Blood Transfusion

Although blood transfusion is widely used, the complexity of the process is sometimes underestimated. All transfusions are in effect a transplantation, and if blood transfusion is not carefully handled, there is a serious risk of fatal consequences. It was in 1900 that Karl Landsteiner demonstrated the ABO blood grouping system. This led to an understanding of the importance of the different groups in the transfusion of blood. In 1927, Landsteiner and Levine described the MN blood group system and the P system. Later, in 1939, the discovery of the rhesus system led to the recognition and cause of haemolytic disease of the newborn (see Chapter 26).

The blood transfusion laboratory is concerned with the cross-matching of blood to ensure that the best possible matches are established between donor blood and the recipient. Cross-matching involves the detection of atypical antibodies that could cause blood transfusion reactions or, in the case of a pregnant woman, cross the placenta and damage the unborn child. Blood transfusion centres are involved in the bleeding and testing of blood donors from which blood and blood products are isolated for the treatment of patients. Blood donors in the UK are not reimbursed, and the stringent procedures of the National Blood Service have insured that the risk of a patient being infected by a blood product is extremely low. All blood donors are required to fill in forms in which an assessment of the risk that they pose to recipients can be determined. Particular concern at the present time is the presence of HIV, which cannot always be detected at the early stages of infection. All blood samples are checked for infectious agents including HIV, syphilis, and hepatitis B (see Chapters 29 and 31).

Blood does not keep well and has to be stored in conditions that are as close to ideal as possible. If the blood is haemolysed or infected, it could be lethal to the recipient, particularly as many recipients of blood transfusions are in poor health. Blood is normally kept in refrigerators at a constant temperature of 4°C, with a maximum range of 2–4°C. If the temperature is outside these limits, damage to the blood will occur. Domestic refrigerators have a wide range of temperatures and blood should never be stored in them.

The types of blood products used in clinical practice, besides whole blood, are frozen plasma, dried plasma, plasma protein fraction, albumin, fibrinogen, cryoprecipitate, factor VIII concentrates, platelets, and white blood cells.

CELL BIOLOGY

FURTHER READING

Adrogue HJ, Madias NE (1998) Management of life-threatening acid-base disorders. N Engl J Med 338:26–34.

Burkitt HG, Stevens A, Lowe JS, Young B (1996) Wheater's Basic Histopathology: a Colour Atlas and Text, 3rd edition. Churchill Livingstone, Edinburgh.

Evans DMD (1995) Specific Tests: The Procedure and Meaning of the Commoner Tests in Hospital, 14th edition. Mosby, London.

Fischbach F (1995) Quick Reference to Common Laboratory and Diagnostic Tests. JB Lippincott, Philadephia.

Gaw A, Cowan RA, O'Reilly D St J, Stewart MJ, Shepherd, J (1995) Clinical Biochemistry – an Illustrated Colour Text. Churchill Livingstone, Edinburgh.

Halperin ML, Rolleston FS (1993) Clinical Detective Stories: a Problem-Based Approach to Clinical Cases in Energy and Acid–Base Metabolism. Portland Press, London.

LeFever Kee J (1995) Laboratory and Diagnostic Tests with Nursing Applications, 4th edition. Appleton and Lange, Norwalk, Connecticut, USA.

Majno G, Joris I (1996) Cells, Tissues and Disease. Principles of General Pathology. Blackwell Science, Oxford.

Marshall WJ (1995) Clinical Chemistry, 3rd edition. Mosby, London.

Worthley LIG (1996) Handbook of Emergency Laboratory Tests. Churchill Livingstone, Edinburgh.

GENETICS IN THE CAUSE AND DIAGNOSIS OF DISEASE

LEARNING OBJECTIVES

After studying this chapter you will have a clearer understanding of:
- the structure of DNA and how it acts as a database of inherited information in stretches of genetic code called genes
- the types of genetic mutation that result in an inherited clinical disorder
- the techniques available to screen patients for inherited abnormalities from pre-implantation to adult screening

INTRODUCTION

The science of genetics has long been recognized as important in our understanding of medicine. In recent years, exciting developments in technology have enabled the analysis of molecules that are the basis of genetic inheritance – DNA (deoxyribonucleic acid) and RNA (ribonucleic acid). This has led to an enhanced knowledge of how our genetic make-up is implicated in the cause of diseases. Much of this information has been applied to clinical practice, so early diagnoses and successful therapeutic interventions are now possible for many inherited disorders.

WHAT IS DNA?

The double-helical structure of the DNA molecule is a familiar image, and its discovery in the early 1950s marked the beginning of research into molecular biology. The DNA helices form the molecules of inheritance that contain the 'blue-print' information to be passed from parent to offspring. Such data not only include physical characteristics such as eye colour and skin tone, but also the instructions for physiological processes. Humans are highly complex organisms having many

tissue types with different functions and histological features; furthermore, the cells of the body need to communicate with one another.

DNA contains all this information in the form of a code, namely the genetic code, which is passed on to subsequent generations via the gametes (spermatozoa, oocytes) in reproduction. Additionally, the DNA is replicated during the cell division for growth and repair, but this needs to be precise because an inaccurate copy could lead to a genetic disorder or cell death. As far as possible, DNA must be protected from damage; one obvious way that the body has used to achieve this is to combine the DNA with proteins called histones to form elongated 'chromosomes' which reside in the nucleus of the cell.

DNA is a linear molecule created by two strands linked together, giving a twisted 'ladder-like' structure. Each side of the 'ladder' is constructed by linking sugar rings (deoxyribose) and phosphate groups so it appears as a series of 'sugar–phosphate–sugar–phosphate'. Each sugar is also attached to one of four types of compound, called bases, that link together to make the 'rungs of the ladders'. The bases are adenine, cytosine, guanine, and thymine, better recognized by the abbreviated code letters, A, C, G, and T. These bases bind in a specific manner by way of weak hydrogen bonds, such that A links only with T, and G links only with C – this is known as complementary base pairing. Thus, looking straight at a rung of the ladder, it may appear as either sugar–A–T–sugar or sugar–C–G–sugar. It is this binding that creates the double-stranded appearance of DNA, with any one sugar molecule bound on three sides – to two phosphate groups and one of the bases (Figure 7.1).

There are two principal roles for DNA. First, it holds a set of instructions, in the form of a genetic code, which dictates how a cell should function. Our language uses an alphabet of 26 different characters to create words for communication. DNA has only four characters – the four bases (i.e. A, C, G and T) – and the order of these four bases along the DNA molecule forms the genetic information as a code. In any cell, the sequence (order) of the bases provides the data to direct the manufacture of proteins. So for instance, a beta-cell in the islets of Langerhans is specifically controlled by the DNA in its nucleus to synthesize insulin, and provide the cellular machinery to secrete the hormone out of the cell.

The second major role of DNA is to be a database that may be copied and transferred from one cell generation to the next. The cell division (mitosis) required for growth and cell replacement demands duplications of DNA. However, the creation of gametes for reproduction requires a different type of cell division (meiosis) in order that the chromosome pairs can be separated. The cellular rearrangement of chromosomes during meiosis allows one of each of the 23 pairs of chromosomes to be allocated to a gamete, thereby ensuring the genetic material found in a fertilized ovum is 50 per cent maternal and 50 per cent paternal.

READING THE INSTRUCTIONS ALONG DNA MOLECULES

Once the structure of DNA was appreciated, this led researchers instinctively to the quest for further knowledge about how the molecule functions in directing the growth and development of individual cells and organisms. One of the first advances came when it was recognized that the sequence of bases on the strands of DNA could be related to the order of amino acids in a specific protein. Briefly, the genetic information on DNA must be correctly translated into another language, which is the arrangement of amino acids for synthesizing a functional protein. As ribosomes are the sites of protein synthesis, this information is conveyed from the nucleus to the cytoplasm by a 'messenger'. The genetic sequence is therefore transcribed from the DNA of the gene to produce messenger RNA (mRNA). This type of genetic information bears a single-stranded copy of the data required to synthesize the protein. In any protein, the amino acids are highly specific in terms of their number, order, and variety; the sequence of the bases on mRNA dictates the order of amino acids in the protein chain (Figure 7.2; see Chapter 1). Knowledge of the relationship between the genetic code and an amino acid sequence was followed by investigations that sought to identify the precise location of different genes on chromosomes (e.g. the gene coding for sickle cell haemoglobin). The importance of these findings for biological and medical science is evident from the fact that many of the researchers responsible for these discoveries have been awarded Nobel Prizes!

DNA has another role, as a regulator of when genetic information should be dispensed and how much should be dispensed; this ultimately determines how and when proteins are manufactured. Both types of information are encoded in the sequence of the bases within the DNA molecules. The language that encodes for amino acid sequences in proteins was deciphered first and is usually referred to as the genetic code. The second language is more complex and is still being deciphered, and this may be considered as the regulatory language.

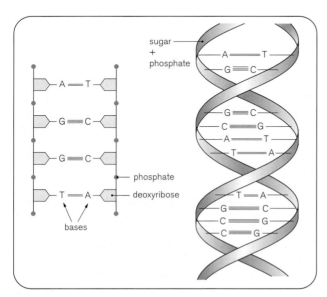

Figure 7.1 Structure of DNA. Note the positioning in the DNA helix of the nucleotide bases in relation to the deoxyribose (sugar) and the phosphate. (A: adenine; C: cytosine; G: guanine; T: thymine.)

The Genetic Code – the Language of Translation
Proteins are generally highly complex polymers of amino acids which are bound together in a specific sequence. For protein synthesis to occur, the genetic

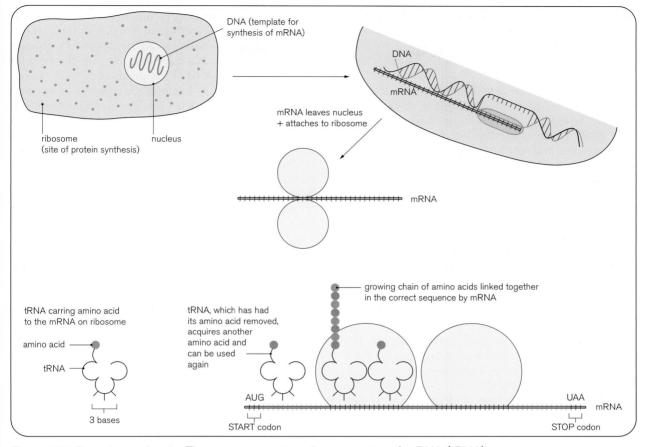

Figure 7.2 Protein synthesis. The process requires ribosomes; transfer RNA (tRNA) – the link between the genetic code and the amino acid; and messenger RNA (mRNA) – the copy of the genetic code stored as DNA in the nucleus.

sequence that is coded by the four different bases in DNA and mRNA must be translated into a different language – the amino acids sequence of the protein being synthesized. For this, a system is used in which the four bases, A, T, G, and C, are assorted into groups of three, and these triplets are termed 'codons'. In producing codons, any base can be used more than once (a codon could be AAG or TTA, for example), and consequently a total of 64 different codons are available; this is more than the minimum number needed to specify 20 amino acids. Nearly all the possible combinations of the four bases are used because most of the 20 amino acids are coded by more than one codon. However, some codons are needed for signalling the termination ('stop') of the translation process. As messenger RNA always has a few extra bases in front of the actual protein-coding region, it is necessary to include a 'start' instruction as well (Box 7.1).

WHAT ARE GENES?

The information found in DNA is organized into discrete sections called genes. Some disorders (e.g. muscular dystrophy) may be associated with the inheritance of a single gene, but many common human features (e.g. height) result from the interaction of a number of genes.

What is meant by the word gene in terms of DNA? Genes fall into three main categories – the common approach is to define a gene as a segment of the DNA on a particular chromosome responsible for the production of a single protein (e.g. actin, insulin). This definition is adequate for many purposes; however, it is imprecise. Large sections of DNA coding for the production of RNA molecules, other than mRNA, are also sometimes referred to as genes, i.e. coding regions of DNA for transfer RNA and ribosomal RNA used in protein synthesis. Likewise, there are stretches of DNA which are the regulator or controller;

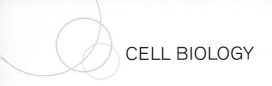

BOX 7.1   WHAT ARE RECOMBINANT PROTEINS?

- Molecular biological techniques are used to analyse the structure of nucleic acids (DNA and RNA) and to find out gene sequences. There are commercially prepared reagents and enzymes that may be utilized to synthesise DNA in the laboratory.
- Human DNA encoding for a specific protein can be synthesized *in vitro*, and subsequently incorporated into a microbe (e.g. bacteria or yeast) by a technique called transfection. Then, using its intracellular organelles and the 'foreign DNA', the microbe can manufacture the protein. Thus, in these circumstances, recombinant proteins are human proteins made by a microbe that can later be extracted and purified for use as therapeutic agents.
- Microbes can be grown in culture on an industrial scale for the synthesis and purification of proteins to be used in therapy (e.g. insulin, recombinant vaccines, cytokines, erythropoietin) (see Chapters 21, 25, and 36).
- A significant advantage of recombinant protein technology is that the proteins produced have not been isolated from human body tissues or fluids. Therefore, there is no risk of contamination with blood-borne infections such as hepatitis B or human immunodeficiency virus (HIV), or with the tissue-derived prions that cause Creutzfeld–Jakob disease.

these are found adjacent to specific protein-coding sections. It must be appreciated that proteins are not necessarily being synthesized all the time, only when they are needed. Thus, when considering the definition of a gene, it is probably reasonable to include these regulatory sections as well, because proteins would not be made without them. Furthermore, there are large parts of the human genome that appear to have no known function, and which have sometimes been termed 'junk' DNA. However, it is perhaps dangerous to ascribe such a derogatory term in the absence of a complete understanding of how the entire genome operates.

Why do humans have more DNA than is apparently needed to provide for all the genes present? One possible answer is that it has given us the potential to produce new genes, which is advantageous in evolutionary terms. Nonetheless, it is not without its disadvantage, for each time a cell divides, the DNA must be copied; this takes time and uses up the cellular resources in terms of DNA production and energy. Other cells, such as bacteria, have more rapid rates of cell division (provided they are in an environment with an adequate supply of nutrients) because they have much less DNA to copy in order to create new daughter cells.

Genes May Be Present in Single or Multiple Copies

Since we have a nearly equal contribution of DNA from both parents, it might be supposed that there are two copies of every gene (one maternally-derived and one paternally-derived). In fact, some genes are represented in multiple copies; for example, there are between 10 and 20 copies of the gene for the histone proteins. It is the histone molecules that aggregate with DNA to construct the chromosomes. There are also several hundred copies of the gene for manufacturing the molecules of ribosomal RNA.

One explanation given for the persistence of multiple copies of a gene is that it enables their products to accumulate more rapidly, which is particularly significant for an active secretory cell. Another reason could be that it is a major form of survival in the process of evolution. Our genes are open to attack to be damaged or mutated. Therefore, if there are two or more copies, one of the genes can mutate and produce a protein with slightly altered function while the other gene remains viable and normal. In succeeding generations, the forces of 'natural selection' that operate on the altered copy eventually produce a new protein. This process has occurred with the haemoglobin gene family, in which there are a number of haemoglobin genes, each with a very similar gene sequence that has apparently become mutated. Sickle cell disease is a classic example of disease caused by an abnormal haemoglobin which must have arisen by a modification process through mutation and natural selection. The sickle cell haemoglobin offers protection against malaria, so it is not surprising that the incidence of the sickle cell gene is between 5 and 20 per cent in central and west Africa where this parasitic infection is endemic (see Chapter 31).

There are extra copies of genes that no longer produce any protein, and this is thought to be because the controlling mechanisms have mutated and no longer allow the genes to work. Again, some of the extra haemoglobin genes fall into this category. The subsequent damage to the sections of DNA that code for the protein means it is difficult to see how they could ever become functional again. These sections of DNA would be correctly classified as 'junk'.

Gene Structure Gets More Complex

The original concept of a gene was that of a continuous 'string of bases' along the part of the DNA molecule that corresponds to the appropriate mRNA molecule. However, the organization for many of the human genes is rather more complex than this. Although DNA is still seen as a 'string of bases' in sequence, the genetic information encoding the order of amino acids in a protein is actually split into sections, with these coding sections separated by stretches of intervening DNA. The term 'exon' is applied to the sections of DNA that are ultimately used to encode an amino acid sequence, and the intervening portions are called 'introns'.

In the initial stage of mRNA production, a copy of the original DNA template is formed that includes both the exons and introns. In the next stage of the process, the segments of the RNA molecule representing the introns are cut out, and the remaining coding sequences (exons) are then spliced together to create the completed mRNA molecules. Finally the mRNA molecule is exported from the nucleus to the cytoplasm, to be translated in protein synthesis. The procedure of physically altering the sequence of the initial RNA molecule (called the primary transcript) into the usable form, mRNA, is known as RNA processing (Figure 7.3).

How does the cell know which sections of the series of continuous bases to cut out to produce readable mRNA? The correct cuts are guided by the genetic code found at the beginning and end of the introns. Some mutations can arise in the DNA within the introns that will not necessarily cause serious damage to the processing stage. The number of introns certainly varies widely in different genes – in the haemoglobin genes, there are just two intervening sequences, but in the genes coding for the collagen molecule (which is a major constituent of connective tissues) there can be as many as 50 intervening sequences.

Why are the genes in a split format? Again, the reason is probably connected with evolutionary history. More new proteins could be made when exons were shuffled to create novel genes relatively quickly. Again, this is not without its disadvantage, because the splicing process leads to more opportunity for serious mistakes to occur through mutations.

Genes Must Be Regulated

Every nucleated cell in the human body contains all the genetic information found in the human genome. However, not all genes are 'switched on' to operate in every cell; rather, only those genes that are required for that particular cell to fulfil its physiological role are operative. Highly controversial experiments in sheep have again proved that the genetic information for the whole animal is in every nucleated cell. Using techniques similar to the ones used for *in vitro* fertilization ('test tube baby'), a nucleus from an adult sheep cell was substituted for the nucleus in a sheep egg and put into a ewe for 'incubation', thus producing a lamb. All the DNA information was available in the adult cell, the genes just needed to be selectively activated. Hence a neurone in the brain possesses the same genes as a cardiac muscle cell, but each has its own characteristic functions by virtue of its working genes; this is known as differential gene expression.

Consider the example of insulin production by the pancreatic cells. Clearly, no other cells in the body take over the production of insulin once these cells have been destroyed, hence people with type 1 diabetes require daily injections of insulin to survive (though clinical trials are evaluating an oral form of insulin) (see Chapter 35). Essentially, the insulin genes in the pancreatic cells are the only ones that take part in manufacturing this hormone. Nevertheless, they must be under some sort of control because insulin is not produced continuously, but in response to blood glucose levels – this regulation is a short-term process. Alternatively, genes can be 'turned off' for long periods, and an extreme example of this can be seen with nerve cells in the brain. They do not divide after birth,

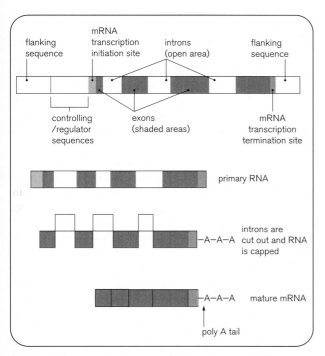

Figure 7.3 Overall structure of a gene and its processing to produce messenger RNA (mRNA) transcript.

so presumably none of the genes that direct the process of cell division are used in brain neurones between birth and death.

How is this regulation of gene activity achieved? The process is complex in human cells and depends on the interaction of special regulatory molecules (generally proteins themselves) whose prime function is to bind to the DNA and influence the rate and production of mRNA for protein synthesis.

How does the regulatory system understand where on the DNA molecule it should operate? There are stretches of DNA near the start of genes that form binding sites for these regulatory molecules to attach to directly. Here, another type of 'genetic language' is used, which also involves the four bases (A, T, G, and C), but in this instance they are not in the codon formation that is required for protein production.

Gene Regulation is an Essential Part of Development

When spermatozoon and oocyte unite to form a diploid embryonic cell, the subsequent cell division creates two identical cells by mitosis, followed by a fundamental modification that is essential for development. With the successive cell divisions, many cells are formed, and these cells begin to assume individual roles – a process known as differentiation. These cells have different shapes and patterns of cell division. Although the DNA within all the cells is identical, these changes are brought about by different genes being activated to direct their diverse structures and functional roles.

Differentiation is amply illustrated by the haemoglobin genes, because they are activated at different sites in the adult and the fetus. It is an elegant process that is able to occur because adult haemoglobin (HbA) and fetal haemoglobin (HbF) genes are regulated to be either 'switched on' or 'switched off', depending on the stage of human development. HbA and HbF are slightly different in structure because they are products of different genes which are decoded and translated to form intact haemoglobin. HbA is primarily composed of two alpha-chains and two beta-chains, (i.e. it is made up of four protein chains), which are synthesized by the precursors of red blood cells in the bone marrow.

Now look at this principle, but at the same time consider the requirements of the fetus. It requires an oxygen transport mechanism that is able to attract oxygen from the maternal red blood cells; therefore, fetal haemoglobin (HbF) has different oxygen-carrying capacities to the adult form, and these differences are of benefit to the fetus. It is also structurally different from HbA in that it is composed of two alpha-chains and two gamma-chains, so alternative genes must be 'switched on' for it to be produced.

Furthermore, HbF is synthesized in the liver rather than in the bone marrow, and until about 6 months' gestation it is the most common form of haemoglobin. Eventually the production of HbF is closed down in favour of HbA made by cells of the bone marrow.

WHAT ARE CHROMOSOMES?

The DNA molecules combine with proteins called histones to form elongated bodies called chromosomes, which are found in the cell nucleus. The number and size of the chromosomes are characteristic of each species. Normal human nucleated cells have 46 chromosomes; in apes, with which we are thought to share a common ancestor, there are 48 chromosomes. An analysis of the appearance of chromosomes suggests that there has been no major loss of useful information during the evolution of humans, rather it has been redistribution among a smaller number of chromosomes.

The maternal oocyte provides 23 of these chromosomes, with the other 23 coming from the paternal spermatozoon. They are arranged in pairs. The chromosome pairs 1–22 are known as the autosomal chromosomes. The 23rd pair of chromosomes is responsible for determining the sex of the person and are called the sex chromosomes – XX codes for females, and XY codes for males. Each pair of human chromosomes is different from all the other pairs – first, each pair has a distinctive structure (e.g. chromosome 1 looks different from chromosome 2), and secondly, each pair has different genetic information contained in its DNA molecules. The genes are found at specific locations (loci); so for instance, the gene that codes for insulin is expressed on chromosome 11, but the gene for prolactin, another hormone, is found on chromosome 6. Similarly, many of the genes that code for inherited disorders have been identified, characterized, and pinpointed as a specific chromosomal anomaly – for example, the gene that predisposes a patient to retinoblastoma (an inherited tumour) is found on chromosome 13.

Genes that predispose a person to a disease may be described as either autosomal or sex-linked, depending on their location within the genome. An autosomal genetic disorder may arise in males or females because the gene is located on one of the autosomal chromosome (chromosomes 1–22). A sex-linked inherited disorder is one where the gene is located on one of the sex chromosomes (chromosome 23, X or Y).

There is an interesting genetic feature of the sex chromosomes. It might be assumed that females, who have are two X chromosomes, would have a double dose of many genes compared with males, who only have one X chromosome. As the genes on the X chromosomes are not merely associated with sex determination (e.g. the gene for haemophilia is on the X chromosome), it might be presumed that females expressed these genes at half the rate of the male X chromosome.

This situation does not arise, however; in the early stages of development in the female, one X chromosome in every cell is 'shut off', a process known as 'X chromosome inactivation'. It is noteworthy that the inactive X chromosome appears different when viewed microscopically – it is known as a Barr body, after the Canadian cytologist who first described it. In any cell it is apparently random as to whether the paternal or the maternal X chromosome is affected. As a result, a female is actually a mosaic with parts of the body expressing the maternal X genes and other parts expressing the alternative copies from the paternal X chromosome.

One of the most beautiful examples of this inactivation is seen in tortoiseshell cats, all of which are females (XX). The gene for their coat is on the X chromosomes, with one X chromosome having the gene for yellow hair and the other having the gene for black. With the random inactivation of the X chromosome in their skin cells, these females have mottled coats, whereas the males (XY) have a single colour. This X chromosome inactivation is fine where both genes are normal, but it may have important implications where one of those genes is defective.

GENETIC DISORDERS – A CONSEQUENCE OF MUTATIONS IN THE GENOME

Mutations are changes in the DNA sequence of the bases. These may be quite small, involving a change in just one single base in the whole of the human genome. Alternatively they may be so large that they are visible when examining the chromosomes using the light microscope (e.g. Down's syndrome, caused by a trisomy on chromosome 21) (Figure 7.4). Chromosomal anomalies tend to affect a considerable number of genes and are generally more serious.

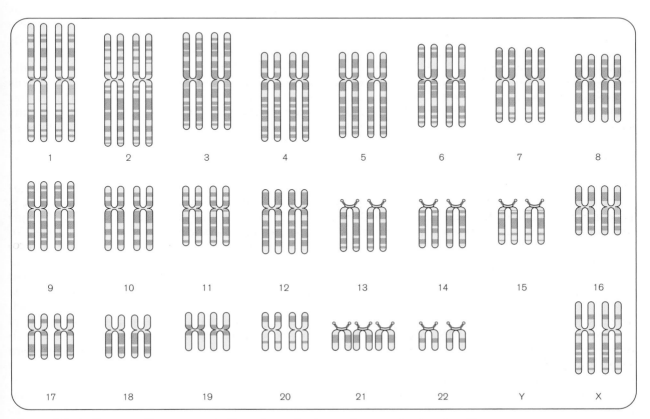

Figure 7.4 A diagramatic representation of an electron micrograph showing the chromosomal spread (karyotype) at metaphase of a female with Down's syndrome.

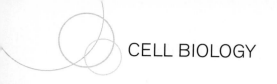

PERSON-CENTRED STUDY: CYSTIC FIBROSIS

Tracy was diagnosed with cystic fibrosis at about 2 years of age. In her young life, she had a medical history of recurrent chest infections and failure to thrive, typified by an inadequate body weight. A malabsorption syndrome had been investigated because she passed foul-smelling, frothy stools containing excess fat (i.e. steatorrhoea) (see Chapter 6). Her mother had also detected that Tracy's skin tasted rather salty when she was kissed; a sweat test was performed and this gave a positive result (i.e. an abnormally high chloride content in the sweat was found).

Because cystic fibrosis is an inherited disorder, Tracy's family was offered genetic screening. The results confirmed that both her parents were carriers of the gene; however, they did not suffer the disorder because it has a recessive genetic inheritance. Her siblings (two brothers and one sister) were also tested, and this revealed that one of her brothers and her sister were carriers of the defect, but the other brother was not (see Chapter 33).

However, even small mutations of a single gene can have grave consequences if the gene codes for a protein with a vital function (e.g. sickle cell haemoglobin). Many mutations are not significant because they occur outside the protein-coding and regulatory regions of the DNA and so do not affect the DNA coding for gene expression.

Many factors have been implicated as causes of mutations. They sometimes occur spontaneously during cell division, since errors in DNA replication happen regularly. Part of a gene may be deleted, inverted, or even copied twice. Chromosomes are particularly vulnerable to damage by environmental factors, such as drugs, chemicals, and viruses, during mitosis and meiosis because they are exposed on the spindle (see Chapter 4). A number of chemical agents are able to enter cells and damage DNA, some having dual effects in being carcinogenic as well as mutagenic. Similarly, heavy doses of radiation are known to cause DNA damage and induce embryonic and fetal abnormalities. Thus, the widespread use of X rays in clinical diagnosis deserves ample consideration, and its use must be balanced against the chance of inducing DNA mutations.

Single Gene Defects may be the Result of Minor Changes to the DNA Sequence

Single gene defects are caused by minor changes to the DNA sequence; a mutation in DNA that codes for a protein may well alter its amino acid composition. For example, consider the modification of the codon, GAG, to a different codon, GTG; in this case a point mutation has changed the second base in the codon from adenine to thymine. Harmless? Not at all; this is the mutation that is responsible for producing the abnormal haemoglobin found in patients with sickle cell dis-

ease. It results in a different amino acid at the sixth position of the beta-globin chain (valine instead of glutamic acid) and significantly affects the function of the haemoglobin molecule as an oxygen transporter, especially at low oxygen levels. Despite this mutation having serious clinical implications in the homozygous condition (sickle cell disease), people who are heterozygotes (and have 'sickle cell trait') are better protected against malaria than normal people.

Sickle cell haemoglobin is caused by a specific change of one codon, but there are literally hundreds of different mutations to the haemoglobin genes that provoke the many diseases collectively termed the haemoglobinopathies. These genes can be mutated at many different sites along their base sequence, with any one of the multiple mutations viewed as a different syndrome, and named accordingly.

The mutated cystic fibrosis transmembrane regulator (CFTR) gene, which results in cystic fibrosis, is another example of single gene mutation (Person-Centred Study: Cystic Fibrosis) (see also Chapter 33). However, although most carriers and sufferers of cystic fibrosis have the same codon error, in total there are about 300 different mutations that have been described in the CFTR gene; even so, the syndrome is collectively known as cystic fibrosis. Nevertheless, each of the mutations have their own characteristic effects on the expression of the gene or the protein produced, hence it is not surprising that the condition is more severe in some sufferers than in others.

In the diseases just discussed, one base has been substituted for another. Now consider the situation in which a base is removed (base deletion) or added (base addition) to the sequence of the gene triplets. The effect is likely to be much more serious because all the codons would be altered from the point where the base is removed or added. Consequently the amino acid sequence of the rest of the protein will be changed owing to a change in the reading frame of the gene. Take as an analogy the following phrase made up of well-known three-letter words, and see that when one of the letters is either removed or added, the sense is lost:

Normal   THE CAT AND FOX HAD JAM FOR TEA
sequence

Base removed   THE CAT AND FOH ADJ AMF ORT EA

Base added   THE CAT AND FOX CHA DJA MFO RTE A

In a DNA sequence, changing the bases within codons may not only modify the amino acids, it may also affect the start or termination of protein translation. If a 'stop' codon is created or destroyed by changing a base, the result would be the protein that was either too short or extended. Almost certainly it would be non-functional, for it is unlikely that the modification would allow the protein to fold into the unique shape required for its physiological function, such as forming the active site of an enzyme (see Chapter 2). Therefore, these mutations, although very simple in nature, may effectively destroy the function of the gene involved.

Mutations that change the DNA sequence of the regulatory region of the gene should also be considered. Such alterations are problematic because, unlike the protein-coding regions, where the sequence order of the bases must be precise, a certain degree of flexibility or 'misspelling' is acceptable. For instance, if the affected area is a stretch of DNA that binds regulatory proteins and regulates the production of actin (a muscle protein), the attachment could be either enhanced or depleted by the mutation – the 'knock-on' effect would be reflected in the amount of actin ultimately produced.

CHROMOSOMAL ERRORS

Some chromosomal abnormalities may result in there being more than 46 chromosomes or fewer. However, the number of chromosomes is generally maintained because losing or gaining an extra chromosome is usually lethal, resulting in cell death. Of course, errors can arise in which part of the chromosome structure is drastically modified (deleted, copied twice, or turned around); this usually involve many genes, implying serious consequences for the individual. These errors often arise at cell division, where chromosomes may break, be rearranged or even be lost or gained by the cells. There is only one condition in which a loss of a whole chromosome from all the cells in the body is compatible with life – Turner's syndrome.

> ### BOX 7.2 ISOLATION OF CHROMOSOMES
>
> - Using a relatively simple procedure, chromosomes can be isolated from cells (e.g. blood cells, skin cells, bone marrow cells) and then stained and viewed using a microscope. This allows any gross abnormalities to be characterized.
> - Each chromosome can be distinguished by its unique structure, it can be ascertained whether the person has the correct number of pairs of chromosomes, and whether part of a specific chromosome is either missing or extended.
> - Since this technique looks only at the whole chromosome; in order to delineate a specific gene defect, closer examination of the DNA is required.

Turner's syndrome affects 1 in 2500 live female births and seems to be independent of both ethnicity and country of domicile. All the 44 autosomal chromosomes are present but there is only one copy of an X chromosome. Usually it is an error arising in the male gamete for in 75 per cent of cases it is the maternal X chromosome that is present. Females with Turner's syndrome display a number of symptoms, including ovarian dysgenesis, stunted growth, and lack of development of secondary sexual characteristics. Oestrogen therapy can correct the lack of secondary sexual characteristics.

About 60 per cent of spontaneous miscarriages appear to be associated with a large-scale chromosomal disorder. Many are due to an additional chromosome, a condition termed trisomy. It is possible that an equivalent number of conceptuses have fewer than 46 chromosomes, but are lost before pregnancy is recognized. There are a number of conditions in which additional sex chromosomes are found – XYY (male), XXY (male), and XXX (female) all appear with a frequency of about 1 in 1000 live births. XYY often causes no obvious clinical symptoms (although there may be a lower level of intelligence than would be expected) possibly because the Y chromosome is small and has relatively few active genes. However, in XXY (Klinefelter's syndrome), the symptoms are more severe; they include infertility and learning disabilities; this extra X is acquired from the mother in 60 per cent of cases. Females with an extra X chromosome (i.e. XXX) appear clinically normal and most are fertile, but generally they

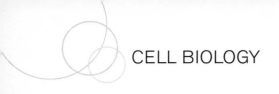
display some learning disability. An intriguing but rare variant is the XX male (1 in 20 000 live births); this has been identified as the translocation of DNA from the Y chromosome to the X chromosome during gamete production, resulting in the X chromosome possessing Y genes. Intelligence is normal but there are features similar to those seen in Klinefelter's syndrome, including infertility.

Apart from the X and Y chromosome abnormalities, Down's syndrome is the most well-documented trisomy that permits long-term survival; this may be in part attributable to the relatively small number of genes on chromosome 21, which is one of the smaller chromosomes. When a more detailed map of human genes to all the chromosomes is known, this theory will be confirmed or disproved. The trisomic condition is normally caused by an unequal division of chromosomes between the haploid cells formed in meiosis when gametes are produced. It is generally associated with maternal age, for the rise in trisomy 21 is seen in women in their mid-30s; hence prenatal screening is offered to older mothers. There is also a rare form of Down's syndrome in which there appears to be the normal number of chromosomes in the affected individual. However, closer inspection reveals that, although there is one normal chromosome 21, an additional pair of chromosome 21 genes are attached to another chromosome, which looks disproportionately large when viewed microscopically.

CHROMOSOMES ARE MOST VULNERABLE DURING CELL DIVISION

During meiosis the chromosomes are separated from their pairs (diploid) into single chromosomes (haploid). In this process, a certain degree of gene mixing occurs along each chromosome pair, so that genetic variation is achieved in the offspring – without this, all the children of a particular pair of parents would look identical. This crossover involves the swopping of genetic material between adjacent sequences on the chromosomes. This is when errors are most likely to happen, for part of the chromosome may be lost, misaligned, or copied twice, giving an extended section to the chromosome.

For instance consider chromosomes with the genes A, B, C, D, E, F, G, H. The following anomalies may occur in addition to the normal chromosome:

Normal chromosome	A B C D E F G H
Gene D is lost	A B C E F G H
Gene F misaligned	A B C D E G H F
Inverted gene F G H	A B C D E H G F
Duplication of genes B and C	A B C B C D E F G H
Translocated genes C D E	C D E A B F G H

Loss of a Gene

Red–green colour blindness is an example of crossing-over resulting in the loss of a gene that affects around 8 per cent of Caucasian males. It is an inability to distinguish between different wavelengths of light (colours) within the red and green parts of the spectrum. The detection of different wavelengths of light depends on three types of opsins (red, blue, and green); opsins are light-sensitive proteins found in the retina. The genes responsible for producing the red-detecting opsins and the green-detecting opsins are very similar in structure and are adjacent to each other on the X chromosome, whereas the gene for the blue opsin is located on chromosome 7. When unequal crossover occurs between the adjacent genes for red and green opsins, a chromatid can be produced that carries just one of the two genes, so colour blindness results. Unlike females, males do not have the extra X chromosome to compensate and provide a replacement gene.

Multiple Copies of a Genetic Sequence

When part of a gene is copied multiple times by mistake, it can also lead to a genetic disorder. This is likely to have resulted from an error in the precision with which DNA is replicated during the meiotic process of gamete production. Where a gene contains several copies of the repeat sequence, there is an increased chance of further repeats being slipped in. Huntington's disease is a consequence of multiple copies being made of one codon (also known as trinucleotide repeats). The disease was formerly called Huntington's chorea because of the jerky movements of those severely afflicted with this neurodegenerative syndrome. DNA analysis has shown that, near the beginning of the gene, there is a surprisingly long run of CAG triplet codons. In a normal person there are between 11 and 34 of these triplet repeats, but in those with Huntington's disease there may be up to 100 copies. The increased number of triplet codons is found within the protein-coding section of the gene, and so it gives rise to an abnormal protein. Unfortunately, the disease does not normally present clinically until after 35 years of age, by which time the patient will have almost certainly had children. It is therefore psychologically distressing for families at two levels:

(i) seeing the progressive decline of a close relative, and

(ii) being faced with the decision of whether to be screened for the defective gene or just to 'wait and see' (see also Chapter 38).

Fragile X syndrome is a similar genetic mutation, but in this case the fault affects gene regulation rather than producing a malfunctioning protein. It is one of the major inherited forms of learning disability and, as its name implies, it is caused by an X chromosome acquiring a fragile end section with a long run of the triplet codon CGG located adjacent to the gene. The number of these trinucleotide repeats is highly variable; normal people have fewer than 50 of these repeated codons, but the symptoms and signs of the disorder present in people with above 230 copies on their X chromosome. In between the two extremes (i.e. under 50 and above 230 copies of CGG), people remain unaffected but may be classed as genetic carriers of the disease.

SCREENING FOR INHERITED DISORDERS

ASSESSING WHETHER A PATIENT WITH A FAMILY HISTORY OF A DISEASE IS CARRYING THE DEFECTIVE GENE AND THE EFFECTS ON HEALTH

In the case of single gene defects, the likelihood of a patient having the genetic disorder can often be evaluated by taking a family history. A person who has acquired a defective gene from both parents is said to be homozygous and will present with the genetic disorder. However, a person who has acquired the gene from only one parent is said to be heterozygous, and clinical presentation depends on whether the disorder is caused by a dominant or recessive gene.

Diseases caused by dominant genes will present in both heterozygous and homozygous people. All children of the affected person who is homozygous will have the disease, but there is a 50 per cent chance that the children of a heterozygous person will be affected. Conversely, in a recessive disorder, the mutated gene must be acquired from both parents for the disease to present clinically. A person who is heterozygous for a recessive gene is merely a carrier with a 50 per cent chance of passing the defective gene to his or her children. People who are homozygous for the recessive gene will always pass one defective gene to their children. Although the children should not suffer the adverse effects of the disease, they are considered as genetic carriers.

It has been suggested that virtually everyone is a carrier of at least one gene defect, but since each defect has such a low incidence in the population, homozygotes occur very rarely. Therefore, only common defects need counselling. It is advisable that known carriers of genetic disorders, as well as those who have the disease, should receive genetic counselling. People who are carriers are at risk of producing children with the defect if their partner either has the disorder or is also a carrier (see also Box 7.3).

When a genetic disorder is encoded on one of the sex chromosomes, it is said to be sex-linked. A classic example is haemophilia, in which the defect is carried on the X chromosomes. Therefore males carrying the haemophilia gene suffer the clotting disorder. Females are merely carriers of the disease because their additional X chromosome compensates, so the severe clotting defect is not presented, although their plasma levels of factor VIII may be reduced. As the father's gamete determines the sex of the child, males acquire the Y chromosome from their father, and the X chromosome from the mother. Thus all sons of a haemophiliac would be free of the disease as they received the Y chromosome from him and not the X chromosome, which carries the genetic defect. However, all the daughters of a haemophiliac would inherit this gene from their father's X chromosome and would therefore be carriers of the clotting disorder.

> **BOX 7.3 WHAT IS THE DIFFERENCE BETWEEN AN INHERITED GENETIC ABNORMALITY AND SIMPLY HAVING A PREDISPOSITION TO A DISEASE?**
>
> - People who have an inherited genetic disease have a defective gene. They may present with the signs and symptoms from birth or soon after, or they may have carrier status depending on whether their inheritance is dominant, recessive, or sex-linked.
> - People who are predisposed to a genetic disorder, such as cancer, carry a defective gene, which in the case of cancer is known as an oncogene. In order to produce an oncogene, the gene must be changed or mutated into its dangerous form by mutagens (e.g. drugs, radiation, or chemicals), which modify the genetic information. The person will not necessarily develop the disease but can still pass on the predisposition to his or her children.

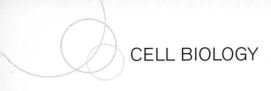
GENETIC SCREENING

Genetic screening is a general term for the examination of a person's genetic constitution. Screening is currently performed to identify the presence of selected genes or gene variants that may give rise to a known genetic disease. However, there is a major drawback in that inherited disorders can only be easily screened for if the DNA sequence is known. The advent of techniques available to sequence DNA has led to the establishment of the Human Genome Organization's (HUGO) project.

HUGO is a major international effort that entails sequencing all the bases of the DNA in the human genome. It is scheduled to be completed in the first few years of the new millennium. This is eagerly awaited by biologists because it will supply the sequences for all genes and assign them a location on specific chromosomes. Vital evidence will then be at hand to ascertain the causes of genetic diseases, to give an insight into how cancer cells behave, and above all to offer the possibility of new therapeutic measures. Such information will also be of value to anthropologists in providing clues about the process of evolution itself.

In particular, it may well illuminate the nature of the inter-relationships between different populations around the world.

MOLECULAR BIOLOGICAL TECHNIQUES USED IN SCREENING

Molecular biological techniques are used to identify the presence or absence of a particular gene, and whether the gene is normal or faulty. Several methods are available for routine diagnostic genetic screening, and the choice depends on the source of DNA and the quantity available. All methods rely on the intrinsic property of DNA molecules, namely that heat-treatment causes them to separate into their individual strands, but when they are cooled down again they reunite because of the complementary base pairing (A–T and G–C). Furthermore, reagents are available to synthesize DNA *in vitro*. Therefore, if the DNA sequence that codes for the genetic disorder is known, a synthetic copy can be prepared. This laboratory-made DNA can then be used as a probe (indicator) to detect whether the patient possesses the abnormal gene.

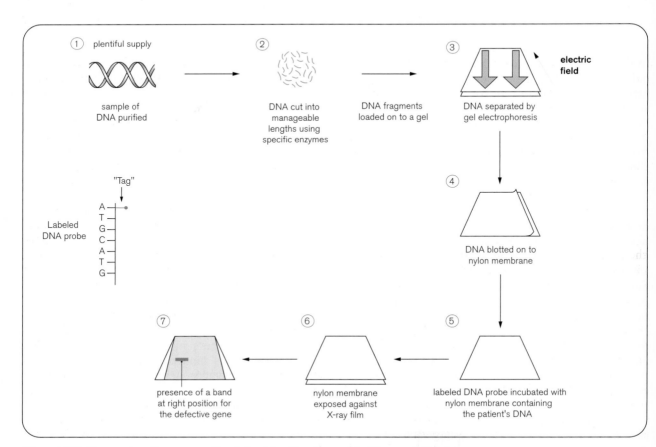

Figure 7.5 Screening for a genetic defect by Southern blotting.

Southern Blot Analysis

Southern blot analysis is a technique used to detect different stretches of DNA. It can be performed on DNA isolated from lymphocytes in a 20 ml sample of venous blood or other body tissues and fluids (e.g. semen, hair, skin). Once a pure sample of DNA has been prepared, these very large molecules are cut into manageable lengths with specific enzymes. The presence or absence of a particular base sequence that is unique to the genetic disorder being investigated can be demonstrated as follows:

- The DNA fragments are separated via gel electrophoresis. The electric current causes them to migrate through the gel at different rates according to their size, with small DNA fragments moving faster along the gel than longer ones.
- For the DNA of interest within the gel to be visualized, it must go through a number of stages of preparation because the gel is delicate and can break easily. Therefore the DNA is blotted on to a stronger material, such as nylon membrane (like blotting a page of writing).
- Simultaneously, in a test tube, a specific DNA probe is labeled with a radioisotope or fluorescent "tag" so that it is detectable. The probe will have been designed in order to be the DNA sequence that is complementary to the defective gene.
- The labeled probe is then incubated with the nylon membrane containing the patient's sample of DNA. If a defective gene is present, the stretch of the DNA that is complementary with the probe will bind together, and because the probe is labeled with a tag, this stretch of DNA is detectable.
- The nylon membrane containing the patients DNA is placed against autoradiographic film. If the DNA and labeled probe are bound together it will show up as a dark band (rather like an X-ray film), indicating the defective gene is present (Figure 7.5).

Polymerase Chain Reaction

The polymerase chain reaction (PCR) is useful when the supply of DNA is limited, because it permits a specific stretch of DNA to be copied over 1 million times (amplified). Within a few hours, a large quantity of DNA can be prepared, and this is easier to handle for the investigation of a mutant gene. The genetic sequences of the normal and abnormal genes are different, and these anomalies can be uncovered by cutting the DNA prepared by PCR with commercially-prepared enzymes that recognize well-defined base sequences. The resultant DNA fragments produced from cutting the normal and abnormal genes are of different lengths. This may be visualized when the enzyme-digested DNA samples are run on a gel, because they appear as a distinctive ladder. Thus the patient's DNA ladder can be compared with that of a normal and abnormal ladder. Unlike Southern blot analysis, which takes up to 1 week to produce a result, PCR processing of a sample usually takes no more than 2 days because the fragment patterns can be visualized under ultraviolet light after the gel has been stained with ethidium bromide.

Genetic Fingerprints

What is a genetic fingerprint, and how is it that every person is unique? The genes, or at least the arrangement of genes on a chromosome, exhibit very slight variation between individual humans, and in between the genes, some of the DNA is arranged as repetitive base sequences. Some of these repetitive units have a common sequence and are therefore called variable number tandem repeats' (VNTRs). As yet the function of the VNTRs is unknown. Each person's 'junk' DNA is unique to that person because the VNTRs may be arranged adjacent to one another (multiple units) or as single units, and they may occur at several different positions in the genome. Genetic fingerprinting is now well established and highlights these repetitive units of DNA so that they can be compared with those of other individuals. There is so much variation between one person and another that it can be used to identify individuals within a population.

DNA is extracted and digested by enzymes using techniques similar to those described for Southern blotting and PCR. In this case, however, the probe is not part of a gene; rather it is a labeled synthetic copy of a VNTR [e.g. AGAGGTGGGCAGGTGG (a known repetitive sequence)]. The digested DNA is mixed with the probe; where there is a match, the complementary sequences will combine. Just as in the Southern blot, the resultant image will have a ladder-like appearance corresponding to the VNTRs of the individual – this constitutes the genetic fingerprint.

How does one genetic fingerprint differ from another? One person's DNA might have five VNTRs in one fragment, for example, but another person's DNA might have 25 VNTRs. Because the number of VNTRs varies so much, the enzyme-digested fragments of DNA will be of various sizes, and this causes the formation of a ladder along the gel with a unique pattern.

Genetic fingerprinting has been invaluable to forensic scientists investigating samples of body fluids found at the scene-of-the-crime. Another use for genetic finger printing has been in sorting out those rare but unfortunate cases when a newborn baby has been given to the wrong parents in hospitals. The correct assignment is possible because the positions of the DNA bands in the baby's genetic fingerprint has equivalent band positions as that seen in samples from either the mother or the father.

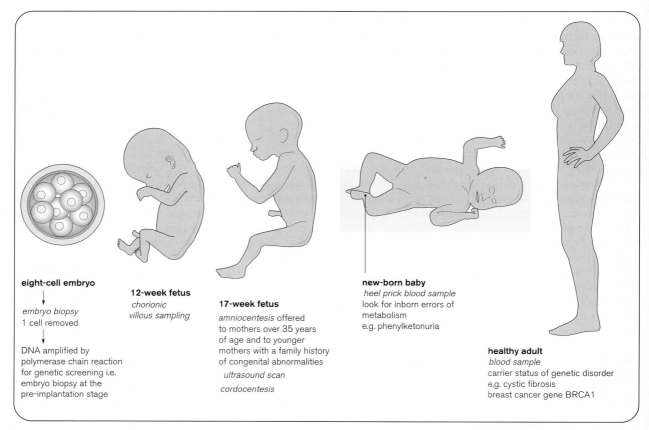

eight-cell embryo
↓
embryo biopsy
1 cell removed
↓
DNA amplified by
polymerase chain reaction
for genetic screening i.e.
embryo biopsy at the
pre-implantation stage

12-week fetus
*chorionic
villous sampling*

17-week fetus
amniocentesis offered
to mothers over 35 years
of age and to younger
mothers with a family history
of congenital abnormalities

ultrasound scan

cordocentesis

new-born baby
heel prick blood sample
look for inborn errors of
metabolism
e.g. phenylketonuria

healthy adult
blood sample
carrier status of genetic disorder
e.g. cystic fibrosis
breast cancer gene BRCA1

Figure 7.6 Genetic screening through life.

GENETIC SCREENING AT DIFFERENT AGES

Genetic disorders affect people of all age groups and just about every tissue and organ. Some of these diseases are visible and obvious at birth (e.g. the characteristic features of Down's syndrome), whereas others may be delayed and present later in life (e.g. an inherited immunodeficiency such as lazy leukocyte syndrome (see Chapter 28), or Huntington's disease). Different procedures are advised at different stages of human development. Screening for genetic diseases is not generally practised on the population at large but is focused on individual people thought to be at risk of a genetic disease because of known familial links (Figure 7.6).

Screening During *In Vitro* Fertilization

Screening during *in vitro* fertilization (IVF) is possible because the first few divisions of the human embryo produce cells that are identical and have not yet begun the process of differentiation. Moreover, the removal of a single cell from the embryo at this early stage of development (embryo biopsy) is possible without affecting the viability of the fetus. Once removed, the DNA from the nucleus of the embryonic cell can be amplified using PCR and examined for the presence of disease-causing genes.

In practice an even simpler procedure may be adopted. For example, if the disease is sex linked, the chromosomes can be examined to identify the sex of the embryo. When the disease is passed through the male line, female embryos may be selected for implantation in preference to male ones.

In Utero Screening

In utero screening is a well-established practice that offered to all pregnant patients; some of the techniques are invasive but others are not. Ultrasound scans are performed at around 16–18 weeks' gestation. A probe that emits high-frequency sound waves is applied. These sound waves are converted into an image to visualize the unborn fetal tissues.

Measurement of the size of the fetus and the location of the placenta are possible, and certain abnormalities are detectable with this technique. It can be used for the *in utero* diagnosis of conditions such as spina bifida, hydrocephalus, and congenital defects of the skeleton and major organs (e.g. heart, gastrointestinal tract). With this information and the appropriate counselling, the parents can then make a decision whether or not to continue with the pregnancy. Alternatively where the condition is treatable with surgery, evidence gleaned from the scan allows the obstetrician to plan for either an *in utero* manipulation or an elective delivery, by induced labour or a Caesarean section, so that corrective surgery may be performed.

At the same antenatal visit as the one at which the ultrasound scan is performed, a sample of maternal blood is taken to estimate the plasma alpha-fetoprotein level. Alpha-fetoprotein is a protein made by the fetal yolk sac early in gestation, and later by the fetal liver. An elevated level in the maternal circulation indicates that there is a greater risk of a neural tube defect in this pregnancy. In addition, the levels of human chorionic gonadotrophin, alpha-fetoprotein, and unconjugated oestradiol may be measured and evaluated as a crude screen for Down's syndrome.

Amniocentesis

Amniocentesis is offered to older mothers (those conceiving after the age of 35 years) because these mothers have an increased risk of carrying a fetus with a genetic defect. It is also offered to younger mothers with a family history of a congenital abnormality. It is generally performed between 16 and 20 weeks' gestation and involves the removal of amniotic fluid surrounding the unborn child. The fluid contains fetal cells which may be analysed for the presence of specific genes, or a simpler karyotype analysis of the number of chromosomes may be performed (see Box 7.2).

Chorionic Villous Sampling

Chorionic villous sampling carries a greater risk of loss of the conceptus than amniocentesis, but it may be performed at an earlier gestational age of about 12 weeks. It is essentially a biopsy of a defined part of the placental tissue. The chorionic villi are generally retrieved using an intrauterine catheter, which is guided to the correct location via the cervix using an ultrasound scan. The cells obtained may be used for chromosome, DNA, or biochemical analysis. The DNA from tissues retrieved by amniocentesis or chorionic villus sampling allows for the early diagnosis of an inborn error of metabolism.

Cordocentesis

Cordocentesis, as the name implies, is the taking of a fetal blood sample from an umbilical artery in the umbilical cord. It can be performed at about 16–20 weeks' gestation. The fetal cells can be used to identify the presence of abnormal haemoglobin (e.g. prenatal diagnosis of sickle cell disease, beta-thalassaemia major), as well as other metabolic and haematological disorders.

Neonatal Screening

Some neonatal screening is performed on the infant soon after delivery – a well-known example is the Guthrie test, in which a heel-prick blood sample is used to screen for phenylketonuria, an inborn error of metabolism (see Person-Centred Study in Chapter 2). In many ways, this test is simple, because evidence of the inherited metabolic disorder is confirmed by an elevated blood level of the amino acid, phenylalanine. It does not require an examination of chromosomes or the DNA itself.

Screening in Adults

Screening in adults evaluates whether an apparently healthy person is carrying defective genes that might cause a genetic disorder. For example, the incidence of cystic fibrosis is around 1 in 2500 (see Chapter 33). As this is an autosomal recessive, inherited condition, people with a family history of a disease can be screened for carrier status. By contrast, the high incidence of thalassaemia in Cyprus has prompted a national programme in which all couples are required to be tested for their thalassaemia gene status before they are allowed to marry.

When a dominant gene codes for a disease, only one copy of the mutated gene is required for the condition to develop. An inherited predisposition to breast cancer is an example of this. Although there are thought to be at least three mutated genes that can predispose to breast cancer, it is now possible to screen for a gene that molecular biologists have named BRCA1; this gene may be responsible for some 5 per cent of cases of breast cancer.

ETHICAL ISSUES ARISING FROM SCREENING

The major consideration arising from genetic screening is what to do with the information once it has been obtained. Although the advantages in disease prevention are indisputable, there is no doubt that a sense of professional responsibility regarding these sensitive issues is mandatory. Ethical committees have therefore been established at local and national levels to protect both patients and clinicians. Likewise, health care professionals must be mindful of and respect the views of the patients who being offered counselling for genetically related disorders.

Prenatal Screening

When the outcome of *in utero* screening unveils a congenital disorder in the developing fetus, the parents must decide whether to continue with the pregnancy or opt for a termination. Obviously this creates moral and religious difficulties for some people and some sections of society. In future, it may be feasible for gene therapy to be offered as an alternative to elective termination of pregnancy for treating some genetic diseases. Initial attempts are already being made at alleviating conditions such as cystic fibrosis.

Meanwhile, the *in vitro* methods for screening preimplanted embryos eliminate the need of aborting an implanted fetus. However, this technique is only possible if IVF is being used, and financial constraints mean it is not likely to be used as a routine procedure for all women who are at increased risk of a fetal abnormality. For some parents, it presents the dilemma of 'playing God' by selecting some embryos for implantation while discarding others in an effort to produce a 'perfect human race'. Undoubtedly some patients have considered these assisted reproduction techniques as a way of ensuring they have the desired gender of baby. However, these are the negative sides of these issues; in cases where there is a favourable diagnosis found during prenatal screening, couples can carry on with the pregnancy. Previously, individuals with a family history of a genetic disorder might have chosen to remain childless; at least screening gives such couples a chance of having a healthy child. The obvious advantage that follows prenatal screening is the sense of optimism that this information engenders for the rest of the pregnancy.

Postnatal Screening

Early diagnosis of conditions such as phenylketonuria poses few ethical issues; in the case of phenylketonuria, an inborn error of metabolism is identified in the neonate, and this can be treated with a phenylalanine-restricted diet. Dietary control can effectively solve the problem of having the defective gene, although genetic counselling and dietary intervention must be offered to women with phenylketonuria before they conceive (see Chapter 2 Person-centred study).

There are, however, some genetic disorders in which adult screening has significant personal and ethical implications; patients with a family history of Huntington's disease are prime examples. Some may not want to live with the positive result, knowing they will ultimately develop this incurable and distressing condition. Equally, the knowledge that a woman is carrying the BRCA1 mutant gene has resulted in requests for elective mastectomies in the absence of any sign of the disease being present. Although this is a preventive safeguard, it is a drastic strategy to eliminate the risk of breast cancer.

As the HUGO project expands our knowledge of the human genome, the ethical issues become more crucial. Currently, when genetic screening is carried out *in utero*, we are dealing with the identification of genes that will lead to serious disease in which the quality of life of the offspring may be seriously affected. How will society react if people wish to terminate a pregnancy because genetic testing has identified that the offspring will have marginal characteristics, such as a particular hair colour or an IQ of less than 120? Certainly the effects of having this information can be significant – India is one of the rare countries in which there are markedly fewer girls than boys. Until recently, there were clinics that allowed prenatal sex determination, and some couples opted for the termination of a pregnancy if the fetus was found to be female.

From another perspective, what will happen if genetic screening for a number of genes that predispose to various malignant conditions becomes routine? Such information could be highly sensitive if it became available to, or was required by, potential employers. Some people may then find employment, mortgages, and insurance policies difficult or impossible to obtain. However, the 'genetic genie' is out of the bottle and there is no doubt that as this kind of genetic information becomes available, society will have to develop mechanisms for controlling the ways in which it is utilized.

KEY POINTS

- DNA is a linear molecule created by two strands linked together, giving a twisted 'ladder-like' structure. This is constructed by linking sugar rings (deoxyribose), phosphate groups, and bases together. The bases are adenine, cytosine, guanine, and thymine, better recognized by their abbreviations, A, C, G, and T.
- The principal roles of DNA are providing a set of instructions in the form of a genetic code, which is essentially the order of these bases along the DNA molecule; and acting as a data base that may be copied and transferred from one generation to another.
- The information found in DNA is organized into discrete sections called genes, some of which are represented in multiple copies within the human genome.
- The organization for many of the human genes is rather more complex. The genetic information encoding the order of amino acids in a protein is split into sections – the exons. The coding sections are separated by stretches of intervening DNA – the introns.
- Not all genes are 'switched on' to operate in every cell; only those required for that particular cell to fulfil its physiological role are operative.
- The DNA molecules combine with proteins called histones to form elongated bodies called chromosomes, which are found in the cell nucleus. They are arranged in pairs: chromosome pairs 1–22 are known as the autosomal chromosomes; the 23rd pair is responsible for determining the sex of the person, and are called the sex chromosomes.
- Mutations are changes in the DNA sequence of the bases. These may be quite small, involving a change in a single base, or so large that they are visible when the chromosomes are examined under a light microscope (e.g. in Down's syndrome).
- In the process of meiosis, a certain degree of gene mixing occurs along each chromosome pair so that genetic variation is achieved in the offspring. This crossover involves the swopping of genetic material between adjacent sequences on the chromosomes.
- When part of a gene is copied multiple times by mistake, it can lead to a genetic disorder (e.g. Huntington's disease, Fragile X syndrome).
- In the case of single gene defects, the likelihood of a person having the genetic disorder can often be evaluated by taking a family history.
- Molecular biological techniques are used to identify the presence or absence of the gene and whether it is normal or faulty. Techniques used include Southern blotting, polymerase chain reaction, and genetic fingerprinting.
- Genetic screening for genetic diseases is not generally practised on the population at large, but is focused on individuals thought to be at risk of a genetic disease because of known familial links.

FURTHER READING

Bove CM, Fry ST, MacDonald DJ (1997) Presymptomatic and predisposition genetic testing: ethical and social considerations. Semin Oncol Nurs 13:135–40.

Council for International Organizations of Medical Science and the World Health Organization (1993) International ethical guidelines for biomedical research involving human subjects. CIOMS and WHO, Geneva.

Crandall BF, Corson VL, Goldberg JD, Knight G, Salafsky IS (1995) Folic acid and pregnancy. Am J Med Gen 55:134–5.

DeMichele A, Weber BL (1997) Recent advances in breast cancer biology [Review]. Curr Opin Oncol 9:499–504.

Farkas DH (1997) DNA Simplified: a Hitchhiker's Guide to DNA. AACC Press, Washington DC.

Hart CR, Burke P. eds. (1992) Screening and Surveillance in Medical Practice. Churchill Livingstone, Edinburgh.

Havens DM, Kovner R (1997) Genetic testing: how it is transforming the role of health professionals and the implications for pediatric nurse practitioners. J Pediatr Health Care 11:193–7.

Jackson JF (1995) Genetics and You. Chapman and Hall, London.

Jenkins J (1997) Educational issues related to cancer genetics. Semin Oncol Nurs 13:141–4.

Müller S, Simon JW, Vesting JW (1997) Interdisciplinary Approaches to Gene Therapy: Legal, Ethical and Scientific Aspects. Springer-Verlag, London.

Paintin D (1997) Ante-natal Screening and Abortion for Fetal Abnormalities. Birth Control Trust, London.

Rasko I, Downes CS (1994) Genes in Medicine. Chapman and Hall, London.

Rendine S, Calafell F, Cappello N, et al. (1997) Genetic history of cystic fibrosis mutations in Italy. I. Regional distribution. Ann Hum Genet 61:411–24.

Savulescu J, Chalmers I, Blunt J (1996) Are research ethics committees behaving unethically? Some suggestions for improving performance and accountability. BMJ 313:1390–3.

Stone PG, Blogg CE (1997) Local research ethics committees. BMJ 315: 60–1

Stoppa-Lyonnet D, Laurent-Puig P, Essioux L, et al., (1997) BRCA1 sequence variation in 160 individuals referred to a breast/ovarian cancer clinic. Am J Hum Genet 60:1021–30.

Turner G, Robinson H, Wake S et al. (1997) Case finding for the Fragile X syndrome and its consequenes. BMJ 315:1223–7.

Wallace DC (1997) Mitochondrial DNA in Aging and Disease. Sci Am 277:22–39.

Pharmacology

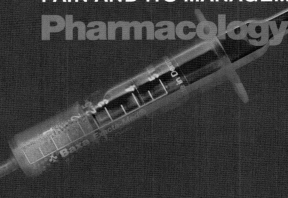

INTRODUCTION TO PHARMACOLOGY

LEARNING OBJECTIVES

After studying this chapter you will have a clearer understanding of:
- the historical perspective of pharmacology
- generic terminology
- the progressive phases of a clinical trial, from drug synthesis to general therapeutic use
- the complexities of prescribing

INTRODUCTION

The science concerned with the physical and chemical properties of drugs is known as pharmacology. It includes the detailed consideration of the mechanisms by which drugs exerts their therapeutic outcome as well as their undesirable side-effects. The part of pharmacology which deals with the mechanisms of drug action is called pharmacodynamics. Pharmacokinetics considers dose regimens and how drugs are processed by the body (drug absorption, distribution, metabolism, and modes of excretion). These factors determine the dose of the drug and how often it should be given.

Clinical pharmacology confines itself to the study of the action of drugs in humans, both in healthy subjects and in patients. Therapeutic studies evaluate the clinical use of all interventions; it thus embraces drug therapy, surgery, and radiotherapy and their actions on each other.

HISTORICAL PERSPECTIVE

It is only comparatively recently (within the last 100 years or so) that many drugs have been constructed from synthetic materials within the confines of a laboratory. Previously, drug treatment came exclusively from naturally occurring substances in plant or animal materials. Drugs were also bound up with folklore and religion. One of the oldest concepts of disease concerned itself with the idea that within every person was a special 'life force or energy', a hypothesis known as Animism. When a person became unwell it was thought that the life force had deserted him or her. Plants, animals, and even certain minerals were all thought to contain varying degrees of this life force. Therefore, by giving them to the sick, it was believed the life force could be transferred, and even that the disease could be cured merely by placing the patient near to the plant or animal. Sometimes it was deemed necessary for the plant or animal to be eaten or rubbed into the skin to obtain a cure. One might smile, but some of the bizarre alternative medicines of today use a similar strategy!

Hippocrates, the ancient Greek physician, taught that disease was not a fate determined by the gods, but a condition that could be diagnosed and treated with natural medicines. This view took many centuries to become accepted but eventually it led to a rational development of new drugs. Clinical doctors today sometimes take the Hippocratic oath that they will observe a code of medical ethics derived from that of Hippocrates.

As we have seen, the common substances used to treat disease in the middle ages were extracted from plants, animals, or minerals. Synthetic chemical preparations found increasing application but they did not revolutionize either the range or the use of the therapeutic agents. It should be emphasized that most physicians were convinced of the infallibility of authority until well into the 18th century; consequently official pharmacopoeias (books that list the chemical and physical properties of drugs) were loath to include or acknowledge any new drugs.

In 1541, Paracelsus introduced the idea of extracting the active compound from the crude drug. He can be considered the true founder of pharmaceutical chemistry. He was also an advocate of the doctrine of signatures. One principle was that a plant that had the shape of an organ or even a human form would be beneficial to that organ or to the body as a whole. Thus, for example, a plant with heart-shaped leaves would be thought to be beneficial to the heart. Another principle of this doctrine was that the cure for a disease lay in close proximity to its cause. For example, salicylates from willow bark were used to improve aches and joint pain; this theory seemed logical since arthritis can be made worse by a damp climate which the willow tree thrived in. Similarly, in areas where malaria is endemic, the cinchona tree, which has an extractable substance in its bark, happened to grow well. The substance was quinine, which was found to be a useful treatment for fevers and malaria.

The 18th century saw rapid advances in the science of botany and chemistry. In 1771, the eminent Swiss scholar, Albecht von Haller, insisted (in his preface to the *Pharmacopoeia Helvetica*) that traditional remedies should be tested on healthy and sick people and only introduced into the pharmacopoeia if their action tallied with the traditional indication.

By the early part of the 19th century, natural sciences had become less empirical, and botany, zoology, chemistry, and physics became integral parts of medicine and pharmacy. By the late 19th century, well-known scientists such as Louis Pasteur and Robert Koch had revolutionized the understanding of disease processes, which led to different approaches to treatment and preventative medicine. Up until 1880, medicines were mostly prepared from natural sources (both animal and plant), but the development of synthetic techniques vastly extended the range of drugs available. The trend was to base therapeutics on the results of experiments and observation of patients, rather than on unproven theories and speculation. With the development of new laboratory techniques, the active principles from crude extracts of plant and animals were purified into a crystalline form – quinine was isolated in 1820 and cocaine in 1885. The introduction of anaesthetics such as ether and chloroform into clinical practice, and the production of drugs from coal tar in the late 19th century were important in the development of analgesia (Figure 8.1). The 20th century brought yet greater advances in this field, with the explosion of modern therapeutics as a real industry.

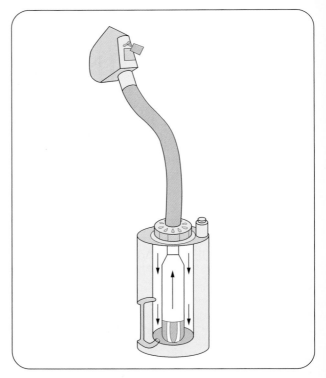

Figure 8.1 Apparatus used in the 19th century to administer chloroform.

DRUGS

Any chemical agent that alters a living process is broadly defined as a drug. There are many different modes of drug action and target areas within the body. Many drugs act by manipulating a physiological mechanism or control system (e.g. nerve, hormone) within the body in order to bring about their effect. Other drugs modify the action of a specific enzyme with an integral function. Certain drugs elicit their effect by mimicking an endogenous substance (a substance that is normally synthesized by the body; see Chapter 10).

Clinical pharmacodynamics examines how a drug exerts its effects in humans; in other words, what the drug does to the body. This can be produced in a variety of ways, and pharmacodynamics therefore includes both the therapeutic and the adverse effects. For informed prescribing, a comprehensive knowledge of the mechanisms of drug action and the full medical history of the patient are required. Nonetheless, even when all this is known, there are other factors that can influence the success or failure of treatment, such as the route of administration.

Drugs are frequently perceived as being distinct from poisons or toxic agents because their effects are generally considered to have a therapeutic outcome. This differentiation is rather artificial. A drug may be beneficial to one patient, but if it is given to another patient it may be harmful. This anomaly can be due to:

- a difference in dosage, or
- a difference in patient susceptibility induced by the underlying disease, or
- an interaction with another drug preparation that has been given concurrently.

Furthermore, despite the efficacy of many drugs, the word 'drug' itself has come to have negative connotations because of substance misuse. Any drug if used inappropriately can be dangerous.

The toxicity of a drug must always be thoroughly ascertained before it can be licensed and marketed. Safety and tolerance are evaluated in early-phase drug trials, which are highly costly. Even when the drug has eventually been given governmental approval, there are still potentially undiscovered risks, as in the tragic cases of the pregnant women in the 1960s who took the anti-nausea drug, thalidomide.

Pharmacokinetics follows the drug from the route into the body (e.g. via injection, orally, rectally) to the way it is distributed throughout body tissues and fluids, the metabolism of the drug, and finally the excretion of the drug metabolites. There are numerous factors that influence drug pharmacokinetics, not least the wide variation between individual patients in gastrointestinal, liver, and kidney function. Thus clinical pharmacodynamics and pharmacokinetics may be viewed as the clinician looking at the action of a drug from two different points of reference.

CHOICE OF DRUG

Choosing the most suitable drug for a disease or symptom is not an easy process. The number of drugs available is continually increasing as pharmaceutical manufacturers compete to produce the best product. It is no longer a matter of prescribing *the* anti-hypertensive drug to cure high blood pressure since there are so many different preparations available. The nature of the drug action requires ample consideration; because different drugs may elicit the same net effect in rather different ways, one may be beneficial and the other harmful.

Increasingly, the cost of drugs influences the choice made by the clinician, and pharmaceutical companies produce different varieties of the same generic compound in different forms and at different prices. Drug sales representatives target hospital doctors and general practitioners to recommend and explain advantages of their product compared with similar formulae supplied by other companies. General practice surgeries are expected to keep within a certain budget and not overspend on the drugs that they prescribe, so naturally this encourages the doctor to use the cheaper drugs on the market whenever possible. Problems can arise when a patient is discharged from hospital on a drug that is expensive even though a cheaper formulation is readily available and may be just as good. Patients may not be happy to have their drug changed. Hospital pharmacies are sometimes provided with new formulation drugs at a cheaper rate in order to encourage doctors within the hospital to prescribe them.

However, changing the drug formulation can lead to unwanted side-effects or loss of efficacy if more or less drug is absorbed than is the case with the standard preparation. Enteric coating on a tablet for example, prevents gastric irritation, but it may also delay the absorption of the drug and thus the onset of the therapeutic effect.

CLINICAL DRUG TRIALS

One of the main reasons why drugs are generally so expensive is that they must undergo exhaustive safety testing before they can be licensed and made available to the public. The time taken from the original formulation of the drug in a laboratory to its arrival on a pharmacist's shelf could be anything up to 20 years, if it arrives at all. Less than 1 per cent of drugs identified as active compounds in the laboratory ever reach the stage of being used in routine clinical practice. Obviously, if a drug fails at the final stages of the clinical trial it can be catastrophic for the drug company. The amalgamation of drug companies in recent years is partly due to this – the larger the company, the greater the number of possible drugs that can be produced and tested (Figure 8.2).

Preclinical research involves the synthesis of a new drug within a laboratory, then the testing in *in vitro* cell lines and laboratory animals. Extensive animal testing is mandatory before the drug can be given to human volunteers for assessment of its safety and tolerability. Laboratory animals are given various doses of the drug and the effects on the different body systems and organs are studied, together with an evaluation of the level of drug that causes toxicity and death.

Phase I Drug Trials

Once safety has been established in animal models, the drug then proceeds to the next phase, that of testing in human volunteers. Phase I drug trials are primarily concerned with drug safety, metabolism, and bioavailability. They involve the use of human volunteers in relatively small numbers (usually between 20 and 80 subjects, often healthy young men). These trials are also concerned with ascertaining the acceptable single and multiple dose regimens in which the drug should ideally be given.

Therefore volunteers are given low doses and carefully monitored for undesirable pharmacological effects and adverse reactions. Regular blood samples are taken for pharmacokinetic analysis of the plasma in order to assess the distribution of the drug within body fluids and the time taken for it to be excreted. Whole blood samples are also taken from subjects in order to analyse the effects of the drug on the body organs, such as the liver and the kidney.

If the drug is considered safe, then phase II and phase III trials can be implemented.

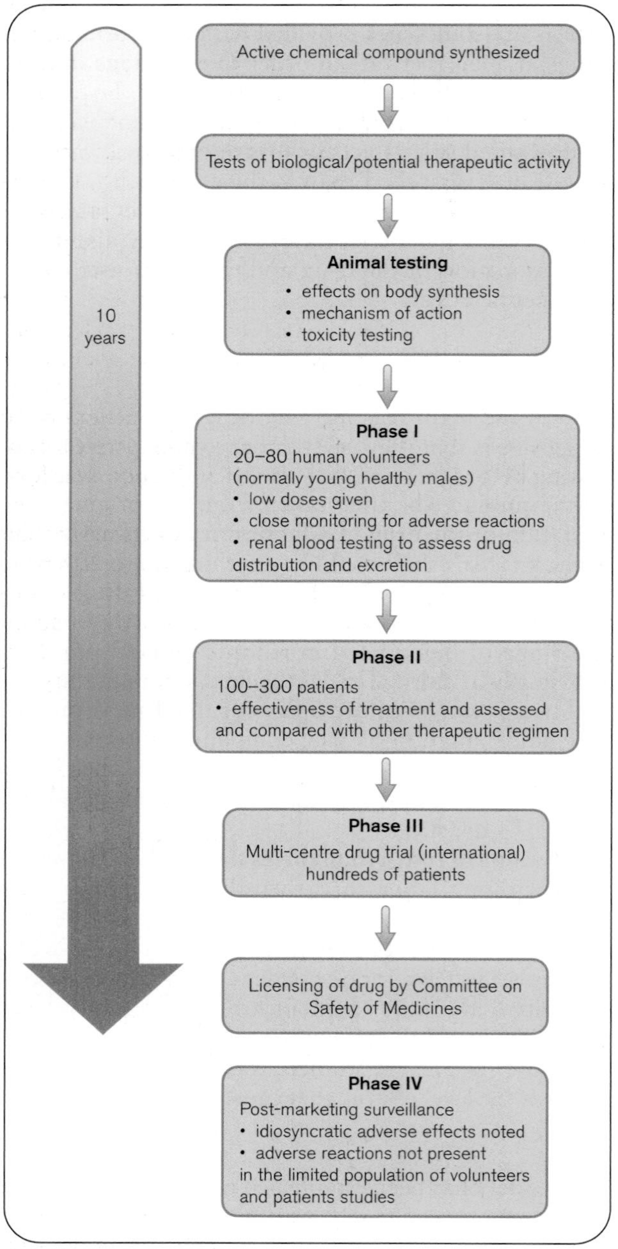

Phase II Drug Trials

Phase II drug trials are also performed on a relatively small number of patients (100–300 people) and are concerned with establishing the effectiveness of the treatment, together with further safety assessment – only drugs with definite therapeutic potential proceed to Phase III testing.

Phase III Drug Trials

Phase III drug trials are carried out on a much larger scale and involve a full evaluation of the drug, together with comparisons with current standard treatment. It is common for the trials to be multi-national and involve many hundreds of patients. Drugs that make it to this stage have proven efficacy, but they still need to show that they have attributes that either match or outperform current conventional treatments.

In all three initial phases, various methods of design are used; these include randomization and the use of placebo as a control. Placebo control means that patients are given either a placebo (dummy drug) or the actual drug under trial (see below). Sometimes the use of a placebo would be unethical (e.g. in drug trials for the treatment of cancer). In such instances, a conventional therapeutic drug is given. However, the assignment of the treatment is random and neither the patient nor the researcher knows which of the two drugs has been given. At the end of the trial the true nature of the treatment is made known, and the efficacy and safety of the drug is compared directly with the performance of the placebo. Obviously, drugs that are highly toxic cannot be tested in healthy volunteers (again, chemotherapy agents are a good example) so they are given directly to patients in Phase II trials.

The actual licensing of a drug is carried out by national authorities such as the Committee on Safety of Medicine (CSM) in the UK and the Federal Drugs Authority (FDA) in the USA. These authorities study all the results of the drug trials and ensure that the trials have been approved ethically and carried out under the correct guidelines.

Phase IV Drug Trials

Phase IV of a drug trial involves monitoring the drug once it has finally been marketed (i.e. post-marketing

Figure 8.2 Stages in the development of a drug from synthesis to the clinic.

surveillance); many adverse side-effects are not noted until this stage. This is not entirely surprising, because in the initial phases of a trial a drug may only be tested on about 3000 people at the most. If a side-effect affects only 1 in 4000 people, for example, it is quite likely it would not have been detected in the smaller group studied. Occasionally, a side-effect is rather idiosyncratic, such as the cough that affects some people when taking drugs such as captopril (an ACE inhibitor), which is given for hypertension (see Chapter 10). In these cases it may make several years for the connection to be realized.

THE USE OF PLACEBO DRUGS IN MEDICINE

Inert or inactive substances are occasionally given to patients for their psychological effect. These are called placebo drugs; the word 'placebo' is derived from the Latin word meaning 'I please'. Placebos were first used in medicine when physicians were unable to provide the actual drug needed, so an apparently identical pill or medicine was prepared from sugar and water or some other harmless substance. Such compounds, by definition, have no adverse effects and their use leads to an improved sense of well-being in many patients. Although this might seem dishonest, placebos in conjunction with psychological counselling can be extremely helpful. However, despite placebos being harmless, they cannot be given to patients without a prescription. Investigations into post-operative pain have shown that such drugs may provide relief in 36 per cent of patients.

This so-called 'placebo effect' is not limited to drugs, however, for a similar observation is found in patients who are adequately educated in advance of treatment. Apparently, patients required less analgesia (therefore one assumes they suffer less pain) if they are adequately informed of possible post-operative complications and if they are encouraged to ask for analgesics for pain relief.

Contrary to popular opinion, patients who respond well to placebo drugs are not necessarily more irrational or demanding than other patients. Placebos seem to provide psychological comfort and alleviate the fear that can exacerbate symptoms. It would therefore be expedient to evaluate the efficacy of some alternative therapies (e.g. the use as crystals in healing) in conventional randomized clinical trials, because it is likely that many of the benefits experienced by patients could be due to a placebo effect (see Chapter 14). Drugs with known pharmacological activities are not generally used as placebos because of their potential adverse effects. The use of a placebo drug in a clinical drug trial enables the clinician to separate the psychological effect of giving a therapy from the true pharmacological effect of the drug.

MATCHING DRUGS TO DISEASES

It is readily acknowledged that drugs can have both harmful and therapeutic effects. So often they are mistakenly regarded as only having anti-disease activity, an unfortunate misconception arising from the names given to certain classifications of drug (e.g. anti-hypertensive, anti-diabetic, anti-emetic). Sometimes a drug may oppose the pathological process, such as an antibiotic that eliminates a microbe causing an infection. More frequently, though, drugs produce the desired outcome by a rather different mechanism (see Chapter 10). Moreover, as they are potential poisons, monitoring of therapy is essential to ensure that the patient has derived a beneficial and not an adverse effect.

In therapeutics, the aims of treatment need to be defined before prescribing the drug (Figure 8.3). For instance, the main purpose of treating an infection is to ameliorate the disease, but often the appropriate antibiotic can only be selected when the causative microbe has been isolated and classified (see Chapter 17) – a broad-spectrum antibiotic would not have any effect on a viral or fungal infection, for example. Sometimes treatment involves giving an exogenous source of treatment in order to cure an endogenous deficiency. Patients with Parkinson's disease are prescribed L-dopa, which can cross the blood–brain barrier to maintain dopamine levels and prevent the adverse signs of tremor.

However, when the aim is to suppress undesirable symptoms such as pain, the use of analgesics is a palliative treatment. Pain control is one of the most compassionate clinical decisions for a patient with terminal cancer; it is neither a cure nor does it prolong life, but it does provides comfort and an improved quality of

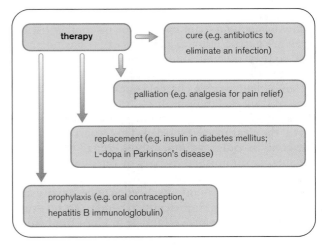

Figure 8.3 Aims of drug treatment. The aims of drug treatment should be defined before prescribing the drug.

life. Likewise, immunosuppressant drugs (e.g. corticosteroids) are prescribed for autoimmune diseases, such as rheumatoid arthritis, and for patients undergoing transplantation to prevent the rejection of the donated tissue or organs. These preparation do not cure the disease, they simply reduce the immune cell activities to avert an aggressive reaction and adverse symptoms (see Chapters 27 and 29).

Some drugs are commonly used in the prevention of disease or pregnancy – this is prophylactic treatment. Chloroquine tablets given to people travelling to areas with a high incidence of malaria is an example of this. Similarly, health care professionals who regularly come into contact with patients' body fluids are at increased risk of hepatitis B. Therefore, many occupational health departments demand that hospital workers be immunized against hepatitis B. Regrettably, a significant minority of people do not become immune even after repeated immunizations. In the event of an accident in which they come into contact with the disease (e.g. a needle stick injury), these people may be offered passive immunization with hepatitis B immunoglobulins (see Chapter 20).

Clearly, for a safe prescription, a sound knowledge of the patient's characteristics is required, along with an evaluation of how these might affect the pharmacological mechanism of the drugs given. When making the choice of drug, an assessment of the benefits versus the risk is an obvious consideration; it would be unacceptable to prescribe a drug if the side-effects were more severe than the disorder being treated. For example, selecting a beta-adrenoreceptor blocking drug (beta-blocker) such as propanolol may be an appropriate treatment for high blood pressure, but it is a potentially lethal choice for a patient with asthma. Similarly, a non-steroidal anti-inflammatory drug may provide adequate pain control for osteoarthritis, but they are gastric irritants that can cause haemorrhage and so they are contraindicated in patients with a history of gastrointestinal ulcers (see Chapter 10).

In patients with a clinical condition that alters the rate of drug metabolism or clearance from the body, drug levels can rapidly accumulate and provoke toxicity if the clearance is retarded. This is particularly significant in older adults, whose renal function is frequently diminished as part of the ageing process even though there may be no evidence of specific renal disease. Similarly, in infants, liver enzyme activity may not have developed sufficiently to handle certain drugs, which could thus prove fatal (e.g. chloramphenicol given to the neonate) (see Chapter 12).

Considerable patient variation in the handling of drugs may be found, which has implications for the effects of the drug actions in treating disease. Genetic differences can profoundly influence drug metabolism, and clinical pharmacogenetics is the study of anomalies that may affect pharmacodynamic or pharmacokinetic aspects of drug activities. Racial differences may be perceived as an external manifestation of genetic variation; for example, the hepatic acetylation of isoniazid is different in the Inuit people (Eskimos) to those whose origins are in Africa. Similarly, people of Mediterranean origin may not produce certain enzymes in the same quantities as a Caucasian person.

Clearly, the most suitable route of administration has to be chosen. When the therapeutic effects need to be attained quickly, the intravenous route provides a more rapid access to the systemic circulation than the oral route. Other factors, such as nausea or inability to swallow, may affect drug absorption, and these conditions would be contraindications to oral administration; an alternative, such as the rectal administration (giving drugs in suppository form), may need to be considered. (In some European countries, rectal administration is generally favoured over the oral route.) Drugs can also be inhaled, taken sublingually, or injected (e.g. subcutaneously) (see Chapter 9).

The mode of administration influences the effectiveness of the treatment. Most out-patients are prescribed oral medications, because it is an uncomplicated route for self administration of drugs. However this is not feasible with certain preparations; for instance, insulin is given by subcutaneous injection rather than orally because it is destroyed by the gut enzymes. Likewise, patient compliance is essential; therefore the advised drug regimen should take into consideration the personal characteristics of the patient being treated (e.g. impaired vision, poor memory, arthritic hands). When a patient has a disability, it is more expedient to prescribe drugs to be given in a minimum number of doses, and the drugs should be dispensed in clearly labelled containers that are easy to open. Patient care does not end once the prescription has been dispensed; patients need educating regarding the taking of the medication, and they should be closely monitored to ensure that the desired therapeutic outcome is attained and that any possible adverse effects of treatment are reported and dealt with (see Chapters 11 and 12).

CULTURAL BACKGROUND AND RELIGIOUS BELIEF

Differing cultures and religions show considerable variation in their attitudes to illness and treatment, and this may be highly significant when prescribing for a patient (Figure 8.4). Cultural factors influence views to conventional medicine, and members of some ethnic groups may prefer to exhaust all traditional herbal

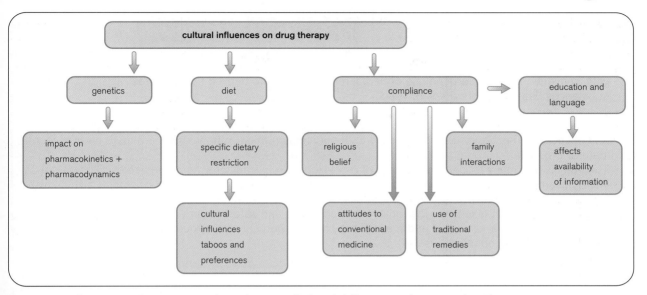

Figure 8.4 Cultural influences on drug therapy. Cultural differences that may alter the effectiveness of drug therapy.

remedies before approaching a clinician who practises Western medicine (see also Box 8.1). Ideally, attempts should be made to establish the extent of the patient's understanding of their disease. If traditional remedies have been previously tried, it is better to respect these attempts but at the same time provide a rationale for replacing them with conventional medicine.

The persistent use of medical jargon can be a source of confusion and may result in the patient not fully appreciating the reasons for treatment or how frequently the drugs should be taken. Clear and simple explanations encourage compliance; a confused patient may not feel able to adhere to the prescribed regimen. Similarly, where there is a language barrier, every effort should be made to find an interpreter – preferably a relative or friend of the patient. Some hospitals provide printed information for patients who do not speak English and have compiled a list of staff with proficiency in specific languages, who may be used as interpreters.

When medical treatment necessitates extended hospitalization, patients may not receive a diet they are used to eating. Many hospitals have recognized the existence of multicultural dietary requirements and have sought to provide a wider choice of food. However, if the hospital is unable to accommodate these cultural differences (and provided a dietary restriction has not been prescribed), relatives may be allowed to bring in food for the patient. This could be quite significant and should be encouraged because an adequate diet influences recovery. Furthermore, some

ethnic groups believe their own cultural diet is a vital part of rehabilitation.

Religious belief can pose ethical difficulties both for patients and for carers. Some conventional treatments are not acceptable for certain religious groups. Jehovah's Witnesses may not receive any human blood products because they believe the sins of man are carried in the blood; this may pose a clinical dilemma where an emergency blood transfusion is refused. Intravenous saline and intravenous iron supplement may be given instead of blood for minor transfusion needs, but inevitably the time taken for rehabilitation is prolonged. Ultimately the decision of an adult patient must be respected, but in a life-threatening situation when the patient is under 18 years of age, the clinician can apply for a court order to enable treatment to go ahead against the wishes of the parents.

OVER-THE-COUNTER MEDICATION

There are a growing number of medications that are sold 'over the counter' and do not require a medical prescription. They tend to be fairly basic drugs, such as analgesics, cold remedies, and vitamins. The availability of these first lines of treatment have certain advantages in that they save time both for the patient and for the doctor. Since many illnesses are short lived and not serious, it is often an inconvenience to attend a general practice surgery. Certainly the pharmacist is available to offer advice, provided the patient asks for

BOX 8.1 HERBAL REMEDIES

- Some patients may chose to self-treat with alternative therapies either independently of, or concurrently with, conventional therapies. The use of herbal remedies that are derived from plant extracts and animal substances dates back hundreds of years.
- There is the popular conception that herbal remedies are somehow 'more healthy', perhaps arising from the fears that have followed bad publicity regarding the widespread use of preservatives, food additives, and pesticides. This trend has therefore led to the perception that synthetic drugs are more harmful than 'natural' products.
- The irony is that many modern medicines were developed from traditional herbal remedies. Digoxin is a classic example of this; it originated from extract of foxglove used in the treatment of cardiac arrhythmias. Similarly, the vinca alkaloids, a group of cytotoxic drugs, are derived from the periwinkle plant.
- Regrettably, the strict guidelines that govern the marketing and safety testing of conventional medicines do not apply to herbal remedies, and their efficacy has not been proved through clinical trials. Indeed, herbal remedies are not always 'safe'.

it and supplies full information about the drugs that he or she is using concurrently.

Nevertheless, it is possible that the use of over-the-counter drugs may mask a more serious medical condition because the medication has improved the symptoms, or act as a placebo for a person who is too frightened about the possible diagnosis to consult a doctor. Ultimately, when the condition is finally discovered, the treatment may be both costly and prolonged, or life-threatening.

A further disadvantage is that a patient may take two non-prescribed medications that contain the same active drug. Taken alone, either medication may be relatively harmless, but taken concurrently they could lead to toxicity because the recommended dose is exceeded. For example, excess paracetamol is hepatotoxic, and unfortunately it tends to be one of the drugs chosen by a depressed patient who takes an overdose as a cry for help rather than a serious suicide attempt. Yet liver failure and death can follow a relatively small overdose if it is not immediately detected and treated – hence the strategy to sell paracetamol tablets in smaller numbers to prevent this occurrence.

Legislation has been introduced to maximize safety, rather than to restrict drugs that can be sold over the counter. Drugs that require a prescription tend to be more powerful, although recently drugs such as ibuprofen (a non-steroidal anti-inflammatory drug) and cimetidine (an H_2-blocker used in the treatment of duodenal ulcers) have been made available without a prescription. The law requires that over-the-counter medications have basic information printed on the packaging (i.e. the name of the product, the name and address of the manufacturing company, the net weight and ingredients of the contents, relevant warnings of possible side-effects, and directions for therapeutic use).

KEY POINTS

- Pharmacodynamics is the detailed scientific consideration of the mechanism of drug action.
- Pharmacokinetics evaluates how the body processes a drug (i.e. the absorption, distribution, metabolism, and the modes of excretion).
- Any chemical agent that alters a living process is broadly defined as a drug.
- Preclinical research involves the actual synthesis of a new drug compound within a laboratory followed by testing in the *in vitro* cell lines and laboratory animals. Once safety has been established in animal models, the drug then proceeds to the next phase of testing in human volunteers (Phase I); then to a relatively small number of patients (100–300 people) to establish the effectiveness of the treatment (Phase II), with evaluation of the treatment on a larger scale (Phase III) before the final post-marketing surveillance (Phase IV).
- A placebo, which is a substance without any direct pharmacological effect, may be given to a patient. By definition, a placebo has no adverse effects, and their use often leads to an improved sense of well-being.
- Cultural differences influence views to conventional medicine; some groups may prefer to exhaust all traditional herbal remedies before approaching a clinician who practises Western medicine.
- The use of over-the-counter drugs may mask a more serious medical condition, which then may remain undetected because the medication has improved the symptoms. Ultimately, when the condition is finally discovered, the treatment is likely to be both costly and prolonged.

FURTHER READING

Appelbe GE, Wingfield J (1997) Pharmacy Law and Ethics. Pharmaceutical Press, London.

Brody BA (1998) The ethics of biomedical research, an international perspective. Oxford University Press, Oxford.

Brown WA (1998) The placebo effect. Sci Am 278:68–73.

Chow S-C, Liu J-P (1998) Design and analysis of clinical trials. John Wiley & Sons, Chichester.

De Smet PAGM, Keller K, Hänsel Y, Chandler RF (1997) Adverse Effects of Herbal Drugs, volume 3. Springer-Verlag, London.

Gilberthorpe J (1996) Consent to Treatment. Medical Defence Union, London.

Hoyte P (1997) The dilemma of the incapacitate patient who has previously refused consent for surgery. BMJ 315:1530–2.

Klees JE, Joines R (1997) Occupational health issues in the pharmaceutical research and development process. Occup Med 12:5–27.

Martin J (ed) (1991) Handbook of Pharmacy Health Education. Pharmaceutical Press, London.

McCaffrey M, Ferrell BR (1997) Pain and placebo – ethics and professional issues. Orth Nurse 16(5):8–11.

Newall CA, Anderson LA, Phillipson JD (1996) Herbal Medicines – A Guide for Health-Care Professionals. Pharmaceutical Press, London.

Plunkett MJ, Ellman JA (1997) Combinatorial chemistry and new drugs. Sci Am 276:54–9.

Raybuck JA (1997) The clinical nurse specialist as research coordinator in clinical drug trials. Clin Nurse Spec 11:15–19.

Skinner S (1996) The world according to homeopathy. J Cardiovasc Nurs 10:65–77.

Spitzer WO (1997) Balanced view of notes of oral contraceptives. Lancet 350:1566–7.

Swayne J (1997) Homeopathic Method. Churchill Livingstone, London.

UK Health Department (1997) Guidelines on Post-Exposure Prophylaxis for Health Care Workers Exposed to HIV. UK Health Department.

PHARMACOKINETICS

INTRODUCTION

Pharmacokinetics is a term that describes the precise effect that the living system has on a drug. It encompasses the rate at which drug molecules cross cell membranes to enter and distribute throughout the body and the rate at which they are finally excreted. The term also includes the structural changes (metabolism) to which the drugs are subjected. The route of administration is of vital importance because numerous factors affect absorption.

A part of the role for a health care practitioner involves explaining to the patient:
- why certain routes of administration have been chosen;
- why blood samples are taken to check drug concentrations; and
- why certain drugs are given more frequently than others.

Some drugs, if given by mouth, are metabolized (chemically transformed) and rendered inactive even before they enter the bloodstream, and they therefore have to be given by an alternative route [e.g. intravenously, intramuscularly, or sublingually (under the tongue)].

The different physical properties of a drug, such as electrical charge and solubility, affect its distribution in body tissues and fluids. Most drugs exist in two forms in the blood compartment. The drug that is bound to the plasma proteins is known as the bound form, and the drug that is dissolved in the plasma is known as the unbound or free form. It is the unbound drug that has the pharmacological effect, and only the unbound fraction can be cleared by the liver or kidneys. Some drugs deposit into fat (adipose tissue), and they tend to be stored there and therefore cleared from the body rather more slowly. The liver is the major site where drugs are metabolized and modified to render them water soluble for excretion. Some drugs (e.g. propanolol and oestrogens) are substantially metabolized as they pass through the liver, the so-called 'first pass effect'. In such cases, only a small fraction of the drug absorbed from the gut enters the systemic circulation to be of therapeutic use.

The molecular size of water-soluble drugs or metabolites governs the route by which they are excreted. If they are sufficiently small, the drug metabolites are disposed of in the urine, but larger molecules (above a molecular weight of 300) are excreted in the bile via the biliary tree and the faeces.

Considerable variations exist between patients in their handling and metabolism of drugs. No two patients are the same and therefore the ways in which they react to, or metabolize, a drug may differ. For example, if warfarin (an anticoagulant drug) were to be given in a fixed dose to several patients, some may become excessively anticoagulated while others may be insufficiently anticoagulated and require a higher dose. Hence, the plasma prothrombin levels are estimated regularly in warfarinized patients to monitor the effects of the drug on haemostasis (see Chapter 10).

Patient compliance is essential if the treatment is to be successful; a drug may be ideally suited in theory, but if taken incorrectly, infrequently, or not at all, then not only will the benefits be lost, but it could also be hazardous. It is therefore desirable to educate patients as to why they have been prescribed the drug as well as making sure that they understand the recommended dose and the frequency and route of administration.

PASSAGE OF DRUGS ACROSS MEMBRANE BARRIERS

For a drug to produce the desired therapeutic effect, it must be present in a sufficiently high concentration at the site of action. This concentration is influenced by the dose, the rate and amount of absorption, how the drug is distributed in the body, the rate at which it is metabolized by the liver, and, finally, how rapidly it is excreted. In order to understand how this occurs, the physical and chemical properties of molecules and the structure of membranes must be considered (see also Chapter 1).

For a drug to penetrate into a cell it must cross the cellular plasma membrane, which is a bilayer of lipid molecules and 'islands' of protein. A drug taken orally must pass through a series of these membranes to enter the bloodstream; the first of these barriers is the gut mucosa. Since the plasma membrane is largely made up of lipid molecules, it does not represent an impediment to the entry of lipid-soluble substances (e.g. diazepam) because they are able to pass easily across the membrane. However, water-soluble substances are repelled by the non-polar components of the plasma membrane. They can, however, enter cells via pore-like structures in the cell membrane, but there is a size limit, so only small molecules, such as urea, pass through by this route.

PASSIVE DIFFUSION

Passive diffusion is the major mechanism by which lipid-soluble drugs pass through membranes (see Chapter 1). This type of transport is dependent on the concentration difference on either side of the membrane and the lipid solubility of the drug. A lipid-soluble drug diffuses across the membrane much more rapidly if the concentration on one side of the membrane is much greater (i.e. if there is a big concentration gradient). This difference promotes the passage of the drug across to the side of the membrane where it is less concentrated.

THE IMPORTANCE OF WATER AND LIPID SOLUBILITY

Many drugs are weak acids or weak bases, therefore the pH (measure of acidity and alkalinity, or the hydrogen ion concentration) of the environment in which the drug molecule exists will have a marked effect on the degree of ionization (i.e. formation of positively or negatively charged ions). For example, just as sodium chloride is made up sodium (positive) ions and chloride (negative) ions, many drug compounds also form positive and negative ions in solutions like plasma. Acidic drugs become proportionally less ionized in an acidic environment, whereas basic drugs become less ionized in a basic (alkaline) environment. Conversely, acidic drugs become more ionized in a basic medium, and basic drugs become more ionized in an acidic medium. The extent to which the drug is ionized influences its ability to diffuse across membranes – non-ionized drugs are lipid soluble and diffusible, whereas ionized drugs are lipid insoluble and less able to diffuse. A drug that is a weak base (e.g. amitriptyline) and is in a basic medium, such as blood, will not dissociate into positive and negative ions, and so will tend to behave more as a lipid-soluble substance. Equally, an acidic drug (e.g. aspirin) will behave as a lipid-soluble substance in acidic urine. A weakly basic drug in the acidic medium of the gastric juice will be highly dissociated into ions, as will an acidic drug in the basic medium of the small intestine.

As a general rule, basic drugs tend to concentrate in an acidic medium, such as the inside of cells or breast milk, and acidic drugs tend to concentrate in a basic medium. The amount of a basic drug that is lost in breast milk is so small it is not significant to the mother. However, even a tiny amount could be significant if ingested by an infant whose drug metabolizing and eliminating mechanisms are not yet fully developed. It is therefore advisable that mothers avoid taking drugs while breast-feeding, if possible. In any event it is essential to consult the *British National Formulary*, which highlights the drugs that are dangerous for a mother to take if she is breast-feeding (see also Chapter 12).

Once a drug is in the bloodstream, the major route across most capillary endothelial membranes is via the pores between cells. The main exception is the central nervous system, where there are tight junctions – this is the blood–brain barrier, which may only be crossed by lipid-soluble compounds (or water-soluble compounds of very low molecular weight). However, in times of infection (e.g. meningitis), the blood–brain barrier becomes leaky and more readily allows drugs across it; this is advantageous in that it allows antibiotics to work where they are needed. In most vascular beds, however, the intercellular gaps are sufficiently large for drug diffusion to occur across the capillaries. This transit is limited by blood flow rather than the lipid solubility of the drugs or the pH gradient, and blood flow is an important factor when considering distribution of drugs after parenteral administration.

LIPID-SOLUBLE DRUGS

Lipid-soluble drugs have the following characteristics:
- they are easily absorbed from the gastrointestinal tract;
- they penetrate readily into cells;
- they pass through the blood–brain barrier and are able to affect the central nervous system;
- they pass the placental barrier easily; and
- they need to be converted into water-soluble compounds before they can be excreted by the kidneys, a process carried out by the liver.

WATER-SOLUBLE DRUGS

Water-soluble drugs have the following characteristics:
- they are poorly absorbed from the gastrointestinal tract (unless they are of small molecular weight);
- they do not readily cross the blood–brain barrier;
- they do not penetrate the cell walls, and it is unusual for them to exert direct intracellular metabolic effect;
- they are excreted unchanged by the kidneys; and
- they do not pass across the placenta easily (unless they are of a small molecular weight).

ROUTES OF DRUG ADMINISTRATION

Drugs can be administered via a number of different routes, and the choice of route deserves consideration. When prescribing, it is vital to consider carefully by which route the drug will be most effective. For example, if a response is required immediately, then the intravenous route is usually the most effective. It is also necessary to consider the patient's physical state; for instance a patient with nausea is at risk of vomiting a drug that is taken orally (see Box 9.1).

BOX 9.1 INJECTION VS ORAL MEDICATION

Patients who feel nauseated following surgery benefit from an injection of anti-emetic drug (e.g. metoclopramide) rather than an oral form of the drug, for two reasons. First, if they do vomit an oral tablet might be lost or only partially absorbed; second, the drug will be more rapidly absorbed if given intramuscularly, thus relieving the symptoms more rapidly.

One route of administration is by injection, which can be intramuscular, intradermal, subcutaneous, or intravenous (Figure 9.1). Although these routes can be uncomfortable, decisions must be made as to the advantage in certain situations. Insulin is given subcutaneously rather than orally because it is a polypeptide that would be rapidly destroyed by the gut enzymes.

With both intramuscular and subcutaneous routes of administration, the absorption of the drug is not dependent on its lipid solubility because there are large aqueous (water-filled) channels for their transport across membranes (see Chapter 1). Drugs injected into an aqueous solution are more rapidly absorbed than those in an oily solution. Some drugs given by intramuscular injection are rapidly absorbed and can reach peak levels in 10–15 minutes (e.g. lignocaine). Lipid-soluble drugs may be absorbed extremely slowly if they

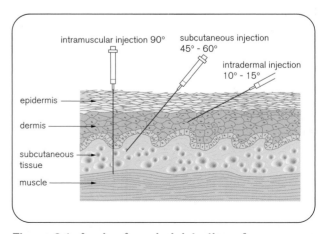

Figure 9.1 Angles for administration of intramuscular, subcutaneous, and intradermal injections.

are contained in an oily substance. Accordingly, the action of the drug is prolonged and it can therefore be given less often – this is often exploited to good effect with patients who may not be compliant. For example, patients with schizophrenia can be given infrequent (e.g. every 2–4 weeks) 'depot' injections of antipsychotic drugs, such as flupenthixol decanoate.

The blood circulation around the site of absorption is another factor that may affect the rate of drug distribution throughout the rest of the body – where the blood flow is poor, absorption will be slower. Absorption from the deltoid muscle is faster than from the gluteus, probably because of a difference in blood flow (Figure 9.2).

ABSORPTION FROM THE GASTROINTESTINAL TRACT (ORAL ADMINISTRATION)

After oral administration, disintegration of the tablet or capsule with subsequent dissolution of the drug (the physical change from solid to solute) are essential preludes to absorption. The science of pharmaceutics has advanced considerably, and thus the rate and site of absorption can now be altered by the way a tablet or capsule is constructed. An example of this is the invention of enteric coating; an analgesic can be made available in a slow-release, enteric-coated formulation.

This means that:
- the tablet is more easily swallowed and tastes more pleasant;
- the drug bypasses the stomach; and
- the drug is slowly absorbed in the intestine, thus avoiding both local irritation to the stomach lining and the destruction of the drug by gastric acid.

Drugs that are unstable in gastric acid should be given on an empty stomach.

Most drugs are absorbed from the proximal third of the small bowel, owing to its vast surface area. The rate of gastric emptying is of fundamental importance in determining drug absorption; a delay might significantly decrease the speed at which the drug is absorbed. Gastric emptying may be retarded by factors such as pain, fear, nausea, and fatty food, and it results in the drug being delayed in arriving at the portion of the gut where it is actively absorbed.

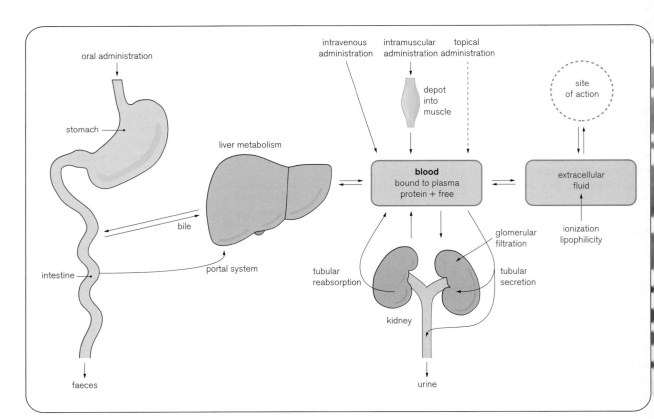

Figure 9.2 Distribution and fate of a drug following oral, intravenous, intramuscular, and topical administration.

(Theoretically, a health care practitioner may, by allaying a patient's fear effectively, help to shorten the time before a drug starts to work.)

If there is a delay in gastric emptying, the plasma drug concentration may fail to achieve a therapeutic level. This is one reason why, ideally, many drugs should be taken before a meal, although this is not advisable for drugs that cause gastric irritation, which should be given with food. Moreover, some foods actually increase the rate at which a drug is absorbed, probably owing to the increased blood flow serving the gut. (The subsequent rise in the rate of blood flow through the liver affects the bioavailability of drugs subject to first pass metabolism.) A drug given to treat nausea, such as metoclopramide, can increase the rate of gastric emptying and may be of value in permitting the rapid absorption of other drugs (e.g. an analgesic).

It is noteworthy that patients with a malabsorption syndrome, such as Crohn's disease, may fail to achieve a therapeutic level owing to their diminished capacity for gastrointestinal absorption. When the disease is severe, it may be necessary to consider other routes of administration. The rate at which the therapeutic level is achieved is particularly important when therapy is intermittent (e.g. in treatment for the relief of occasional pain), and it can also be significant when a high concentration is necessary to achieve tissue penetration (e.g. in antibiotic therapy). Factors such as a rapid intestinal transit rate, disease of the gastrointestinal tract (as with Crohn's disease), and poor blood supply to the gut (as in cardiac failure) may affect the efficacy of treatment. For example, the decreased absorption of oestrogens following gastroenteritis in a woman taking the oral contraceptive pill could lead to loss of the contraceptive effect.

For most drugs, the amount absorbed is usually more important than the rate of absorption, especially for drugs given over a long period of time. Drugs may be broken down by gastrointestinal flora (bacteria normally living in the gut), which results in poor net absorption. Some drugs can also be broken down by enzymes in the intestinal mucosa and liver and thus fail to reach a therapeutic concentration in the systemic circulation. Obviously such drugs are not given by mouth.

Some drugs cannot be given by mouth, despite the fact that they are well absorbed, because they are metabolized so rapidly by the liver that they never enter the rest of the circulation in sufficient concentration to be of therapeutic use. In some cases, a sizeable percentage of the drug is removed on its initial passage through the liver, a process referred to as the 'first-pass effect' (Table 9.1). Unless an oral drug is absorbed directly into the systemic circulation via the sublingual route, it passes through the liver via the hepatic portal circulation.

Common Drugs Subject to First-Pass Metabolism

• Aspirin	• Morphine
• Chlormethiazole	• Nortriptyline
• Chlorpromazine	• Oral contraceptives
• Glyceryl trinitrate	• Paracetamol
• Imipramine	• Pentazocine
• Isosorbide dinitrate	• Prazosin
• Labetalol	• Propranolol
• Levadopa	• Salbutamol
• Lignocaine	• Terbutaline
• Metoprolol	• Verapamil

Table 9.1: Some common drugs which are subject to first-pass metabolism.

THE SUBLINGUAL ROUTE

The sublingual route of administration is used to aid the absorption of a drug that is subject to a high first-pass effect, such as glyceryl trinitrate, which is used in the treatment of angina pectoris, and nifedipine, which is an antihypertensive. Drugs are placed under the tongue and allowed to dissolve; consequently they enter the venous circulation without passing through the gut and liver. The veins drain via the superior vena cava to the heart, and thus initial hepatic breakdown (first-pass effect) is avoided. Blood concentration, potential surface area, and blood supply are important factors in determining the rate of absorption from the sublingual route. The patient should be instructed not to chew or swallow the tablet and not to drink water, since these activities all interfere with the effectiveness of the medication.

RECTAL ADMINISTRATION

Drugs may be administered rectally to avoid gastric irritation and to decrease the first-pass effect. Blood concentration, surface area, and blood supply all affect absorption of drugs from the rectal mucosa. Usually 50 per cent of the drug will pass through the liver before entering into the systemic circulation; the other 50 per cent escapes the first-pass effect. If, however, the drug is inserted too high into the rectum, all may pass into the hepatic portal circulation and be subject to first-pass metabolism. Drugs given as suppositories may sometimes precipitate adverse effects, such as local rectal bleeding. Suppositories are also available as slow-release formulations, which can be especially advantageous for pain control. Indomethacin suppositories administered morning and night may offer steady pain control over 24 hours because they are absorbed slowly through the rectal mucosa. Likewise, administering a drug rectally

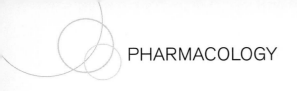

is useful when the patient has a traumatized gut or is unable to retain a tablet because of nausea or vomiting, or if the drug has an unpleasant odour or taste. However, other routes should be considered in a patient with rectal bleeding or diarrhoea.

TOPICAL APPLICATION

Drugs for topical application are available in many different types of preparation (ointments, creams, pastes, dusting powders, and lotions). Oral irrigations and gargles also come under this category. Ointment is the most suitable medium for a drug to be applied to a specific site without contaminating the surrounding areas (e.g. steroids usually come as an ointment). Antifungal foot applications often come in the form of a powder because excessive moisture would encourage the growth of fungi.

In general, drugs are absorbed more slowly through the skin than through mucosal surfaces. The epidermis itself forms a lipid barrier, but the dermis is freely permeable to many solutes, so any degree of excoriation of the skin would tend to increase absorption. Factory workers handling stilboestrol (a synthetic oestrogen) have been found to suffer undesirable side-effects, such as the development of female secondary sexual characteristics in males, owing to drug absorption through the skin. Indeed, the dermal route is now favoured for the administration of natural oestrogen in the form of patches and gels (e.g. hormone replacement therapy for menopausal women). Again, drug concentration, surface area, and the blood supply to the skin are important factors affecting absorption.

Certain medications are available in the form of mouthwashes or gargles, which can be directly administered to the mouth or throat provided they are not swallowed. For instance, antifungal mouthwashes are available for the treatment of oral *Candida albicans* (see also Chapter 18). Likewise, it is a fairly common practice to treat a cold or sore throat with an antiseptic gargle, but this often damages sensitive tissues and destroys the natural immune defences of the throat and mouth. A lozenge is just as effective in soothing a sore throat as many of the expensive over-the-counter preparations.

Inhalation

The direct inhalation of drugs may be used to treat diseases of the respiratory tract, such as asthma or chronic obstructive pulmonary disease (see Chapter 33). The drug formulation and mode of inhalation influence the effectiveness of the therapy. Inhaled particles larger than 10–20 µm have a tendency to adhere to the upper respiratory tract, and only the smaller particles reach the bronchioles and alveoli. There are various ways of ensuring that the particles arrive at their intended destinations. Asthma preparations often come in small aerosol cans, which dispense the medication in pressurized bursts. If the medication is given by a nebulizer, the drug is pre-mixed with water or saline, then it is converted to a vapour by the passage of a gas through the solution, and then it is inhaled through a mask.

The advantage of inhalation is that it ensures the drug arrives directly at the site of action to provide a rapid effect. Disadvantages include local irritation to the respiratory tissues, and occasionally bronchospasm is induced by the preservatives and antimicrobials present in the aerosol solutions. It is important to teach patients the correct technique for using their inhalers to co-ordinate inhalation with depressing the aerosol. For people with asthma, nebulized medication is more effective than an inhaler, since the particle size is much smaller. Therefore, the drug reaches the smaller bronchioles and penetrates the mucosal surface much better.

Vaginal Administration

Vaginal absorption of a drug in the form of pessaries is dependent on the exact preparation and on vaginal pH. Surface area and vascularity are also important factors. Virtually none of the drug passes through the liver before entering into the systemic circulation, so first-pass metabolism is avoided. Drugs such as bromocriptine for the treatment of hyperprolactinaemia can be given by the vaginal route, which obviates the adverse gastrointestinal side-effects, which are assumed to be due to a local action on the gut mucosa (see Chapter 37).

INTRAVENOUS INJECTIONS

Intravenous injections provide direct access to the bloodstream (vascular compartment) and may be given as a continuous infusion or as a bolus. Because the drug is not subject to first-pass metabolism, it is able to go directly to highly perfused organs, such as the brain and heart. It is also easier to control the plasma concentration of a drug, because absorption of the drug from the gut can be erratic. Intravenous administration of drugs is usually only required in the short term when a patient is acutely ill. They may also be given prophylactically; for example, intravenous antibiotics may be given following bowel surgery for patients who are unable to eat or drink, to prevent post-operative infection.

The intravenous route is certainly the most efficient and desirable route of administration in an emergency situation. But drugs given via the intravenous route must be injected slowly to reduce the risk of an adverse cardiac or respiratory effect (see also Chapter 13).

The disadvantages include the high cost of treatment, the increased risk of side-effects, and the possibility of damage to the tissues if extravasation occurs. When giving more than one drug via an intravenous giving set, care must be taken to flush the line with saline to avoid the mixing of two chemically incompatible drugs. The resultant precipitate could result in tissue damage by causing occlusion of small blood vessels.

INTRAMUSCULAR INJECTIONS

Intramuscular injection may be painful, but it provides a route for achieving a more rapid therapeutic effect than the oral route. Fairly large volumes of solution may be administered and absorbed via the aqueous channels in the membranes of muscle. There is, however, a slight difference in the rate of absorption depending on the site of injection – drugs are more rapidly absorbed from the muscles in the upper arm (deltoid) than from the gluteal muscles and thigh. Furthermore, the rate of absorption may vary depending on the fitness of the patient, because fit people generally have a greater blood supply to their muscles.

The disadvantages of intramuscular injection are that self-administration by the patient is rather difficult, and local irritation at the injection sites may arise. Many hospital trusts have strict protocols regarding the sites used for the administration of intramuscular injections. One hazard of gluteal injections is the risk of hitting the sciatic nerve and causing paralysis.

SUBCUTANEOUS INJECTIONS

Self-administration of a drug is more feasible by a subcutaneous injection – it is a daily task for many insulin-dependent diabetics. This route is also much less painful than the intramuscular one; the technique requires a small needle to be inserted vertically through the skin and injected slowly. However, because this mode of drug administration is limited by the need for a good blood supply it is not effective for patients in shock, because their low blood pressure means that they do not readily absorb drugs from a subcutaneous site. Similarly, repeated injections in the same area can cause lipoatrophy (wasting of fatty tissues); therefore injection sites need to be 'rotated' regularly. People with diabetics are particularly at risk from peripheral circulatory failure, which can affect the absorption of insulin.

DISTRIBUTION OF DRUGS

Generally, drugs that are readily absorbed from the gastrointestinal tract are rapidly distributed to other body compartments. The proportion of the dose given which then becomes available at the site of action is called the 'bioavailability' of the drug.

This property is affected by rate and extent of absorption, and therefore it is governed to some degree by the route of administration. The bioavailability of a drug is assessed by evaluating the plasma drug levels following identical dosing via the intravenous and oral routes. Graphs are then produced showing the changes in plasma concentration with time corresponding to the two routes of administration. From these data, the fraction of the dose that is available for therapeutic effect in a given time may be estimated and the two routes can be directly compared. The different ingredients that make up the medicine and the methods of manufacture are often responsible for variation in drug bioavailability and thus therapeutic activity (see Figure 9.3).

It would be difficult to measure the drugs levels in every different part of the body, so the blood plasma is used as an indicator. By estimating the plasma levels, it is possible to establish how much drug has remained in the general circulation and how much has apparently distributed into the tissues. The relationship between the initial dose administered and the plasma concentration is called the volume of distribution (Vd). This makes the assumption that the drug is dispersed equally throughout the whole body at the same concentration in the plasma (analogous to adding a drop of ink to a tumbler of water, where the ink becomes evenly dispersed). If a drug remains predominantly in the bloodstream, it will have a small Vd. However, if it distributes widely into other tissues or organs, then its volume of distribution will be much greater.

A knowledge of Vd is highly significant for calculating the loading dose to achieve an initial therapeutic plasma concentration. Likewise, it is invaluable for the management of a patient who has taken an overdose, because drugs that remain predominately in the blood (low Vd) can be removed easily by plasmapheresis or haemodialysis. However, these procedures are of little use for a drug that has a large volume of distribution, because this drug will have passed into cells. When drugs remain in the plasma at a high concentration, they have a small 'apparent volume of distribution'. With drugs that readily enter cells, the blood concentration is thereby reduced, so they tend to have a large 'apparent volume of distribution' (Figure 9.4). Drugs that are concentrated in tissues such as body fat stores are said to be 'sequestrated'.

The site at which a drug is given can influence the proportion found in the plasma.

- An oral drug that is easily absorbed may still be found only in low concentrations in the plasma if it

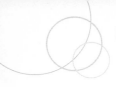

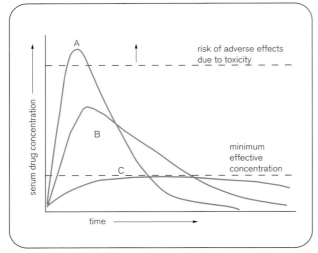

Figure 9.3 Bioavailability of a drug following oral administration. The bioavailability of a drug depends on the rate and extent of its absorption. Three drugs are shown here. With drug A, the therapeutic concentration is attained extremely rapidly and with the risk of toxicity. With drug B, therapeutic concentration is attained more slowly than drug A but sustained over a longer period and without the risk of toxicity. With drug C, sub-therapeutic concentration is slowly achieved.

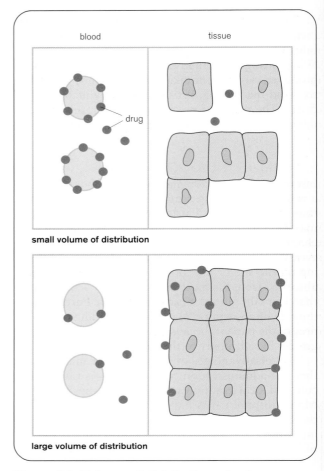

Figure 9.4 Volume of distribution of a drug. A drug with a small volume of distribution remains predominantly in the blood compartment. A drug with a larger volume of distribution disperses at a greater concentration into body tissues.

is substantially metabolized as it passes through the liver.

- A drug given intravenously will be 100 per cent available in the systemic circulation before hepatic processing.
- Acidic drugs are often substantially bound to albumin, which is the main plasma protein for the binding of many natural substances and drugs. Such drugs therefore have a smaller Vd, usually similar in fact to the plasma volume.
- Certain basic drugs, such as propranolol, bind to another protein in plasma called alpha-1-acid glycoprotein, which is an acute-phase protein whose concentration is increased in the inflammatory response.
- The fraction of a drug bound to protein depends upon its concentration, its avidity (greediness) for binding sites on the protein molecule, and the number of sites available.

Drugs can compete for plasma proteins, and one drug can displace another that has already bound to a site. This 'knock-off effect' then increases the concentration of free unbound drug in the systemic circulation and results in an enhanced pharmacological effect. It is the unbound portion of a drug that is pharmacologically active and available for breakdown in the liver or able to be excreted by the kidneys.

THE ROLE OF THE LIVER IN DRUG METABOLISM

The liver has a major role in the metabolism and clearance of drugs. Although liver enzymes are responsible for metabolizing most drugs, there are other sites available, such as the gastrointestinal tract, the kidneys, the lungs, and blood. The breakdown of drugs by the liver is called 'biotransformation' – it converts lipid-soluble compounds (which pass readily into liver cells) into water-soluble ones, thus rendering them liable to excretion.

Lipid-soluble drugs pass readily into liver cells, and their biotransformation into water-soluble metabolites occurs in two phases. Phase I reactions bring about a change in the drug molecule by oxidation, reduction, or hydrolysis. Oxidation is the most important of these, and this process is catalysed by an enzyme called cytochrome P_{450}.

The product of the phase I reactions is then subjected to further modifications in phase II. As a result, a larger molecule is generated; this larger molecule is more water soluble. Together, phase I and phase II reactions result in the inactivation and modification of the drug for excretion. The microsomes located in the smooth endoplasmic reticulum of the liver play an important part in these processes. Microsomal enzymes are responsible for most oxidation reactions (Figure 9.5). The rate of biotransformation can vary six-fold or more between patients, and it is thought that these differences in the metabolic processes are at least in part genetically controlled (see also Box 9.2).

The function of the liver is affected by malnutrition, and severe liver cirrhosis also diminishes its capacity to metabolize drugs. In these conditions, the first-pass effect is reduced and availability of active drug in the circulation is increased. Patients affected are at risk from an exaggerated response to normal doses of drugs which are ordinarily cleared by the liver, so toxicity is likely to occur.

ENZYME INDUCTION

Enzymes were developed in the process of evolution to deal with lipid-soluble substances that are taken in as food. In a modern society, these enzymes are required to deal with ever more complex drugs and environmental hazards, such as tobacco smoke and hydrocarbons (e.g. charcoal grilled food products). When the body is exposed to large quantities of these substances, it responds by increasing the amount and activity of the enzyme system – i.e. the enzymes are induced. Conversely, as the exposure lessens, so the production of these enzymes is reduced.

A typical example may be found in someone who finds that drinking two glasses of wine occasionally has a favourable effect on his or her mood. If that same person were to drink two glasses of wine every night, the liver enzymes would become more active and his or her tolerance would be enhanced. Therefore, the person would not necessarily experience the change in behaviour, because two glasses of wine consumed regularly would be rapidly metabolized, and more wine would be required to produce the same initial effect.

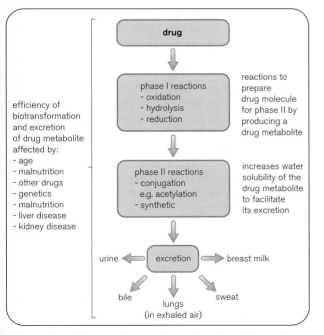

Figure 9.5 Biotransformation of a drug. Phase I and Phase II reactions to render a drug liable for excretion. The efficiency of biotransformation and excretion of drug metabolites can be affected by age, malnutrition, other drugs, genetic factors, liver disease, and kidney disease.

BOX 9.2 PRO-DRUGS

- Some drugs are manufactured as the inactive form and must be subjected to metabolism by the liver or bacterial flora in the gut or other organs to be rendered active.
- These drugs are called pro-drugs and need to be converted into an active drug by the body.
- Sometimes pro-drugs have an advantage over the parent drug. For example, pivampicillin is a pro-drug; it is converted to ampicillin following absorption.
- Pivampicillin does not have the same antibacterial activity as ampicillin, it does not alter the gut bacterial flora, and therefore diarrhoea, one of the most troublesome side effects of ampicillin, is less likely to occur.

Competition between drugs for the same enzyme does not necessarily slow down their clearance. In fact, if two drugs metabolized by the same enzyme system are given over the same time period, it can increase the activity of the enzyme, so the clearance of one or both of the drugs may be increased. For example, if the anti-epileptic drug, carbamazepine, is given with the anticoagulant, warfarin, the enzyme activity induced by the carbamazepine increases the metabolism and clearance of warfarin. Less warfarin is now available and the patient may no longer be satisfactorily anticoagulated; a larger dose of warfarin would therefore be required to secure anticoagulant control. However, if carbamazepine were suddenly stopped in favour of a different anti-epileptic drug, the patient would be liable to become over anticoagulated. Therefore the warfarin therapy would have to be adjusted again to compensate.

Although enzyme induction must be considered an important factor, not all drugs are broken down in the liver microsomes. Some are broken down at other sites in the hepatic cell. The enzyme systems involved are not usually inducible. The inhibition of drug metabolism by another drug is usually of limited clinical importance, but an interaction between phenytoin (prescribed for epilepsy) and warfarin is one important exception. Warfarin slows down the metabolism of phenytoin by the liver, causing a build up in plasma concentrations that results in severe phenytoin toxicity (poisoning).

GENETIC FACTORS IN DRUG METABOLISM

Some differences in patient response to drug therapy are due to metabolic variations that are under genetic influence (and therefore inherited). Acetylation is an important route of metabolism that is controlled genetically. The UK population can roughly be divided into what are termed 'slow acetylators' and 'fast acetylators', depending on their ability to metabolize drugs by acetylation. This distinction is mainly due to genetic differences in the activity of the enzyme N-acetyl transferase. Drugs that are subject to acetylation may therefore be cleared from the body either quickly or slowly. Approximately 45 per cent of the UK population are slow acetylators, whereas less than 5 per cent of Canadian Inuit (Eskimos) are in this category.

The existence of slow and fast acetylators is now known, and the clinical relevance of these differences in relation to prescribing is established. Those who are fast acetylators inactivate drugs quickly; as a general rule the incidence of side-effects in these subjects is less, but they do not derive as much therapeutic benefit from the drug as slow acetylators do. Slow acetylators benefit more from the drugs because they are not rendered therapeutically inactive so quickly, but these individuals tend to experience more side-effects. For example, peripheral neuritis as a side-effect of isoniazid is more common in slow acetylators (Table 9.2).

HEPATIC CLEARANCE

In order to evaluate the dose and the time interval in a drug regimen, an overall consideration of the rapidity with which a drug is absorbed, distributed, metabolized, and excreted is required. If pharmacological activity is prolonged, the time between doses may have to be extended. Many drugs are processed at a rate that is proportional to the quantity administered; as the amount given is increased, so the rate of processing is faster. However, in the same way, as the concentration in the body falls as a result of the processing, so the rate of elimination decreases in parallel – this is known as 'first-order kinetics'.

In the case of drugs such as alcohol, the situation is rather different – the liver can detoxify only a fixed amount in a set time interval. Therefore, as more alcohol is consumed, the longer it takes for it to be removed from the body. The limiting factor here is that alcohol-metabolizing enzymes are easily saturated. Therefore, a high concentration may be metabolized slowly – this is an example of zero-order kinetics.

All drugs are processed by first-order kinetics until a certain quantity is present in the blood stream. If the level of drug goes above this amount, then zero-order kinetics comes into effect. For most drugs, zero-order kinetics does not come into effect because the dose would be too toxic at this level. There are exceptions as in the case of phenytoin, for example, if the dose is doubled, then initially the rate of metabolism doubles commensurately and the dosage is reflected in the plasma concentration. However, above a certain dose, the metabolizing process becomes overwhelmed and the rate of metabolism reaches saturation. Thus the plasma level is disproportionately elevated compared to the dose because the eliminating capacity is less proficient at that level of administration. A small increase in dose can then cause a huge increase in plasma concentration.

Many drugs are rapidly cleared by the liver and pass into the bile in a modified and more water-soluble form. As a general rule, larger water-soluble compounds of a molecular weight of over 300 are excreted in the bile, whereas smaller compounds under 300 tend to be excreted in the urine. Some drug metabolites excreted in the gut may be modified by bacterial activity, which renders them more lipid soluble and therefore liable to re-absorption back into the circulation.

Drugs that are rapidly cleared by the liver are sometimes referred to as 'high-extraction-ratio drugs'; exam-

Examples of Slow and Fast Acetylator Effects on Drugs

Drug Name	Fast or Slow	Effect(s)
Isonizid - antimicrobial drug used for tuberculosis	Slow acetylators	Develop collagen diseases more easily Peripheral neuritis is common More prone to hepatitis as the acetylated metabolite is responsible for causing hepatitis by an immunological mechanism
Procainamide - used for cardiac dysrhythmia	Slow acetylators	Develop antinuclear antibodies more frequently
Hydralazine - antihypertensive	Slow acetylators	Develop antinuclear antibodies more frequently
	Fast acetylators	Higher doses required to control hypertension
Sulphasalazine - anti-inflammatory drug used for ulcerative colitis	Slow acetylators	More haematological side effects
Phenelzine - monoamine oxidase inhibitor antidepressant (MAOI)	Slow acetylators	More side effects Headaches
	Fast acetylators	Less effective treatment of depression

Table 9.2: Slow and fast acetylators – possible adverse side-effect experienced.

ples include chlorpromazine, diltiazem, imipramine, morphine, propranolol, and oestrogens. The clearance of these drugs is almost entirely dependent on liver blood flow, so if the flow of blood through the liver falls, their clearance falls to a similar extent. If all the drug coming to the liver is cleared, the extraction is 100 per cent and the extraction ratio is 1. If half the drug delivered to the liver is cleared, then the extraction is 50 per cent and the extraction ratio is 0.5.

Drugs that are not rapidly cleared are said to have a 'low extraction ratio'. In these cases, the fraction of the unbound drug (free drug) plus the inherent drug metabolizing capacity of the liver become important variables in determining their hepatic clearance.

When the capacity of the liver to metabolize a drug is greater than the rate at which it is being delivered, then its clearance is limited by the blood flow – this is called 'flow-limited clearance'. Thus, when the hepatic blood flow is high, the drug is rapidly cleared. However, when blood flow to the liver is slow (e.g. in shock or cardiac failure), drug clearance is impaired.

When drug delivery to the liver is greater than its metabolic capacity, then the degree of detoxification will not be determined by blood flow, but rather by the clearance efficiency of the liver. This is called 'capacity-limited clearance'. Inevitably the proportion of unbound fraction in plasma that is free and available for metabolism will influence clearance (Figure 9.6).

RENAL CLEARANCE

Drugs are eliminated from the kidneys once they have been partly or completely metabolized to a water-soluble metabolite. The renal clearance of drugs is determined by three mechanisms:
• glomerular filtration;
• renal tubular excretion; and
• renal tubular reabsorption.

Glomerular Filtration
The rate at which a drug enters the glomerular filtrate depends on the concentration of free drug in the plasma and on its molecular weight. Low protein binding tends to accelerate filtration because a greater proportion of the drug is free and soluble in the plasma and so available to be filtered. High protein binding will decrease the amount that is filtered at the glomerulus because less drug is free and soluble in the plasma.

Renal Tubular Secretion
Active secretion of a drug depends primarily on adequate kidney function, but again the proportion bound to protein must also be taken into consideration. Drug metabolites with a high electrical charge may be actively transferred from the plasma and through the cells of the proximal renal tubule into the tubular fluid. There are two such systems, one for acids and one for bases.

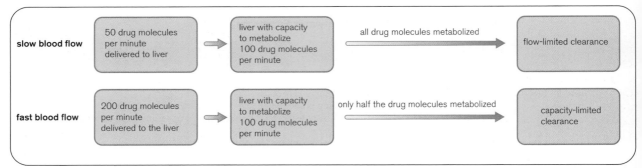

Figure 9.6 Flow-limited clearance and capacity-limited clearance of a drug by the liver. Flow-limited clearance of a drug occurs in a situation of slow blood flow (e.g. as in cardiac failure) when the liver can metabolize the drug at a faster rate than it is being delivered. Capacity-limited clearance of a drug occurs in a situation of faster blood flow, when the drug is being delivered to the liver at a rate faster than the liver can metabolize the drug.

Renal Tubular Reabsorption

Reabsorption of drugs from the renal tubule back into the plasma can be an active or passive process. Changes in urinary pH can make a significant difference to the clearance of certain drugs by altering their water- and lipid-soluble properties.

Changing urinary pH in order to counteract a drug overdose

Aspirin is more rapidly cleared in alkaline urine because it is then more highly water soluble. Alkalinizing the urine with sodium bicarbonate is an effective treatment for aspirin overdose. In a large overdose involving the anti-epileptic drug, phenobarbitone, forced alkaline diuresis with sodium bicarbonate may again be considered.

Conversely, a weakly basic drug, such as amphetamine, in an alkaline medium will behave as a lipid-soluble substance and be reabsorbed back into the bloodstream along a concentration gradient. Its excretion can therefore be hastened by causing an acid diuresis, and this procedure may be carried out in the case of a patient who has overdosed with amphetamine.

HALF-LIFE AND STEADY-STATE CONCENTRATION

The rate at which a drug is eliminated from the body is denoted by its half-life, which is the time taken for the plasma concentration of the unmodified drug to fall by half (e.g. the time interval between a plasma concentration being reduced from 500 units/ml to 250 units/ml). The half-life of every drug is different and, within certain limits, it is not dependent on dose. For example, if 500 units of a drug with a half-life of 6 hours is given,

then after 6 hours its concentration will be reduced to 250 units, and 6 hours later 125 units, and so on. This is an important factor for evaluating the time interval between doses – a drug with a long half-life does not need to be administered as often as a drug with a short half-life. These figures are sometimes considered academic because they rely on normal hepatic and renal function. When there is impairment in hepatic or renal function, the half-life is prolonged.

When a drug is given by a continuous intravenous infusion, the plasma concentration gradually rises until a plateau (i.e. the steady-state concentration) is reached. At this point, the rate at which the drug is being eliminated equals the rate of the infusion. With oral drugs, there is delay between taking the drug and its entering the circulation because it must surmount a number of membrane barriers. Once in the plasma, the concentrations fluctuate between elevated peaks and low troughs. Even so, the same principle applies, and within the time interval of four or five half-lives an oral drug should reached a concentration at which the peak and trough levels are within its therapeutic range. Similarly, when the treatment is withdrawn it would take the same time interval of four or five half-lives for the drug to be finally eliminated.

Depending on the nature of the drug action, the time fluctuation between doses caused by lack or changes in patient compliance may or may not be acceptable. For instance, varying the time between drug administration is sometimes safe enough in the treatment of infection with antimicrobial agents, but in the case of a drug being given to control coagulation, deviations from the advised regimen could lead to haemorrhage or thrombosis, depending on whether the patient was underdosed or overdosed.

Plasma concentrations are not always good indicators of the effects of treatment. The amount of drug needed to provide the same therapeutic effect differs considerably from patient to patient. If a physiological parameter is being modified, then it is more expedient to ascertain whether the drug is producing the desired change. For instance, to provide the same anticoagulant control to a range of patients, the dose regime for warfarin may be very different.

It is noteworthy that effects of some drugs persist even after the treatment has been withdrawn; for example, the anti-aggregation effect of aspirin on platelets can last for weeks after the drug was last taken. Similarly, the enzyme monoamine oxidase must be resynthesized after drug-induced inhibition with monoamine oxidase inhibitors (see Chapter 10). Drugs that continue to exert an effect long after they have been cleared from the body are often colourfully known as 'hit-and-run' drugs.

CALCULATION OF DOSE AND FREQUENCY OF DRUGS

The main aim when prescribing a drug is to achieve a desired effect without causing toxicity. The initial dose may be calculated after having ascertained the plasma concentration needed to produce the therapeutic outcome and the volume of distribution of the drug. Naturally if the drug is given intravenously, the advised plasma concentration will be achieved more rapidly than if it is given by the oral route. A knowledge of the drug's half-life is essential for calculating dose and frequency of administration. When an immediate therapeutic effect is necessary, a larger 'priming' dose may be given for the required plasma concentration to be attained quickly. This is called a loading dose; it must be followed by smaller doses (the maintenance doses) given at regular intervals to maintain the drug levels. If immediacy of action is not required, no loading dose is given and similar doses are given on each occasion.

As previously mentioned, the half-life of a drug is the time taken for the plasma level to fall by 50 per cent. If the time interval between administration of the drug is the same as its half-life, then half the loading dose may be given as the maintenance dose (e.g. first dose = 500 mg, second dose = 250 mg).

However, the half-life of the drug may be prolonged if drug elimination is less efficient (e.g. in renal failure or in elderly patients), and the dose must therefore be adjusted. In practice, it may be more convenient to keep the same time intervals in the drug regimen and simply reduce the dose. Conversely, if the dose remains the same, the dosing interval needs to be prolonged to match the increased half-life. Generally, drugs given on a 6-hourly, 12-hourly, or daily basis afford the patient greater freedom and improved compliance than drugs given more frequently.

THERAPEUTIC INDEX

The therapeutic index is an indicator of the margin of safety between the dose that produces the desired therapeutic effect and the dose that is toxic. If a drug has a large safety margin, a change in dose can be prescribed with relatively low risk of an adverse side-effect. However, if a drug has a tendency to accumulate in the body, it may have a low therapeutic index. The dose that ensures efficacy is often specific to the patient, since considerable individual variation is exhibited in patient handling of drugs and reactions to drugs.

The antibiotic, gentamicin, which is widely used to treat Gram-negative infections, is one example of this (see Chapter 19). It has a low therapeutic index, for the level of drug that causes adverse side-effects in the ear (ototoxicity) and kidney (nephrotoxicity) is only slightly greater than the amount required to kill the bacteria causing the infection. Regular blood tests are therefore advised to monitor drug levels so that the dose can be adjusted accordingly. Unfortunately, with some therapies, the side-effects of the drug imitate the disease they have been prescribed to treat. For instance, an increased frequency of epileptic fits is a noted side-effect of phenytoin toxicity, and this could be exacerbated if more phenytoin was prescribed in an effort to reduce their incidence. Regular evaluation of plasma drug levels allows the prescriber to distinguish between a symptom that is being caused by the disease and a side-effect that is being caused by the drug.

A knowledge of the patient's body weight is often required when calculating dosage because it influences drug distribution – with increased body weight there is a commensurate rise in total body water (i.e. water found intracellularly, extracellularly, and in the circulation). Consequently, there is a greater volume of distribution, and a dilution of drug concentration may be found. Body surface area may also be used, but again this relates to weight because obese patients have a greater surface area than their lean counterparts.

Anaesthetic dosages are generally calculated using the body surface area of the patient, because the amount of drug administered has to be exactly proportionate to its expected distribution within the body. This is vital in order to ensure that the level of anaesthesia achieved is deep enough yet easily reversible at the end of surgery. Chemotherapy drug regimens are also calculated using the patient's surface area because a balance must be achieved to ensure that the dose destroys the tumour with minimal toxicity to other tissues.

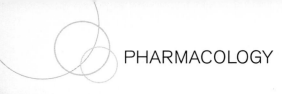

RULES GOVERNING CONSTANT INFUSION OR CONSTANT DOSING

When a constant intravenous infusion is administered (i.e. when no loading dose is given), the plasma level of drug circulating in the body gradually increases from zero until it becomes constant or steady-state when the amount of drug entering the body is equal to the amount excreted or removed. Hence, the rate of infusion may be calculated thus:

Rate of infusion = Plasma concentration × Clearance

This is true for nearly all drugs; moreover, it can be shown that the time taken to reach this plateau (or steady-state) plasma concentration is between four and five half-lives (i.e. it takes one half-life to attain 50 per cent of the plateau, two half-lives to attain 75 per cent of the plateau, three half-lives to attain 87.5 per cent of the plateau, and so on). Similarly, when the infusion is stopped it will take the same amount of time (four to five half-lives) for the drug to be fully cleared from the plasma. The same general rule governs repeated oral dosing, although the plasma concentration obviously rises and falls with individual doses. Drugs given by constant dosing have to be given sufficiently frequently for accumulation to occur. If the drug is given once a week accumulation is not likely, but if it is given every hour it most probably will. Accumulation of a drug within the body arises only when drugs are administered inappropriately. It cannot occur if the dosage interval is greater than 1.44 times the drug's half-life. (This is about 18 hours with a once-daily dosage and 9 hours with a twice-daily dosage).

KEY POINTS

- Drugs can enter the body through a number of routes to achieve either a local or systemic effect.
- Drugs that are primarily metabolized as they pass through the liver are subjected to the 'first-pass effect'.
- Drugs may be water-soluble or lipid-soluble substances.
- Passive diffusion is the most important mechanism by which a drug can pass through a membrane.
- Drugs circulate in the blood either bound to plasma proteins (the bound fraction) or unbound (the free portion of the drug) which is pharmacologically active.

- The liver has a major role in the metabolism and clearance of drugs; this is called biotransformation, in which lipid-soluble drugs are converted to a water soluble form to render them liable for excretion.
- Renal clearance of drugs is determined by three mechanisms: glomerular filtration, renal tubular secretion, and reabsorption.
- The rate at which a drug is eliminated from the body is denoted by its half-life.
- Therapeutic index is the margin of safety between the dose that produces the desired effect and the dose that is toxic.

FURTHER READING

Burman WJ (1997) The value of *in vitro* drug activity and pharmacokinetics in predicting the effectiveness of antimycobacterial therapy: a critical review [Review]. Am J Med Sci 313:355–63.

Cheek J, Gibson T (1996). The discursive construction of the role of the nurse in medication administration: an exploration of the literature. Nurs Inq 3:83–90.

Cowan T (1996). Nebulisers for use in the community. Prof Nurse 12:215–20.

Foster RW (1996) Basic Pharmacology, 4th edition. Butterworth-Heinemann, Oxford.

Gilman AG, Rall RW, Nies AS, Taylor P (eds) (1992) Goodman and Gilman's The Pharmaceutical Basics of Therapeutics, 8th edition. McGraw-Hill, London.

Gladstone J (1995) Drug administration errors: a study into the factors underlying the occurrence and reporting of drug errors in a district general hospital. J Adv Nurs 22:628–37.

Heinzer M, Beitz JM, Dreher HM, Ambrose MS, *et al*. (1997) A program evaluation approach to drug administration education. Nurse Educ 22:4 25–31

Jeffers LA (1996) Anesthetic considerations for the new antiobesity medications. AANA J 64:6 541–4.

Nie GY, Butt AR, Salamonsen LA, Findlay JK (1997) Hormonal and non-hormonal agents at implantation as targets for contraception [Review]. Reprod Fertil Dev 9:65–76.

Saivin S, Pavy-Le Traon A, Soulez-LaRiviere C, Guell A, Houin G (1997) Pharmacology in space: pharmacokinetics. Adv Space Biol Med 6:107–21.

Schneider NG, Lunell E, Olmstead RE, Fagerstrom KO (1996) Clinical pharmacokinetics of nasal nicotine delivery. A review and comparison to other nicotine systems. Clin Pharmacokinet 31:65–80.

Taylor CA III, Abdel-Rahman E, Zimmerman SW, Johnson CA (1996) Clinical pharmacokinetics during continuous ambulatory peritoneal dialysis. Clinical Pharmacokinetics 31:293–308.

van den Anker JN (1996) Pharmacokinetics and renal function in preterm infants. Acta Paediatrica 85:1393–9.

10

PHARMACODYNAMICS – HOW DRUGS EXERT THEIR THERAPEUTIC EFFECT

LEARNING OBJECTIVES

After studying this chapter you will have a clearer understanding of:
- the interactions of drugs with physiological molecules in body fluids and cells
- receptor-mediated interactions of drugs to elicit a therapeutic effect
- modifications to metabolic activities that can summon a change of symptoms and even cellular death
- the use of replacement therapies
- how drugs affect membrane channels to modify a physiological mechanism

INTRODUCTION

Pharmacodynamics is concerned with the precise activities of a drug which ultimately leads to a therapeutic outcome but which, on occasions, can lead to toxicity and adverse side-effects. In Chapter 9, the various barriers to be overcome by the drug were discussed, as was the time delay between drug administration and the onset of a beneficial effect. Whatever the route of administration, most drugs modify a physiological or pathological process either by interacting with a cellular component or by influencing a chemical reaction in the body. This chapter discusses how some of these mechanisms operate to treat a disorder or, at the very least, to alleviate undesirable symptoms.

HOW DO DRUGS ACT?

Many forms of biological communication rely on the release of chemical messengers (e.g. hormones, neurotransmitters, cytokines) that disperse through body fluids to influence the activity of a target cell or organ. Such molecules mainly operate by binding to receptors located on the outer cell membrane, although some penetrate and attach to intracellular receptors in the cytoplasm or on the nucleus (see Chapter 1).

A substance that binds to a receptor may be referred to as a ligand. Accordingly drug-receptor binding provides a stimulatory or inhibitory signal to promote a change in cellular function. Many synthetic drugs have been designed to mimic a naturally occurring molecule in order to modify a disease process. Thus, an in-depth knowledge of the normal physiological as well as the pathological mechanisms is essential when designing a drug.

Drugs may also elicit change by interfering with a metabolic reaction associated with the disease or one that could modify the disease. Some drugs have been synthesized to act as bogus, non-functional metabolites. Thus, when incorporated into part of a metabolic pathway, they form a block and halt the progress of metabolism along that pathway. Moreover, as these reactions are catalysed by enzymes, an alternative strategy has also been contrived for a drug-induced stimulation or inhibition of enzyme activity. Specificity is one of the important issues with these types of drug activities so that a drug targets or modifies only the precise enzyme system intended. If a drug affects other metabolic pathways, it could result in undesirable side-effects.

Cellular metabolism operates effectively when the precise ionic composition of the intracellular environment is maintained and when there is an adequate supply of nutrients. Therefore, the plasma membrane has a fundamental role in the selective transport of ions and molecules between the intracellular and extracellular fluids. Accordingly, membrane-bound ion channels control the concentration of ions (e.g. hydrogen, sodium, potassium, chloride, calcium), which are required in physiological processes, including metabolic pathways.

Some drugs can indirectly modify a physiological function by their influence on ion channels by:
• blocking the channels completely;
• preventing the channels from opening or closing; or
• inhibiting a functional component of the channel.

DRUGS THAT MODIFY RECEPTOR MECHANISMS IN CELLULAR MEMBRANES

A great number of drugs act by binding to membrane receptors located on the cell surface. However, these receptors have evolved to respond to naturally occurring signal molecules, such as neurotransmitters, hormones, and cytokines, not to synthetic drugs; it is by chance there is a reaction in response to drug–receptor binding. Receptors are coupled to various types of cellular functions. Some changes occur within milliseconds, like muscle contraction following release of the neurotransmitter acetylcholine into the synapse of a neuromuscular junction. Other physiological changes occur much more slowly. For example, thyroxine-induced effect on metabolism occurs several minutes or even hours after its release from the thyroid gland.

In summary, then, communication via nerve impulse transmission is rapid (Figure 10.1), and communication via hormone release is slower but the effect is longer lasting (Figure 10.2).

EVIDENCE OF CHEMICAL MESSENGERS IN THE BODY

In the 1920s, a German pharmacologist, Otto Loewi, was interested in understanding the mechanism by which the vagus nerve controls the heart rate. He went on to provide some of the first irrefutable evidence to suggest that chemical messengers were an integral part of nerve impulse transmission. In one of his experiments he took two hearts, which he immersed in separate tissue culture baths and stimulated them to maintain continuous beating. The vagus nerve was still attached to one of the organs, and when the nerve was activated, the heart slowed and finally stopped beating. Loewi examined his results and considered that, if a chemical messenger was responsible, then it could have been released into the tissue culture fluid.

Therefore, he removed the culture medium from the bath containing the heart that had stopped, and added it to the bath containing the second heart which was still beating – the outcome was that the second heart stopped. About 5 years later, Loewi demonstrated that the chemical messenger released by the vagus nerve was acetylcholine.

There are various neurotransmitters, which are classed as monoamines, amino acids, or peptides. Information from the study of their structure and role in normal cell functions has been used to synthesize drugs that bind to their specific receptors. Accordingly, these compounds are tested in biological systems to evaluate their potential use in therapy. However, there are multiple receptor subtypes for certain neurotransmitters, and the subsequent outcome of receptor binding varies, depending on the tissue being modified. For instance, when adrenaline is released into the peripheral circulation and binds to alpha-adrenoreceptors on the blood vessels, it causes vasoconstriction. This results in blood flow being reduced to areas such as the skin because of the hormone-induced stimulation of smooth muscle contraction in the endothelium. However, adrenaline also has a vasodilatory effect on the cardiac circulation and respiratory tract, because when it binds to their beta-2-adrenoreceptors, the smooth muscle relaxes. Yet another receptor subtype, the beta-1-adrenoreceptor, stimulates the heart rate in response to adrenaline. Clearly, binding of the same hormone to these three types of adrenaline receptors provokes different physiological effects (Figure 10.3). Therefore, in the development of a drug to mimic the effect of a naturally occurring substance like adrenaline, it is essential to design a molecule that will specifically target the receptor subtype of interest in order to limit the chances of an unwanted side-effect.

DRUGS THAT ARE RECEPTOR AGONISTS

When a drug binds to the receptor and causes a measurable change in the cellular function, it is called an 'agonist', a term which was derived from the Greek word meaning 'to act'. When an agonist binds to a receptor, it may bring about a transformation in symptoms by direct action. For instance, salbutamol is a bronchodilator drug used in the treatment of asthma. It is an agonist that binds to the beta-2-adrenoreceptor (an adrenaline receptor subtype) and stimulates dilation of the bronchi via the action on smooth muscle. Salbutamol is a topical drug given via an inhaler or nebulizer, and in effect relieves the bronchoconstriction experienced in an asthma attack. However, because the drug 'mimics' adrenaline, excess use can provoke a marked tremor, which resembles the natural response

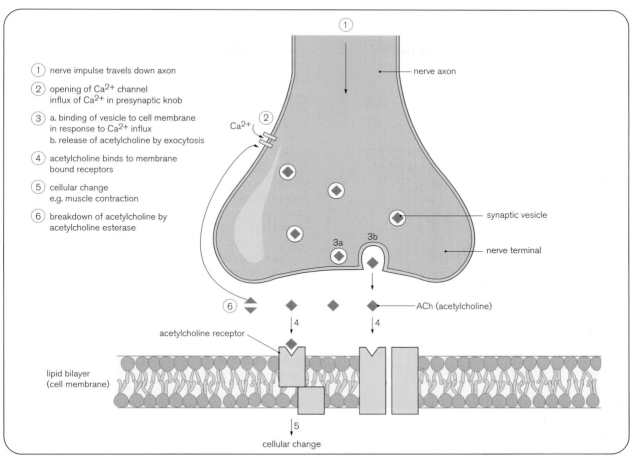

Figure 10.1 Transmission of nerve impulses.

found in excitement or panic. Adrenaline is an endogenous hormone, but it is also an agonist given intravenously in certain medical emergencies, and one of the first lines of treatment for patients in anaphylactic shock (see Chapters 13 and 26). It is also added to local anaesthetic drug preparations because of its vasoconstrictive properties. The anaesthetic effect abates as the blood flowing through the area removes the drug, therefore vasoconstriction by adrenaline assists in prolonging the pain control.

Opium has been used as a drug and narcotic since 4000 BC, and its effects are produced as a result of opioid receptor-binding. These receptors are found on different organs and tissues, thus ensuring that the reaction to a narcotic or natural opiate is tissue-dependent. Drugs such as morphine have opiate-like properties and are prescribed for effective control of pain, for instance in terminal cancer. Morphine and its derivative diamorphine (heroin) may be given as an oral preparation, or

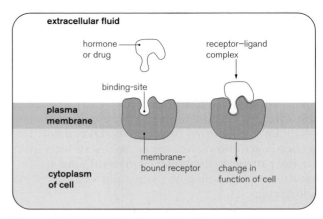

Figure 10.2 Modification of cell function by a hormone or drug. Hormone or drug may bind to a cell-surface receptor to form a receptor–ligand complex and thus cause a change in the function of the cell.

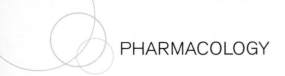

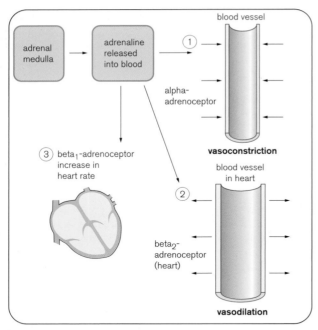

Figure 10.3 Effects of adrenaline. Adrenaline is released from the renal medulla and, depending on the subtype of receptor, exerts various effects.

by injection (intramuscular, intravenous, or subcutaneous) since both drugs are rapidly metabolized by the liver (see Chapter 14).

In an attempt to study the mechanisms by which morphine provides pain control, drugs with a chemical structure that is similar to the naturally occurring compound have been synthesized – the so-called synthetic derivatives or analogues. However, having prepared these analogues, it has been found that only specific forms of morphine actually relieve pain. Methadone is a morphine analogue with prolonged opiate-like activity; it has been used in detoxification programmes for heroin addiction, but regrettably, some patients become dependent on methadone. A well-known oral preparation, kaolin and morphine, is available without prescription for gastrointestinal disturbances, because of the inhibitory effect of morphine on gut motility. Another opiate, codeine, has analgesic and antitussive activity, but exerts little effect on the gastrointestinal tract. Patients do not tend to misuse codeine, unlike the situation with morphine and heroin.

DRUGS THAT ARE RECEPTOR ANTAGONISTS

Antagonists are drugs that bind to a receptor and prevent other molecules from binding there. Propanolol

is one example. It is prescribed for angina pectoris and cardiac arrhythmias. As a receptor antagonist, it brings about a decrease in heart rate, cardiac output, and myocardial contractility. It is sometimes referred to as a beta-blocker because it opposes the action of adrenaline and noradrenaline by blocking the active site of beta-1-receptors and beta-2-receptors. Therefore, because the beta-blocker is bound to the receptor, it prevents the tissue's active response to adrenaline and noradrenaline. However, it only competes for binding so the effects of propanolol are reversible provided the receptors can be flooded with sufficient natural neurotransmitter or an agonist to dislodge the drug. For instance, dobutamine is an example of a beta-1-agonist that is used to improve cardiac function in patients with congestive cardiac failure.

Similarly, the antidote for heroin overdose, naloxone, is a receptor antagonist which may be given intravenously to produce a rapid effect – heroin is a powerful agonist that binds to opiate receptors and can induce potentially fatal respiratory depression. Naloxone is therefore an extremely useful opiate receptor antagonist to displace heroin (Figure 10.4). Thus, by occupying the receptors, the adverse consequences of high doses of heroin may be negated.

Metoclopramide is frequently the anti-emetic of choice and may be given orally or as an injection (intramuscular or intravenous). It is particularly effective for patients receiving the chemotherapeutic drugs that cause nausea (e.g. cisplatin). *How does metoclopramide alleviate the symptoms of nausea?* As a dopamine receptor antagonist, it targets the chemoreceptor trigger

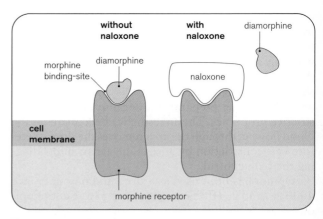

Figure 10.4 Effects of naloxone. Naloxone is a competitive antagonist of morphine and its derivative, diamorphine (heroin). It competes for the binding sites of morphine receptors, and remains bound for longer than morphine and diamorphine, thus blocking their effects on the cell.

zone in the brain and blocks the vomiting reflex. In addition, metoclopramide acts locally within the gut to enhance motility and promote gastric emptying; hence it has a practical use for preparing patients for certain radiological procedures. However, there are some adverse side-effects to be aware of, including fatigue, dizziness, and diarrhoea.

The antihistamine drugs utilized in the treatment of allergies must be some of the best-known receptor antagonists. When mast cells are triggered in an allergic reaction, they degranulate and release histamine, which disperses through body fluids (see Chapters 13 and 26). When histamine binds to the histamine receptors on blood vessels and in the external surfaces, uncomfortable symptoms are produced (e.g. sore eyes, rhinitis, rash, and occasionally anaphylactic shock, which is extremely serious). There are two different types of histamine receptor, H_1 receptors and H_2 receptors. Antihistamine drugs do not block all histamine activity within the body; rather, they inhibit only the actions mediated by the H_1 receptors, and thereby reduce itching, inflammation, vascular permeability, and vasodilatation. Certain antihistamines have a sedative effect. One preparation, terfenadine, is no longer available as an over-the-counter medication because there have been cases of cardiac arrest and death following treatment (see Chapter 26).

In contrast, the H_2 receptors are responsible for the signalling effects of histamine on cardiac acceleration and gastric secretion, which are not generally affected by antihistamine drugs. However cimetidine binds specifically to H_2 receptors in the stomach to reduce the secretion of gastric acid, because it is a competitive receptor antagonist; it is often prescribed to patients with peptic ulcers.

REVERSIBLE AND IRREVERSIBLE RECEPTOR ANTAGONIST EFFECTS

Receptor antagonists may be loosely divided into two classes: reversible antagonists and irreversible antagonists. A reversible antagonist competes with the natural ligand (or an agonist drug) for the receptor binding site. Therefore, if sufficient ligand or agonist is available, the effects of the antagonist can be counteracted. So, for example, an agonist drug that is prescribed at a sufficient dose will alleviate the effects of the antagonist. With more agonist molecules available to 'flood the system', the antagonist is dislodged. Cimetidine and naloxone are examples of competitive receptor antagonists.

Conversely, the effects of a drug that is an irreversible receptor antagonist are prolonged, for once bound it is not dislodged from the receptor by even high doses of the agonist (i.e. it is non-competitive). In fact, in many instances the receptor is 'wrecked', and becomes inactive. Phenoxybenzamine is an irreversible antagonist of alpha-adrenergic receptors and is prescribed to control hypertension. However, as the drug is non-competitive, the therapeutic effects are perpetuated even after cessation of treatment, and they only subside as the cells synthesize more receptor molecules. Thus

---

PERSON-CENTRED STUDY: THE EFFECTS OF ADRENALINE

Joseph was an ice cream vendor aged 52 years. He had complained of intermittent headache, tremor, palpitations, and anxiety. He noticed that when he took codeine tablets they only succeeded in making his headaches worse. Finally, Joseph went to his general practitioner. On two separate appointments it was found that his blood pressure was extremely variable and very high on occasions (it ranged from 135/70 to 240/160). Therefore he was referred to the local hospital where a high urinary level of adrenaline was detected. The presence of an adrenal tumour was confirmed by computerized tomography. It was explained to Joseph that the codeine tablets had promoted the release of more adrenaline from the adrenal glands, hence his headaches had become worse when he had taken them. Whilst awaiting surgery, his symptoms were treated with beta-blockers and the alpha-blocker, phentolamine, in order to reduce the adverse effects of the excess adrenaline. However, because his blood pressure was so difficult to manage, his alpha-blocker had to be changed to phenoxybenzamine. The rationale for this change was that the influence of phenoxybenzamine on blood pressure is generally more prolonged because it is an irreversible receptor antagonist. However, in order to maintain a strict control on his erratic blood pressure during surgery, Joseph was given phentolamine as an infusion because the effects are reversible since it is a competitive receptor antagonist.

hypotension may be precipitated in patients who are overdosed. Hence, many clinicians prefer to use another drug, phentolamine, which is a reversible antagonist of alpha-adrenergic receptors (see Person-Centred Study: The Effects of Adrenaline).

DRUGS AND HORMONES THAT BIND TO INTRACELLULAR RECEPTORS

Steroid hormones, such as cortisone, oestrogens, progesterones, and androgens, mediate a response by penetrating the cell. Unlike peptide hormones, steroids bind to a cytoplasmic carrier and are then transported as a complex into the nucleus. In turn, the transcription of specific genes is regulated by steroids. It is recognized that some malignant breast tumours are hormone-dependent and rapidly divide in the presence of oestrogen. Thus the anti-oestrogen drug, tamoxifen, has an inhibitory influence on tumour growth by competing with the endogenous hormone for nuclear receptors. Once bound to the oestrogen receptor, the drug is not readily dissociated. Treatment with tamoxifen has been particularly effective in postmenopausal women. However, it is contraindicated during pregnancy and can cause vaginal bleeding and dizziness.

AFFINITY AND EFFICACY

The main physiological function of a receptor is to relay a signal after binding to a ligand (or to a drug). If it is a reliable signal, the cell is programmed to react accordingly. However, more than one drug preparation or ligand may bind to a given receptor, and some bind with greater affinity than others; this has implications for drug dosage. The affinity is determined by the chemical bonds that couple the drug and receptor together. A larger dose of a drug that binds with low affinity is needed in order to produce the same therapeutic effect as a drug exhibiting high affinity. Hence, the therapeutic responses of different drugs may be compared – the maximum dose is attained when all receptors are occupied. Where a drug is highly potent, a lower dose may achieve the same therapeutic outcome as a much higher dose of a drug which is not as potent. This property has certain implications for drugs with a low therapeutic index, such as gentamicin and cyclosporin A, which have a narrow margin of safety. If a drug can be given at a lower dose to achieve the desired outcome, then the incidence of adverse side-effects may be reduced.

Predicting the Therapeutic Response to a Drug Dosage
In order to predict the response to a drug, one must evaluate the relationship between the dosage and the

therapeutic effect. In cases when the drug interacts with a receptor, this is relatively straightforward. Since there is only a finite number of receptors on a cell, there will be a maximum dose when all the receptors are full, and any increase in dosage at this point will have no effect. If the number of receptors is reduced, the response is diminished; conversely, if the number of receptors is increased, then the response is enhanced. Empirically, many agonist drugs demonstrate a relationship between the dose and response which can be plotted on a graph. The response is calculated as a percentage (the maximum is obviously 100 per cent) and compared with the drug concentration. When the same data is plotted on a logarithmic scale for concentration, a sigmoidal curve is produced, with a linear portion between 30–70 per cent response, and ultimately a plateau. This type of curve is known as a log dose response curve (Figure 10.5).

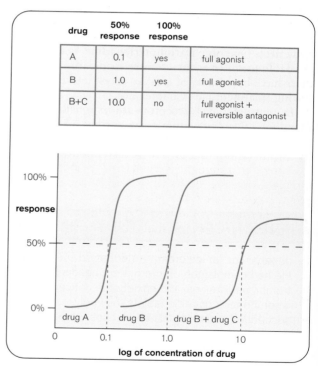

drug	50% response	100% response	
A	0.1	yes	full agonist
B	1.0	yes	full agonist
B+C	10.0	no	full agonist + irreversible antagonist

Figure 10.5 Log–dose response curve of agonists. The log–dose response curve of an agonist (drug A) is shown on the left of the graph. A 10-fold greater dose of another agonist (drug B) is needed to produce the same response as drug A. If an irreversible antagonist (drug C) is given with drug B, the full response is not achieved. This is because of the irreversible binding of the antagonist, which permanently removes the ability of the receptor to respond.

Therapeutic Effects as Direct or Indirect Consequence of Drug Action

If a drug is a receptor agonist or antagonist, its effects are likely to elicit a direct response by the cell. However, an indirect effect may be achieved in which the drug induces a modification in the activity or level of the endogenous substance (e.g. a neurotransmitter or hormone) that acts at the receptor.

Neostigmine is an obvious example – it indirectly elevates the level of acetylcholine in the synaptic cleft of neuromuscular junctions (see below). Similarly, cromolyn sodium, prescribed as a drug for inhalation, has an indirect action. It blocks the release of histamine and other inflammatory mediators from mast cells within the respiratory tract that would otherwise precipitate an asthma attack. Theophylline is an alternative treatment for asthma; it inhibits mast cell degranulation by another strategy – it inhibits the metabolism of cyclic AMP and so elevates the intracellular concentration of this compound, which encourages bronchiolar muscle relaxation (see Chapter 26).

Previous studies have shown that a reduced serotonin level in the brain is linked to depression. Some antidepressant drugs maintain the level of this neurotransmitter by one of a number of mechanisms; for example, by preventing the breakdown of the neurotransmitter (monoamine oxidase inhibitors work this way); or by preventing the re-uptake of the released neurotransmitter by the presynaptic nerve ending. Fluoxetine is a specific serotonin re-uptake inhibitor that leads to an increase in serotonin levels.

However, although some drugs have proved to be effective treatments, their precise mode of action remains undefined. Lithium carbonate, used to relieve manic episodes in patients suffering from bipolar depression, is one such example. Its main effect is to reduce the mood swings seen in this disease by indirectly modifying neurotransmitter levels in the brain.

DRUGS THAT INTERFERE WITH METABOLIC PATHWAYS

CHEMOTHERAPEUTIC DRUGS FOR INFECTIONS AND MALIGNANCIES

Generally anti-tumour regimes use a combination of drugs that target the malignant cells at differing stages of cell division and nucleic acid metabolism. Thus, cell death is induced by adding chemical groups to DNA to render it useless (e.g. busulphan causes alkylation). Other drugs are designed to be a 'phoney' metabolite that is subsequently incorporated into RNA and blocks its metabolism; 5-fluorouracil is an example of this type of drug. Some cytotoxic drugs inhibit a phase of mitosis by binding to the mitotic spindle (e.g. vincristine, which is cell-cycle specific). Regrettably, normal tissues that have a rapid cell division are often adversely affected by such treatments (e.g. the skin, gut, hair, and mouth). Problems caused because of this are shown in Box 10.1.

Certain antimicrobial drugs modify metabolic activities and may be highly specific for a particular microorganism. Some antibiotics interfere with bacterial wall formation (e.g. cephalosporins); others act intracellularly and inhibit protein synthesis (e.g. gentamicin) (see Chapter 19).

DRUGS THAT ALTER ENZYME ACTIVITY

Most drugs that have been designed to target an enzyme within a specific metabolic pathway elicit a therapeutic effect by enzyme inhibition. Some drugs achieve their effect by attaching to the enzyme molecule. In particular, they have been synthesized to compete with a naturally occurring substance and block the active site of the enzyme. Accordingly, such binding may directly influence one or more cell types. Other drugs have an indirect effect, in which the production or metabolism of an endogenous substance, such as a neurotransmitter or a hormone, subsequently modifies a number of body systems.

Generally, where the drug-induced enzyme inhibition is reversible, the duration of the therapy is governed by the dose and how long it takes for the drug to be

> ### BOX 10.1 CYTOTOXIC THERAPY OFTEN PRODUCES UNDESIRABLE SYMPTOMS
>
> - gastrointestinal disturbances (e.g. nausea, vomiting, mouth ulcers, changes in taste acuity);
> - hyperuricaemia, which is caused by the increased breakdown of DNA, resulting in the release of larger quantities of purines; uric acid is the end product of purine metabolism, and it crystallizes and causes gout and uric acid renal stones;
> - hair loss;
> - impaired bone marrow function, leading to anaemia, increased risk of infections (owing to a reduced number of available immune cells) (see Chapter 20) and depleted platelet numbers (which can cause easy bruising).

inactivated by metabolism and excreted (i.e. its half-life). However, when the drug-induced inhibition is irreversible, the therapeutic influence may persist long after treatment has been withdrawn, until more enzyme can be synthesized. Such drugs are often referred to as 'hit-and-run drugs'.

Aspirin

Aspirin is well known for its anti-inflammatory, antipyrexic, and analgesic properties, which are elicited because it suppresses the activity of cyclo-oxygenase. This enzyme acts at one of the crucial steps in the synthesis of prostaglandins, which are chemical mediators of inflammation, fever, and pain. Thus, drug-induced inhibition of cyclo-oxygenase leads to a reduction in prostaglandin production and release, and so these adverse symptoms are alleviated. The effect of aspirin on cyclo-oxygenase is reversible in most cells, but not in platelets, where enzyme inhibition is irreversible. Consequently, because the prostaglandin metabolite thromboxane A_2 is required for platelet aggregation, the clotting mechanism is impaired by aspirin and persists for the life of the platelet. However, the overall effects are relatively short-lived because new platelets arise from the bone marrow and replenish the modified ones.

Patients who have suffered a cerebral vascular accident (stroke) or myocardial infarct (heart attack) are frequently prescribed aspirin therapy to prevent further thromboembolic episodes. Obviously, aspirin should not be given to patients with clotting disorders, such as haemophilia. Moreover, since aspirin is a gastric irritant, it is contraindicated for patients with peptic ulcers. Children under 12 years should not be given aspirin because of the risk of Reye's syndrome, which has a mortality rate of about 50 per cent. Reye's syndrome presents with evidence of acute encephalopathy, with cerebral oedema and fatty liver.

Captopril

Captopril is a reversible inhibitor of angiotensin converting enzyme (ACE), which catalyses the conversion of angiotensin I to angiotensin II (part of the renin–angiotensin–aldosterone pathway). Hence captopril is classed as an ACE inhibitor. It is used to treat hypertension, because angiotensin II is a vasoconstrictor and blood pressure falls as its synthesis is inhibited by this drug. Clinical trials have demonstrated that changes in blood pressure in response to captopril therapy are more pronounced in hypertensive patients than healthy subjects.

Angiotensin II also influences the release of the adrenal hormone, aldosterone, and thus sodium and water retention by the kidney tubules. However, it has not been confirmed that changes in electrolyte and water balance with captopril therapy contribute to the fall in blood pressure. Nonetheless, when other drugs that modify renal function are prescribed (e.g. loop diuretics), close observation is required with the first dose of the ACE inhibitors because there is the potential risk of hypotension. High, non-clinical doses of captopril can also cause proteinuria.

Neostigmine

Neostigmine indirectly increases the level of acetylcholine at the synapse of neuromuscular junctions. It is one of the treatments for myasthenia gravis, in which symptoms such as drooping eyelids, double vision, respiratory distress, and swallowing difficulties are caused by an autoantibody block in nerve impulse transmission (see Chapter 27). In healthy people, a muscle responds to a nerve impulse because acetylcholine diffuses across the synaptic cleft to bind the acetylcholine receptors on the postsynaptic membrane of the neuromuscular junction. However, in people with myasthenia gravis, there is a relative lack of acetylcholine at the synapse owing to antibodies binding to the acetylcholine receptors. Neostigmine is prescribed because it inhibits the enzyme acetycholinesterase and increases the concentration of acetylcholine in the synaptic cleft. As a result, the nerve impulse at the neuromuscular junction is propagated, and muscle tone is improved.

Phenelzine

Phenelzine is a monoamine oxidase inhibitor (MAOI). MAOIs, as the name suggests, impede the activity of the enzyme, monoamine oxidase. Consequently, the metabolic pathway that inactivates monoamine neurotransmitters such adrenaline, noradrenaline, dopamine, and serotonin is suppressed. Thus MAOIs are invaluable for increasing neurotransmitter concentrations in the brain, and are particularly useful in the treatment of neurological disorders in which abnormal levels of one or more of these monoamines have been implicated in the disease mechanism. Examples of such neurological disorders are depression and Parkinsonism (see Chapter 38).

The effects of phenelzine persist even after treatment has been withdrawn because it is an irreversible inhibitor; it takes 2 weeks or so to restore normal enzyme levels because the enzyme must be re-synthesized. Foods containing tyramine are contraindicated for patients who are taking MAOIs. It is essential that a tyramine-free diet is maintained, because the interaction between tyramine and MAOIs stimulates the production of noradrenaline and results in severe hypertension which could prove fatal (Box 10.2).

> ## BOX 10.2 SOME OF THE FOODS THAT CONTAIN TYRAMINE AND INTERACT WITH MONOAMINE OXIDASE INHIBITORS
>
> wines
> beers, including the low-alcohol and alcohol-free varieties
> broad beans
> ripe bananas
> avocados
> mature cheese
> some smoked, dried, or salted meats (e.g. salami)
> soy sauce
> pickled herring
> foods that have been allowed to decompose and could contain yeast

Warfarin and Heparin

Two of the most commonly prescribed anticoagulants, warfarin and heparin, are both enzyme inhibitors. They modify different areas of the clotting cascade (see Chapter 31) to achieve the same net result.

Warfarin

Warfarin is an oral anticoagulant which produces a drug-induced block of the enzyme vitamin K epoxide reductase. As a result, a proportion of the vitamin K-dependent clotting factors (Factors II, VII, IX, and X) are synthesized in such as way as to be non-functional. The inhibitory effect is dose-dependent, and higher doses of warfarin give rise to longer clotting times because a greater percentage of the clotting factors manufactured are ineffectual.

When an overdose has led to haemorrhage, patients can be treated with vitamin K. By flooding the system, vitamin K competes with warfarin, so more functional clotting factor molecules are synthesized.

Warfarin doses are monitored and adjusted according to how the treatment affects the patient's pro-thrombin time. The results are compared with the prothrombin time of normal, healthy adults and reported as the international normalized ratio (INR). An INR of 2–4 is considered the therapeutic range for anticoagulation.

Heparin

Heparin may be given as a subcutaneous or intravenous injection to assist antithrombin III, a naturally occurring anticoagulant in plasma. In effect, antithrombin III has a 'housekeeping' function to inhibit the enzyme thrombin and thus prevent clot formation. In the absence of heparin, antithrombin III activity is slow, but in the presence of heparin it is increased by a factor of 1000. Heparin itself is an endogenous substance synthesized by mast cells and detectable in the endothelium lining of blood vessels (see Chapter 22). However, for clinical use, the drug is extracted from the lungs of cattle or the intestinal mucosa of pigs.

Protamine sulphate is an antidote to treat patients who haemorrhage following heparin therapy. A 1% solution is given intravenously; this forms a complex and inactivates the anticoagulant.

The haematological tests used to monitor heparin anticoagulation vary from hospital to hospital; some clinicians use the thrombin time, and others prefer the activated partial thromboplastin time.

DRUGS THAT MODIFY ION CHANNELS IN CELLULAR MEMBRANES

Certain biological systems depend on the appropriate supply of ions to provide the optimum environment for their physiological functions. Therefore, the selective ion channels or pores are essential for the movement of ions (particularly sodium, potassium, calcium, and chloride ions) across membranes (see Chapters 1 and 2). One way of modifying certain biological and pathological processes is to alter these channels (usually by blocking them). The intracellular environment is changed when the movement and exchange of ions are impeded.

A classic example is the local anaesthetics that block the transmission of a nerve impulse. The axons rely on the sequential opening and closing of selective membrane-bound ion channels to propagate an action potential or nerve impulse (see Chapter 1). Loss of nerve function arises with local anaesthetics like lignocaine and cocaine because they act as a 'plug' for sodium channels in the axon membrane. Accordingly the passage of nervous stimuli to the central nervous system from the periphery is blocked, and the sensation of pain is not experienced (Figure 10.6).

Similarly, ion channels have a fundamental role in muscle functions, because calcium is essential for muscular contraction. Verapamil is a calcium channel blocker that prevents an influx of calcium ions; its main influence is on heart muscle and smooth muscle. It may

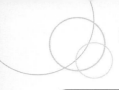

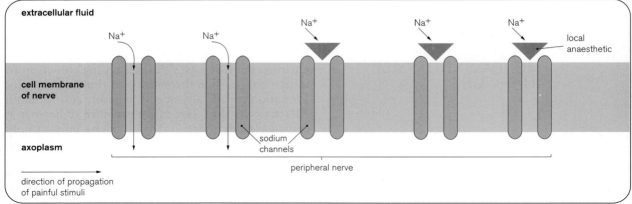

Figure 10.6 Mechanism of action of local anaesthetics. Local anaesthetics impede the transmission of the nerve impulse by blocking the sodium channels in the axon, thus blocking the transmission of sensory impulse to the brain.

be given orally or as an intravenous infusion and is prescribed for cardiac patients (e.g. in angina pectoris, cardiac arrhythmias). It acts by aiding muscle relaxation to slow and lengthen the cardiac cycle. Some of the unwanted symptoms of verapamil (such as hypotension, headaches, flushing, and gastrointestinal disturbances) are caused by the effects of verapamil on smooth muscle.

Certain diuretics increase the volume of urinary output by inhibiting the normal mechanism for concentrating urine within the ascending loop of Henle. Normally, the counter-current exchange in this part of the nephron entails:

- the export of sodium from the lumen of the loop into the surrounding renal medulla via ions channels.
- thus the movement of sodium out of the ascending loop creates a hypertonic environment in the surrounding interstitial fluid.
- this encourages the movement of water molecules out of the lumen of the loop by osmosis, so the water is not lost in the urine and body water is conserved.

Diuretics such as frusemide block the transport of sodium and potassium ions in the ascending loop of Henle. Thus:

- the sodium and potassium ions that are retained create a hypertonic environment inside the loop of Henle.
- so water molecules do not move out into the renal medulla. As a result, a greater volume of urine is produced (Figure 10.7).

Frusemide and other loop diuretics are prescribed for heart failure and renal and hepatic disease, par-

ticularly where there are symptoms of oedema. These drugs are short acting and may be given orally or as an intravenous infusion to encourage the sodium and potassium excretion. As this drug alters the homeostatic mechanisms in the renal medulla, more water and electrolytes are excreted. Therefore, regular monitoring of serum electrolytes is necessary. Potassium supplements may be needed to prevent the unwanted side-effects of hypokalaemia and consequent cardiac arrhythmias.

DRUGS USED TO REPLACE AN ENDOGENOUS DEFICIENCY

It might be judged a misnomer to consider replacement regimes as drug therapy, but in certain disorders they are essential. This class of therapy encompasses treatment where an exogenous source is required because the endogenous substance either is no longer produced or is inaccessible. A classic example is the use of subcutaneous injections of insulin for the control of blood glucose in insulin-dependent diabetics (see Chapters 27 and 35). Certain medications for the restoration of an adequate nutritional status may be included in this category; iron supplements (given orally or intramuscularly) are prescribed for patients with iron-deficiency anaemia. Regular intramuscular injections of vitamin B12 are required for pernicious anaemia; oral supplements would be of little value owing to the impairment in gastric absorption that is caused by an autoimmune mechanism (see Chapter 27).

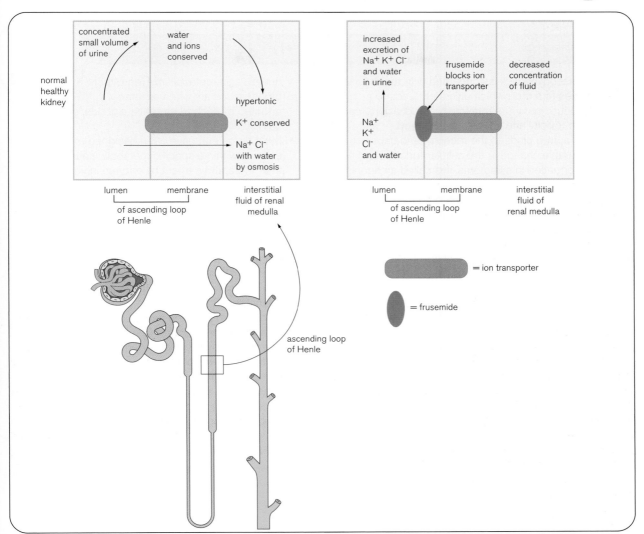

Figure 10.7 Mechanism of action of frusemide. Frusemide blocks the ion channels in the ascending loop of Henle, thereby increasing the excretion of water with the sodium, potassium, and chloride ions.

PHARMACOLOGY

KEY POINTS

- Pharmacodynamics is concerned with the precise activities of a drug which ultimately leads to a therapeutic outcome but which, on occasions, can lead to toxicity and adverse side-effects.
- When a drug binds to the receptor and causes a measurable change in the cellular function and a transformation in symptoms, it is called an agonist (e.g. the bronchodilator, salbutamol, is an agonist that binds to beta-2-adrenoreceptors).
- Drugs that bind to a receptor and prevent other molecules from binding are called antagonists, and may be loosely divided into two classes: reversible antagonists and irreversible antagonists.
- A reversible antagonist competes with the natural ligand or an agonist drug for the receptor binding site (e.g. naloxone, the antidote for heroin, is a competitive receptor antagonist).
- The effects of an irreversible receptor antagonist are prolonged, because once bound, the drug is not dislodged from the receptor even by high doses of the agonist (i.e. it is non-competitive). In many instances, the receptor is 'wrecked', and becomes inactive.
- Anti-tumour regimens generally use a combination of drugs that target the malignant cells at differing stages of the cell cycle and nucleic acid metabolism. Regrettably, other tissues are often adversely affected by such treatments (e.g. skin, gut, hair).
- Most drugs that have been designed to target an enzyme within a specific metabolic pathway elicit their therapeutic effect by enzyme inhibition.
- Where the drug-induced enzyme inhibition is reversible, the duration of the therapeutic effect is governed by the dose and the half-life, as with the ACE inhibitor, captopril, for example.
- In irreversible drug-induced inhibition, the therapeutic influence may persist long after treatment has been withdrawn, until more enzyme can be synthesized, as is the case with the MAOI, phenelzine, for example.
- Certain biological and pathological processes alter membrane ion channels (usually by blocking them), thereby eliciting a change in the intracellular environment by impeding the movement and exchange of ions. Local anaesthetics such as cocaine work in this way.
- Replacement regimens encompass treatments in which an exogenous source is required because the endogenous substance either is no longer produced or is inaccessible.

FURTHER READING

Ebling WF, Levy G (1996) Population pharmacodynamics: strategies for concentration- and effect-controlled clinical trials. Ann Pharmacother 30:12–19.

Garg R, Yusuf S (1997) Overview of randomized trials of angiotensin converting enzyme inhibitors on mortality and morbidity of patients with heart failure. JAMA 273:1450–6.

Hunt D (1998) Low-molecular-weight heparins in clinical practice. South Med J 91:2–10.

Kennedy MJ (1997) Systemic therapy for breast cancer. Cur Opin Oncol 9:532–9.

Laurence DR, Bennett PN, Brown MJ (1997) Clinical Pharmacology, 8th edition. Churchill Livingstone, Edinbugh.

Melethil S (1995) Pharmacokinetics and pharmacodynamics of maternal-fetal transport of drugs of abuse: a critical review. NIDA Res Monogr 154:132–51.

Moyle JT (1997) Correct choice of anti-emetic (letter). Anaesthesia 52:(11)1117.

Page CP, Curtis MJ, Sutter MC, Walker MJA, Hoffman BB (1997) Integrated Pharmacology, Mosby, London.

Tanner HA (1995) Bioenergetics in the pathogenesis, progression and treatment of cardiovascular disorders. Med Hypotheses 44:347–58.

PRINCIPLES OF PRESCRIBING DRUGS

INTRODUCTION

About 65 per cent of consultations with a general practitioner involve the writing of a prescription. Many factors influence the decision to prescribe medication; obviously the patient's health-related disorder is the major component. However, motivation for the choice of drug prescribed in some situations could be affected by the attitudes and expectations of the patient as well as by possible financial constraints. In this chapter, the various stages of drug prescribing are discussed in relation to the choice of drug, the mode of delivery, and dose regimes for providing the most beneficial therapeutic outcome. The roles of the nurse and clinicians in this process are evaluated.

INITIAL STEPS BEFORE PRESCRIPTION

PURPOSE OF THE TREATMENT

Before prescribing, it is necessary to decide the exact purpose of the treatment. Although this may seem obvious, it is surprising how often this basic decision can be the source of confusion. The aim is to treat or prevent the pathology arising in the first place,

whether it is a cure, prophylaxis or palliation. If the patient has an infection, the aim is a cure by the use of appropriate antimicrobial therapy to eliminate the micro-organisms. Yet the same drug may be prescribed as prophylaxis, to prevent the pathology arising (as is the case when antibiotics are given before surgery to reduce the risk of postoperative infections). Similarly, oral contraceptives are used to prevent pregnancy. It is not uncommon for a multivitamin or a mineral preparation to be prescribed to a patient complaining of feeling generally 'under the weather' when there is no clinical evidence of a nutritional deficiency – this is essentially a placebo to promote a feeling of well-being.

NATURE OF DESIRED CHANGE WITHIN THE PATIENT

Having determined the rationale for treatment, it follows that the next consideration is the nature of the change within the patient this intervention hopes to achieve. If the patient is hypertensive, the hoped-for modification is the lowering of the blood pressure. Nevertheless, the physician must also consider the magnitude of desired change and how rapidly this should be achieved – i.e. to what extent does the blood pressure need to be lowered and how quickly?

CHOICE OF FORMULATION OF THE DRUG

The available choice and formulation of the drug to be selected is vast, because drug companies have provided a wide range. Even when the group of drugs to be given has been chosen, it still remains to be determined which is the most appropriate individual drug with respect to the patient and the cost of treatment. This judgement is made in light of further information; questions to be asked include:

- Are there any predictable adverse drug reactions with this drug that could arise in this patient?
- Is the patient on any other drug preparations?
- Could the new drug adversely interact with on-going treatments?
- If so, is there an alternative drug available?

PERSONAL CHARACTERISTICS OF THE PATIENT

The personal characteristics of the patient as well as the underlying pathology being treated are essential criteria to be evaluated when judging which drug and which route of administration to use. Obviously, the oral route is by far the most straightforward; however, it is contraindicated where the patient is unconscious, nauseated or vomiting, or has a malabsorption syndrome such as coeliac disease (gluten-sensitive enteropathy). In these cases an alternative route is advised to ensure the adequate delivery of the drug. It is also important to realize that certain drugs can not be given by mouth as they are destroyed in the stomach, gut or liver before they get to the site of action. Therefore, these drugs must be given by another route.

The use of an intravenous line also allows the effects of drugs to be achieved more rapidly and this is especially useful in emergency situations, but it is an invasive technique. The intravenous route should be used only by a clinician or health care professional with specialist training. Certainly, when giving any injectable drug it is essential to verify whether the drug preparation is available in a vial that is immediately ready for injection. If the drug is lyophilized and requires reconstituting, the manufacturer's instructions must be strictly adhered to; for example, is mixing water for injections or saline advised?

Although an oral drug may not produce an immediate therapeutic effect, this can be advantageous for the clinical management of the disease. A slow-release oral preparation of an antihypertensive drug given for 24-hour control ensures blood pressure control is maintained throughout the night. Patients suffering from cancer who have chronic pain are often prescribed a slow-release morphine preparation, which can provide better 24-hour pain control and therefore give pain-free nights. When treating acute pain, drugs that work very quickly such as glyceryl trinitrate (for the treatment of angina attacks) come in a formula that, when placed under the tongue (sublingually), are rapidly absorbed; this means that relief from the chest pain is almost instantaneous.

Personal characteristics of the patient, such as the body weight, are often significant. A good example of this is the administration of an anaesthetic to infants and children. The main problem an anaesthetist must overcome is the assessment of depth of anaesthesia, and knowledge of the patient's body weight allows an accurate calculation of the dose.

The age of the patient also influences prescribing. For example, an older adult patient whose eyesight and memory have deteriorated, the number of drugs prescribed should be kept to a minimum to avoid confusion. Changes in the efficiency of drug metabolism and excretion must also be taken into account to avoid an overdose (see Chapters 9 and 12).

The effect of other medication that the patient is taking must also be considered. For example, prescribing carbamazepine, an anti-epileptic drug, to a patient who is already on anticoagulant therapy with warfarin could result in a thrombosis. This is because carbamazepine causes enzyme induction in the liver (see Chapter 9), with the result that warfarin is cleared more rapidly, so the anticoagulant effect is diminished.

WRITING THE PRESCRIPTION

On any prescription form, the patient's name and address are required, together with the age if the patient is under 12 years old. (This is because the dose for the drug is likely to be less in a child than in an adult.) It is the duty of the pharmacist to check the prescription and inform the doctor of any errors. Pharmacists should also check for any signs that the prescription has been tampered with, especially if the drug prescribed is potentially addictive or a controlled drug. It is a criminal offence to tamper with a prescription (see Person-Centred Study: Prescribing for a Known Methadone Addict).

All drug names should be written in capital letters. To some extent this is the counsel of perfection and is not always followed, yet illegible prescriptions are not only time-wasting but can be dangerous if the wrong drug is dispensed by the pharmacist. We all tend to think that our own handwriting is legible compared with everybody else's, but for a prescription to be worthy, it is essential that the writing is clearly legible. The strength of the tablets, capsules, or mixture must be written on the prescription, the dose frequency clearly indicated, and the total quantity to be dispensed written down.

Prescriptions are generally signed by a fully registered medical practitioner but there are increasing signs that other health care practitioners may be able to prescribe from a limited list of drugs. Pre-registration house officers can prescribe more or less any drug for hospital in-patients, but they are not allowed by law to prescribe controlled drugs (such as morphine for pain) for patients to take home on discharge – a fact that is frequently forgotten, which wastes a lot of ward and pharmacy time. There are special regulations pertaining to controlled drugs (see below).

The name of the prescriber and the address of the clinical practice or the institution must be given clearly on the prescription, preferably with a telephone number so the prescriber can be contacted by the pharmacist. Writing instructions in Latin does not create a good prescription; English is more satisfactory and clearer on the whole. Yet there are a number of Latin abbreviations that are often used by the prescriber:

- *NP* stands for *nomen proprium* ('the correct name') and means that the bottle will be labelled with the name of the drug. If the prescriber does not wish the patient to know the nature of the drug that is being taken, he or she may cross out the printed *NP* sign on the form, although it is most unusual to encounter this on a family practitioner's prescription form.
- *od* stands for *omne die*; this indicates that the medication is to be taken once a day.
- *bd* stands for *bis die* ('twice a day').
- *tds* and *tid* both mean 'three times a day'.
- *prn* stands for *pro re nata* and really means 'as necessary'. Although a drug might be prescribed 'as necessary', it is essential to specify exactly what the drug is for (e.g. for pain or nausea), and the prescriber should provide advice on the maximum dose and the minimum dose interval. This information may be required by the patient or by a third party who will be administering the medication (e.g. a family member, carer, health care professional).

For simplicity, it may be better to select a drug that only needs to be given once or twice a day, though dose frequency rather depends on the pharmacokinetic properties of the drug. Instructions should be as straight-forward as possible for the patient taking the therapeutic agents in order to promote compliance. With multiple prescriptions, the practice of giving one drug 8-hourly and another 6-hourly should be avoided since this can be disruptive to the patient's life and may be especially difficult for an older adult patient. The importance of completing the course of treatment and medication exactly as instructed must also be stressed; it is generally emphasized when antibiotics are dispensed. Often, however, when the physical symptoms of a disease are no longer apparent the patient forgets to take the drug, which may result in the recurrence of symptoms a week or two later. It can also provoke a drug-resistant infection, which could be a threat to the community (see Chapter 19).

THE NAMING OF THE DRUG ON THE PRESCRIPTION
Proprietary Name versus Approved Name

Once a decision regarding the type of drug to be prescribed has been made, it remains for the doctor to choose whether to use the proprietary name or the approved (generic) name of the drug on the prescription. The advantage of using the proprietary name is that they are often catchy and easy to remember. It is one of the marketing strategies used by drug companies to find the most suitable, pronounceable, and memorable names. As a patient who is already taking a particular drug will probably know it by its proprietary name, it is easier to continue with this preparation simply to avoid confusion. Otherwise the approved name should usually be used.

However, proprietary drugs also come in precise formulations that are sometimes unique to the manufacturer, which is a reason for continuing to prescribe them. Problems can arise when hospital pharmacies do not stock certain brands. Hospital pharmacies are more likely to stock approved-name drugs simply because they are less expensive, so although they might dispense the same drug, it may be one which is marketed under a different name. This could be a source of confusion and lead to delay in dispensing the drug if the doctor needs to be contacted to confirm its acceptability.

COMMUNICATION

Having written a prescription, it is advisable to fully explain the reasons why the patient requires a particular treatment. To encourage patient compliance it may be advantageous to take more time with certain patients (such as older adult patients) to ensure they have understood; it may also be helpful to acquaint a relative

PHARMACOLOGY

PERSON-CENTRED STUDY: PRESCRIBING FOR A KNOWN METHADONE ADDICT

Simon, aged 24 years, started injecting heroin at the age of 15 and supported his ever-increasing habit by burgling houses on his estate and stealing from shop tills. Most of his drugs were bought from dealers on the street, but Simon was also able to forge his own prescriptions using a pad he had stolen from his general practitioner. He was able to prescribe drugs correctly without arousing suspicion because he copied earlier prescriptions. At the age of 22 Simon had seroconverted and become HIV-positive; he had often resorted to using hypodermic needles with other addicts. He has since been attempting to control his heroin habit by going on a methadone programme. He is, however addicted to methadone and finds that his need for the drug is increasing rather than decreasing. Methadone is a synthetic drug that is closely related to morphine but it produces much less sedation, euphoria and doesn't produce the same levels of respiratory depression.

Methadone had been prescribed for Simon to try to prevent him from injecting heroin from the streets which could be potentially contaminated with another substance that had been added by the dealer in order to save money. Substances such as baking powder or even washing powder are sometimes used. In addition, the methadone programme is designed to wean addicts off their addiction by gradually decreasing the amount prescribed. The programme is cautiously structured with dosage regimes estimated to minimize heroin withdrawal symptoms.

In the case of Simon, great care must be taken to monitor his progress and the length of time he has been taking methadone. A common problem with methadone addiction is that, in order to satisfy the addiction, the addict might visit more than one doctor, to acquire prescriptions for maintaining an illicit supply of drug. Simon's GP needs to ascertain whether Simon is tolerating a reduction in his methadone. If the programme is successful then Simon should require a smaller dosage. If he seems drowsy or becomes aggressive when given his prescription then the likelihood is that he is having too much.

Simon's GP decreased the dose of methadone steadily and in order to prevent Simon from taking all of the dose at once, he issued daily prescriptions for small amounts.

---

or carer accompanying the patient with the reason why the drugs are prescribed and how often they should be taken. For patients who are confused or have poor eyesight, it may be necessary to enlist a district nurse to administer the drugs. Although all doctors would prefer to think that patients take all the medication as directed, it is realized that this is not the case. Statistical evidence has shown that something like 40 per cent of medicines prescribed are taken as instructed, and of the other 60 per cent, some are taken as the patient wants rather than as the doctor advises, and quite a sizeable proportion are not taken at all.

Physical disability may also present a problem – for instance, it is necessary to inform the pharmacist if the patient has arthritic hands so that childproof bottles are not used. These bottles may be excellent in preventing medicines being taken inadvertently by young inquisitive children, but for some patients they may be difficult to open.

MONITORING THE EFFECTIVENESS OF A DRUG

When commencing treatment, certain drugs need to be regularly monitored, particularly those with a narrow margin of safety. Measurement of the drug concentration or that of its metabolite in plasma is the most precise means of evaluating the therapy. Assessing the effectiveness of a drug is straightforward if the aim is to produce a response such as the lowering of blood pressure. This is a physiological variable that can be measured before and after treatment. Sometimes, however, selecting the dose and monitoring of its effect may not be so straightforward. When treating a patient suffering from depression with antidepressant drugs, the outcome is more difficult to evaluate.

The duration of treatment requires attention: should the drug only be given while the symptoms occur, or should it be given for a fixed period? Ampicillin, an antibiotic that may be used to treat a urinary tract infection, is usually prescribed for 5 or 7 days (see Chapter 19), whereas anti-epileptic drugs may be given for a lifetime.

Counting the remaining tablets at the next clinic appointment is one option, but it only assesses the number of tablets taken, not whether the advised dose regimen has been observed. It is good practice to encourage the patients to bring their medicines along to the clinic, and they should also be questioned about any side-effects of the treatment they might have experienced. By careful monitoring, the effect of the drug can be evaluated as to whether the desired therapeutic effect has been achieved. If this is not the case, there is the opportunity either to modify or to stop the treatment. Although this seems like obvious logic, it is seldom done, and it is surprising just how many drugs are given in insufficient dosage.

Many drugs cause side-effects; if these are likely to be relatively trivial, it is the responsibility of the health care practitioner to forewarn and reassure the patient. If the side-effects are more severe, a change to a drug that has a similar therapeutic effect without the adverse symptoms would be preferred. Inevitably there will be situations when this is not possible, and another drug may be required to combat the side-effects. Generally, this is not regarded as good practice but it may be the only answer on occasions, as, for instance, when anti-emetics are given to relieve nausea experienced with cytotoxic therapy (Figure 11.1).

In certain circumstances it may be in the best interest of the patient to prescribe a combination therapy, giving more than one drug. This is frequently advised with antituberculous drugs, where the prescription of one drug alone would almost certainly result in bacterial resistance. Therefore the usual practice is to commence treatment with at least three drugs to avoid drug resistance occurring (see Chapter 20).

THE ROLE OF THE NURSE IN PRESCRIBING

At present, most drugs must be prescribed by a doctor, but it is becoming increasingly likely that nurses and other health care professionals will be able to prescribe certain drugs in the future. At present, the law in the UK does not permit nurses to prescribe drugs. However, some hospital trusts are prepared to accept responsibility and have trained emergency nurse practitioners who are authorized to supply drugs from a limited formulary according to stringent protocols. Within these guidelines, instructions are in place regarding the indications for treatment, the drug dosage the nurse is allowed to supply, and the route of administration of drugs.

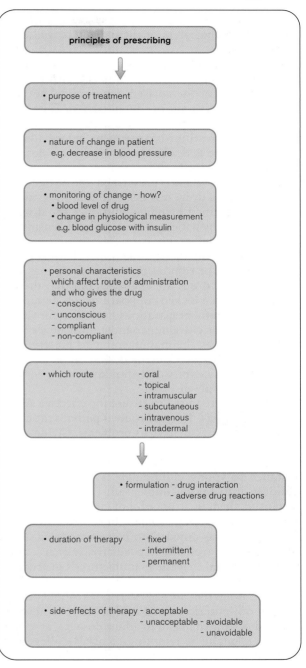

Figure 11.1 Principles of prescribing. These principles need to be considered to ensure that drugs are prescribed safely and effectively.

When a patient is admitted to a ward, the nurse is required to perform a thorough assessment of the patient's physical, psychological, and social needs; all these factors are potentially relevant when estimating patient compliance with any prescribed drug regimen.

When making this assessment, it is helpful to include reports from the carers of the patient as well as the doctor's notes.

Ward nurses are responsible for giving the correct drugs prescribed to their patients and ensuring that they are given at the advised time interval and dose and by the correct route of administration. They should be aware of the potential side-effects, drug interactions, and contraindications of treatment before administration. If there is doubt about the correct dosage it should be discussed with a pharmacist or with the doctor who originally prescribed the drug. When administering a drug, it is essential that the patient is correctly identified by name, and once the drug has been given to the patient, the nurse should ensure that the patient actually takes it.

Some wards do not have their own pharmacy clerk, so nurses may be responsible for ensuring that stock and non-stock drugs are available and that they are safely stored in a locked cupboard or refrigerator. All drugs and harmful preparations (including the various lotions used for cleaning wounds) must be stored as recommended by the manufacturer to preserve their therapeutic activity. Containers that are damaged or are beyond their expiry date should be returned to the pharmacy for safe disposal.

Nurses are required to ensure the effective administration of drugs. The oral route is perhaps the easiest route, but even it can have its problems. Giving a drug in tablet form to a co-operative adult is straightforward, but it can prove more difficult in some situations – for instance in young children. It is possible to coax children into taking unpleasant-tasting tablets by disguising them in a spoonful of jam or by offering a reward. Alternatively, some tablets are available in elixir form or as powders to be reconstituted. Many antibiotics are available in paediatric suspensions.

It is essential that the manufacturer's instructions are followed when administering oral medications. For example, drugs that are gastric irritants should be given with food; enteric-coated tablets should never be crushed or broken in half to adjust dosage. If the ward is busy it might be tempting to ask a colleague to prepare a drug; however it is vital that nurses do not administer medications that they have not personally prepared. In this way, the actual dosage and precise drug is known; after all, it is the nurse who administers the medication who is legally liable, not the one who prepared it.

THE ADMINISTRATION OF ORAL DRUGS

The administration of oral drugs to a patient who has a nasogastric tube *in situ* can be difficult. Therefore, before dosing by this route, the correct position of the tube within the stomach must be checked. This may be clarified by aspirating and testing the fluid with litmus paper to ensure that it is acidic. Alternatively, the injection of a small amount of air while using a stethoscope to listen for a 'swooshing' sound is an indicator of the correct location of the tube. However the introduction of excessive air into the stomach should be avoided. A common ward practice is to crush tablets and mix then with water, then to use a syringe to feed them down the nasogastric tube. Care must be taken when crushing together more than one drug preparation for it is possible the two drugs may react together and the therapeutic effect be modified. Alternatively stomach contents could render the drug inactive e.g. if an enteric coated tablet is crushed. When in doubt it is essential that the ward, hospital or community pharmacist is contacted for advice.

THE ADMINISTRATION OF DRUGS BY INJECTION

Caution is essential when administering drugs by injection. Therefore, health care practitioners should be familiar with the most effective and safe injection sites, together with the potential side-effects that are likely to be caused. An aseptic technique is required, both in the preparation of the drug for injection and in its administration. The correct needle gauge must be selected for the particular type of injection. A needle inserted and withdrawn quickly minimizes pain. In the case of intramuscular and subcutaneous injections, it is important to ensure the needle is not within a blood vessel. Therefore aspiration is advised before injecting the drug.

The solution should be injected slowly to prevent discomfort and damage to the surrounding tissues. Injection sites should be checked regularly for any evidence of local irritation (in most cases the patient can be encouraged to do this). People with diabetes who inject subcutaneous insulin on a daily or twice-daily basis should 'rotate' their sites of injection to conserve the integrity of the skin and underlying tissues.

Anaphylaxis is a potential hazard when injecting into an intradermal site (as is often used for allergens and immunization); therefore, it is advisable to keep emergency drugs close at hand. Adrenaline and other emergency drugs should be readily available on an emergency trolley or in a specially marked cupboard out of the reach of children (see Chapter 13). On wards where such drugs are not frequently used, a check should be made periodically to ensure that the expiry date has not passed.

PRESCRIBING CONTROLLED DRUGS

There are special regulations pertaining to the prescription of controlled drugs, such as morphine and diamorphine. The prescription for controlled drugs must be signed and dated by a fully registered medical practitioner. A provisionally registered practitioner can prescribe controlled drugs only in hospital, since house officers are not permitted to prescribe any controlled drugs for patients being discharged from hospital. For all prescriptions, the specific form and strength of the preparation must be given and the total quantity written in both words and figures. It is also necessary to write the precise dose; it is an offence for a doctor to issue an incomplete prescription.

THE MISUSE OF DRUGS ACT

This Act was passed in 1971 in order to provide tighter controls over the misuse of drugs (it superseded the earlier Dangerous Drugs Act). The Act prohibits certain activities in relation to the manufacture, supply, and possession of controlled drugs. The penalties relating to the abuse of particular drugs are broadly categorized according to the harmful effects that ensue. Controlled drugs are therefore graded into three classes:

- class A includes diamorphine (heroin), lysergide (LSD), methadone, and morphine;
- class B includes oral amphetamines, barbiturates, cannabis, cannabis resin;
- class C includes certain amphetamine-related drugs, such as mazindol, and most benzodiazepines.

A clinician who suspects, or has reason to suspect, that a patient is addicted to any of the fourteen drugs listed within the Act must report the patient to the Chief Medical Officer. The Misuse of Drugs Regulations (1985) stipulate that only specially licensed medical practitioners may prescribe diamorphine, dipipanone, or cocaine for known addicts. Most hospitals have their own standard regulations regarding the storage and administration of controlled drugs, and nurses should familiarize themselves with these. Generally, two nurses are required to check these drugs before they are administered to a patient, and both nurses must sign the 'controlled drugs book' after administration.

PRESCRIBING FOR PATIENTS WITH IMPAIRED RENAL FUNCTION

One of the kidney's functions is to filter water-soluble waste products for their disposal in the urine. Much of the initial metabolism of drugs carried out by the liver render the substances more polar (charged) for clearance by the kidney. Hence, elimination of drugs may be reduced in patients with impaired renal function.

Renal function is particularly crucial for drugs with a low therapeutic index (i.e. drugs that produce a toxic effect at a dose only slightly higher than the normal therapeutic dose). With these drugs, it can be difficult to achieve a balance between underdosing and overdosing the patient because of the narrow margin of safety. Therefore, plasma concentration must be regularly monitored in conjunction with an evaluation of renal function by measuring creatinine clearance.

However, this is only significant for patients with established chronic renal failure, rather than those with acute renal failure (as may happen after surgery, for example). It is a parameter that can be calculated by comparing the level of creatinine excreted with the level of creatinine in the plasma. When the renal clearance is impaired, it is advisable to adjust the drug regimen either by a decrease in dosage or a prolonged dose interval.

DECREASED PROTEIN BINDING

Reduced plasma albumin is one of the clinical features of chronic renal failure because impaired glomerular filtration leads to excess excretion of albumin. This particularly affects the acidic drugs that bind to albumin in plasma. As a result, a smaller proportion of the drug is in the bound form, giving effectively more free drug available within the plasma. The decrease in binding is often correlated with a degree of renal impairment. The effects of this are two-fold; initially the increased amounts of free, unbound drug are able to produce a greater pharmacological effect. However, this tends to be offset by the greater amount of drug being free and available to be metabolized by the liver. In practice, although the total amount of drug in plasma is reduced, the free component remains at the normal level because the excess amount has been available for hepatic and renal clearance.

It is therefore essential to prescribe with caution. Consider, for instance, the prescribing of phenytoin to a patient with impaired renal function. A therapeutic concentration of phenytoin of 10–20 mg/l is appropriate when the plasma albumin level is normal. However, in renal failure, when plasma albumin is lower, a reduced plasma concentration of 5–10 mg/l is required to achieve the same therapeutic control – in both the normal patient and the patient in renal failure the amount of free drug is likely to be at a similar level.

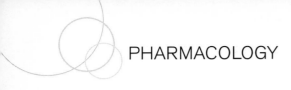

PHARMACOLOGY

INCREASED TISSUE SENSITIVITY

In patients with renal failure there is the possible complication of an increased sensitivity of the brain to a whole variety of drugs, even when these agents are not excreted principally by the kidney. Again, one of the main reasons is the reduced protein binding that results from renal failure. In addition, the build-up of endogenous substances can themselves have a direct effect on the brain. For example, opioid analgesics have a greater influence in renal failure. Similarly, antihypertensive drugs are more likely to cause postural hypotension in patients with renal failure (see Chapter 36).

DRUG THERAPY AS A CAUSE OF CLINICAL DETERIORATION

When prescribing drugs that are capable of causing quite severe and unwanted side-effects, their therapeutic benefit must be balanced against the negative outcome. Certain drugs are known to be nephrotoxic (e.g. cyclosporin A and penicillamine), and these may cause clinical deterioration by further impairing renal function. Others may be considered as relatively harmless, such as the non-steroidal anti-inflammatory drugs. However, they may not only cause sodium and fluid retention but may also lead to acute renal failure in older adult patients who have a degree of renal impairment (see Chapters 12 and 40). Drugs that affect protein metabolism may increase the urea load on the kidney and lead to uraemia and renal failure. Tetracyclines are one such example, and this is a contra-indication for their use in renal impairment (see Chapter 19).

PRESCRIBING FOR PATIENTS WITH LIVER DISEASE

When prescribing for patients with liver disease, the pharmacokinetic and pharmacodynamic properties of the drug need particular attention. It is expected that in hepatocellular disease there is a decreased efficiency in drug clearance. Nonetheless, the measured changes are not as great as might be predicted from the degree of impaired liver function. It would appear that the drug-metabolizing enzymes in liver cells that are unaffected by the disease process are capable of being induced. In other words, there may only be half the number of active cells, but they are more efficient, so in effect there would be less change in clearance than expected. Nevertheless, sedative drugs should not be given to patients with liver disease since the brain seems to be more sensitive than normal to their effects – this is sometimes known as an end-organ increase in responsiveness.

Drugs that are subject to the first-pass effect are very much influenced by changes in liver blood flow. In patients with hepatic bypass of blood (which occurs pathologically in patients with cirrhosis, or surgically as in a portocaval anastomosis), the plasma concentration of these drugs is likely to be raised because they have escaped metabolism in the liver – chlormethiazole, labetolol, pentazocine, pethidine, propranolol, nortriptyline, and morphine are examples. Conversely, in patients with acute hepatitis, in whom there is an increased liver blood flow, plasma drug concentration could fall more rapidly than expected owing to an increased rate of clearance.

Patients with hepatocellular disease often have a low plasma albumin because the liver is the site of synthesis. Inevitably this affects the therapeutic activity of the drug because of the subsequent decrease in acidic drug binding. The increase in free unbound plasma concentration of the drug can cause problems of toxicity. The liver is a major source of clotting factors, and factors II, VII, IX, and X are often abnormal in liver disease, which leads to prolonged clotting times. Measurement of the prothrombin time is a useful indicator of the severity of the disease (see Chapter 31). As a general rule, anticoagulant agents should be withdrawn because haemorrhage is common in patients with hepatocellular disease.

PHARMACODYNAMIC ALTERATION

Hepatic coma can be produced by centrally acting drugs or drugs that cause respiratory depression. Hyperventilation is common problem in patients with hepatic encephalopathy, and it can provoke a respiratory alkalosis. At one time, carbon dioxide was given to correct the alkalosis, but in fact this only exacerbated the problem. In effect the hyperventilation is a compensatory response; therefore, if it is prevented by drugs that depress respiration, the condition of the patient deteriorates.

Hepatic coma can also be provoked by a low level of plasma potassium, which can be precipitated by the diuretics that are given to combat fluid retention and ascites found with liver disease. In fact, any drug that promotes fluid retention should be avoided; non-steroidal anti-inflammatory drugs are an example of drugs with this effect. Obviously, hepatotoxic drugs are contraindicated, not only by virtue of the resultant decrease in hepatic reserve, but also because there is evidence that hepatotoxicity is far more easily provoked in patients with liver disease.

KEY POINTS

- The aim of prescribing can be preventative, curative, or palliative.
- The selection of an appropriate formulation and route of administration must take into account the physical state and personal characteristics of the patient.
- The prescriber should generally use the approved name, but there are certain occasions when the proprietary name has to be used.
- The number of tablets prescribed and the frequency of the dose should be kept to a minimum.
- Monitoring treatment for therapeutic outcome and possible adverse side effects is essential, particularly when prescribing drugs with a narrow margin of safety (e.g. gentamicin).
- All prescriptions for controlled drugs must be signed and dated by a fully registered medical practitioner. A provisionally registered practitioner can prescribe these only for patients in hospital; house officers are not permitted to prescribe any controlled drugs for patients being discharged from hospital.
- When prescribing for patients with impaired hepatic or renal function, it may be advisable to adjust the drug dose regimen (e.g. by decreasing the dose or prolonging the dose interval) in order to prevent adverse side-effects.

FURTHER READING

Bloor K, Freemantle N (1996) Lessons from international experience in controlling pharmaceutical expenditure. II: influencing doctors BMJ 312:1525–7.

British National Formulary March 1998. Pharmaceutical Press, London.

Buetow SA, Sibbald B, Cantrill JA, Halliwell S (1996) Prevalence of potentially inappropriate long term prescribing in general practice in the UK, 1980–95: systematic literature review. BMJ 313:1371–4.

Dodds C (1995) Anaesthetic drugs in the elderly. Pharmacol Ther 66:369–86.

Edwards C, Stillman P (1995) Minor Illness or Major Disease? 2nd Ed Pharmaceutical Press, London.

Fuller D (1995) Simplifying the system. Assessing drug administration method. Prof Nurse 10:315–17.

Kelly J (1997) Prescribed drugs and iatrogenic disease. Prof Nurse 12:552–4.

Lesar TS, Briceland L, Stein DS (1997) Factors related to errors in medication prescribing. JAMA 277:312–17.

McMaster P, Mirza DF, Ismail T, Vennarecci G, Patapis P, Mayer AD (1995) Therapeutic drug monitoring of tacrolimus in clinical transplantation. Ther Drug Monitoring 17:602–5.

Majeed A, Evans N, Head P (1997) What can PACT tell us about prescribing in general practice? BMJ 315:1515–19.

Mason BJ (1996) Dosing issues in the pharmacotherapy of alcoholism. Alcohol Clin Exp Res 20:10–16A.

Medicine Control Agency, Committee on Safety in Medicines (1997) Prescribing systemic corticosteroids safely. Curr Probl Pharmacovigilance 23:4.

Misuse of Drugs (1997) BMA. Harwood Academic Publications, London.

Oliver D (1993) Ethical issues in palliative care – an overview. Palliat Med 7(supp 4):15–20.

Page CP, Curtis MJ, Sutter MC, Walker MJA, Hoffman BB (1997) Integrated Pharmacology. Mosby, London.

Schuckit MA (1997) Science, medicine and the future. Substance use disorders. BMJ 314:1605–8.

Soumerai SB, Lipton HL (1995) Computer-based drug-utilization review – risk, benefit, or boondoggle? N Engl J Med 332:1641–5.

Wills S (1997) Drugs of Abuse. Pharmaceutical Press, London.

Zermansky AG (1996) Who controls repeats? Br J Gen Pract 46:643–7.

THE USE OF DRUGS IN PREGNANCY AND AT THE EXTREMES OF AGE

LEARNING OBJECTIVES

After studying this chapter you will have a clearer understanding of:
- why drugs might be prescribed during pregnancy, and the possible health risks to both the mother and fetus
- the direct effect of drugs excreted in breast milk, and the effects of drugs on lactation
- how changes in body composition affect drug handling in pregnant women, infants and older adults
- the factors affecting drug use and compliance in older adults

INTRODUCTION

All drugs are poisons – there is none that is not a poison. The right dose differentiates a poison from a remedy. **Paracelsus (1493–1541)**

The demand for drugs has never been greater than it is now in our society. Consumers and health care professionals alike share reliance on drugs, to treat a wide spectrum of problems, which is encouraged by powerful advertising. Patients obtain drugs from a number of different sources including:

- doctors' prescriptions;
- over the counter from a pharmacist;
- through complementary medicine; and
- as 'street drugs'.

Regrettably, the use of drugs carries risks as well as benefits because they can cause unpleasant and adverse ill effects. This chapter discusses particular problems that may arise when drugs are used to treat pregnant women, neonates, infants, and older adults, and it describes the special considerations that should be made when drugs are used in these vulnerable patient groups (Figure 12.1).

USE OF DRUGS IN PREGNANT WOMEN

The use of drugs during pregnancy is remarkably common. In the UK, nearly 40 per cent of women take at least one drug during pregnancy in addition to vitamin and mineral supplements. Despite the possibility that drugs may cause damage to the fetus, pregnant women take more drugs than non-pregnant women of the same age. In this section we consider why drugs are used, what effects they may have on the mother and fetus, and the guidelines that should be followed by the mother and health care professionals when using drugs in pregnancy or prescribing drugs for use in pregnancy (Box 12.1).

WHY DRUGS ARE USED IN PREGNANCY

Drugs prescribed or taken under the advice of a doctor are generally given because they are essential for the health of mother and baby. However, some are also used in pregnancy by the mother to seek relief from unpleasant symptoms, or because of an addiction.

Treatment of Maternal Illness

Drugs may be required for treatment of pre-existing illness affecting the mother. It is important that the mother remains healthy during the pregnancy because ill health could adversely affect the developing fetus. Women may also require drug treatment for conditions such as urinary tract infections, hypertension, or pre-eclampsia. Examples of chronic illnesses that may be present in women of child-bearing potential and that

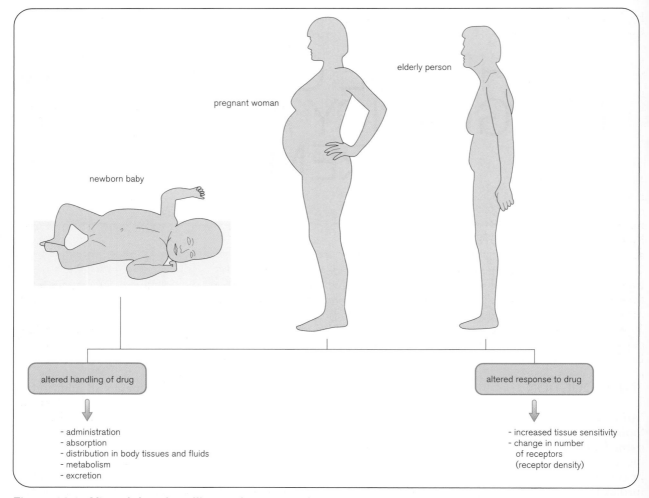

Figure 12.1 Altered drug handling and response in neonates, pregnant women, and the elderly.

need to be controlled during pregnancy include asthma, epilepsy, diabetes, and valvular heart disease.

Maternal asthma
Fetuses carried by asthmatic mothers may become distressed if the asthma is not well controlled and are more likely to die around the time of birth. During pregnancy, the mother should continue to take her usual treatment for asthma (e.g. inhaled cortico-steroids to prevent asthma and salbutamol to treat symptoms).

Maternal epilepsy
Epileptic fits may put both the mother and fetus at risk, and therefore anti-epileptic medication should be continued during pregnancy.

Maternal diabetes
If a mother is diabetic she is more likely to become ill during pregnancy. Fetuses of diabetic mothers may become too large (macrosomic), which can lead to premature delivery or problems during labour. Babies born of diabetic mothers are also three or four times more likely to have an anatomical abnormality than those born of non-diabetics. Maternal and fetal ill

---

BOX 12.1 WHY DRUGS ARE USED IN PREGNANCY

to treat illness in the mother
to treat illness in the fetus
to improve the outcome of pregnancy
to relieve the discomforts of pregnancy
because of addiction

health can be reduced by careful regulation of blood sugar by insulin treatment.

Maternal valvular heart disease

Women with artificial or diseased heart valves may require treatment with anticoagulant drugs to prevent life-threatening blood clots from forming on the heart valve – this treatment must be continued during pregnancy.

Treatment of Illness in the Fetus

Most drugs cross the placenta, and on rare occasions those given to the mother may also treat the fetus. For example, one of the complications in pregnancy of a mother with Grave's disease (an autoimmune form of hyperthyroidism) is that the fetal thyroid gland may also become overactive (see Chapter 27). Evidence of tachycardia and fetal distress may be demonstrated by fetal heart and ultrasound scans. The overactive thyroid can be treated by giving the mother carbimazole. This drug crosses the placenta, reducing the amount of thyroxine produced by the fetal thyroid gland and thus reducing the adverse symptoms. However, care must be taken, for overtreatment can result in fetal goitre.

Treatment to Improve the Outcome of the Pregnancy

Some mothers require drug preparations that are essential for their own health. For example, diabetic mothers must continue their treatment during pregnancy. However, careful control of diabetes with insulin injections is also important to prevent fetal loss and fetal malformations. Similarly, nutritional supplements of folic acid are offered as part of ante-natal care to maintain the maternal health by reducing the chances of anaemia. Recent evidence has also shown that folic acid taken before conception and during the first 8 weeks of pregnancy can help prevent neural tube defects, such as spina bifida. It has been proposed that 200 mg of folic acid per day of folate as a dietary supplement will reduce the risk of neural tube defects.

Treatment to Relieve the Discomforts of Pregnancy

In the early stages of pregnancy women may suffer from morning sickness. As pregnancy continues, they may suffer heartburn, haemorrhoids, and ankle swelling (oedema), which may prompt the use of medicines to gain symptomatic relief. Some of these drugs may be obtained over the counter without a prescription; others may be obtained from the midwife, doctor, or other carer. Women may be addicted to alcohol, cigarettes or 'street drugs' such as heroin. They may continue to take these substances during pregnancy with risk to their own health and the health of the baby.

PROBLEMS ASSOCIATED WITH TAKING DRUGS IN PREGNANCY

The use of drugs during pregnancy requires special consideration – not only may the drugs have an effect on the fetus, but pregnancy itself may alter the therapeutic effects of the drug on the mother.

Effect of Drug Use on the Embryo and Fetus

All drugs must be considered capable of having some effect on the fetus, whether directly or through effects on other structures such as the placenta or uterus. The outcome depends not only on the drug given, but also on the stage of development of the embryo and fetus (Figure 12.2).

- Fertilization and implantation of the embryo may be affected by drugs given from before conception to around 17 days gestation.
- Organ formation (organogenesis) may be affected by drugs given to the mother during weeks 3–11 of intrauterine embryonic life.
- Growth and development of the fetus may be affected by drugs given from week 11 onwards.
- Drugs given around the time of delivery may affect the newborn baby and are discussed in the next section.

Effects of Drugs on Fertilization and Implantation

The effects of drugs on fertilization and implantation of human embryos are poorly understood because damage at this time usually results in fetal loss (as a spontaneous abortion), usually before the woman knows she is pregnant. It is possible for some drugs to have a damaging effect even before conception is attempted. Anticancer drugs, for example, may alter the genetic material carried by the spermatozoa and oocytes, which could cause abnormalities of the fetus if conception then occurs.

Effects on Organ Formation (Organogenesis)

During early pregnancy, organ structures are forming, and certain drugs given at this stage can cause major anatomical abnormalities. This deforming effect is known as teratogenesis, a word that comes from the Greek words *teratos*, meaning 'monster', and *genesis*, meaning 'production'.

The best known example of a teratogenic drug is thalidomide, which was commonly used in the late 1950s by pregnant women to treat morning sickness. Its adverse effects were only discovered when a large number of babies with phocomelia were born in the early 1960s. Phocomelia (meaning 'seal extremities')

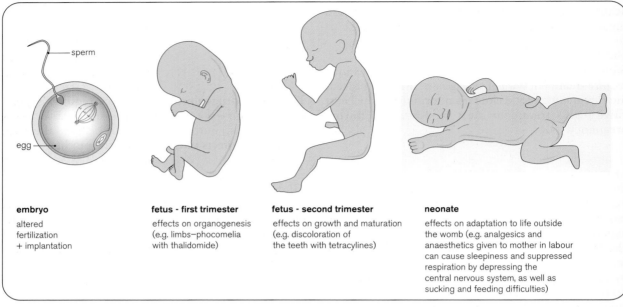

embryo
altered
fertilization
+ implantation

fetus - first trimester
effects on organogenesis
(e.g. limbs–phocomelia
with thalidomide)

fetus - second trimester
effects on growth and maturation
(e.g. discoloration of
the teeth with tetracylines)

neonate
effects on adaptation to life outside
the womb (e.g. analgesics and
anaesthetics given to mother in labour
can cause sleepiness and suppressed
respiration by depressing the
central nervous system, as well as
sucking and feeding difficulties)

Figure 12.2 Adverse effects on the fetus of drugs given to mother in pregnancy. Drugs given to the mother during pregnancy can adversely affect the growing conceptus and hinder adaptation to life outside the womb.

describes the deformities that result from failure of development of the long bones, so that the hands and feet are attached near the trunk of the body like flippers. Thalidomide was withdrawn from the UK market in December 1961 once its terrible impact on fetal development had been recognized. Regrettably, however, the teratogenic effects of this drug have re-emerged in countries such as Brazil, where thalidomide is prescribed for the treatment of leprosy.

Other examples of known teratogens include stilboestrol, which causes vaginal adenosis and adenocarcinoma in female offspring when they reach early adulthood, and warfarin, which can cause abnormalities of the bones and absence of the spleen. Warfarin, a small molecule that crosses the placenta, should therefore be avoided in pregnancy; heparin, an ionized, larger molecule that does not cross the placenta, should be used instead if anticoagulation is required (see Chapter 11).

Any drug may be teratogenic, even at doses that are considered harmless to the mother. Since between 1 and 2 per cent of all babies are born with a deformity, it is difficult to determine the influence of a particular drug on the fetus. The effects of thalidomide, warfarin, and stilboestrol were relatively easy to identify because the abnormalities they caused were:

- anatomical (and therefore easily identified);
- similar in each affected baby; and
- very uncommon in the absence of the drug.

However, the teratogenic effects of other drugs may be less easy to determine, particularly if the abnormalities they produce are:

- non-anatomical (e.g. an alteration of brain biochemistry);
- non-specific; or
- relatively common even in the absence of the drug.

Thus it is preferable to assume that no drug is completely safe when taken during early pregnancy, and to avoid all drugs whenever possible. A significant problem is that during the first weeks of pregnancy, when the embryo is most vulnerable, some women may not even realize that they have conceived. Hence it is very important that a woman of childbearing age is advised to avoid taking drugs while she is trying to conceive or that the couple should ensure that an effective method of contraception is used when the woman is taking drugs that are known to be teratogenic.

EFFECTS ON GROWTH AND DEVELOPMENT

Drugs given in later pregnancy are less likely to cause anatomical abnormalities in the fetus, because by this stage the major body structures have been formed. However, their development and function can still be adversely affected. For instance, tetracycline antibiotics given to pregnant women may delay bone growth and discolour teeth in the offspring. Hormones such as androgens or progesterone can affect the fetal genitalia. Similarly, antithyroid drugs, such as carbimazole, given as treatment for the mother may cross the placenta and reduce the activity of the fetal thyroid gland. Angiotensin-converting enzyme inhibitors (used to treat high blood pressure) can damage fetal kidney function.

Effects of Pregnancy on Drug Administration

Effective treatment of chronic conditions such as epilepsy and heart disease must continue during pregnancy, because illness in the mother may have serious consequences both for her own health and for the health of the growing fetus. Nonetheless, physiological changes occur in pregnancy which alter drug handling by the body, and these must be taken into consideration when prescribing drugs (Box 12.2). Body composition varies during pregnancy. There is an increase of up to 8 l in the volume of plasma and extracellular fluid, and the components of blood are therefore diluted, which accounts, at least in part, for the fall in plasma albumin and in haemoglobin concentrations that are seen in pregnancy. Blood flow to certain body structures (notably the placenta and kidneys) is increased. Around 4 kg of body fat is stored as energy in preparation for lactation, and liver enzyme activity is increased, possibly because it is stimulated or induced by high circulating levels of progesterone.

GUIDELINES FOR PRESCRIBING IN PREGNANCY

Vigilance by health care professionals and an awareness of the risks of drug use in pregnant women and women of a child-bearing age should minimize drug-induced fetal abnormalities (Box 12.3). However if a woman is exposed to a teratogen during early pregnancy, she should be counselled about the risks to the embryo. She may subsequently wish to be screened for possible abnormalities so that postnatal treatment may be considered (e.g. treatment of a cleft lip induced by phenytoin, or a severely affected fetus may be terminated) (see Chapter 7).

It is important that fetal abnormalities are reported to the UK Committee on Safety of Medicines if there is any suspicion that they are drug-related, so that information on the effects of drugs in pregnancy can be improved.

DRUGS AND NEONATES

A neonate is defined as infant in the first month after delivery. Babies are particularly susceptible to ill effects of drugs at this time because their drug-metabolizing and drug-eliminating mechanisms are immature. Exposure to medications may be unavoidable if they are required as treatment for a neonatal illness; however, drugs given to the mother during labour or while she is breast-feeding may be inadvertently passed to the baby. Adverse effects of drugs may be particularly severe in the neonatal period if they interfere with the

---

BOX 12.2 PHENYTOIN TREATMENT IN PREGNANT WOMEN WITH EPILEPSY

The body changes that occur in pregnancy alter the distribution and handling of drugs; this can be illustrated by their effects on the anti-epileptic drug, phenytoin. In non-pregnant epileptics, a large proportion of phenytoin is bound to albumin and inactive in the plasma (because only a small percentage is in the free and pharmacologically active form). Thus the reduced plasma albumin concentration that occurs in pregnancy means there are fewer sites available for drug-binding, so a greater proportion of the phenytoin is unbound in the plasma.

Although the pharmacologically active concentration of phenytoin in the blood is increased, other changes of pregnancy prevent an increase in toxic effects. The free form of phenytoin is distributed throughout the greater volume of body water and it is more rapidly metabolized in the liver owing to the raised liver enzyme activity.

Thus the therapeutic effects of a given dose of phenytoin should remain the same in pregnancy, but the effects may be unpredictable. The overall concentration of phenytoin measured in the blood falls owing to the increased volume of distribution. As a result of all these changes, it is a complex task for the clinician to prescribe the appropriate dose of phenytoin in such cases.

BOX 12.3 GUIDELINES FOR PRESCRIBING IN PREGNANCY

Drug use may be necessary in pregnancy, but it is always associated with some risk to the fetus. The risk to the fetus can be minimized by remembering the following rules when any woman of child-bearing potential starts drug treatment:
- check that she is not pregnant
- advise of the risks of getting pregnant while on the drug
- avoid all drugs, if possible, in the first 12 weeks of pregnancy
- only use drugs in pregnancy if the expected benefit to the mother (and fetus) is thought to outweigh the risks to the fetus (and mother)
- only use drugs that have previously been used extensively in pregnancy and usually appear to be safe; avoid drugs that have recently been introduced or those that are known teratogens
- use the smallest effective dose of any drug given

---

ability of the newborn baby to establish life outside the womb or if they prevent healthy growth and development.

HOW NEONATES ARE EXPOSED TO DRUGS

Direct Use of Drugs to Treat Neonatal Illness

Neonates may require drugs for treatment of illness developing in the first month of life. Babies born prematurely are particularly likely to become unwell, not least because of a naïve immune system (see Chapter 23). Examples of neonatal illnesses requiring drug treatment include:

- infections, which may be treated with antibiotics;
- fits which may be treated with diazepam or anti-epileptic drugs; and
- bleeding, which may require vitamin K therapy (Box 12.4).

Indirect Exposure of the Fetus to Drugs Given to the Mother

Drugs given at the end of pregnancy

Some drugs given to the mother around the time of delivery may cross the placenta and affect the ability of the baby to adapt to life outside the womb once it is born. Certain drugs prescribed for labour may prevent the newborn baby from starting to breathe properly after delivery by causing depression of the central nervous system. For example, pethidine is commonly administered during labour to relieve pain. Although it is usually given in the early stages so that the drug can be metabolized and eliminated from both the mother and the baby before the baby is born, if labour proceeds more quickly than expected, the baby may be delivered while the pethidine is still at a concentration that is high enough to suppress respiration. Similarly, general anaesthetics given to mothers who require a Caesarean section, and benzodiazepines taken by the

---

BOX 12.4 VITAMIN K THERAPY

Newborn babies are at risk of bleeding shortly after birth. Bleeding around the brain (intracranial haemorrhage) may be fatal or cause severe brain damage. To prevent this, neonates have been given vitamin K at birth since the 1940s.

Evidence derived from investigations of neonates receiving intramuscular injections of vitamin K at birth had indicated that this treatment doubled the risk of cancers during childhood. However, there appear to be some inconsistencies in the published epidemiological data, because recent studies have not been able to confirm these data, and it is likely that the risks, if any, are much smaller than was previously suggested. Therefore, the best current advice is that intramuscular vitamin K should be given only to infants with a high risk of bleeding owing to vitamin K deficiency, and that all other infants should receive oral preparations.

---

mother as sleeping tablets or for anxiety, can produce similar effects. In addition to being sleepy, babies affected by depressants of the central nervous system may also be less able to suck and feed properly.

Drugs given to the mother which alter the clotting mechanism have been known to cause bleeding into the brain (intracranial haemorrhage) in the neonate around the time of birth. For instance, non-steroidal anti-inflammatory drugs taken for pain can cause bleeding in the newborn because they have an inhibitory effect on platelet aggregation (see Chapter 10).

Antibiotics prescribed for the mother may also make the newborn baby unwell. For example, chloramphenicol causes low blood pressure and collapse in neonates. Sulphonamides can precipitate jaundice by binding to plasma proteins and displacing bilirubin. This is particularly dangerous in neonates because they have an immature blood–brain barrier, and bilirubin can therefore more readily cross into the nervous system and cause kernicterus, a type of brain damage that is characterized by abnormal writhing movements (choreoathetoid movements) and deafness.

Drugs of addiction

Women who are addicted to alcohol, nicotine, or street drugs such as opiates may continue to take these drugs throughout their pregnancy. The use of such drugs may directly damage the fetus. Babies of women who misuse alcohol during pregnancy do not grow to their full capacity and, if exposed to large amounts of alcohol in the womb, may be born with fetal alcohol syndrome. Symptoms of this include characteristics such as learning disabilities, small size, poor co-ordination, and facial abnormalities. Mothers who smoke are also more likely to deliver a baby with a reduced body weight, and there is a higher risk of death in these babies around the time of birth. The fetus of an addicted mother who takes heroin invariably becomes physically addicted *in utero* and may well suffer symptoms of drug withdrawal after birth. An added complication for babies of mothers who inject street drugs is the risk of viral infections such as hepatitis B or human immunodeficiency virus.

DRUGS AND BREAST-FEEDING

Most drugs in a mother's plasma appear to some extent in breast milk, and they may either affect the suckling neonate or alter the breast-feeding process.

Direct effects on the neonate of drugs excreted in breast milk

The drugs that are most likely to cause ill effects in a breast-fed baby are the ones that reach high concentrations in the breast milk. Iodine (found in contrast media used in X-rays or in seaweed preparations from health-food shops) and iodine-containing drugs (e.g. amiodarone used in the treatment of abnormal heart rhythms) are particularly prone to concentrate in breast milk, and can affect the thyroid gland of the baby, causing underactivity (hypothyroidism) and swelling (goitre).

Highly toxic drugs can adversely affect the neonate even at low concentrations in breast milk. For this reason, patients receiving anticancer drugs are advised not to breast-feed. Some reactions to drugs are idiosyncratic, which means that they are unpredictable and not related to the dose to which the patient is exposed. Neonates may have idiosyncratic reactions to drugs present at low levels in the breast milk. For example, neonates exposed to aspirin in the breast milk may develop Reye's syndrome, with fatty infiltration of the liver and brain swelling.

Effect of drugs on lactation

Drugs can disrupt breast-feeding by interfering with milk production. Diuretics such as bendrofluazide in large doses may reduce the volume of milk produced. Androgens, oestrogens, and progesterones, as well as bromocriptine, alter levels of the hormones that control lactation and therefore they can suppress the normal production of milk. Drugs that have sedative properties (e.g. phenobarbitone and benzodiazepines) may cause poor suckling in the neonate and interfere with the establishment of breast-feeding. Some drugs deter the baby from feeding because they make the milk taste unpleasant (Figure 12.3).

FACTORS THAT AFFECT THE HANDLING OF DRUGS BY NEONATES

Children before puberty differ from adults in their response to drugs. In particular, their variable body size requires that the dosage administered to each individual child is carefully calculated according to weight or surface area. The handling of drugs in neonates differs to that in older children and adults because of their different body composition and underdeveloped organ functions; this is especially true when birth has been premature. Both size and maturity must be taken into account when prescribing in the first month of life, and tables are available that use all these factors to determine the appropriate dose of drugs to give to individual neonates.

Body Composition of Neonates

Neonates have a higher body water composition (80 per cent of body weight) than older children (65 per

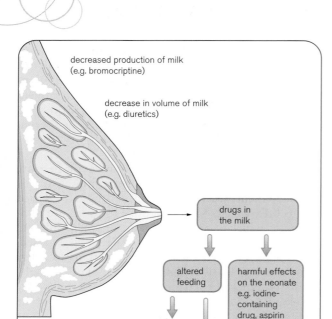

decreased production of milk
(e.g. bromocriptine)

decrease in volume of milk
(e.g. diuretics)

drugs in
the milk

altered
feeding

harmful effects
on the neonate
e.g. iodine-
containing
drug, aspirin

sucking
reflex
e.g. CNS
depressants

altered
taste

Figure 12.3 Effects of drugs on lactation and the breast-fed baby.

cent of body weight) and a relatively low proportion of skeletal muscle and fat. This increases the volume of distribution of water-soluble drugs such as aminoglycosides (see Chapter 9). Therefore a larger dose per unit body weight is given to neonates than is given to older children. Drug distribution is also different in neonates because there is less extensive binding of drugs to plasma proteins and increased penetration of drugs into the brain owing to immaturity of the blood–brain barrier.

Body Function in Neonates

Absorption from the intestine is slower in neonates than in older children, although the proportion of drug ultimately absorbed may be similar. Furthermore, absorption of drugs given by intramuscular or subcutaneous injections is unpredictable in newborn infants owing to the low proportions of skeletal muscle and fat. However, delivery of topical drugs through the skin is increased in neonates because, in the first month of life, the skin has a thin, well-hydrated stratum corneum, which is less effective as a barrier. Thus, compounds applied to the skin, e.g. in dusting powder, may be inadvertently absorbed by the neonate, leading to toxicity.

Metabolism

Metabolism by the neonatal liver enzymes is less efficient, especially by those responsible for oxidation

and conjugation reactions (see Chapter 9). Drugs inactivated or excreted through liver metabolism should be given in reduced doses and at less frequent intervals in neonates to prevent build-up of the drugs and adverse events. Chloramphenicol, which is inactivated by hepatic conjugation, should be avoided completely in neonates, in whom accumulation results in the fatal 'grey baby' syndrome; symptoms include muscular hypotonia and circulatory collapse. Liver enzyme activity increases greatly over the first few weeks of life.

Excretion

Neonatal renal function is immature, and excretion of drugs is poor on account of low renal blood flow and tubular function. Drugs that are excreted by the kidney, such as aminoglycosides or frusemide, should be given less frequently and in reduced doses per unit body weight to limit the risk of adverse events. Renal function reaches adult values in relation to body surface area between 2 and 5 months of age.

GUIDELINES FOR AVOIDING ADVERSE DRUG REACTIONS IN NEONATES

Drugs should be used with caution during:
- the last trimester of pregnancy;
- labour; and
- breast-feeding.

When drugs are given to neonates directly, it is important to:
- calculate the dose according to age and body surface area;
- use established drugs with known safety record in neonates; and
- monitor carefully for adverse events

DRUGS IN OLDER ADULTS

The aim of treatment with all drugs is to produce a therapeutic effect without causing morbidity or premature mortality. However this may be more difficult to achieve in older adult patients, who often take large numbers of drugs and who have poor drug metabolizing and eliminating capability. People over the age of 65 make up approximately 16 per cent of the UK population, but are recipients of over 40 per cent of all prescriptions for drugs. In the USA, Sweden, and the UK, it has been shown that more than 70 per cent of all people over the age of 65 receive at least one doctor's drug prescription each year. In addition to prescribed medicines, older adult people tend to take a larger number of medicines from other sources, including over-the-counter drugs, herbal or alternative remedies, and drugs previously prescribed for themselves (or another person) and stored in a medicine cabinet.

Drug taking can lead to adverse reactions and unwanted effects in anybody, but older adults are particularly at risk. Bad reactions to a drug are between two and three times more common in older adults than in younger adults. Up to one-quarter of medical hospital admissions of older adult patients are directly related to drug treatment, and drug-related illnesses also result in many hospital outpatient appointments and general practitioner consultations.

The interaction of the physical, mental, emotional and social changes associated with ageing put these patients at risk of ill health from drug use. In this section these changes are described, as are their effects on drug action and side-effects. Health care professionals must be aware of these changes and effects when prescribing drugs for older adult patients.

FACTORS THAT AFFECT THE USE OF DRUGS IN OLDER ADULTS

Factors that affect the use of drugs in older adults include:
- multiple illnesses, which are common in older adult patients, and often result in polypharmacy (multiple drugs being taken by the patient);
- altered handling of drugs by the patient (i.e. reduced absorption, altered distribution in body tissues and fluids, and diminished ability to metabolize and eliminate drugs);
- altered effects of the drugs on the patient; and
- altered compliance, which is affected by physical disability, reduced mental agility, or the attitudes of health care professionals.

MULTIPLE ILLNESS IN OLDER ADULT PATIENTS

One of the features of getting older is that it is more likely that several diseases will develop at once (see Chapter 40). Certain drugs that are helpful in improving one condition may worsen or even precipitate another illness in the same patient. For example, a patient given a pain killer such as ibuprofen for arthritis is more likely to develop gastric bleeding if they already have a peptic ulcer or stomach cancer.

POLYPHARMACY

Patients who suffer from more than one disease are likely to be prescribed different drugs for each condition. Hence older adults are often taking a number of different drugs at the same time. This can lead to difficulties in the patient remembering which drugs to take and when to take them. If the patient takes extra doses of a drug by mistake, then side-effects are more likely; conversely, if the patient forgets to take the drugs, then obviously they will not work. The use of several drugs at once may also lead to interactions that may either put the patient at more risk of side-effects or reduce the therapeutic effectiveness of one or more than one of the drugs (see Chapter 13).

ALTERED HANDLING OF DRUGS BY THE PATIENT

Many changes occur within the body during the transition from middle age to old age. In particular, blood flow to organs tends to become more sluggish and the overall number of functioning cells making up each organ falls. The outcome is that function of organs (e.g. the gut, liver and kidney) is reduced, and consequently the handling of drugs by the older adult patient is altered (Figure 12.4).

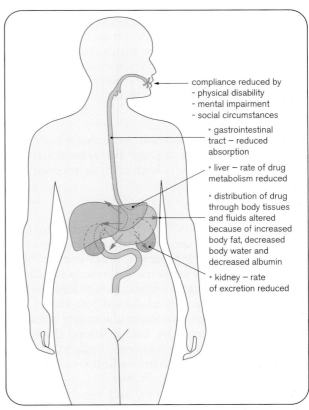

compliance reduced by
- physical disability
- mental impairment
- social circumstances

• gastrointestinal tract – reduced absorption

• liver – rate of drug metabolism reduced

• distribution of drug through body tissues and fluids altered because of increased body fat, decreased body water and decreased albumin

• kidney – rate of excretion reduced

Figure 12.4 Alteration of drug handling in older adults. Drug handling is altered in older adults due to changes in compliance, body composition, and organ functions.

PHARMACOLOGY

Absorption

The effects of ageing on the gastrointestinal tract include a reduction of blood flow to the gut, a reduction in gut motility, and a reduction in the amount of acid produced by the stomach. As a result, drugs may be less well absorbed by the older adult patient. Nonetheless, this has not yet been shown to make a significant difference in the clinical use of drugs.

Distribution of drugs

Body composition changes with the ageing process. Older adults have decreased lean body mass, which means that standard adult doses deliver an increased amount of drug per unit body weight. They also have an increased proportion of body fat, which leads to increased storage of fat-soluble drugs, such as diazepam, (used for treatment of anxiety and insomnia). This can ultimately lead to a delay in the elimination of fat-soluble drugs so prolonging their effects. Additionally, the increase in body fat results in a decrease in body water, which reduces the volume into which water-soluble drugs such as digoxin can be distributed. Thus, water-soluble drugs become more concentrated in the remaining body water.

Most drugs circulate in the blood partly bound to proteins such as albumin. Problems can arise when protein levels fall, which often happens if older adult patients become unwell. Consequently, more active drug is free and available in the blood, increasing the risk of a side-effect from the therapy.

Elimination of drugs

Effects of drugs may be terminated either when a drug is metabolized to an inactive form, or when it is removed from the body. Both of these processes are slowed by ageing.

Liver metabolism

Both the blood flow to the liver and the number of functioning hepatocytes decrease with age, and hence the liver becomes less able to remove drugs from the body. Older adult patients are particularly likely to suffer ill effects from drugs that are subject to high levels of first-pass metabolism (e.g. propranolol and benzodiazepines). The concentration of these drugs is normally limited by extensive metabolism in the liver following absorption from the intestine. If liver function is reduced, a greater proportion of the drug is active in the body and adverse effects are more likely (see Chapter 9).

Renal excretion

In old age, there is a reduction in blood flow to the kidneys, and the number of functioning glomeruli and renal tubules also falls. The glomerular filtration rate, a sensitive measure of renal function, has been shown to decline by 30 per cent or more with normal ageing even in the absence of kidney disease. Older adult people are also susceptible to sudden deterioration in kidney function, for example, if they become dehydrated or develop a urinary tract infection (see Chapter 36). Poor renal function means that drugs that are normally removed by the kidneys are excreted less efficiently and therefore accumulate in the body. Drugs that are commonly taken by older adults and excreted by the kidneys include digoxin and aminoglycoside antibiotic, such as gentamicin. Hence the blood levels of these drugs should be monitored and the dosage prescribed is generally lower in older adult patients than in younger adults in order to limit the likelihood of adverse events.

ALTERED EFFECTS OF DRUGS ON THE PATIENT

Some drugs have greater or lesser effects in older adult patients than they do in younger adults; this makes the goal of effective treatment with few adverse events even more difficult to achieve. The response of older patients to drugs may be altered directly because of changes in 'tissue sensitivity' to the drug, or they may be altered indirectly because of a loss of regulation of normal body functions.

Effects of changes in sensitivity on drug response

Older adult people are particularly sensitive to effects of drugs that act on the central nervous system. Drugs that reduce anxiety or are used as sleeping tablets, such as diazepam and other benzodiazepines, produce more sedation than might be expected from the dose given and cause a pronounced hangover effect. Conversely, drugs that affect the autonomic nervous system, especially beta-agonists, such as salbutamol, and beta-antagonists, such as propranolol, often have a lesser effect in older adults. This anomaly may be attributed to a diminished number of receptors for these drugs to act upon (see Chapter 10).

Effects of loss of regulation of normal body functions on drug response

Cardiovascular postural reflexes normally prevent the blood pressure from dropping when a person rises to a standing position. These reflexes become less effective as part of the ageing process, so the older adult patient is at risk of low blood pressure on standing (postural hypotension). Drugs that lower blood pressure either as a deliberate effect, such as nifedipine (a calcium channel blocking agent) or as a side-effect, such as amitryptiline (a tricyclic antidepressant), may therefore make this postural hypotension worse and put the patient in greater danger of suffering accidents from falls (see Chapters 32 and 40).

COMPLIANCE

For drug use to be safe and effective it is important that the treatment is administered in the correct amounts and at the right times. However, consideration of the ability of the patient to follow instructions is sometimes neglected in a busy clinical practice. Compliance can be affected by many different factors, including physical disability, mental impairment, and social factors.

Physical disability

Physical disabilities such as arthritis or a stroke may hinder the patient from removing the drug from the packet, especially if the tablets are dispensed in bubble packs or childproof containers. This is a significant problem, as shown by a study in Australia in which about 40 per cent of older adult patients tested were unable to get at least one of their usual medications out of the packaging.

Physical disability may also make the effects of tablets difficult to tolerate. For example, diuretic drugs such as frusemide may cause incontinence and distress in patients with bladder problems or immobility which prevents them from getting to the toilet 'in time', so leading to non-compliance.

Patients with poor eyesight may be less able to comply correctly with treatment if they cannot read instructions. Likewise, patients with a dry mouth or dysphagia may have difficulty swallowing drugs in tablet form.

Mental impairment

Mental impairment becomes increasingly common with age, affecting one-quarter of all people over the age of 85 years. Dementia, memory loss, depression, and other disorders may all impair the ability to follow a prescribed treatment regime. Multiple prescriptions considerably increase the risk of mistakes. Studies have indicated that if a patient is taking three drugs they have a 20 per cent chance of making an error; if ten drugs are being taken, then there is almost a 100 per cent likelihood that the patient will take the treatment incorrectly.

Social circumstances

Social circumstances of older adult patients are as significant as the physical factors just described in having an impact on the effectiveness and safety of drug use. General feelings of ill health arising from isolation, poverty, loneliness, or other factors associated with ageing may be treated inappropriately and unsuccessfully with increasing numbers and doses of drugs which have few beneficial and many adverse effects. Older adults have the highest suicide rate of any age group, and it should not be forgotten that some of them may attempt to kill themselves with prescribed drugs.

Successful treatment requires a good relationship between patient and carer. Older adult patients are among those most at risk of the breakdown of this relationship, particularly when they are not perceived as capable of making a decision about their own care. Patients who have not been allowed to have an opinion may refuse treatment. Occasionally these patients may be denied effective or appropriate therapy if they are seen to be 'too old'. Because some clinical trials exclude the data on drugs used for older adult subjects, there is often little information to help carers decide what treatment is best.

GUIDELINES FOR GOOD PRESCRIBING IN OLDER ADULTS

Many of the problems seen with drug use in the older adults can be avoided if a few simple rules are followed. New drugs should only be started in older patients if the answers to all of the following questions are yes!

- Is the drug really necessary?
- Is it the right drug?
- Is it safe and the dose correct for the older patient?
- Can the patient comply with treatment?
- Is the use of the drug to be kept under review?
- Has other treatment been reviewed and stopped if possible?

Is the Drug Really Necessary?

Many complaints in old age may be treated more effectively and safely using physical or social therapy rather than drugs. For example, physiotherapy and provision of aids for daily living may be of greater help to a patient with osteoarthritis than yet more drugs. If these measures are used in conjunction with analgesia they could help the patient to manage on a lower dose of drugs, thus reducing the risk of side-effects.

Is it the Right Drug?

Drugs are often given to treat non-specific symptoms in the older adult. Their use may help the carer to feel they are doing something but there may be no benefit to the patient. It is therefore crucial that an accurate diagnosis is made before commencing drug treatment in older adult patients to improve the chance of success. As with other patient groups, for a safe prescription it is necessary to be aware of any other drugs being taken.

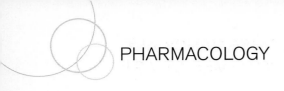

PHARMACOLOGY

Is it Safe and is the Dose Correct for the Older Patient?

Any drug can be dangerous, and those most likely to cause severe side-effects include preparations with a long half-life or a narrow therapeutic–toxic ratio. Drugs with a long half-life are eliminated from the body slowly, so if an adverse reaction occurs it may last a long time. Therefore (when possible), preparations with a shorter half-life should be prescribed for older patients. For example, older adults with diabetes who are treated with oral anti-diabetic drugs are at risk of a hypoglycaemic attack, which could lead to falls and unconsciousness. Therefore, a drug such as tolbutamide, which stays in the body for about 8 hours, is preferable to chlorpropamide, which stays in the body for about 36 hours (see Chapter 35).

Most older patients require a lower dose of drugs than younger patients because of the reduced rate at which they are eliminated from the body and the increased sensitivity to the effects of drugs. Therefore drug regimens should be commenced at a lower dose, and preparations with a low therapeutic index (see Chapter 9) should be avoided when possible since the dose producing the therapeutic effect is only slightly less than the one likely to cause adverse reaction. Small changes in drug levels (e.g. caused by altered kidney function) are enough to cause severe side-effects. Examples of drugs that fall into this category include digoxin, aminoglycoside antibiotics, and lithium. However, it is not always feasible to avoid using these drugs; therefore, if they are prescribed their level in the blood must be carefully monitored and doses adjusted accordingly.

Can the Patient Comply with Treatment?

A few simple measures can be implemented to ensure that the patient is able to comply with treatment. Medication should be given in a form the patient is able to swallow; for example, syrups may be necessary instead of tablets, and medications should be dispensed in containers that the older adult patient is able to open. Instructions should be clear and in writing and language that the patient can both read and understand. Treatment regimens should be simplified, with the number of different drugs prescribed and frequency of dosage kept to a minimum. Patients suffering from mental impairment that makes them unable to follow a treatment regime may need the help of a friend, family member, carer, or district nurse.

A tablet dispenser may be helpful in reducing mistakes and improving compliance. This is a shallow box which is divided into seven columns (one for each day of the week) and several rows (representing the times of the day when tablets are to be taken). The tablets to be taken can be set out in the box at the beginning of the week, for example by a district nurse. The patient then takes the tablets laid out at the appropriate time.

Is the Use of the Drug to be Kept Under Review?

Once a drug has been started, the patient should be monitored carefully to ensure that the drug has the desired therapeutic outcome without producing serious side-effects; for example, blood pressure should be measured regularly in patients on antihypertensive treatment.

Has Other Treatment Been Reviewed and Stopped If Possible?

All medication should be reviewed each time any change is made to the patient's regimen. It is important to consider whether a drug is causing the illness. If it is, it should be changed if possible rather than giving an additional drug to treat the adverse effect (see Person-Centred Study: Polypharmacy).

An example of an unavoidable situation in which one drug is prescribed to prevent side-effects of another might occur in a patient with very painful arthritis who has a medical history of peptic ulcers. The patient may be given a non-steroidal anti-inflammatory drug, such as ibuprofen, to help the pain and stiffness, and misoprostol to protect the gut mucosa and prevent peptic ulcers, which are a side-effect of the ibuprofen.

PERSON-CENTRED STUDY: POLYPHARMACY

Vivienne, who has high blood pressure, is given nifedipine to lower the blood pressure. However, this causes ankle swelling, for which she is prescribed bendrofluazide, a diuretic. The diuretic in turn causes gout, for which she is is given allopurinol, and brings on diabetes, for which she is given tolbutamide. All of these drugs could have been avoided if the drug prescribed for the hypertension had been changed in the first place.

KEY POINTS

DRUGS IN PREGNANCY
- The use of drugs is remarkably common in pregnancy; drugs are used to treat maternal or fetal illness, to improve the outcome or to relieve the discomfort of pregnancy, and to satisfy an addiction.
- In the period of gestation when organ structures are being formed, drugs can have teratogenic effects. The consequences of thalidomide were relatively easy to identify because the abnormalities in the affected babies were anatomical and very uncommon in the absence of the drug. However, the adverse effects of other drugs on fetal development may be less well defined.
- Physiological changes occur in pregnancy that alter drug handling by the body; these include an expansion in the volume of plasma and extracellular fluid, increased blood flow to vital organs, extra body fat storage, and raised liver enzyme activity.

DRUGS IN NEONATES
- Some drugs given to the mother during labour and lactation may pass to the baby and affect the newborn baby's ability to establish life outside the womb or its growth and development. However, exposure to drugs may be unavoidable if they are required for the treatment of neonatal illness.
- The offspring born to women who are addicted to alcohol, nicotine or 'street drugs' often have a reduced body weight, and there is a higher incidence of birth defects and perinatal mortality in these infants.
- Breast-feeding may be affected by drug therapies that suppress milk production. The baby may not be fed effectively if drugs given to the mother affect the suckling reflex or deter the child from feeding by making the milk taste unpleasant.

DRUGS IN OLDER ADULTS
- Older adults tend to take a large number of medicines from sources other than those prescribed by a clinician, including over-the-counter drugs, herbal or alternative remedies, and drugs that were previously prescribed for themselves (or another person) and stored in a medicine cabinet.
- One of the features of old age is that several diseases are likely to develop at once; therefore such patients are likely to be taking multiple drug preparations at the same time. Consequently there is an increased incidence of adverse side-effects and a likelihood of reduced therapeutic effectiveness of one or more of the drug preparations being taken.
- Changes in body composition, blood flow, and vital organ function alter the way older patients are able to absorb and distribute drugs throughout body tissues and fluids.
- The metabolism and excretion of drugs are slower in old age, which means that they are liable to remain in the body for longer. Therefore, careful monitoring of symptoms and blood levels of drugs are required to reduce the risk of an overdose.
- Compliance with treatment can be affected by physical disability, mental impairment, and the social circumstances. A good relationship between patients and health care professionals is essential for compliance, so that older patients feel they are able to contribute to the decision making about their care.

FURTHER READING

Bartnicki J, Saling E (1994) The influence of maternal oxygen administration on the fetus. Int J Gynaecol Obstet 45:87–95.

Berlin CM Jr (1995) Advances in pediatric pharmacology and toxicology. Adv Pediatr 42:593–629.

Bonassi S, Magnani M, Calvi A, *et al.* (1994) Factors related to drug consumption during pregnancy. Acta Obstet Gynecol Scand 73:535–40.

Colie CF (1996) Medications in pregnancy. Curr Opin Obstet Gynecol 8:398–402.

Daly S, Mills JL, Molloy AM, *et al.* (1997) Minimum effective dose of folic acid for food fortification to prevent neural-tube defects. Lancet 350:1666–9.

Corlett AJ (1996) Aids to compliance with medication. BMJ 313:926–9.

Lau HS, Beuning KS, Postma-Lim E, Klein-Beernink L, de Boer A, Porsius AJ (1996) Non-compliance in elderly people: evaluation of risk factors by longitudinal data analysis. Pharmacy World Sci 18:63–8.

McKinney P, Juszczak E, *et al.* (1998) Case-control study of childhood leukaemia and cancer in Scotland. Findings for neonatal intramuscular vitamin K. BMJ 316:173–7.

McNinch A (1997) The vitamin K story (Review). Midwives 110(1310):56–8.

Miller JM Jr, Boudreaux MC, Regan FA (1995) A case-control study of cocaine use in pregnancy. Am J Obstet Gynecol 172:180–5.

Monane M, Avorn J (1996) Medications and falls. Causation, correlation, and prevention. Clin Geriatr Med 12:847–58.

O'Connor TZ, Holford TR, Leaderer BP, Hammond SK, Bracken MB (1995) Measurement of exposure to environmental tobacco smoke in pregnant women. Am J Epidemiol 142:1315–21.

Offerhaus L (1997) Drugs for the Elderly, 2nd edition. WHO Reg Publ Eur Ser 71:1–145.

Primatesta P, Del Corno G, Bonazzi MC, Waters WE (1993) Alcohol and pregnancy: an international comparison. J Public Health Med 15:69–76.

Passmore S, Draper G, *et al.* (1998) Case-control studies of relation between childhood cancer and neonatal vitamin K administration. BMJ 316:178–83.

Roberts E, Snyder D, Friedman E (1996) Handbook of Pharmacology of Aging. CRC Press Inc, Boco Raton, USA.

Sannerstedt R, Lundborg P, Danielsson BR, *et al.* (1996) Drugs during pregnancy: an issue of risk classification and information to prescribers. Drug Saf 14:69–77.

Tripp JH (1997) Vitamin K: mandatory prevention for breast fed infants (Review). Modern Midwife 7(10):22–5.

van der Put NM, Thomas CM, Eskes TK, *et al.* (1997) Altered folate and vitamin B12 metabolism in families with spina bifida offspring. Q J Med 1997 90:505–10.

13

ADVERSE DRUG REACTIONS

LEARNING OBJECTIVES

After studying this chapter you will have a clearer understanding of why an adverse drug reaction may arise as a result of:
- abnormal rates of absorption and the extent to which a drug is absorbed
- inappropriate activities of the immune system
- impaired liver, heart, and kidney function
- the way in which drugs can influence the behaviour of certain enzymes
- genetic factors and their influence on drug metabolism

INTRODUCTION

Between 3 and 5 per cent of all hospital admissions are due to adverse drug reactions (ADRs), and these figures exclude self-poisoning (drug overdoses). Evidence also suggests that between 10 and 20 per cent of patients in hospital suffer from some form of ADR. The exact percentage cited depends on the population studied and the precise definition of ADR that is used. Some studies limit ADR to life-threatening events whereas others include minor ADRs in which the mild side-effects present merely as an uncomfortable inconvenience (as recorded in patient questionnaires), and could affect compliance with treatment.

Although there is no agreed definition of an ADR, perhaps it is best defined as an unwanted action of a drug which does the patient harm. Several factors influence the likelihood of an individual suffering an ADR. Age is a significant determinant – the incidence increases with age because the capacity to metabolize and excrete drugs is somewhat depleted in older adults. Moreover, they may be prescribed a number of drugs concurrently because of the increased incidence of health-related disorders that occurs with age (see Chapters 12 and 40).

There is considerable variation between individual patient physiological responses to a specific drug and

its dose, some patients being less tolerant than others to a change in dose regimen. Between 70 and 80 per cent of ADRs are predictable because they are dose-dependent. Sometimes the drug concentration within the body increases, causing an ADR because the organs normally responsible for metabolism or clearance (notably the liver and kidneys) are diseased. Alternatively, a retarded drug clearance may be due to a genetic factor. These are examples of pharmaco-dynamic adverse drug reactions. Pharmacodynamic ADRs may also arise because certain diseases provoke a change in the sensitivity of target tissues to the drugs; examples of this are asthma and inherited predisposition to epilepsy.

Between 20 and 30 per cent of ADRs are unpredictable because they are not dose related, but have a well defined immunological basis (e.g. allergy to penicillin). These are referred to as immunological ADRs. Another crucial issue that demands attention is that of drug interactions: the ability of one drug to affect the pharmacological activity of a second drug. Although drug interactions represent only a small fraction of ADRs encountered, they are a key factor to be aware of when treating patients who have been prescribed a number of different preparations (Figure 13.1).

In theory, drug reactions that are predictable should also be avoidable, and there is no doubt that the

PHARMACOLOGY

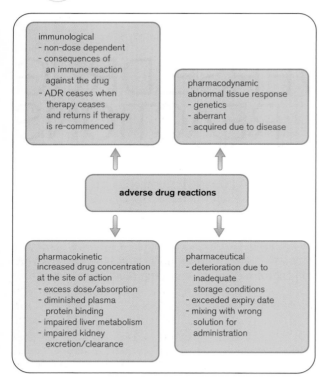

immunological
- non-dose dependent
- consequences of
  an immune reaction
  against the drug
- ADR ceases when
  therapy ceases
  and returns if therapy
  is re-commenced

pharmacodynamic
abnormal tissue response
- genetics
- aberrant
- acquired due to disease

adverse drug reactions

pharmacokinetic
increased drug concentration
at the site of action
- excess dose/absorption
- diminished plasma
  protein binding
- impaired liver metabolism
- impaired kidney
  excretion/clearance

pharmaceutical
- deterioration due to
  inadequate
  storage conditions
- exceeded expiry date
- mixing with wrong
  solution for
  administration

Figure 13.1 Adverse drug reactions. Features of pharmaceutical, pharmacokinetic, pharmacodynamic, and immunological causes of adverse drug reactions.

incidence of ADRs could be reduced if more thought were given to prescribing. It is potentially hazardous to adopt a 'cook-book attitude' to prescribing, in which a drug preparation is given simply because its group has the prefix 'anti', without taking heed of the pharmacological effect of the drug or the health profile of the patient being treated. For example, when prescribing for a patient with depression who suffers symptoms of anxiety, it may be appropriate to give one of the tricyclic antidepressants that have a sedating and anxiety-relieving effect. However, the same antidepressant may be unsuitable if it causes undue sedation for someone who needs to operate machinery. Patients with identical diagnoses may display very different responses to the same drug, even when the preparation and dose regime is the same. Thus, for an informed prescription, an evaluation of the personal characteristics of the patient is necessary; these characteristics include the age and body weight of the patient as well as the patient's pathological disorder.

In the interests of safety, a basic knowledge of the following issues must be considered in relation to the health profile of the patient:

- the mechanisms by which the drug causes its pharmacological effect;
- the mode by which it is metabolized and excreted; and
- the potential contraindications to its use.

PHARMACEUTICALLY INDUCED ADVERSE DRUG REACTIONS

Most drugs have a finite shelf-life; furthermore, deterioration during storage may result in reduced efficacy or an increase in the toxic effect of the drug. Drugs should be handled and stored as advised by the manufacturer (e.g. the avoidance of exposure to light or heat) in order to prevent unnecessary ADRs. All drug packaging is clearly marked with an expiry date, which must be checked before a drug is administered; if the expiry date has passed, the batch should be disposed of. Although manufacturers give expiry dates that have a safety margin, there could be serious medico-legal consequences of giving a drug beyond its expiry date.

Care should also be taken when administering intravenous drugs via an infusion. Intravenous fluids such as saline and glucose should be checked to ensure that they are within their expiry date and have not leaked or become contaminated. Some antibiotics that are designed to be given over an extended period may be added to intravenous saline. However, the process of mixing the drug requires knowledge of and skill in aseptic techniques, because intravenous infusions that become contaminated with pathogens can cause fever and infection.

When administration of a drug is the sole responsibility of the patient, compliance is often a problem. Some patients do not take the full prescription; others may not take the advised dose. For instance, if the full course of an antibiotic treatment is not completed, a drug-resistant strain of pathogen may emerge, and this strain is likely to be difficult to eradicate (e.g. methicillin-resistant *Staphylococcus aureus* (see Chapters 16 and 20).

ADRs have arisen when the manufacturers' change in drug formulation has not been adequately communicated to prescribing clinicians. An example of this occurred when a drug company changed the formulation of digoxin without effectively alerting the prescribers. The new product dissolved more slowly in the gastrointestinal tract and so was not as efficiently absorbed, resulting in lower plasma concentrations. Clinicians increased the dosage to compensate for what was believed to be resistance to the medication. When the manufacturer reverted to supplying the old formulation and did not circulate this information to clinicians, it resulted in an increased incidence of digoxin poisoning.

Legislation has now been implemented to make a recurrence of these events unlikely. However, it is important to be aware of this potential dilemma, since cheap medicines with a different pharmacokinetic profile are being imported from overseas. Moreover, not all countries are as stringent as the UK in maintaining consistency of formulation in their products.

PHARMACOKINETIC DRUG REACTIONS

These reactions arise because the concentration of drug at the site of action is too high. A number of factors may increase the level and retention of drug activity:

- an increased level of dosage and absorption of the drug;
- decreased protein binding of the drug (a low amount of protein binding means that there is more free drug available);
- decreased rate of metabolic breakdown by the liver; and
- impaired renal clearance.

The drugs implicated in pharmacokinetic ADRs are generally those with a low therapeutic index. Consequently it is more difficult to achieve a balance between desired therapeutic effect and toxicity. Nonetheless, when deciding the frequency and dosage, care must be taken that an exaggerated fear of toxicity does not leads to underprescribing. Regular blood tests are therefore advocated with some drugs to ensure that the drug does not accumulate and cause toxicity; gentamicin, an antibiotic with a low therapeutic index, is an example of such a drug (see Chapter 19).

ABNORMAL ABSORPTION

Drugs are absorbed in the small intestine because of its large surface area. Thus, the rate of gastric emptying is an important factor in determining the rate of absorption. Gastric emptying is slowed by fear, nausea, and certain drugs such as opiates and tricyclic antidepressants, and this in turn slows the rate of absorption. The reduced rate of absorption leads to a lowering of peak plasma concentration and a possible loss of therapeutic effect.

Certain diseases of the gut lead to a reduction in the total amount of drug absorbed. A reduced total surface area following a surgical resection of the small bowel can also affect drug absorption. Similarly, alcohol misusers tend to have damaged gut mucosa, which can indirectly reduce the effectiveness of drug therapy. Pathological disorders that increase the rate of transit through the gut (e.g. hyperthyroidism) can

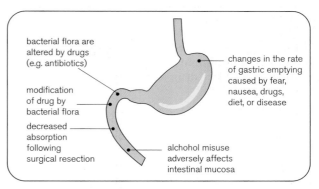

bacterial flora are altered by drugs (e.g. antibiotics)

modification of drug by bacterial flora

decreased absorption following surgical resection

changes in the rate of gastric emptying caused by fear, nausea, drugs, diet, or disease

alchohol misuse adversely affects intestinal mucosa

Figure 13.2 Causes of an adverse drug reaction following the oral administration of a drug.

also affect drug absorption. Furthermore, the normal bacterial flora are an important part of the environment within the gut, and some drug preparations are metabolized by these micro-organisms, resulting in altered pharmacological efficacy. Oral antibiotics can alter the balance of these bacteria – this potentiates the effect of oral anticoagulants on the one hand, yet may be responsible for contraceptive failure if the absorption of the oral contraceptive pill is affected due to changes in gut motility (see Figure 13.2).

ABNORMAL DISTRIBUTION AND BINDING

The distribution of drugs can be affected by diseases that alter the level of plasma albumin. The proportion of free, unbound drug is modified in these diseases. With a reduced serum albumin, drug binding is decreased, therefore a greater proportion of unbound form is available, so the pharmacological effect is enhanced. Nevertheless, to a certain extent the potential danger of an overdose is counterbalanced by an increased availability of the unbound drug for clearance. A low plasma albumin may be found in older patients, in patients with liver disorders, and in patients with certain kidney diseases such as nephrotic syndrome (a protein-losing syndrome). A further complication when prescribing for patients with impaired renal function is the possible availability of more endogenous substances to bind plasma proteins, with the result that they compete with the drug for binding sites; this may lead to an increased level of free (and pharmacoactive) drug.

Most drugs obey first-order kinetics, in which there is a direct relationship between the dose of the drug and its plasma concentration – within limits. Therefore, if the dose is doubled, the plasma concentration doubles. However, unexpected problems may arise; for instance, an overdose can occur in epileptics on phenytoin with a low plasma albumin level. The unbound drug may be within therapeutic limits, even though the overall plasma concentration is low because the bound fraction is reduced. A small increase in the dose of phenytoin may cause a large increase in the plasma level of free drug (see Chapter 9).

ABNORMAL METABOLIC BREAKDOWN

The liver is the organ mainly responsible for the metabolic conversion of drugs. Genetic variation can account for a number of problems but the other important issues are liver disease and environmental factors. For most drugs, the rate of metabolic breakdown is influenced by genetic as well as environmental factors. For instance, identical twins may have the same rate of clearance provided that environmental factors are exactly the same. When the environment differs, their ability to metabolize drugs may vary commensurately.

Acetylation is a common route of drug detoxification; it uses the enzyme N-acetyl transferase. Individual variation in the levels of this liver enzyme alters the rate at which drugs are acetylated. Some people are 'slow acetylators' and others are 'fast acetylators' (see Chapter 9). In the slow acetylators, there is the increased risk of ADRs because the activity of some drugs is retained for longer. Other metabolic pathways are also under a genetic influence; for example, about 10 per cent of the population are slow hydroxylators of the drug debrisoquine, an antihypertensive agent that blocks the release of noradrenaline from the adrenergic nerve terminal and tends to produce marked postural hypotension; this ADR is most obvious in patients who metabolize debrisoquine slowly.

Liver Disease

Most lipid-soluble drugs must be converted into water-soluble form, usually by the liver, before they can be excreted. Drugs that modulate the central nervous system are often lipid-soluble. Thus effects of sedative drugs, such as opiates and tranquillizers, may be greatly enhanced in patients with liver disease if they are unable to metabolize them adequately, because the drug will remain active for longer. The problem is exacerbated because liver damage also renders the brain much more sensitive to the depressant effects of these drugs.

The therapeutic effect of some drugs is modified in liver disease, and although these modifications are correctly thought of as being due to pharmacodynamic changes, they are considered here for convenience. Severe liver damage impairs the production of several vital coagulation factors. A healthy liver requires vitamin K for the synthesis of certain coagulation factors – factor II (prothrombin) and factors VII, IX, and X. However, the prothrombin time becomes abnormal only when the plasma concentration of any one of these factors falls to below 30 per cent of normal, a level that is likely to correspond with severe liver damage. Patients with vitamin K deficiency may be treated with replacement injections, and these are often required in cases of biliary obstruction. Particular care is needed in prescribing for these patients, because some drugs may exacerbate the problems of abnormal clotting. For example, non-steroidal anti-inflammatory drugs should be avoided because they affect platelet aggregation and further increase the risk of gastric bleeding.

Since first-pass metabolism is dependent on hepatic blood flow, changes in cardiac function can alter the clearance of certain drugs. Those drugs that are subject to a high degree of first-pass metabolism tend to be cleared more slowly in patients with heart failure and 'shock', because such conditions cause a fall in hepatic blood flow. Conversely, drug clearance may be more rapid in the initial stages of hepatitis owing to an increased blood flow, leading to reduced plasma drug levels. The normal blood flow bypasses hepatic cells when there has been a surgical shunt constructed, as it does in cirrhosis. Therefore, in these circumstances, an overdose may occur when a drug escapes metabolism by the liver and so reaches a higher concentration in the systemic circulation.

Ascites is a complication of cirrhosis with portal hypertension. Liver failure leads to a decrease in renal blood flow and glomerular filtration, together with electrolyte and water retention. The combination of liver failure and decreased renal function leads to an electrolyte imbalance, which must be corrected, usually by restriction of fluid intake and the administration of diuretics and potassium supplements. In addition, these patients should be closely monitored for drug toxicities because their ability to metabolize and excrete drugs may be greatly reduced. Hypo-kalaemia (low plasma potassium) often provoked by excessive diuretic therapy, is particularly likely to cause hepatic coma (see also Chapters 10 and 34).

ABNORMAL RENAL CLEARANCE

The kidney is responsible for the excretion of all water-soluble drugs, and, indeed, for the excretion of the majority of drugs once they have been partly or completely converted into inactive water-soluble metabolites. Disturbances in renal function may thus affect drug excretion; furthermore, the administration of certain drugs can cause further deterioration. For instance, once tetracyclines have been metabolized in the liver they are excreted in the urine, but if there is renal insufficiency the resultant accumulation of drug

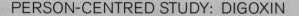

PERSON-CENTRED STUDY: DIGOXIN

Robert, aged 74 years, was admitted to hospital as an emergency following a ' collapse' at home. On arrival in the Accident and Emergency department he was paralysed down his right side and was unable to communicate with the medical staff. His previous medical notes showed a history of heart disease, chronic obstructive airways disease, and peripheral vascular disease. He also had a history of heavy cigarette and alcohol consumption. He could not tell the hospital staff about what medication he was currently taking, although the ambulance staff had found a bottle of digoxin in his house. Robert was diagnosed as having suffered a stroke and admitted to a ward for the care of older adult medical patients.

He could have been prescribed quinidine to treat his cardiac arrhythmias. However, Robert had been given digoxin for his cardiovascular disease: because of his age the blood levels of drug were estimated regularly, so the dose could be adjusted to prevent its accumulation, and reduce the risk of digoxin toxicity. Quinidine was contraindicated because it increases plasma digoxin by an unknown mechanism. On Robert's admission to hospital he was found to be hypertensive. In the acute phase following the stroke, his blood pressure was carefully monitored and no antihypertensive drug was given. Once he stabilized in hospital, the doctor prescribed an appropriate antihypertensive drug. Beta-blockers were not used because of his history of heart failure and because of his peripheral vascular disease.

---

leads to further renal damage. Thus, in patients with renal impairment, it is preferable to use an alternative drug with similar pharmacological action which may be excreted by another route, such as in the bile; doxycycline may be chosen as an alternative treatment.

Variation in urinary pH can alter drug elimination, and diet can exert an influence here. For instance, a patient consuming a largely vegetarian diet produces urine that is more alkaline than a meat eater, who consumes large amounts of protein. If the urine is more alkaline, weakly basic drugs, such as amphetamines and quinidine, are excreted more slowly and the plasma drug concentration rises commensurately.

Water-soluble drugs and drugs subject to tubular excretion are likely to accumulate in renal disease. Older patients have diminished renal function, and glomerular filtration rate can be around half that of healthy young adults. This is often due to the normal ageing process rather than to a specific renal disease. With certain therapies e.g. digoxin, the renal function of the patient must be considered when prescribing (Person-Centred Study: Digoxin; Box 13.1).

PHARMACODYNAMIC ADVERSE DRUG REACTIONS

Pharmacodynamic ADRs are the result of an abnormal tissue response to the drug; this may be congenital or acquired.

CONGENITAL CAUSES OF ADVERSE DRUG REACTIONS

This group of reactions is rather disparate, but of significance are the drug-induced haemolytic anaemias found chiefly in Mediterranean and Afro-Caribbean patients with an inherited deficiency of the enzyme glucose-6-phosphate dehydrogenase. Preparations such as the sulphonamides, aspirin, and anti-malarial drugs affect the integrity of red blood cells in these patients, which results in haemolysis. Other inherited disorders, such as porphyria (a rare disease caused by an abnormality in haemoglobin synthesis), may be provoked by drugs that cause enzyme induction (e.g. barbiturates). The disease is characterized by the urine turning red when it is left to stand; this is caused by the excretion of porphobilinogen. Patients also suffer attacks of intermittent abdominal pain and mental health disturbances. The 'madness' of King George III is now thought to have been caused by porphyria.

Some of the congenital causes of ADRs are associated with aberrant tissue responses; some of them are potentially fatal. Malignant hyperpyrexia is a rare syndrome in which there is defective calcium release from muscle. Consequently, when suxamethonium, a muscle relaxant used in anaesthesia, is administered, the patient develops an extremely high temperature with lactic acidosis. Therefore, in view of the high mortality rate of malignant hyperpyrexia, patients with a family history of death during surgery must be properly investigated.

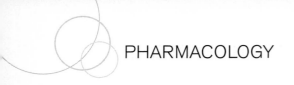

PHARMACOLOGY

ACQUIRED DISEASES AS CAUSES OF ADVERSE DRUG REACTIONS

ADRs caused by an acquired disease are much more frequently encountered, and they are often avoidable (Box 13.2).

Cardiovascular Disease

Patients with advanced cardiac disease commonly have secondary abnormalities of metabolism and endocrine function, which may be partly attributed to the cardiac failure and partly the result of concomitant therapy. With the subsequent diminished cardiac output, blood flow to the kidneys and liver is reduced, resulting in a corresponding decrease in drug clearance. These factors require adequate consideration when prescribing for such patients. Furthermore, some drugs given for heart failure cause a loss of electrolytes (e.g. frusemide and some other diuretics increase the renal excretion of potassium). Accordingly, changes in electrolyte balance can lead to an increased sensitivity to certain drug preparations and thus precipitate an ADR. Digoxin toxicity is a common outcome of treating cardiac failure with digoxin in patients with impaired renal function.

With cardiovascular disease, even some seemingly harmless drugs (which are available without prescription) can induce an ADR. Heart failure can be provoked by non-steroidal anti-inflammatory drugs such as naproxen because they cause sodium retention. Likewise, hypertension can be exacerbated by drugs containing sodium and by drugs that may cause sodium retention. Similar effects may be seen in patients receiving a large quantity of sodium (e.g. from treatment with intravenous saline or certain antacids, or from excessive consumption of beer). It is well known that a family history of hypertension contraindicates the use of the synthetic oestrogens in the contraceptive pill; hence blood pressure is routinely checked before it is prescribed owing to the risk of a cerebrovascular accident (stroke).

A heart damaged by a recent myocardial infarction may be particularly sensitive to certain drug preparations – digoxin is much more likely to cause dysrhythmias in these patients. If there is bradycardia, certain calcium antagonists (e.g. verapamil, used in the treatment of hypertension) and digoxin may cause cardiac slowing and even arrest. Peripheral vascular disease is exacerbated by beta-blockers or by antimigraine preparations containing ergotamime.

Angiotensin-converting enzyme inhibitors (ACE inhibitors), such as captopril and enalapril (see Chapter 10), or one of the new angiotensin II receptor antagonists can cause a further deterioration in renal function if given to patients with renal artery stenosis. In healthy people, there are mechanisms to ensure that blood flow to the brain remains constant despite fluctuation in blood pressure, but these are not as efficient following a stroke. Attempts to lower blood pressure in acute stroke patients can provoke further infarction; this is a fairly common occurrence.

Respiratory Disorders

Where a patient has decreased lung function, care must be taken not to prescribe drugs that might exacerbate the condition and cause respiratory distress or failure. Patients with asthma or chronic obstructive airways disease must not be given opiates or sedative drugs, which depress ventilation. Beta-blockers should never be prescribed for asthmatic patients because they can cause massive bronchospasm. Cases in which death has followed within half an hour of taking these drugs have been reported.

Neurological and Psychiatric Disorders

Narcotics, such as morphine, and centrally acting sedatives are invaluable when an effective palliation of severe or chronic pain is required. Yet these drugs are potentially dangerous in patients with raised intracranial pressure, as may result from a space-occupying lesion or a head injury. In addition, such drugs may depress ventilation and provoke a further rise in intracranial pressure. The consequent rise in blood carbon dioxide concentration is a powerful cerebrovascular vasodilator.

Symptoms of rigidity and bradykinesia in Parkinson's disease can be exacerbated by certain types of drugs (e.g. phenothiazines). Drug-induced parkinsonism often presents in patients given chlorpromazine for psychotic illness. Similarly, an increased risk of seizures may result if tricyclic antidepressants, such as amitriptyline, are prescribed for a patient with epilepsy. Acute psychotic illness has been documented following the prescription of tricyclic antidepressants, steroids, and isoniazid in a patient with a history of psychiatric instability.

ADAPTIVE CHANGES AND REBOUND PHENOMENA

When a drug is taken for an extended period of time, adaptations in physiological mechanisms can occur which may lead to an adverse reaction – a 'rebound phenomenon'. For instance, alcohol misusers can tolerate large quantities of alcohol which could prove fatal to a moderate drinker. However, in the heavy drinker, sudden withdrawal of alcohol may lead to delirium tremors. Similarly, patients can develop a tolerance to opiate analgesia, and so with time, require increasing amounts to control their pain. In the same way, barbiturate-dependent patients who suddenly cease treatment experience severe withdrawal symptoms (e.g. restlessness, sleeplessness, convulsions, and confusion); these may last for several days, until the dependence is broken. An alcohol misuser in the initial stages of detoxification faces similar withdrawal symptoms and may experience frightening hallucinations and fits. Drugs such as chlormethiazole may be prescribed to counteract these severe symptoms, but since these too can be addictive, it is inadvisable for them to be given in the long term.

These rebound phenomena do not only apply to addictive drugs; patients on long-term steroid therapy may experience an ADR if treatment is withdrawn abruptly. Corticosteroids disrupt normal feedback control mechanisms of the hypothalamus, pituitary, and adrenal gland because of the continual stimulation by the exogenous source of hormones. Sudden withdrawal of steroids should therefore be avoided; the dosage should be reduced gradually to allow the atrophied glands to recover and regain their original functional ability. A patient who has been on long-term steroid therapy requires an extended time for drug withdrawal.

When clinical trials are carried out to ensure the safety and tolerability of a drug, only the most common ADRs are discovered initially, because of the relatively small number of people on which the drug has been tested (approximately 5000). It is only when the drug is licensed and given to much greater numbers of patients that other serious ADRs are discovered. Some ADRs may be discovered years after the drug has been licensed.

Perhaps the most feared side-effect of drugs is the possibility that they may eventually cause cancer. Since relatively little is understood about the aetiology of some cancers in humans, this type of ADR can only be proved from epidemiological evidence. Take the example of hormone replacement therapy (HRT): there is slightly higher incidence of breast cancer in women prescribed these drugs. On the other hand, HRT greatly reduces the incidence of cardiovascular disease and protects against osteoporosis. Carcinoma of the uterus may be caused by oestrogens given as HRT if it is not accompanied by progesterone (see Chapter 37).

Oral contraceptives have also been open to scrutiny since their use has become wide-spread. A higher frequency of benign liver tumours has been noted; however, the link between breast cancer and oral contraceptives is still unproven. Such information needs to be disseminated wisely to the general public. Unfortunately, recent data suggesting that women prescribed the modern low-dose oestrogen contraceptive pills were more at risk of developing thrombosis gained media coverage. The panic and thus the abrupt cessation of treatment that ensued led to some unwanted pregnancies.

IMMUNOLOGICAL ADVERSE DRUG REACTIONS

Most drug preparations are compounds that are not synthesized naturally by the body, so they may be considered as 'non-self'. The immune system offers protection against a multitude of antigens, but it can not distinguish between a 'foreigner' that causes harm and one that might have a desirable therapeutic effect. When the immune system mounts an assault against drugs, this constitutes an immunological ADR. A well-known example is allergy to penicillin.

Most ADRs are dependent on the dose of the drug, whereas most immunological ADRs are not dose-dependent. In an immunological ADR, the patient's symptoms are the consequence of the aggressive immune cells responding to the drug that is discerned as being non-self or dangerous. Therefore, once the stimulus for the immune cells is no longer there, the reaction ceases –

therefore, if the drug is stopped, the ADR disappears; if the drug is started again, the ADR returns. Some patients are more at risk of an immunological ADR than others; patients to be aware of are those known to have allergic diseases (e.g. hay fever, asthma, eczema) and those with a history of other ADRs.

The immunological ADRs are categorized according to the specific type of response of the immune system. Some are caused by a specific class of antibody (immunoglobulin) raised against the drug (i.e. IgM, IgE, or IgA; see Chapter 24 for more information about the antibodies produced by the immune system), others by the direct action of immune cells. It is therefore possible to classify them accordingly into type I, II, III, or IV hypersensitivity. There are many substances and treatments other than pharmaceutical preparations that provoke these reactions; how and by what mechanisms they occur are discussed in more detail in Chapter 26.

Type I Hypersensitivity Reactions

Drug allergies are examples of type I hypersensitivity; these do not generally erupt with the first administration of the drug but with a subsequent course of treatment. In the sequence of events, the drug is identified as foreign by specific immune cells, but even though they release IgM antibodies, the physical symptoms and signs of allergy are not present at this stage. However, when the first dose of the succeeding course of treatment is given, these cells 'remember' the drug and become sensitized (reminded and alerted), so by the time they encounter the second dose supplied a few hours later, they frantically release another type of antibody called IgE. It is this class of antibody that is responsible for provoking the adverse symptoms and signs, because it not only has the capacity to bind its target molecule (the drug) it can also bind to the surface of mast cells or basophils. Once a 'sandwich of mast cell–IgE–drug' is formed, the mast cell responds by releasing histamine and other mediators of inflammation that cause the allergic reaction. The symptoms can be anything from a rather uncomfortable skin irritation (urticaria) to the life-threatening effects of anaphylaxis (Box 13.3).

Mast cells are found in most tissues; if they release histamine in the lungs it can cause constriction of the bronchial smooth muscle and result in an acute asthma attack – aspirin has been known to produce asthma by this mechanism. If a similar reaction occurs in the gut mucosa, diarrhoea and vomiting may present. In extreme cases, anaphylactic shock may follow the administration of certain drugs, including antibiotics, vaccines, intravenous contrast media used in some X-rays, and iron injections. The symptoms include collapse of blood pressure, bronchospasm, and an acutely swollen glottis, which causes respiratory obstruction. As these events are potentially fatal, adrenaline must be given promptly to counteract them. Some hospitals have a policy that the first dose of intravenous drugs should be given by a clinician, as a precautionary measure. However, the patient should be closely observed when the second dose is administered since this carries the greater risk of anaphylaxis.

Type II Hypersensitivity Reactions

When other classes of antibody against a drug are made, quite different symptoms are presented. The drug-induced type II hypersensitivity reactions are generally caused by the immune system mounting an antibody response against drug compounds with a tendency to be rather 'sticky' and adhere to the surface of cells. A huge complex forms when the antibody binds to its target (the drug), which is already attached to a cell, so a cell–drug–antibody complex is formed. This provokes an immunological assault whereby the cell is perforated and destroyed by lysis. Methyldopa, a rather old-fashioned antihypertensive drug, though it is still in use, attaches itself to red blood cells and can cause a haemolytic anaemia. Similarly, when the cell under attack is a platelet, their numbers are then depleted (thrombocytopenia), which leads to bruising and bleeding owing to an inadequate clotting mechanism – the drug quinidine can cause this.

Type III Hypersensitivity Reactions

Antibodies do not operate in isolation; rather, they have a number of proteins to help them, some of which belong to a series of proteins called 'complement' (see Chaptr 25). When a patient makes an antibody against a drug that recruits the assistance of the complement, the outcome is a type III hypersensitivity reaction. An abundance of huge macromolecules are formed; these are drug–antibody–complement complexes. If these are not cleared efficiently, inflammatory damage erupts wherever they lodge and accumulate. If the endothelial lining of blood vessels becomes the 'crevice' where the complexes lodge, a serum sickness-type illness can ensue, characterized by fever, which is often accompanied by joint pains, urticaria, and lymphadenopathy. Penicillins, streptomycin, sulphonamides, and the antithyroid drugs have been known to be responsible for this type of reaction. If the lung is involved, one sees a pneumonia-like picture: the drug nitrofurantoin may provoke a type III hypersensitivity reaction. Other organs, such as the kidney, are candidates for getting the large complex molecules lodged within them. Penicillamine, used in the treatment of rheumatoid arthritis, has been known to provoke a protein-losing state called nephrotic syndrome by this mechanism.

Type IV Hypersensitivity Reactions

All the three major types of immunological ADR discussed so far are mediated by antibodies binding to drug molecules. Type IV hypersensitivity reactions differ from the others in that they are occur when immune cells are activated by a drug (the macrophages and T lymphocytes which provoke an inflammatory response). Contact dermatitis is an example of this type of immunological ADR; it sometimes occurs when patients are given topical drugs such as antihistamine creams, antibiotics, and local anaesthetics.

DRUG INTERACTIONS

Some patients (especially older adults) may have multiple symptoms and pathologies that require several different drugs to be taken at a time. Unfortunately this may provoke an ADR because of the effects of one drug being altered by the presence of another. However, not all drug interactions have undesirable consequences; on rare occasions they can be beneficial. It is useful to classify them according to how they are mediated, i.e. whether the ADR results from the patient's physiological reaction to the drug or from the interaction of two drug compounds. The subject of drug–drug interactions is a vast one. Not all the interactions are important in clinical practice, but some are. A comprehensive list of clinically important interactions is given in the *British National Formulary*. From a practical clinical viewpoint it is advisable to check that a drug interaction is not recorded before prescribing.

One area of concern is the possible interaction of cigarette smoking and drug therapy. Smoking induces the enzymes responsible for drug metabolism, thereby increasing the clearance of certain drugs. Consequently doses of some drugs in smokers may need to be increased to up to twice the normal dose; theophylline used to treat asthma is one such example. Essentially, smokers are more likely to suffer an ADR, as their reactions to certain drugs may differ from those of non-smokers. Women who smoke and take the oral contraceptive pill have a greater risk of developing heart disease or a stroke because of the interaction between cigarette consumption and oestrogens. The absorption and utilization of certain nutrients, such as vitamins C, B12 and B6, are also affected in very heavy smokers, so they may require vitamin supplements or a recommended dietary modification to maintain adequate nutritional status.

Ethanol (alcohol) is well known to react with many medications; hence it is contraindicated under certain circumstances. A survey of the 100 most frequently

BOX 13.3 SIGNS AND SYMPTOMS OF AN ALLERGIC DRUG REACTION

Allergic reactions to drugs are unavoidable and occur in a relatively small proportion of patients. They differ from other drug toxicities because:

- they are not dependent on the dose of the drug given
- the patients have invariably received the drug previously
- they may have a rapid onset, resulting from the explosive release of histamine (and other chemical mediators of inflammation) in response to the drug

Symptoms

Mild reaction
rashes or itching of the skin (urticaria)

Severe anaphylactic reaction
wheezing
chest tightness
abdominal pain
nausea and vomiting
rapid fall in blood pressure
bronchospasm
acutely swollen glottis causing respiratory obstruction

Treatment of anaphylaxis in adults
adrenaline given by intramuscular injection (0.5–1.0 mg) repeated every 10 minutes until recovery is life saving; *this is one of the greatest of all medical emergencies where seconds count*
for children under the age of 12 years, consult the *British National Formulary*

Therefore, when taking a medical history, the ethanol consumption and any smoking habits should be determined and the possible dangers of ethanol interactions with medications explained.

INTERACTIONS OF TWO DRUGS DURING PREPARATION BY THE PHARMACIST MAY ALTER THEIR THERAPEUTIC VALUE

In certain circumstances, an ADR may arise from a pharmaceutical interaction that occurs when two drugs are mixed. If the drugs are prescribed to patients who are not hospitalized, it is the duty of the dispensing pharmacist to ensure that this potential interaction is foreseen and avoided. When treating hospitalized patients, the health care practitioners conducting the drug round must be aware of these types of ADR. For instance, a mixture of slow-acting and fast-acting forms of insulin are prescribed to maintain a realistic control over blood glucose. Accordingly, the two types of insulin are mixed in the syringe to be given as one injection. However, if care is not taken, the vial of fast-acting insulin may be contaminated with the slow-acting form when the mixed injection is being drawn up. Consequently the therapeutic value of the fast-acting insulin will have been altered, which may be significant when the vial is used at a later date – the patient may suffer a hypoglycaemic coma in the night and never regain consciousness, because of the delay in onset of insulin activity whilst they are asleep, for example. This may be avoided by drawing up the fast-acting insulin into the syringe first, before drawing up the slow-acting insulin.

Some intravenous drug preparations are not compatible when administered together, so care must be taken to ensure that they are not mixed. All intravenous drugs come with detailed instructions on how they should be reconstituted, including which fluids are advised and which contraindicated. When reconstituting a lyophilized drug into a solution, it is essential to check for clouding or precipitation, as this is a sign of incompatibility. If two incompatible intravenous drugs are prescribed, it is advisable to schedule administration at different times and flush the intravenous line with saline between administrations to prevent mixing.

INTERACTIONS AT THE SITE OF ENTRY

The rate of gastric emptying (and therefore the speed at which the maximum plasma concentration) is attained is influenced by the contents of the stomach, the pH of the gastric juices, and the action of the drug that is passing through it. Such factors can significantly affect the rate at which the drug is absorbed. High plasma concentrations are necessary with certain antibiotic

prescribed drugs showed that over half contained an ingredient known to interact adversely with ethanol. Such reactions are especially likely if the drug is metabolized in the liver, but the severity of the interaction depends on the frequency and amount of alcohol consumed. Patients should be instructed to avoid alcohol when taking narcotics, tranquillizers, or sedatives because the activities of these drugs can be enhanced, causing respiratory or central nervous system depression.

treatments and in analgesic therapy. Slowing of drug absorption by opiates and drugs having atropinic effects will reduce the maximum plasma concentration. If the drug is an analgesic, adequate pain control may not be achieved. In the case of antibiotics, not achieving sufficient tissue penetration may lead to persistent infection and antibiotic resistance (see also Chapter 19). The absorption of a drug is impeded when it chelates (attaches itself chemically) to another compound; for example, cholestyramine, a cholesterol-lowering drug, reduces the absorption of thyroxine and fat-soluble vitamins by this mechanism (Figure 13.3a).

DRUG–NUTRIENT INTERACTIONS

Certain foods can significantly affect drug absorption by retarding, inhibiting, or (occasionally) enhancing uptake by the gut. For example, dairy products, which contain calcium, reduce the absorption of tetracyclines. Sometimes food causes an adverse effect because of a previously administered drug. Foods containing tyramine (e.g. yeast-containing foods, cheese, processed meats) must be avoided when monoamine oxidase inhibitors are prescribed (see Chapter 10). In this case, the drug–nutrient interaction is potentially fatal because tyramine indirectly increases noradrenaline levels that precipitate hypertension. Consumption of a meal rich in vitamin K (e.g. liver, spinach) can cause a reduction in the effectiveness of certain anticoagulant tablets such as warfarin. Conversely, some foods speed up the absorption of certain drugs; one example of this is ascorbic acid (vitamin C), which increases the absorption of oral iron (see Chapter 31).

Drug preparations that change gut motility may enhance or diminish nutrient absorption. Certain drugs, such as loperamide and metoclopramide, cause changes in gastric and intestinal motility. Liquid paraffin can lead to a decrease in the absorption of drugs because of intestinal hurry. Increased fat in the gut also decreases the absorption of lipid-soluble substances.

Nutritional status may be compromised by long-term treatments. A reduced overall energy intake results from drug-induced appetite suppression (as may occur in amphetamine therapy) or from a decreased dietary intake or absorption caused by the altered taste acuity or gastrointestinal disturbances that occur in cytotoxic therapies.

Some drugs adversely affect the nutritional status of specific nutrients; anticonvulsant therapy affects folate and vitamin D status, so an increased dietary intake is required. Similarly, a number of drug preparations are known to reduce blood vitamin C levels (e.g. tetracyclines, oral contraceptives, aspirin). Patients on long-term diuretic therapy require mineral supplements, for

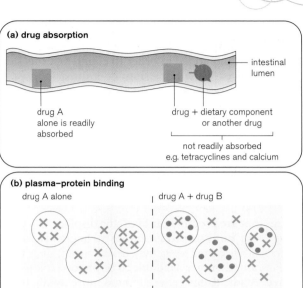

(a) drug absorption

drug A alone is readily absorbed

drug + dietary component or another drug

intestinal lumen

not readily absorbed e.g. tetracyclines and calcium

(b) plasma–protein binding

drug A alone

drug A + drug B

drug A binds to plasma proteins

drug B dislodges drug A from plasma protein so that there is more free drug A in plasma, increasing the risk of toxicity

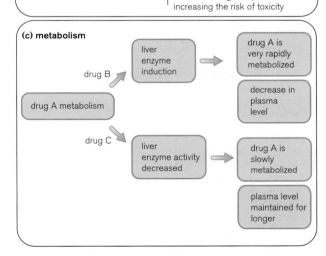

(c) metabolism

drug A metabolism

drug B → liver enzyme induction → drug A is very rapidly metabolized

decrease in plasma level

drug C → liver enzyme activity decreased → drug A is slowly metabolized

plasma level maintained for longer

Figure 13.3 Factors that affect drug absorption. (a) A component in the gastrointestinal tract may retain a drug in the lumen so that it is not readily absorbed. (b) When two drugs (Drug A and Drug B) are given together, if drug B preferentially binds more strongly to plasma proteins and displaces drug A, the amount of free drug A increases, possibly resulting in toxicity. (c) Here, drug B induces activity of drug-metabolizing enzymes, meaning that clearance of drug A from the blood is more rapid than usual, and its therapeutic effect is therefore not sustained. Drug C inhibits the activity of drug-metabolizing enzymes, meaning that retarding the clearance Drug A from the blood is slower than usual, and its therapeutic effect is therefore retained for longer.

they may be at risk of potassium deficiency, which could lead to heart dysrhythmias. Many diuretic tablets now have potassium added in order to counteract this side-effect. However the potassium contained in most of these preparations is not sufficient to make up for the deficit. Potassium salts can cause small bowel ulceration; therefore the combined use of potassium-sparing diuretics with loop diuretics or thiazides is a far better solution (Figure 13.4).

INTERACTIONS DUE TO PROTEIN BINDING

Drugs that are protein bound can be displaced by other drugs that bind to protein more strongly. Thus, the effects of 'dislodged' drug may be enhanced, since more free unbound drug is available to be pharmacologically active. Acidic drugs generally bind more avidly to the plasma protein, albumin; therefore oral anticoagulants, sulphonylureas, and methotrexate can be displaced by drugs such as non-steroidal anti-inflammatory drugs, clofibrate, and bezafibrate. For example, normally

about 5 per cent of warfarin is free and active, but the bound form can be displaced by the non-steroidal drug naproxen (both drugs compete to bind to the same protein), and this could cause up to double the normal amount of warfarin (i.e. 10 per cent of the warfarin) to be free. Therefore, a prescription of naproxen given as an analgesic may cause a haemorrhage in a patient who is normally well-controlled on warfarin anticoagulation (Figure 13.3b).

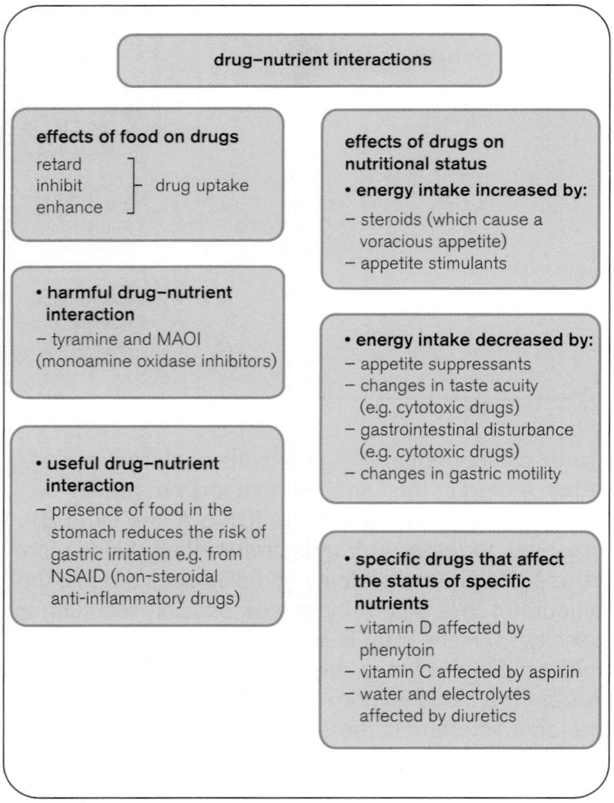

THE INFLUENCE OF ENZYMES ON DRUG METABOLISM

Enzymes influence normal cell function by catalysing metabolic reactions, and they are instrumental in many pathological mechanisms. Indeed, many drugs have been designed specifically to target enzymes in order to modify their level of activity; most such drugs prevent or inhibit the activity of an enzyme in order to exert their own influence. Drug toxicity may follow enzyme inhibition because the rate of drug metabolism is retarded, leading to a slower drug clearance from the body. As an example, warfarin can slow the rate of phenytoin metabolism when the two are given simultaneously, causing fairly rapid phenytoin toxicity and provoking a cerebellar syndrome in which the patient loses the sense of balance. Regrettably, this syndrome may be permanent, even if the offending drugs are withdrawn. Similarly, the tricyclic antidepressants, such as amitriptyline, can retard the breakdown of warfarin and so prolong the anticoagulant effect. Cimetidine also slows the metabolism of drugs like propranolol and diazepam, and the subsequent increased drug levels that result can have potentially disastrous effects. Some antibiotics (e.g. erythromycin and ciprofloxacin) interfere with the metabolism of theophylline (a drug prescribed for asthma). If the level of theophylline is allowed to rise, convulsions and cardiac dysrhythmias may occur.

Enzyme induction can have equally harmful consequences, when the administration of a second drug hastens the metabolism of the first. Rifampicin, an anti-tuberculosis drug, is a powerful enhancer of enzymes and has been found to inactivate the contraceptive effect of the low-dose oestrogen contraceptive pill. It also modifies the anticoagulant action of warfarin (Figure 13.3c).

Drugs that raise the level of enzyme activity in the liver can augment its detoxification capacity. In so doing, the drugs that stimulated the liver are themselves more rapidly cleared from the circulation along with any other drugs the patient is taking. Phenobarbitone induces liver enzymes, and therefore, eventually, an increased dose is needed to compensate because of the more rapid drug clearance.

Figure 13.4 Drug–nutrient interactions. These can alter either: a. the therapeutic effects of drugs; or b. the nutritional status of the patient.

EXCRETION OF DRUGS

Excretion interactions may arise from a drug causing decreased reabsorption or tubular secretion of another drug in the kidneys. Reabsorption of drugs into the plasma from the renal tubule can be an active or passive process. Changes in urinary pH can significantly affect the clearance of certain drugs. An overdose of aspirin (an acidic drug) can be successfully treated with sodium bicarbonate, which produces a more alkaline urine to increase the excretion of aspirin (see Chapter 9). In renal tubule excretion, highly charged molecules are actively transferred by cells from the plasma into the tubular fluid. Probenecid, a drug given to enhance the excretion of uric acid, also decreases the excretion of penicillin. Therefore, when treating a patient suffering from gout (hyperuricaemia) who is taking probenecid and has subsequently developed an infection that can be treated with penicillin, care must be taken to adjust the dose downwards when prescribing penicillin.

PHARMACODYNAMIC INTERACTIONS

These reactions are the result of one drug exerting an effect on the action of another drug; for instance, if an agonist drug is simultaneously prescribed with an antagonist, the effects of one could essentially cancel out the other. These interactions are not encountered regularly, and are invariably caused by the prescriber being unaware of the prescription provided by another clinician. Two drugs with the same clinical outcome can also prove to be a problem if prescribed together; for instance warfarin and aspirin alter haemostasis, albeit by differing mechanisms, but if taken together there is the possible danger of haemorrhage. The anticoagulant effects of warfarin are mediated by modifying the amount of active clotting factors in plasma. Aspirin also has anticoagulant properties, but these are caused by inhibiting platelet aggregation. Similarly, propanolol and digoxin effective slow down the heart, and if taken together, excessive bradycardia may result, leading ultimately to cardiac arrest.

KEY POINTS

- The chance of an ADR increases with age and the dosage of drugs taken.
- Between 70 and 80 per cent of ADRs are dose-dependent and likely to be caused by some underlying abnormality.
- ADR incidence can be due to pharmacokinetic causes such as genetic variation, liver disease or renal disease.
- Pharmacodynamic causes of an ADR include increased sensitivity of the tissues because of asthma and a genetic predisposition to epilepsy or depression.
- Between 20 and 30 per cent of ADRs are unpredictable and usually have a well-defined immunological base.
- Certain drugs, if given together, are incompatible and can precipitate an ADR.

FURTHER READING

Adelsberg BR (1997) Sedation and performance issues in the treatment of allergic conditions. Arch Intern Med 157:494–500.

Chung, Lu H, Parikh PP, Lorber DL (1996) Phenformin-associated lactic acidosis due to imported phenformin. Diabet Care 19:1449–50.

Cook GC (1995) Adverse effects of chemotherapeutic agents used in tropical medicine. Drug Saf 13:31–45.

MacKenzie C (1997) The safety of inhaled corticosteroids in children. Prof Nurse 13:110–12.

Merk HF, Hertl M (1996) Immunologic mechanisms of cutaneous drug reactions. Semin Cutan Med Surg 15:228–35.

Romano A, Pietrantonio F (1997) Delayed hypersensitivity to flurbiprofen. J Intern Med 241:81–3.

Roe DA (1995) Diet and Drug Interactions. Chapman and Hall, London.

Seifeldin R (1995) Drug interactions in transplantation. Clin Ther 17:1043–61.

Stephens MDB, Routledge PA, Talbot J (1998) Detection of new adverse drug reaction. Macmillan Press, London.

Stockley IH (1996) Drug Interactions, 4th edition. Pharmaceutical Press, London.

PAIN AND ITS MANAGEMENT

INTRODUCTION

Pain is an unpleasant response to a stimulus, yet it is essential to survival since it often acts as a warning signal of impending tissue damage. When pain is severe it can provoke symptoms of nausea and vomiting, sometimes even cardiovascular collapse. With chronic pain, the sensation itself is often more intense than one might suppose from the cause alone. This invariably leads to anxiety and depression, and in turn these feelings can exaggerate the person's perception of symptoms. Thus, analgesia is as much part of patient care as the treatment for the underlying pathology.

Pain is such a personal experience that it can only be quantified and described by the patient. Unfortunately, health care professionals are in danger of underestimating the severity of symptoms owing to frequent exposure to all levels of pain in their patients. The result of this is that analgesia may be underprescribed and the pain may remain uncontrolled; yet no one should be allowed to develop break-through pain. Health care professionals should be aware of these potential prejudices, so that rather than using their own value system, the patient's perceptions are considered in the evaluation and treatment of pain.

HOW IS PAIN PERCEIVED?

There are pain receptors (known as nociceptors) in many parts of the body. These can respond to a variety of noxious stimuli (e.g. mechanical stimuli, extremes of temperature, electrical stimuli, pressure). When nociceptors have been stimulated they release chemical substances that either produce the pain response directly or sensitize the nerve endings. Bradykinin and prostaglandins are two notable chemical mediators of pain; others include histamine, serotonin, and substance P. Bradykinin in particular is likely to be involved in the sensation of acute pain. Prostaglandins both increase pain nerve fibre sensitivity and enhance the pain sensation elicited by bradykinin. Thus, some analgesic drugs act by strategically altering the production, the release, or the pain-stimulating activities of these chemicals. For example, aspirin inhibits the production of prostaglandins.

Pain is also associated with electrical activity in two main types of afferent nerve fibres. Type C fibres are unmyelinated and generate a dull burning pain. Type A fibres are myelinated fibres that conduct more rapidly and cause sharp, well-localized pain. These fibres are bipolar neurones with cell bodies lying in the dorsal root ganglion, through which the nerves pass from the periphery and enter the spinal cord.

The brain is also involved in pain; afferent nerves conduct a nerve impulse in response to a pain stimulus in the periphery and activate the neurones in the dorsal horn. The stimulus is relayed to the thalamus, where the pain is appreciated, though the finer sensations are thought to occur when the stimulus has been transmitted to the cerebral cortex (see Chapter 38). The activity of the dorsal horn neurones may be suppressed by a variety of inputs (Figure 14.1).

The use of the transcutaneous electrical nerve stimulating (TENS) apparatus was introduced into modern clinical practice following the 'gate control theory' expounded by Melzack and Wall in 1965. This theory concerned the mechanism by which the nervous system controls the input and distribution of nerve impulses that are perceived as pain by the brain. The theory described how impulses in the brain could close the so-called 'gate', thereby regulating the levels of pain that a person actually experiences.

Another important factor in pain perception is the descending inhibitory tract in the central nervous system. A key part of the descending system is found in a section of the midbrain, the periaqueductal grey (PAG) matter. When this area is stimulated, it virtually abolishes pain appreciation without interfering with other sensory modalities. PAG receives many inputs from other areas of the brain, including the cortex and thalamus, which are capable of altering its signal output. The main neuronal pathway activated by PAG stimulation runs first to the nucleus raphe magnus (NRM), an area of the medulla close to the midline.

From the NRM the pathway runs via fibres to the dorsal horn. Two of the major neurotransmitters in these areas of the brain are enkephalin and serotonin. It is well documented that a low level of serotonin in the brain has a role in depression. Low doses of anti-depressants that act by increasing the functional amount of neurotransmitters in the synapse are now well-established treatments for chronic pain. Tricyclic antidepressants increase both serotonin and nor-adrenaline levels; the newer serotonin uptake inhibitors such as fluoxetine (Prozac) increase only serotonin. These agents are effective in patients with pain who do not appear to be particularly depressed, and in those patients with pain who are depressed, the treatment has an additional benefit. Unfortunately, there is a marked difference in the time course between their ability to increase the levels of neurotransmitters and the ultimate antidepressant effect. The increase in amines is immediate but the clinical antidepressant effects take many weeks to be realized. The same is probably true for their influence on pain.

ASSESSMENT OF PAIN

The word 'pain' describes a multitude of sensations, so it is important to have an accurate description for making a diagnosis for prescribing analgesia. It is important to remember that there are variations in the level of pain that can be tolerated by different people. Some cultures encourage vocalization of pain, and patients from these culture groups may shout out and cry, whereas other cultures may suffer silently. This does not mean that one person's pain is more severe, simply that their response to the sensation is expressed in different ways.

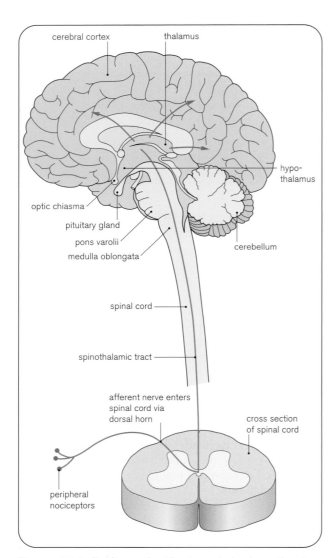

Figure 14.1 Pathway for the transmission of pain from the nociceptor to the brain. The pathway runs from the nociceptor in the periphery via peripheral nerves and the spinal cord to the brain.

Successful treatment requires a thorough evaluation of the patient. The patient should describe the nature, frequency and severity of the pain. Only the person experiencing the pain is able to adequately characterize the unpleasant sensation, because the way pain is perceived varies greatly between individuals. Once a full pain history and pain description have been taken, reassessment of the symptoms is required on a regular basis with the original used as a baseline (Figure 14.2).

However, it is not sufficient simply to record details of the pain itself, because environmental, social, physical, and psychological factors (e.g. inadequate heating in the home, demands of family life) can all have an influence and thus modify the sensation of pain.

date _____

patient's name _____   age _____ ward _____

diagnosis _____

doctor _____

nurse _____

I. location: patient or nurse mark drawing

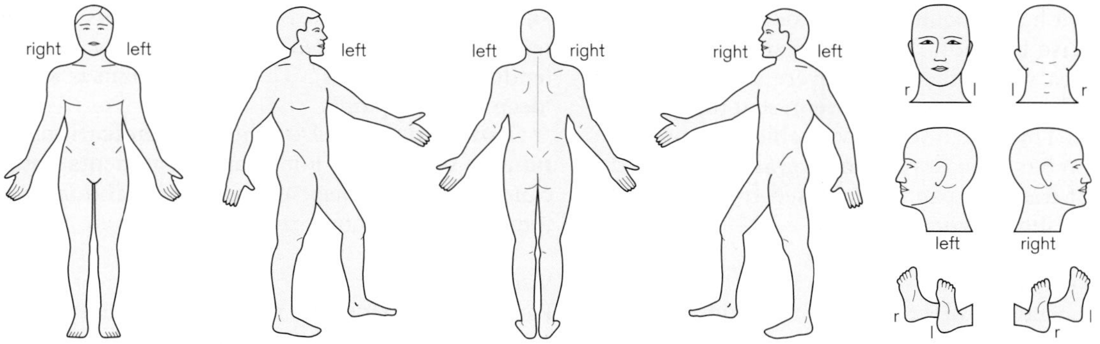

II. intensity : patient rates the pain - scale used _____
present _____
worst pain gets _____
best pain gets _____
acceptable level of pain _____

III. quality (use patient's own words, e.g. prick, ache, burn, throb, pull, sharp) _____

IV. onset, duration variations, rhythms _____

V. manner of expression of pain _____

VI. what relieves the pain _____

VIII. what causes or increase the pain _____

VIII. effects of pain (note decreased function, decreased quality of life)
accompanying symptoms (e.g. nausea) _____
sleep _____
appetite _____
physical activity _____
relationship with others (e.g. irritability) _____
emotions (e.g. anger, suicidal, crying) _____
concentration _____
other _____

IX. other comments _____

X. plan _____

Figure 14.2 Initial pain assessment tool. (From McCaffery M, 1994.)

Initial Onset of Pain

The patient should be questioned about when the pain first presented and the factors (if any) that played a part in the onset. Sometimes patients can be quite mistaken in their concept of the causal elements. For example, a patient who has been diagnosed with cancer may have considered (in the months preceding the diagnosis) that the pain had been caused by a previous injury. Conversely, patients requiring surgery for a hernia repair can usually recall the start of the problem because it was associated with the onset of the pain.

Location of the Pain

It is a useful exercise to provide an anatomical picture of the human body and allow the patient to shade in the area (or areas) where they are experiencing pain. This use of diagrams can be very helpful particularly if the patient has difficulty naming or indeed pointing to the precise location. If the pain seems to radiate from an area where there is a severe sensation, then different colours may be used to represent the intensity of the pain. This visual tool is valuable, because after the diagram has been drawn on several occasions, the progress of the pain can be analysed by referring to the series of illustrations.

Description of the Pain

Having an accurate description of the pain can assist in the diagnosis but, again, obtaining the full picture from the patient may be difficult because each person has a unique perception of his or her symptoms and differing levels of ability to describe it. It is often expedient to offer certain key words and phrases if there is difficulty in describing the pain in words (e.g. 'a burning sensation', 'a deep ache'). Pain questionnaires (such as the McGill Pain Questionnaire) may be used to provide the vocabulary that many patients struggle to find. This can also help the patient to give information about the frequency and duration of the pain and the effects that the pain has on emotional well-being. Some health care teams use visual analogue scores for evaluating the intensity of the pain experienced before and after treatment (Figure 14.3). Such parameters are advantageous for assessing the effectiveness of the analgesia.

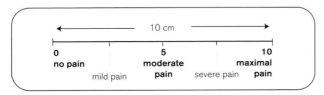

Figure 14.3 The visual analogue score flow diagram.

Superficial somatic pain

Pain that is fast conducting is usually felt as a sharp, pricking sensation, such as occurs when skin touches something extremely hot, resulting in a speedy reaction to retract from the heat. Slow conducting pain is felt as a burning sensation, and this occurs when there is infection and inflammation, for example. The skin that surrounds a wound that has become infected feels hot and tender and often aches. The origins of these types of pain are the receptors in the skin, and fast and slow conducting pains are known as 'superficial somatic pain'.

Deep somatic pain

Patients who suffer from arthritic type illnesses often experience deep aches in their joints and tendons. This is particularly unpleasant because of its relentless nature, which affects the patient's everyday comfort and ability to sleep. The origin of this pain is the receptors in the diseased area (e.g. the knee, other joints, tendons, or muscles). This type of pain is known as 'deep somatic pain'.

Pain may be one of the first indications that a tumour has arisen. For example, patients with liver cancer may feel a deep ache inside the abdomen which they can only vaguely pinpoint.

Visceral pain

Pain resulting from the stimulus of nociceptors in the body's organs is known as 'visceral pain'. This type of pain is particularly disconcerting because it is internal, so the patient is unable to visualize any physical signs of an abnormality.

Referred pain

Pain may arise from pathology at one site in the body but be experienced at another site – 'referred pain'. For instance, a patient who is about to suffer a myocardial infarction may experience pain in the left arm. Similarly, patients with glaucoma often present with pain in the forehead and localized pain in the eye before they actually start to become visually impaired. The size of the area where the pain is perceived is often far greater that the anatomical structure affected.

One of the explanations put forward for referred pain is that the brain receives an impulse via an afferent nerve that shares a common dorsal horn with another afferent nerve from a different area. In the sequence of events the brain misinterprets the message. Another suggestion is that the area that is the source of the pain shares common embryonic origins with the area where the pain is perceived. For example, the pain that occurs in cancer of the testis is sometimes experienced in the inguinal canal.

Phantom limb pain

Phantom limb pain is the sensation felt in the part of the limb that has been amputated. It differs from stump pain, which can be caused by haematoma or osteomyelitis. The intensity of the pain felt in the 'phantom limb' can be very severe and psychologically distressing for the patient.

In the past there was a tendency to disregard phantom limb pain and to consider it as a patient's grief-stricken reaction to the loss of a limb. Fortunately this kind of thinking no longer prevails and there are various treatments for the pain. Phantom limb pain may sometimes be prevented by giving the patient an epidural infusion of diamorphine, clonidine. and bupivacaine before the amputation, but this is not always successful. After the amputation, the patient may be maintained on epidural analgesia for at least 3 days. Once the patient has recovered from the anaesthetic, he or she should be encouraged to mobilize and exercise the stump regularly.

If phantom limb pain remains a problem then alternative methods of pain control should be considered, such as carbamazepine or even acupuncture. TENS may be contraindicated because it has been known to exacerbate rather than relieve the symptoms of phantom limb pain.

FACTORS THAT AFFECT THE PAIN

Assessment of the patient's pain should also include a list of factors that intensify or relieve the sensation.

Certain activities such as climbing stairs or lifting heavy objects may worsen the pain, whereas lying in a certain position or taking a hot bath may soothe it. Certainly, pain is invariably exacerbated at night; one reason for this is that there are less distractions at night than there are during the day, so the pain becomes more of a focus for the patient. Furthermore, the circadian rhythms of hormone release also influence pain.

Lack of Sleep and Anxiety

Lack of sleep may enhance the symptoms, as may anxiety that the intensity of the pain is not believed or appreciated by others. Although it may be presumed that pain is controlled when the patient finally sleeps, the onset of sleep may occur because of sheer exhaustion (Figure 14.4).

Patients who suffer from pain are often frightened and depressed to varying degrees. Therefore it is important to:
- reassure them;
- ascertain the factors that might exacerbate the pain so that they can be eliminated if possible; and
- provide adequate analgesia to relieve the pain.

Previous Experiences of Pain

Previous experiences can influence the patient's perception of the intensity of the symptoms. The oncology patient who has enjoyed a period of remission from their disease may be fearful of every ache and pain because it could indicate a relapse. Indeed, the acceptance of pain may vary considerably depending

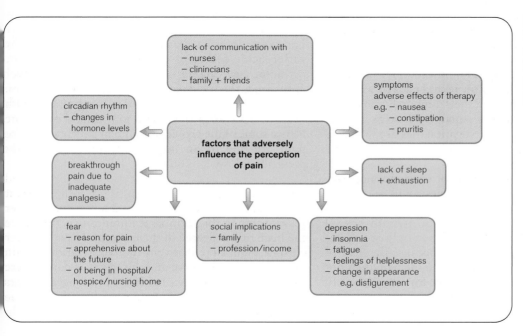

Figure 14.4 Factors that adversely influence the perception of pain.

BOX 14.1 ANALGESIA IN THE FACE OF INJURY

- Patients may arrive in the Accident and Emergency department with acute injuries (e.g. a severed finger) and yet be free of pain. This is known as episodic analgesia. Although the analgesia is often instantaneous it has a limited time course. Pain eventually arrives following psychological awareness about the extent of injury.
- Another anomaly is that some people have a congenital insensitivity to pain; this is known as congenital analgesia. These people do not realize that they are damaging themselves in certain situations. Patients who cannot feel pain are likely to have a shortened life expectancy and suffer frequent injuries, which they are unaware of owing to a lack of pain.
- Certain diseases can reduce the ability of the body to feel pain, such as leprosy and diabetes, in which there is peripheral neuropathy.

on its origins. For instance, pain experienced because of an underlying pathology such as cancer may be of the same intensity as the pain experienced by a woman in labour. However, in the latter context the pain has a reason that may be considered acceptable (see Box 14.1).

Patients may experience pain that is not caused by the main diagnosed disease. For instance, it should not be assumed that the only pain experienced by a patient with cancer is on account of their tumour. For instance, adverse symptoms such as pain may arise as a result of a medical or surgical investigation they are subjected to (e.g. adverse effects of chemotherapy) as part of the management of their disorder.

Pre-operative patients should be warned about post-operative pain, and told that analgesia will be required on a regular basis. It has been demonstrated in clinical trials that pre-operative patients who are fully briefed about what to expect after surgery generally experience less intense pain. This is perhaps because the 'fear of the unknown' has been removed, so the pain does not come as such a shock. It is better for the patient to realize that if any breakthrough pain is experienced it should be reported immediately so the dosage of

analgesia can be adjusted. There is a tendency in some cultures to try to 'grin and bear it', because of the fear of being a hindrance to the carers. Although this type of patient may be more pleasant to look after, this attitude should be discouraged because pain is nearly always preventable.

DURATION OF PAIN

Acute Pain

Acute pain can usually be attributed to a specific cause and is of a relatively short duration. Appendicitis is a well-known example of acute pain; it usually presents with a history of a sudden onset of vague central abdominal pain that shifted to the right iliac fossa after a few hours. Once diagnosed, the conventional treatment is the removal of the organ, and post-operative recovery is normally fast and uneventful.

Following many surgical procedures, most patients are transformed from a state of only moderate pain (pre-operatively) to a state in which they have high levels of severe pain (post-operative pain). Because this post-operative pain is likely to last for only 3–4 days, there is sometimes a tendency to prescribe inadequate doses of drugs to 'tide the patient over' the acute phase of pain. Patients who demand analgesia between the recommended times for administration are sometimes accused of exaggerating their symptoms.

It is important to prescribe adequate post-operative analgesia in order to mobilize the patient, because the immobile post-operative patient is more likely to suffer complications, such as chest infections, urinary tract infections, deep vein thrombosis, and pressure sores.

One of the topical medical issues has been drug-dependence in patients prescribed long-term analgesia. For example, it has been implied that patients who suffer sickle cell crisis often become dependent on pethidine (see Chapter 31). Although it is very much publicized, the incidence of addiction to analgesia is rare; however, overestimation of its occurrence has led some health care professionals to withhold treatment. Hence some of the problems found in patients suffering pain are due to an inadequate allocation of the prescribed dose.

Chronic Pain

The sensation of acute pain bears a reasonably close relationship to the peripheral stimulus (e.g. the size of the burn or the degree of the trauma). However, with chronic pain there is a very indirect relationship (or none at all) between the amount of tissue damage and the peripheral pain stimulus. It has been suggested that in many states of chronic pain, the abnormality must also lie in the central processing rather than in the afferent input alone. Chronic pain, such as that experienced by patients with chronic back conditions or by cancer patients entering the terminal phase of their disease, is pain that has been generally present for longer than 6 months. The symptoms can be intermittent or constant, and they may vary in severity.

Chronic pain differs from acute pain in that it rarely serves as a protective function or warning of injury. Moreover it causes great suffering, is debilitating, affects the patient's quality of life, and costs the National Health Service in the UK vast amounts of money every year.

Chronic pain sufferers also have to contend with the fact that they are sometimes undertreated or misdiagnosed. Analgesia has to be given long term and generally as a combination of drugs. This is certainly fraught with problems (see Chapter 13). Some of the most effective analgesics are those that are known to have addictive properties (e.g. morphine). From another perspective, most non-steroidal anti-inflammatory drugs (NSAIDs) can produce unwanted side-effects. Thus, some patients suffering from chronic pain who are in charge of their own drug administration may decide to take less than the prescribed dose of analgesia, a problem arising from their perception that the possible adverse effects of the drugs could be worse than the pain itself; of course this is not necessarily the case. When a patient is known to have intractable pain, nerve destruction is sometimes the suggested treatment.

Chronic pain is not always a continuous sensation and it may sometimes be described as recurring acute attacks of pain. In sickle cell disease, there are episodes of severe pain followed by long trouble-free periods. In this inherited disorder the red blood cells become distorted (sickle) when the blood has a low oxygen tension. Consequently as the blood becomes more viscous, blood flow is obstructed and this results in a crisis in which the tissues affected become severely painful, swollen, and tender. Infarcts occur, most commonly in bones and the spleen, though they can arise anywhere within the body. Pain is usually most severe for the first 24 hours, and patients should be given regular, strong analgesia. Pethidine or morphine given by continuous infusion tends to afford the most effective pain relief. Factors that precipitate a sickle crisis include dehydration, infection, and extreme cold. Therefore an evaluation of the patient's life-style is necessary in order to advise on how to avoid sickle crises (see also Chapter 31).

Transient Pain
Transient pain is characterized by its extremely brief duration and the fact that it results in little or no damage and therefore is usually of little consequence.

A person exercising in a gym may feel transient muscle pain but this soon passes when the exercise stops.

PHARMACOLOGICAL MANAGEMENT OF PAIN

The control of pain is one of the most important topics in medicine. Drugs that help achieve this (analgesics) fall into three main categories:
- non-steroidal anti-inflammatory drugs (aspirin and related substances);
- morphine-like drugs (opioids); and
- local anaesthetics, which block nerve impulse transmission (see Chapter 10).

Aspirin-like drugs exert their effect by suppressing inflammation in the tissues and thereby decreasing the amount of 'traffic' in the pain fibres. Morphine-like drugs, including codeine, act by suppressing the central awareness of pain. Local anaesthetics directly impair nerve transmission, and modalities of sensation such as light touch are also abolished. Local anaesthetic drugs such as procaine usually need to be given by injection, but some, such as amethocaine eye drops, are applied topically, since they can be absorbed through mucous membranes.

DRUGS USED FOR MILD PAIN
Non-Steroidal Anti-Inflammatory Drugs
Non-steroidal anti-inflammatory drugs (NSAIDs) are a group of drugs with anti-inflammatory, antipyretic, and analgesic properties. They are most effective in the treatment of mild or moderate pain, and most are available over the counter. NSAIDs act by preventing the synthesis of the prostaglandins, which are responsible for inflammation. Unfortunately, these drugs have a number of side-effects, and this limits their use in certain patients. These side-effects are related to prostaglandin inhibition, and include gastrointestinal, haematological, and renal disturbances. Gastro-intestinal side-effects are caused by the drugs irritating the gastric mucosa, and prolonged use potentially causes haemorrhage. Care should be taken when prescribing NSAIDs for patients who have asthma, heart failure, or renal insufficiency because there is an increased risk of worsening these conditions (see Chapter 13).

Paracetamol
Paracetamol is antipyretic but not anti-inflammatory. It is commonly used to reduce pain, and to lower body temperature in patients with fever. The advantage of paracetamol over other non-steroidal anti-inflammatory

drugs (e.g. aspirin) is that it is not a gastric irritant and that it is safe to use in combination with warfarin. However, if the advised dose is exceeded, it may be toxic to the kidneys, and it can cause fatal liver damage even after a relatively small overdose.

Codeine

Codeine (methyl-morphine) is a derivative of morphine, but it does not cause the euphoria that morphine does. It is an effective analgesic and has the additional benefit of being a cough suppressant. However, constipation is a side-effect of prolonged codeine use. Dihydro-codeine is slightly more potent than codeine, but again constipation is a common side-effect. Co-proxamol, more frequently known as distalgesic, is a combination of dextropropoxyphene and paracetamol. It is particularly unsafe to consume alcohol when taking this prescribed drug since this can result in respiratory arrest. In addition, the paracetamol component can cause liver failure if the patient is inadvertently over-dosed because co-proxamol has been given in combination with another paracetamol-containing drug preparation.

DRUGS USED FOR SEVERE PAIN

Morphine

Morphine is an alkaloid of opium (codeine, which is methyl-morphine, noscapine, papaverine, and thebaine are the other main ones). Papaveretum is a preparation of total opium alkaloids standardized to the equivalent of 50% anhydrous morphine. The pharmacological actions of morphine can be divided into central actions and peripheral actions. The central actions include euphoria, sedation, hypotension, vomiting, pupillary constriction, increased release of ADH, and reduced secretion of adrenocorticotrophic hormone (ACTH), follicle-stimulating hormone (FSH), and luteinizing hormone (LH). The peripheral actions of morphine include the histamine release, constipation, and smooth muscle spasm.

After intramuscular injection, the time the drug takes to reach its peak plasma level is approximately 1 hour, and the effects of the drug last for about 4 hours. Morphine is often formulated as an elixir for oral use, but 70 per cent of the drug is subject to first-pass effect in the liver. Morphine and other narcotic analgesics are often given with phenothiazines (often cyclizine) to decrease nausea. Morphine is also available in a slow-release formula, which is an ideal analgesic for patients with chronic cancer pain whose quality of life would be disrupted if they had to take analgesia every 4 hours. Slow-release morphine maintains therapeutic levels when administered on a 12-hourly or a daily basis.

Diamorphine

Diamorphine is less bulky to inject and therefore preferable to morphine in patients with terminal illness. It can be administered subcutaneously or intravenously via a pump. The other advantage it has over morphine is that it causes less nausea and more euphoria, factors that are particularly useful in cancer patients. Some of the disadvantages of diamorphine (also known as heroin) include that it is more addictive than morphine and that it readily crosses the placental barrier. Babies born to mothers who misuse diamorphine are also addicted to the drug and have to undergo detoxification (see Chapter 12).

Other Narcotic Analgesics

Pethidine is a fast-acting analgesic whose effect lasts only a short time. It is sometimes used for women in labour, but it can cross the placental barrier, so the baby is often drowsy when it is born.

Methadone is less sedating than morphine and acts for longer periods. It is a drug most often prescribed in the treatment of heroin addiction.

Buprenorphine is an analgesic for sublingual or parenteral use with a much longer duration of action than morphine; furthermore, its use probably results in less dependence.

Nefopam is a new analgesic unrelated to the narcotic analgesics. Side-effects include a dry mouth, and the precipitation of epilepsy has been noted, though this is a rare event.

Side-Effects of Narcotics

Narcotic analgesics act by binding to opiate receptors in the central nervous system. Opiate receptors are located in the brain, spinal cord, peripheral nerves, ganglia, adrenal medulla, and gut. Respiratory depression, produced when the opiate receptors in the brain are stimulated, is the most serious and unwanted side-effect associated with opiates. This effect is seen when high doses are given, and it can be avoided by careful titration of the dose.

Another common side-effect is mental cloudiness, in which the patient may experience disorientation, dizziness, hallucinations, and nightmares. This is very disturbing to a patient who may well be feeling frightened anyway, especially if the narcotic drug has been given for pain caused by a terminal illness. If these symptoms persist, the drug regimen should be changed.

Some patients suffer from pruritus, which is treatable with oral or topical antihistamine drugs.

Nausea and vomiting are two of the other, less serious side-effects. They are still distressing, nonetheless, and they are aggravated by the fact that opiates reduce gastric motility. Metoclopramide may be prescribed to treat opiate-induced nausea and vomiting because, in addition to its anti-emetic properties, it speeds up the rate of gastric emptying. However, it is not always effective, and some patients would rather have pain than feel sick. Therefore, if the first anti-emetic drug tried does not relieve the symptoms, it should be changed. If the nausea persists, a modified analgesia regimen may be required (e.g. combination therapy using a reduced dose of morphine and another drug such as diclofenac, a non-steroidal anti-inflammatory drug, given per rectum, or paracetamol.)

Constipation is a very common side-effect of narcotics. A prophylactic laxative and a high-fibre diet with increased fluid intake is the most effective way of controlling this problem.

Physical dependence is a pharmacological property of all opioids, and withdrawal symptoms can occur when the drug is stopped abruptly. However, although these have been highly publicized for substance misusers, patients given morphine for pain do not generally suffer from withdrawal when treatment is stopped. Withdrawal occurs because the administration of exogenous opioids suppresses the normal endogenous production. This effect can be prevented by gradual reduction of the dose rather than sudden withdrawal of the drug.

PATIENT-CONTROLLED ANALGESIA

Pump devices for patient-controlled administration of analgesia have been developed to allow the patient (or the carer) to have greater management of the pain relief. For successful patient-controlled analgesia (PCA), it is essential that the patient or the carer (or both) is educated in the use of the device. PCA may be used in the relief of chronic pain, in which analgesic agents can be given as a continuous intravenous infusion, periodically, or as a bolus. PCA may also be used for acute pain; examples include using an intrathecal pump for the management of labour; or intravenous administration for postoperative analgesia.

Patients on PCA require monitoring to:
- evaluate the effectiveness of the pain relief;
- ensure that there are no adverse side-effects of the drugs;
- check that the pump equipment is working optimally.

PCA has the advantages that:
- the patient feels more in control of his or her symptoms;
- it saves nursing time; and
- it may reduce the length of time the patient has to be hospitalized.

NON-INVASIVE TECHNIQUES OF PAIN MANAGEMENT

Pharmacological intervention is not the only option for pain control, for there are many alternative methods available.

Transcutaneous Nerve Stimulation

Electrical nerve stimulation as an aid in the control of pain was used in Roman times – the use of electric eels applied to haemorrhoids and the feet of gout suffers was carried out by physicians over 2000 years ago! The transcutaneous electrical nerve stimulation (TENS) apparatus can be used to treat many different types of pain. One of the major advantages of TENS is there are no side-effects if it is used correctly, although, very occasionally, some patients develop minor skin rashes where the skin pads are fixed.

The apparatus itself is battery operated and may be worn on a belt or held in a trouser pocket (Figure 14.5). The pads are applied to the skin with the aid of a contact electrode jelly, such as KJ jelly, which should be used sparingly. Non-allergic tape can be used to secure the electrodes, but it is advisable to remove them at least once a day to allow the skin to recover.

Acupuncture

Acupuncture was originally practised as part of traditional Chinese medicine, which is now increasing being

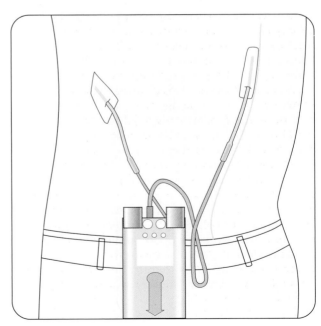

Figure 14.5 Transcutaneous electrical nerve stimulation apparatus.

used alongside Western medical techniques. It involves the insertion of sterilized needles into specific acupuncture points (acupoints) to a depth of a few millimetres. The needles are then left untouched, or manipulated, or heat may be applied to them, depending on the therapy required. The rationale for the success of acupuncture is the belief that meridian lines join the various organs of the body. The important principle is to achieve a balance between two opposing forces flowing between the meridians, the so-called Yin and Yang. When these forces are balanced, the person feels healthy; imbalance results in ill health. If a disorder is due to excess of Yang, which is the most active and dominant force, then Yin, the more 'peaceful' of the two, needs to be stimulated. Acupuncture is used as an alternative or in conjunction with analgesic drugs. Although some patients consider this to be a suitable method of pain control, others find it to be rather painful and cannot tolerate the treatment.

Heat and Cold

The application of sources of heat and cold is an easily accessible method of pain control. Cold causes peripheral vasoconstriction followed by vasodilatation, which is believed to decrease pain by slowing the rate of nerve conduction and decreasing histamine release. A very effective way of administering cold therapy is to apply massage using a block of ice rubbed over the painful area until it becomes numb. Alternatively, an ice pack may be wrapped in a towel and placed over the painful area. There are special cold packs that do not freeze to a solid and can be moulded around bony prominences. Vasocoolant sprays are also capable of providing short-term relief for pain, such as those used in sport injuries. However, cold therapy is contraindicated for some patients, for example those with Raynaud's syndrome. This disorder presents as spasm of the arteries supplying the toes or fingers and symptoms are generally triggered by cold.

The application of heat may have analgesic properties by stimulating an increased blood flow to the skin, making it more 'elastic'. This is useful before massage and stretching exercises. The heat may be applied to the skin as hot packs or paraffin baths to relieve painful joint conditions, such as arthritis of the hands or feet. Many physiotherapy departments now have a hydrotherapy pool, which allows a patient with the chronic pain of arthritis to be gently manipulated. In turn, hydrotherapy helps to maintain muscular activity, for muscle wasting around the

diseased or injured joints is a significant problem in patients who are immobile (e.g. those with osteoarthritis). The movement of the warm water soothes in a similar way to massage, with the added benefit that water can bear the weight of the patient. Because the painful areas may be exercised with less discomfort, hydrotherapy can help preserve muscle mass and makes it likely that benefit from orthopaedic surgery will be achieved more quickly.

Massage and Relaxation Therapies

The earliest records of massage as a therapeutic tool date back to 1800 BC in India, where it was used by yoga cults. Massage is commonly used in pain management today, and there are numerous classical techniques that may be used. One technique involves the application of deep friction massage to assist in the mobilization and separation of adhesions in the muscle (e.g. after strains or minor ruptures). However, it is important to ensure that haemorrhage has not arisen at the site of the injury and that massage is only applied after the episode has passed (e.g. after any oedema has subsided). More and more health care professionals are becoming familiar with the techniques of therapeutic massage, realizing the benefits when it is used in combination with conventional pain control.

Other non-invasive techniques of pain control include the use of relaxation therapy and hypnosis. Relaxation therapies include arranging for patients to listen to tapes of soothing sounds (e.g. music, waves lapping on a beach), or instructing patients about various ways to relax. Some therapists give scenarios to visualize, suggesting to the listener that they imagine themselves to be in these desirable locations. This can provide patients suffering from chronic pain with temporary relief from discomfort by being a useful diversion and a calming influence. Similarly, encouraging patients with pain to take part in conversation or merely to listen to the radio or watch television may also provide them with temporary relief. If the patient feels comfortable, e.g. use of pillows, foot stool, this too can offer some assistance.

Clinical studies have indicated that hypnosis can also be effective for both severe and chronic pain, but it is not widely used. Again, such techniques are ways of distracting patients and encouraging them to concentrate on something other than the pain. There are also thought to enhance the inhibitory processes within the nervous system that attenuate pain.

KEY POINTS

- Pain receptors are present in many parts of the body and respond to a variety of noxious stimuli (e.g. mechanical stimuli, extremes of temperature, electrical stimuli, and pressure).
- Pain is associated with electrical activity via two main types of afferent nerve fibres – type C fibres generate a dull, burning pain; type A fibres conduct more rapidly and cause sharp, well-localized pain.
- The sensation of acute pain bears a close relationship to the peripheral stimulus (e.g. size of burn, degree of trauma). It is usually attributable to a specific cause, and of short duration.
- Chronic pain is pain that has been present for longer than 6 months and may be intermittent or constant and vary in severity. It bears only a very indirect relationship (or none at all) to the stimulus and the amount of tissue damage.
- The perception of pain is a personal experience that can only be quantified and described by the patient. It is significant to remember that people have different pain thresholds and varying levels of tolerance. Some cultures encourage vocalization of pain, whereas patients from other cultures are more likely to suffer silently.
- Successfully treatment requires a thorough evaluation in which the patient describes the nature, frequency, and severity of the pain.
- Patient should be questioned about when their pain first presented and what factors, if any, they feel played a part in the onset (e.g. where the pain is, a description of the pain, factors that exacerbate or relieve the pain).
- Drugs that help control pain other than surgical anaesthesia fall into three main categories – non-steroidal anti-inflammatory drugs (aspirin and related substances), morphine-like drugs (opioids), and local anaesthetics.
- Non-pharmacological interventions may be used in pain control, e.g. transcutaneous electrical nerve stimulation (TENS), acupuncture, the application of sources of heat and cold, massage, hypnosis, and relaxation therapies.

FURTHER READING

Aunvil-Novak SE (1997) A middle-range theory of chronotherapeutic intervention for postsurgical pain. Nurs Res 46:66–71.

Baron R, Maier C (1995) Phamtom limb pain: are cutaneous nociceptors and spinothalamic neurons involved in the signalling and maintenance of spontaneous and touch-evoked pain? A case report. Pain 60:223–8.

Cowan T (1997) Patient-controlled analgesia devices. Prof Nurse 13:119–24.

Dickerson A, Besson JM (1997) The Pharmacology of Pain Handbook of Experimental Pharmacology, volume 130. Springer Verlag, London.

Hawkins RMF (1997) The role of the patient in the management of pain. Psychol Health 12:565–77.

Hopf HW, Weitz S (1994) Postoperative pain management. Arch Surg 129(2):128–32.

Irving G, Wallace M (1997) Pain Management and the Practising Physician. Churchill Livingstone, Edinburgh.

Jahangiri M, Jayatunga AP, Bradley JW, Dark CH (1994) Prevention of phantom pain after major lower limb amputation by epidural infusion of diamorphine, clonidine and bupivacaine. Ann R Coll Surg Engl 76:324–6.

Kitson A (1994) Post-operative pain management: a literature review. J Clin Nurs 3:7–18.

Lander J (1990) Fallacies and phobias about addictions and pain. Br J Addict 85:803–9.

McCaffery M, Beebe A, Latham J (eds) (1994) Pain: Clinical Manual for Nursing Practice. Mosby, London.

McCaffery M, Ferrell BR (1997) Influence of professional vs. personal role on pain assessment and use of opioids. J Contin Educ Nurs 28:69–77.

McCaffery M, Ferrell BR (1997) Nurses' knowledge of pain assessment and management: how much progress have we made? J Pain Symptom Manag 14:175–88.

McQuay H, Moore A, Justins D (1997) Treating acute pain in hospital. BMJ 314:1531–5.

Melzack R, Wall P (1988)The Challenge of Pain. Penguin, London.

Ng B, Dimsdale JE, Rollnik JD, Shapiro H (1996) The effect of ethnicity on prescriptions for patient-controlled analgesia for post-operative pain. Pain 66:9–12.

Nikolajsen L, Ilkjaer S, Christensen JH, Kroner K, Jensen TS (1997) Randomized trial of epidural bupivacaine and morphine in prevention of stump and phantom pain in lower-limb amputation. Lancet 350:1353–7.

Phillips LL (1998) Managing the pain of bone metastases in the home environment. Am J Hosp Palliat Care 15:32–42.

Prevention and Control of Pain in Children (1997). Royal College of Paediatrics and Child Health. BMJ Books, London.

Rampes H, Sharples F, Maragh S, Fisher P (1997). Introducing complementary medicine into the medical curriculum. J Roy Soc Med 90:(1) 19–22.

Tyrer SP (1992) Psychology, Psychiatry and Chronic Pain. Butterworth Heinemann, London.

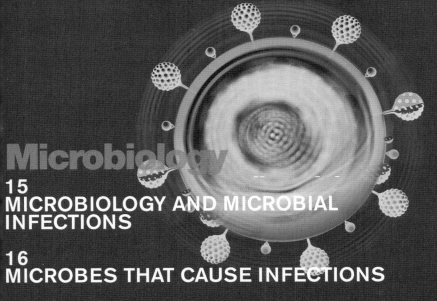

Microbiology

MICROBIOLOGY AND MICROBIAL INFECTION

INTRODUCTION

Microbiology is the study of microbes, many of which are the agents responsible for infections in humans and animals. However, many microbes are present in the immediate environment of the host as commensal organisms. In contrast to the microbe described in the Person-Centred Study (An Influenza Epidemic), which looks at the dynamics of the spread of an infectious disease, commensal organisms are generally harmless and non-pathogenic to the host. They may even be beneficial because they protect against infection and colonization by pathogenic organisms. However, on the very rare occasions when the innate (in-built) resistance to infection is compromised, some of these non-pathogenic commensals can cause disease; they are then referred to as 'opportunistic pathogens'.

PERSON-CENTRED STUDY: AN INFLUENZA EPIDEMIC

A general practitioner noticed that there was an increase in the number of patients attending his surgery with colds and fever. He became concerned that this might be the beginning of an influenza outbreak and enquired from his colleagues whether they were having the same experience. This was indeed the case, and some of the patients were found to have a more severe form of the disease that required hospitalization. The patients requiring hospitalization had higher temperatures, were either elderly or very young, and developed symptoms characteristic of pneumonia with X-ray changes showing lung consolidation. There were also a few reports of deaths. Most of the severe cases occurred in the patients who were residents of homes for the elderly, and the severity of the disease was unaffected by antibiotic treatments. It was also found that the incidence of colds and fever, unresponsive to antibiotic treatment, was rapidly increasing in the community. Most cases, however, were generally of mild or moderate severity and did not require major treatment or hospitalization. Influenza A virus was isolated from throat washings of many of these patients and serological tests showed the presence of an antibody to a particular antigen of influenza A virus, confirming an epidemic caused by a single type of the virus.

A large number of commensals are found within the host and on the surface of the host in direct contact with the external environment. The skin surface harbours organisms such as *Streptococci* and *Staphylococci*; these are easily shed into the air and may settle on raw and open wounds, where they cause wound infections. These organisms are often spread in hospital wards during bed making or dusting.

The throat, mouth, and upper respiratory tract carry a large number of commensal organisms. Sometimes these areas may become colonized with pathogenic (disease-producing) organisms such as *Streptococci*, pneumococci, and *Staphylococci*, and these organisms are dispersed during coughing and sneezing. They can also cause secondary descending infections in the bronchi (causing bronchitis) and lungs (causing pneumonia), especially when the bronchial tract is partially devitalized by the presence of a severe virus infection such as influenza (see Person-Centred Study).

The intestinal tract of humans and animals carries a very large number of commensal organisms. In fact, much of the volume of faeces consists of commensals of the intestinal tract. Two main groups of organisms are generally found:
- aerobic organisms (those which can grow in the ordinary environment containing oxygen), such as the enterobacteria (e.g. *Escherichia coli*); and
- anaerobic organisms (those that are unable to grow or survive in the presence of oxygen), such as *Bacteroides fragilis*.

Since these are normal commensal flora of the gut, they do not usually cause infection of the intestinal tract. When implanted in other sites, however, they are capable of producing infections (e.g. urinary tract infections caused by *Escherichia coli*; postoperative wound or blood infections caused by *Bacteroides fragilis*).

The genitourinary tract of males and females can be colonized by a number of commensal organisms. Commensals in the male genitourinary tract are generally of no clinical significance. Because of the proximity of the perineal region, both the female and male urethra may become colonized with gut organisms. In the female, owing to the shortness of the urethra, some of these organisms often cause ascending infection in the bladder (see Chapter 36). The female genital tract also harbours a number of organisms, some of which may have major implications for infection; particularly notable are the opportunistic pathogens such as *Candida albicans*, which may cause thrush. These occur especially when immunity is compromised as a consequence of prolonged antibiotic or corticosteroid therapy, and in diabetes mellitus (see Chapters 18 and 28).

WHAT IS AN INFECTION?

An infection is a process that occurs when a pathogenic microbe or an opportunistic organism is established in a host, either by an active process in which the host's tissues and organs are damaged, or because of weak innate resistance of the host. Establishment of an infection means that, on implantation, the microbe can multiply in the tissues, invade deeper tissues and blood, and produce poisonous substances (i.e. toxins and enzymes), which precipitate major damaging effects on host functions.

In order to establish an infection, a microbe must enter the host, usually by breaching one of the physical external barriers such as the skin or mucous membrane. This may occur following an accident (e.g. burns, a cut, or the elective incision of a surgical wound). The influenza virus causes injury to the respiratory mucosa during the infection process. The damaged mucosa then allows pathogenic bacteria (such as the pneumococcus and *Haemophilus* species) to establish an infection by multiplying and causing pneumonia through an active pathogenic process. Damage to the respiratory mucosa can also be caused by a number of extraneous and environmental factors. Extremes of environmental temperature, air pollutants, smoking, and debilitation can inflict major damage to the mucosa, permitting secondary bacterial and viral infection to occur.

Other situations in which infections are likely to occur include overcrowding, poor living conditions, malnutrition (see Chapter 28), alcohol misuse, chronic infective conditions, diabetes, and an unhygienic environment. Similarly, a prolonged stay in hospital means that a patient (who is likely to be vulnerable already) is exposed to a number of pathogenic and opportunistic infections; this is a common factor which leads to acquisition of infection in hospital.

An opportunistic pathogen precipitates an infection when the patient's immune and non-immune defence systems fail to prevent the establishment of an infection. A prime example occurs in the use of cytotoxic drugs, which are toxic to the cells. Although they primarily kill cancer cells, they can also damage the host's normal cells (see Chapter 10). Similarly, patients given immuno-suppressive drugs (e.g. after transplant surgery) or prolonged antibiotic and steroid therapy, and those with immunosuppressive diseases such as infection with human immunodeficiency virus (HIV) are vulnerable to opportunistic infections (see Chapters 18 and 28).

15. MICROBIOLOGY AND MICROBIAL INFECTION

THE MICROBES

A large number of microbes are found in the immediate environment of the host. Many are non-pathogenic, environmental organisms that are of little or no clinical significance.

BACTERIA

The microbes that cause disease in humans and animals have been studied in more detail. The pathogenic microbes that predominate in human infections are the single-celled microscopic agents called bacteria. Most bacteria are visualized under a light microscope by staining with a series of dyes.

On the basis of their staining characteristics with the Gram stain, bacteria can be subdivided into Gram-positive bacteria and Gram-negative bacteria. They can be further subdivided on the basis of their morphological appearances (Table 15.1). Bacteria may be spherical (the cocci), rod-shaped (the bacilli), comma-

Classification of Common Pathogenic Bacteria

	Shape and other characteristics	Genus name	Species name
Gram positive	coccus (spherical)	*Staphylococcus*	*aureus* *epidermidis*
		Streptococcus	*pyogenes*
	(diplococcus)	*Streptococcus*	*pneumoniae (pneumococcus)*
Gram positive	bacilli (rod-shaped)	*Corynebacterium*	*diphtheriae*
		Listeria	*monocytogenes*
		Clostridium	*tetani* *botulinum* *perfringens*
Gram negative	coccus (spherical)	*Neisseria*	*meningitidis* *gonorrhoeae*
		Pseudomonas	*pyocyanea*
Gram negative	bacilli (rod-shaped) (aerobic)	*Salmonella*	*typhi*
		Shigella	*sonnei*
		Escherichia	*coli*
	short rods (parvo-bacterium)	*Haemophilus*	*influenzae*
		Bordetella	*pertussis*
		Brucella	*abortus*
	bacilli (anaerobic)	*Bacteroides*	*fragilis*
	vibrio (comma-shaped)	*Vibrio*	*cholerae*
		Campylobacter	*jejuni*
Other pathogenic bacteria	rod-shaped	*Mycobacterium*	*tuberculosis* *leprae*
	spiral-shaped	*Treponema*	*pallidum*
		Leptospira	*icterohaemmorhagica*

Table 15.1 Classification of common pathogenic bacteria.

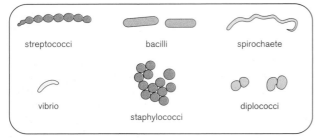

Figure 15.1 **Common bacteria associated with human infection.** This simple diagram shows some of these common bacteria.

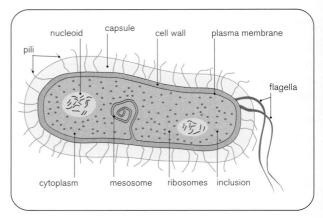

Figure 15.2 **Simplified structure of a bacterial cell.**

shaped (the vibrio), or spiral-shaped (the spirochaetes) (Figure 15.1). A more detailed account of these bacteria and the diseases they cause will be given in Chapter 16.

Bacteria are microscopic agents with a fairly simple structure (see Chapter 1). From outside inwards, they consists of:

- a cell wall, which is organized differently in Gram-positive and Gram-negative bacteria;
- a cell membrane enclosing the cytoplasm of the cell; the cell membrane is very similar in structure to mammalian cell membranes, and it is also involved in the respiratory function of the cell;
- cytoplasm, which contains a variety of cytosolic organelles, such as ribosomes, inclusion bodies of different sizes, and other structures; these organelles have different functions (e.g. storage); and
- nuclear material existing as a disorganized mass of DNA; this is not enclosed by a nuclear membrane as it is in mammalian cells.

Outside the cell wall, a bacteria may have a number of extracellular appendages. These include:

- a capsule, which is a large and loose chemical frame, such as the capsular polysaccharide found in some bacteria (e.g. the pneumococcus), in which it acts as a protective coat against phagocytosis by neutrophils and macrophages;
- flagella, which are complex structures of variable size and distribution; they are generally responsible for movement of the bacterial cells; and
- fimbria or pili, which are hair-like appendages found on the surface of bacteria; they are responsible for bacterial adherence to epithelial cells; some of these (the sex pili) are also involved in the transfer of genetic material between bacterial cells (Figure 15.2).

VIRUSES

The second important group of pathogenic microbes are the viruses. These are extremely minute in size and cannot normally be seen under the light microscope – they require electron microscopy for their visualization. Viruses are structurally very simple, having a small amount of nucleic acid – either deoxyribonucleic acid (DNA) or ribonucleic acid (RNA) – surrounded by a protein coat (capsid). On the basis of the ultramicroscopic capsid arrangement, they are classified as:

- cubical (e.g. adenovirus, poliovirus);
- helical (e.g. influenza virus, measles virus); or
- complex (e.g. poxviruses) (Figure 15.3).

Poxviruses are the largest in size – about 400 nm (0.4 μm) – less than half the size of a *Staphylococcus* organism; polioviruses are some of the smallest viruses – about 20–30 nm.

FUNGI

Some fungi are associated with human infections. Only a small number of these fungal infections are found in the UK, and they occur mostly in patients who are debilitated owing to chronic diseases (e.g. diabetes); immunocompromised owing to treatment with cytotoxic drugs, steroids, or prolonged antibiotic therapy; or infected with HIV. The fungi responsible for deep, systemic infections in these patients are yeast-like fungi, such as *Candida albicans* and other *Candida* species, and *Cryptococcus neoformans*. *Aspergillus* species have also been associated with infections in immunocompromised patients (see Chapter 18). Other fungi that are associated with infection, particularly superficial infection, are those that are associated with ringworm (dermatophytes). Fungi are generally more complex in their structural organization than viruses or bacteria, and they are often multicellular. Figure 15.4 shows the appearances of some common fungi.

PROTOZOAL AND PARASITIC PATHOGENS

Infections caused by these pathogenic organisms are rare in the developed world (Figure 15.5). Some of these infections may be imported into the UK from these area by travellers (e.g. malaria). Protozoal and parasitic infections usually occur in the intestinal tract, in the blood, and in a number of tissues including lung and brain.

In the intestinal tract, the main infections (infestations) are caused by unicellular protozoa (e.g. *Giardia lamblia* and *Entamoeba histolytica*,) and parasitic worms, including roundworm (e.g. *Ascaris lumbricoides*), hookworm (e.g. *Ancylostoma duodenale*), threadworm (e.g. *Strongyloides stercoralis*), and tapeworm (e.g. *Taenia solium*). These infections are transmitted by contaminated food and water and are generally found in poorer countries of the world with inadequate housing and sanitation facilities.

Examples of blood-borne parasitic infections are malaria, filariasis, leishmaniasis, and trypanosomiasis; these are mainly a problem in tropical countries and are transmitted via an insect vector.

Tissue infections are not very common; examples include the infections caused by liver and lung flukes and some worms. A disseminated tissue infection caused by *Toxoplasma gondii*, a unicellular protozoal parasite, is often seen in immunocompromised patients; (see the Person-Centred Study in Chapter 24).

HOW DO MICROBES CAUSE DISEASE?

INVASION OF THE HOST

Before a pathogenic microbe can enter and cause disease, it needs a 'foothold' within or upon the host. This may be established by first adhering to one of the

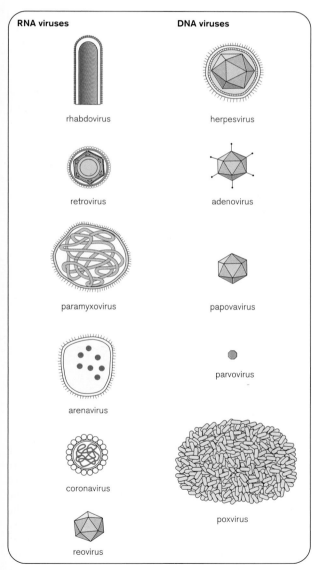

Figure 15.3 Common viruses associated with human infection. This simple diagram shows some of these common viruses.

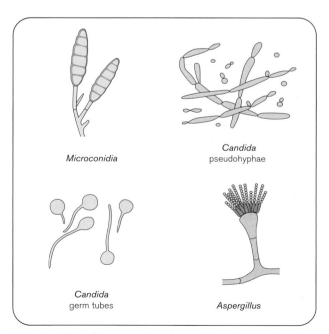

Figure 15.4 Appearance of some common fungi.

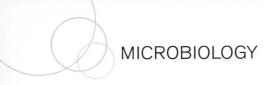

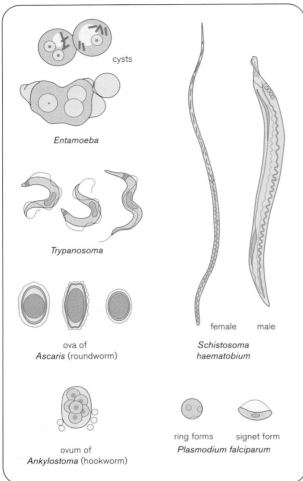

Figure 15.5 Appearance of some common protozoan parasites.

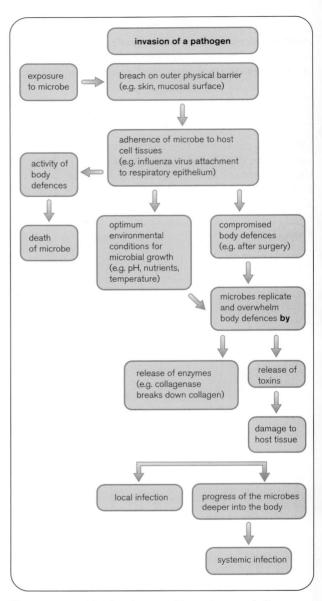

Figure 15.6 Mechanisms of invasion and disease causation by pathogens.

various body surfaces of the host (e.g. a mucous membrane). Adherence of the microbes to the host is facilitated by a number of microbial components that attach to receptors on the host tissue. In the case of influenza virus, for example, haemagglutinin and neuraminic acid, molecules on the surface of the virus particles, have the ability to adhere to the respiratory epithelium because of the presence of receptors (attachment sites) on these epithelial cells. *Neisseria gonorrhoeae* attaches to the urethral epithelium with the help of pili on the surface of these organisms (Figure 15.6).

LOCAL MULTIPLICATION OF MICROBES

In order to initiate a disease process, microbes need to enter the host and multiply in large numbers. If microbes are able to overcome the natural defence mechanism, either because of the overwhelming nature of the infection or because of inadequate resistance of the host, they will begin to replicate. At first, the organisms attack locally; then, with the progress of the infection, they invade more deeply into tissues and spread to other areas, including the blood. The blood can be a vehicle for transmission of infection to other parts of the body.

When the multiplication process is firmly established, rapid growth will occur. During this process, nutrients for growth of the microbes (such as essential amino acids, minerals, carbohydrates, and vitamins) are provided by the patient's tissues. An optimal environment, such as the ideal pH, temperature, and oxygen–carbon dioxide balance is required for exponential growth of the organisms, and this is provided by the host; hence, an infection occurs (Figure 15.7).

RELEASE OF MICROBIAL TOXINS
Tissue Damaging Enzymes

Microbes produce a wide variety of enzymes, which act on different substrates. This results in the structure of the surrounding tissue becoming disorganized in areas where the microbes multiply, thereby allowing the invasion to occur. *Streptococci* and *Staphylococci* are known to produce enzymes such as collagenase, which breaks down the collagen that provides the structural framework of a cell. Similarly, hyaluronidase is an enzyme that splits hyaluronic acid, which is responsible for cementing the cells together to form

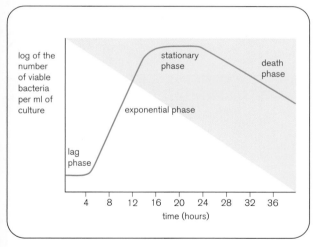

Figure 15.7 Phases of bacterial growth. The lag phase is a period of minimal bacterial growth. In the exponential phase, bacterial growth reaches its full potential and the bacteria make maximum use of the available nutrients. In the stationary phase, bacterial growth is maintained, but there starts to be a gradual retardation in the growth rate because nutrient supplies are becoming depleted. *In vivo*, the stationary phase in bacterial growth occurs when the host defences are active against the infection. In the death phase, bacterial growth ceases as the nutrient supply is exhausted. *In vivo*, the death phase occurs as the host defences eliminate the infection.

tissue. Microbial proteases, lipase, and DNAse metabolize proteins, lipids, and DNA respectively. *Neisseria gonorrhoeae* and several other bacterial and viral agents produce a protease that destroys immunoglobulin A (IgA), the secretory antibodies found predominately at the mucosal surfaces. The IgA antibodies normally have a protective function at the interface between the internal and external environments (see Chapter 24).

Toxins: Exotoxins and Endotoxins

Many microbes are known to produce toxic products (toxins) during their multiplication. These toxins may be actively produced by a living organism (exotoxins), or they may be released as bacteria disintegrate (endotoxins).

The classic examples of exotoxins are those released by the microbes that cause diseases such as tetanus, botulism, and diphtheria. Exotoxins have specific target sites where they exert their damaging effects. Tetanus exotoxin is produced by the anaerobic bacteria *Clostridium tetani*; it interferes with the nerve cells, and this results in intermittent spasm of muscles with repeated convulsion. Botulinum toxin, actively produced by *Clostridium botulinum*, is probably the most powerful toxin. It blocks the release of acetylcholine (a neurotransmitter) at the neuromuscular junctions, resulting in flaccid paralysis. *Clostridium perfringens* is the organism responsible for gas gangrene (see Chapter 4). This organism produces lecithinase, an enzyme that acts on lecithin, which is a major component of the cell membrane of various cells, including red blood cells. Thus, the activities of lecithinase can result in the lysis of red blood cells and other tissues, producing major necrotic changes and hypoxia to aid the survival of the *Clostridium perfringens* organisms which require an oxygen-free environment.

Corynebacterium diphtheriae, the causative agent of clinical diphtheria, produces an exotoxin that binds to the heart muscle. The toxin causes disruption of protein synthesis, resulting in severe damage to the heart muscle. This can lead to cardiac failure. The toxin also acts locally in the throat, where it produces extensive necrosis and tissue damage and leads to the formation of a pseudomembrane. This may cause obstruction of the airway and lead to death by oxygen deprivation (asphyxia).

Staphylococcus aureus is responsible for a wide range of pyogenic (pus-producing) infections, including boils, abscesses, osteomyelitis and deeper blood-borne infection. This bacteria produces a variety of exotoxins. Some of these exotoxins have tissue-destroying activities (e.g. leukocidin, which kills leukocytes). Toxic shock syndrome toxin is a very powerful staphylococcal exotoxin which can result in severe systemic manifestations (see Chapter 25). *Streptococcus pyogenes* produces a similar toxin, which also causes severe systemic effects. Some of the well-known exotoxins produced by micro-organisms and their adverse effects on different target organs are listed in Table 15.2.

The endotoxins are usually produced by the Gram-negative organisms when they die and disintegrate. These are lipopolysaccharides (lipid and sugar molecules) from the cell wall of the bacteria, and they are powerful activators of the monocyte– macrophage series of white blood cells.

Activation of these cells results in the release of a number of cytokines, such as the interleukins (especially interleukin-1 and interleukin-6) and tumour necrosis factor-alpha. Some of these cytokines, when released in excessive amounts in response to an infection, can produce widespread effects by acting on different target sites. The clinical manifestations include septic shock, intravascular coagulation, haemorrhage in internal organs, respiratory distress syndrome, haemodynamic imbalance (resulting in a fall in blood pressure), a destabilizing effect on the body's temperature regulation mechanisms, and other non-specified effects (see Chapter 25). Many of these manifestations are produced classically by *Neisseria meningitidis*, the organism responsible for meningitis, but other Gram-negative bacteria also evoke these symptoms.

Although the mechanisms by which micro-organisms cause disease have been studied in detail for a number of pathogenic bacteria, for other organisms the mechanisms remain unknown. The *Mycobacterium* species are typical examples of this. With the application of newly developed molecular biology technology and the better understanding of the genetic organization of the microbes, it is hoped that the pathogenic mechanisms of many pathogens will soon be successfully elucidated.

Viruses produce disease by infecting various host cells and destroying them. A virus must enter a host cell in order to survive. Thus, viruses utilize the metabolic machinery of the host for their own benefit and incorporate their own genetic material into the host genome and so are able to replicate as the cell divides (see Chapter 28). Viruses also use protein synthetic pathways to synthesize capsid proteins which are then used for producing new virus particles. During this process, a large number of new virus particles are formed, the host cell dies and disintegrates, and the new virus particles are released. These new virus particles then infect other cells and the process is perpetuated. The reproduction process generates a

Some Important Bacterial Exotoxins

Pathogen	Toxin	Disease
Gram-positive organisms		
Corynebacterium diphtheriae	diphtheria toxin	pharyngeal diphtheria, myocarditis
Clostridium tetani	tetanus toxin	tetani (muscle spasm)
Clostridium botulinum	botulinum toxin	botulism
Clostridium perfringens	alpha toxin or lecithinase C, enterotoxin	gas gangrene and tissue necrosis; food poisoning
Clostridium difficile	toxin A	diarrhoea
Staphylococcus aureus	toxic shock syndrome toxin (TSST-1) exfoliative toxin, haemolysins, leukocidin, and cytolysins	toxic shock syndrome kills leukocytes and other cells
Streptococcus pyogenes	scarlet fever toxin (erythrogenic toxin)	scarlet fever – scarlatinal rash
Gram-negative organisms		
Vibrio cholerae	enterotoxin	cholera
Escherichia coli	enterotoxin	diarrhoea
Bordetella pertussis	pertussis toxin	whooping cough

Table 15.2 Some Important Bacterial Toxins

considerable amount of degraded tissue debris, which acts as endogenous toxic products. These stimulate the host immune system to generate cytokines through the macrophage–monocyte cell system, and these cytokines promote the defence mechanism as well as symptoms of infection.

TRANSMISSION OF INFECTIONS

An infection can spread through the community, initially affecting only a few people but rapidly involving large numbers and causing an epidemic (see Person-Centred Study: an Influenza Epidemic). Epidemics may extend beyond national and geographical barriers, causing a pandemic, as has happened with several strains of influenza during the past few decades.

A major potential source of infection is an infectious patient. During the clinical presentation of disease, a patient may be highly contagious and spread the infection to his or her immediate contacts and to health care workers. This is particularly important to remember when an infected patient is being cared for in a hospital ward because there are other vulnerable patients around. It is also notable in institutions such as prisons and homes where people with special needs are cared for. An infected patient may also contaminate inanimate objects, such as items of clothing, bed linen, crockery and cutlery, and reading materials. In certain circumstances (e.g. in the case of infections caused by multiple-drug-resistant bacteria) special attention needs to be given to these items in order to prevent cross-infection in hospital and other settings.

The common mechanisms by which infections are spread are:
- the air-borne route (e.g. influenza, the common cold, streptococcal infections, pulmonary tuberculosis);
- the water-borne route (e.g. cholera, typhoid, dysentery, hepatitis A, enterovirus infections);
- the food-borne transmission (e.g. infections caused by food-poisoning, *Salmonella* infections, *Shigella* infections);
- transmission by hand (e.g. staphylococcal infections, Gram-negative hospital-acquired infections);
- implantation of micro-organisms (e.g. infections in cuts and burns, infections resulting from insect bites);
- transmission by blood and blood products (e.g. blood transmission of hepatitis B in infected needles);
- sexual transmission (e.g. gonorrhoea, syphilis, HIV);
- transmission from animals to humans (zoonoses) (e.g. anthrax, brucellosis); and
- transmission from mother to fetus (congenital infections) (e.g. rubella, toxoplasmosis, cytomegalovirus).

AIR-BORNE ROUTE

Respiratory Infections

Respiratory infections are likely to be contagious owing to the ease with which the infection can spread by coughing, sneezing, and even talking. Infections that are often spread by this route include the common viral infections of the upper respiratory tract, such as the common cold, influenza, measles, mumps, and rubella. Several acute bacterial infections, such as diphtheria, whooping cough, and streptococcal sore throat, may also be transmitted by the air-borne route. An example of a chronic bacterial infection is tuberculosis, which also spreads via the air.

Therefore, patients with respiratory infection require careful management, particularly if they are in a hospital ward because of the relative ease with which they can cross-infect other patients and the health care workers. Factors that perpetuate the spread of respiratory infection are overcrowding and general debilitation of other patients in the ward (see Box 15.1).

Pyogenic Infections

Pyogenic infections, such as staphylococcal skin infection, streptococcal superficial infections, streptococcal throat infection, and pneumococcal infections (these may also be transmitted through the air) are potential sources of hospital cross-infection. Patients with these infections generally shed a large number of the organisms in the immediate environment. These organism are easily spread when there is any major air movement in the vicinity of the patient (e.g. making of beds or moving of newspapers). The organisms may then initiate infections in other patients, either as surface infections (e.g. within wounds) or as respiratory infections (e.g. pneumonia).

Multiple-Resistant and Methicillin-Resistant *Staphylococcus aureus* Infections

In recent years there have been numerous reports of hospital-acquired MRSA (multiple-resistant *Staphylococcus aureus* or methicillin-resistant *Staphylococcus aureus*) infections. Although many of these MRSA infections have been superficial colonizations, there have also been deeper infections (e.g. after hip-replacement surgery) and blood-borne infections. MRSA infections have caused substantial mortality.

WATER-BORNE ROUTE

A large number of infections may be spread via the water-borne route. They are commonly a problem in the developing world, where safe water supplies may not be easily available and people are dependent on unfiltered water sources. Water is a common vehicle

BOX 15.1 TRANSMISSION OF *LEGIONELLA PNEUMOPHILA*

A striking example of rapid spread of a respiratory infection is the outbreak of legionnaires' disease in Philadelphia in 1976. During a convention of the American Legion in a major hotel in the centre of Philadelphia, a large number of participants were struck down by severe respiratory infection, and there were several deaths. The causative organism was found to be a small Gram-negative bacillus, *Legionella pneumophila*, which was transmitted to the participants through the hotel's air conditioning system. The infection spread rapidly to the older people at the convention, particularly those who were heavy smokers and consuming alcohol relatively liberally.

for a large number of intestinal protozoal infections, giardiasis and amoebic dysentery, as well as for organisms that cause diseases like cholera, typhoid, and bacterial dysentery. Sometimes these appear in epidemic proportions and are responsible for high mortality and morbidity. Epidemics of water-borne virus infections are also common, particularly hepatitis A virus (infectious hepatitis). Enteroviral infections, such as those caused by poliovirus and Coxsackie virus, are also spread by this route.

Although water-borne infections are generally rare in the developed world, there have been occasional reports of water supplies being contaminated with tiny parasites such as *Cryptosporidia*, which can cause diarrhoea in vulnerable people (i.e. young children, older adults, and immunocompromised patients).

FOOD-BORNE TRANSMISSION

Poor hygiene and inadequate food storage facilities are generally responsible for contamination of food with infective organisms. As with water-borne infections, these infections are more frequently seen in the developing countries. The infecting agents are much the same as those involved in water-borne infections, although bacterial agents such as *Salmonella*, *Shigella*, and *Vibrio cholerae* (which causes cholera) are more regularly implicated. Travellers returning from developing countries (e.g. in Asia, Africa, South America) are more likely to present with these infections than are other people in the developed world.

Food-borne infections do, however, occur in the developed world, and again poor hygiene and inadequate facilities are generally to blame. Food-borne infections are usually reported in small or large outbreaks in institutions, such as hospitals, homes, and other communal centres. Infections due to a number of *Salmonella* species, *Campylobacter jejuni*, and *Shigella sonnei* are some of the familiar infecting agents. Most of these agents are contracted from poultry, cooked meats, milk and milk products, and food that has been inadequately reheated (see Chapter 16).

TRANSMISSION BY HAND

Infection caused by direct contact with dirty hands is a relatively common occurrence in hospitals. Doctors, nurses, and paramedical workers are frequently responsible for the spread of infection, particularly when there is a breakdown of strict hand washing practice. Gram-negative enteric organisms, such as *Pseudomonas* species, *Klebsiella* species, and *Escherichia coli*, are transmitted from patient to patient in high dependency units (e.g. intensive care units). Staphylococcal infections, including MRSA infections, also spread in hospitals by this method.

Some infections are transmitted by salivary contacts through kissing and biting. Examples include glandular fever (infectious mononucleosis), acute streptococcal infections, and rabies. Certain infections may be caused by direct skin penetration by the infective organism. An example is leptospirosis, which is caused by *Leptospira*. *Leptospira* are found in sewage and polluted rivers; immersion in contaminated water allow the organism to penetrate intact skin.

IMPLANTATION OF ORGANISMS
Infections Acquired Through Cuts and Lacerations
Penetrating wounds
Accidental implantation of infections can occur from dust and foreign bodies containing organisms such as *Staphylococci*, *Streptococci*, and *Clostridia* (both *Clostridium tetani* and *Clostridium perfringens)*.

Iatrogenic infections
Infections can be transmitted in doctors' surgeries and in operation theatres through inadequately sterilized surgical instruments. Most of the infections described above can be transmitted by this means, as can, on rare occasions, blood-borne infections such as hepatitis B , hepatitis C, and HIV infection.

Infections Transmitted by Infected Hypodermic Needles

Blood-borne *Staphylococcus aureus* infection and other blood-borne infections are transmitted by hypodermic needles in intravenous drug misusers. Hepatitis B, hepatitis C, and HIV infection are typical examples of infections in intravenous drug misusers that have arisen because of the sharing of dirty needles.

Infections Implanted by Animal Bites

Rabies can be transmitted by a bite from an infected dog or fox; bats in South America are sometimes infected with rabies virus and transmits the infection by bites.

Infections Implanted by Insect Bites

Malaria is transmitted by mosquito bites. Female anopheline mosquitoes while feeding on a malaria infected patient, acquire malaria parasites in the blood. The parasites survive in the stomach of the mosquitoes and are transmitted to another person when the mosquitoes next feed.

Phlebotomus argentipes (sandfly) transmits microfilaria from infected patients to healthy people. The tsetse fly carries trypanosomiasis from infected patients to healthy contacts.

TRANSMISSION BY BLOOD AND BLOOD PRODUCTS

Various infections have been known to be transmitted by blood and blood products. These include hepatitis B, hepatitis C, HIV infection, syphilis, and malaria. In the 1970s and 1980s, a large number of people with haemophilia who had received the blood product, factor VIII, became infected with HIV. Several cases of hepatitis B and HIV infection related to blood transfusion have been reported. During the past decade, transfusion services across the developed world have instituted testing for HIV, hepatitis B, and other transfusion-related infections in all their blood and blood products (see Chapters 29 and 31).

SEXUAL TRANSMISSION

Several infections are transmitted by sexual intercourse with infected partners. The most common of these are gonococcal infection, caused by *Neisseria gonorrhoeae*, and infection with *Chlamydia trachomatis*. Other infections that are transmitted by this route include syphilis, hepatitis B, hepatitis C, HIV, *Candida albicans*, and *Gardnerella vaginalis*.

TRANSMISSION FROM ANIMALS TO HUMANS

Animal infections are often accidentally transmitted to humans, particularly from infected domestic animals. These infections are called zoonoses and their transmission generally occurs by inhalation or by direct contact. Some examples of zoonotic infections include brucellosis, anthrax, leptospirosis, and some common skin infections such as ringworm fungal infections from infected puppies. Animal infections are often transmitted to humans through insect bites (e.g. plague through bites by fleas parasitising on infected rats, and yellow fever through bites by mosquitoes from infected monkeys).

TRANSMISSION FROM MOTHER TO FETUS

Infections transmitted from mother to fetus *in utero* (congenital infections) include rubella (German measles), toxoplasmosis, cytomegalovirus infections, and syphilis. These infections can cause considerable congenital deformities, miscarriage, or stillbirth (see the Person-Centred Study in Chapter 24).

MICROBIOLOGY

FURTHER READING

Brooks GF, Butel JS, Ornston LN, Jawetz E, Melnick JL, Aldberg EA. (1995) Jawetz, Melnick and Aldberg's Medical Microbiology, 12th edition. Prentice-Hall International.

Collier L and Oxford J. (1993) Human Virology. Oxford University Press, Oxford.

Greenwood D, Slack RC and Peutherer JF. (1997) Medical Microbiology, 15th edition. Churchill Livingstone, London.

Mims PC. (1998) Medical Microbiology, 2nd edition. Mosby, London.

Ryan, KJ, (ed). (1994) Sherris's Medical Microbiology: an Introduction to Infectious Diseases. Prentice-Hall International.

Shansen DC. (1998) Microbiology in Clinical Practice, 2nd edition. Wright, London.

MICROBES THAT CAUSE INFECTIONS

LEARNING OBJECTIVES

After studying this chapter you will have a clearer understanding of:
- the nature and extent of the infections that are caused by microbial agents
- the complexities of infections in different tissues and organs of the body
- the modes available for containing various infections

INTRODUCTION

Our immediate environment is strewn with a wide range of microbes, which are found in the air, water, dust, soil and in or on the other inhabitants of the earth. Most of these microbes are innocuous and are unlikely to pose any major threat. As described in Chapter 15, besides the large population of innocuous microbes in the environment (called saprophytes), people themselves carry a large number of microbes within or on the body surfaces. These microbes are also generally harmless and are called commensals. However, there are large numbers of microbes which, on entering the body, can cause damage to the host. These are called pathogens. When people are infected with such organisms, they becomes a potential source

PERSON-CENTRED STUDY: A CHILD WITH MENINGITIS

Carol is a student nurse. One evening when Carol was on duty, Sarah, an 8-year-old girl, was admitted to the ward with a cold, fever, severe rash, and headache. Sarah was put in a separate room where her mother also stayed. In the early hours of the morning, Sarah's mother anxiously called Carol to come and see the child. Carol found her covered with a rash and not responding readily. She raised the alarm immediately. The on-call doctor came and examined the child and immediately contacted a senior doctor with a diagnosis of provisional meningitis. Blood was taken for microbiological culture and benzylpenicillin was administered intravenously. A lumbar puncture was also performed and the cerebrospinal fluid (CSF) sent to the microbiology laboratory.

The laboratory phoned promptly with the result of the CSF microscopy. The CSF had a large preponderance of white blood cells (polymorphonucleocytes), and Gram stain of the CSF showed Gram-negative diplococci in pairs. The laboratory later confirmed that the blood culture also grew Gram-negative diplococci. Further tests confirmed the isolate to be *Neisseria meningitidis* type C. Following treatment with antimicrobial therapy, Sarah made a full recovery.
Because Carol was closely involved in the care of the child in the early stages, it was felt that she should be given prophylaxis against *Neisseria meningitidis* with the drug, rifampicin. Sarah's mother and a 5 year old sibling were also given rifampicin prophylaxis (see also Chapters 19 and 38).

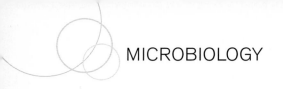
of spread of these pathogens to healthy contacts. Thus, an infected patient is a major source of infection to others in the community (see Person-Centred Study: a Child with Meningitis). The many other sources of infection are discussed in Chapter 15.

INFECTIONS OF THE DIFFERENT BODY SYSTEMS

When a host acquires a microbe from an infected person or from any other source, the microbe multiplies in the host's body and evokes various damaging effects. The many symptoms and signs produced include a rise in body temperature (pyrexia), general weakness and malaise, as well as other more specific symptoms characteristic of the disease (see Chapter 17). An infection may take its own course and lead to further aggravation, resulting in morbidity or death of the host unless interrupted by prompt and effective treatment; or an infection may activate the host's defence mechanisms that promote spontaneous healing.

There are many ways in which to describe infections. One of the simpler ways is to present infection according to the different body systems affected.

INFECTION OF SKIN

These are some of the most common types of infection, and they are often seen in hospital as well as in the doctor's surgery. Infections in these sites are frequently caused by:
- Gram-positive organisms such as *Streptococci* and *Staphylococci*;
- anaerobic bacteria such as *Bacteroides* and *Clostridium*; and
- viral infections causing skin rashes.

Streptococcus Species

These are Gram-positive (appearing dark violet on Gram staining), spherical bacteria (cocci) that are generally found in long or short chains (the Greek word *streptos* means 'chain') in the affected tissues (Figure 16.1). They usually cause pus-producing lesions in the skin and soft tissues. They also produce cellulitis in deeper tissues and often, in association with *Staphylococci*, cause impetigo (superficial skin infections with pus and crust formation). While growing in the tissues the microbes may also produce a number of toxins (poisonous substances), which are responsible for evoking the damaging effects of the infection.

Streptococci can be classified into a number of groups and types on the basis of the chemical structure of the cell wall. Group A *Streptococcus* is the most common pathogen in skin lesions as well as in throat infections (follicular tonsillitis). More than 80 per cent of cases of tonsillitis and sore throat are caused by *Streptococci*, of which group A is the predominant organism; group C and group G *Streptococci* cause a smaller number of infections.

Streptococcal infections of throat and skin may have late sequelae, probably caused by immunological reactions of the host against some components of *Streptococci*. Among the most frequent such sequelae is acute glomerulonephritis, in which immune complexes consisting of streptococcal antigens, and antibodies formed by the patient against the antigens, cause damage to the kidneys. The other sequelae include damage to the heart muscle leading to rheumatic heart disease, the mechanism of which is still not clear (see Chapter 27). This is one of the reasons why these infections should be treated rapidly and effectively.

Streptococcal infections, especially those affecting tonsils and skin, are highly contagious among children. If a health care worker who has direct patient contact gets a streptococcal infection, he or she must stay away from work until the infection is clear in order to reduce the risk of cross-infection to patients and other staff. In hospital wards, patients with streptococcal skin or throat infections should be isolated to prevent dissemination of the infection to other patients.

Streptococcal infections can be diagnosed in the laboratory by taking swabs from the infected sites and culturing them (see Chapter 17). *Streptococci* are susceptible to penicillin, which remains the drug of

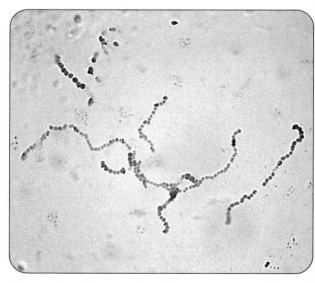

Figure 16.1 Gram stain of *Streptococcus*. These bacteria occur, for example, in the throat or skin (as in impetigo).

choice. In severe, deep-seated infections, the drug is given intravenously. About 10 per cent of the population is allergic to penicillin, and in these people an alternative drug, such as erythromycin, is generally used.

Other groups of *Streptococci*, such as enterococci *(Streptococcus faecalis)* and Group B *Streptococci*, will be discussed in the relevant sections of this chapter. *Streptococcus pneumoniae* (pneumococcus) will be dealt with in the section on respiratory infection.

Staphylococcus Species

Staphylococci appear as Gram-positive clusters of spherical cocci in the infected tissues (Figure 16.2). Like *Streptococci*, they also produce pyogenic lesions in the skin and other tissues, which often develop into small or large abscesses, such as styes in the eyelids, boils, carbuncles, and large abscesses following wound infections. Staphylococcal infections of the deeper tissues may take the form of blood-borne infections (e.g. septicaemia and endocarditis) or bone infections (e.g. osteomyelitis).

Staphylococci may be further classified into *Staphylococcus aureus* and *Staphylococcus epidermidis* (also called coagulase-negative *Staphylococcus*) on the basis of the coagulase test. This test examines the ability of the organism to coagulate plasma. *Staphylococcus aureus* produces coagulase, an enzyme that causes co-agulation of plasma; *Staphylococcus epidermidis* does not produce this enzyme. *Staphylococcus aureus* is generally responsible for most of the clinical diseases

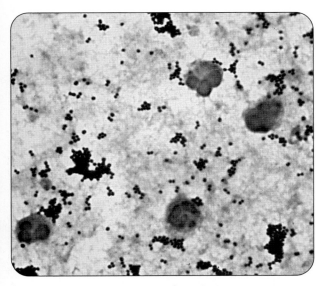

Figure 16.2 Gram stain of *Staphylococcus aureus*. These organisms are associated with the production of pus (e.g. as occurs in *S. aureus* abscess).

described above. *Staphylococci* can be isolated from clinical material by culturing on simple laboratory media (see Chapter 17).

Staphylococci are generally susceptible to a variety of antibiotics. The majority of the isolates of *Staphylococcus aureus* are sensitive to flucloxacillin as well as erythromycin and fusidic acid, and these antibiotics are generally used for the treatment of this infection. Only a small percentage of isolates are sensitive to penicillin.

Staphylococcal wound infection in hospitals can pose significant cross-infection problems, especially if the strain of *Staphylococcus* is multiple resistant or, more importantly, methicillin resistant. Methicillin-resistant *Staphylococcus aureus* (MRSA) is presently causing major clinical and management problems, and infections with this organism can cause prolonged hospital stays of infected patients and the need for ward closures (see Box 16.1).

Anaerobic Infections

The two most frequently seen types of anaerobic infections are those due to *Bacteroides* species and *Clostridium* species. *Bacteroides* are Gram-negative, rod-shaped organisms that are usually present in large numbers in the gut as commensals. These commensals may be implanted in other tissues during surgery. Although most *Bacteroides* infection occurs in deeper tissues following gut operations, they may produce infection elsewhere, particularly in the lower extremities. *Bacteroides fragilis* is the species most often associated with the infection.

Clostridia are Gram-positive anaerobic rods. They have been allied with both superficial and deep infections. These are also gut-derived organisms and both *Bacteroides* and *Clostridia* establish themselves in hypoxic conditions, which are often found in major tissue damage (e.g. necrotizing injury) and in post-operative sites. There are a number of different types of *Clostridia*, but the one commonly associated with tissue infections is *Clostridium perfringens*, the organism that causes gas gangrene (Figure 16.3).

Bacteroides fragilis is sensitive to metronidazole, and this is the mainstay of treatment for this organism. *Clostridium perfringens* is sensitive to a variety of antibiotics, but either metronidazole or penicillin, to which these organisms are generally susceptible, is invariably used for the treatment.

Viral Infections Causing Rashes

Viruses frequently produce rashes of different types, including vesicular or maculopapular rashes; the rash may be pustular if it is secondarily infected with bacteria such as *Staphylococci* or *Streptococci*. The rashes are most frequently caused by:

MICROBIOLOGY

BOX 16.1 COMMON CLINICAL PROBLEM – MRSA

- Incidence of MRSA in hospitals has increased many-fold during the last few years and has caused major infection control and management problems, with additional financial burden on hospitals. Although MRSA has, in most cases, been implicated only as a colonizing agent (i.e. present only on body surfaces, including wound surfaces), it has, on occasions, been involved in deep-seated infections such as septicaemia and infections of lung, bone, and joint.
- High-dependency units, such as intensive therapy units, cardiothoracic postoperative units, and orthopaedic units, have often been affected. Whether colonised or infected, patients with MRSA are generally not welcome in other units and other hospitals. As a consequence, such patients block beds in these expensive-to-run units and put extra pressure on the resources, and they are sources of further cross-infection in these units.
- Systemically infected patients also pose treatment problems. Some strains of MRSA are very stubbornly resistant to many antibiotics that are effective against other strains of *Staphylococci,* and therefore it is often difficult to find a useful antibiotic.
- Resistant strains, including MRSA, are generally susceptible to vancomycin, and this is commonly used for the treatment of MRSA systemic infection. If the patient is colonized with MRSA, as evidenced by the presence of these organisms on superficial sites, only a localized eradication programme is employed (see Chapter 20).
- Infection-control measures and nursing care of these patients are matters for concern. Although isolation of MRSA patients is generally recommended, it is not always possible to arrange isolation when larger numbers of patients are affected. Cohort nursing has often been tried with some success, but this is very much dependent on the availability of good and adequate nursing facilities.

- herpes simplex virus;
- varicella–zoster virus;
- enteroviruses;
- rubella; or
- rubeola.

Herpes simplex virus causes papular rashes in muco-cutaneous junctions, such as the mouth and gums. These rashes often occur in children. The rashes may become vesicular and ulcerated, and they can be very painful. Vesicular lesions also develop in infections of the genitalia – the vulva, penis, and the cervix; such infections are often sexually transmitted. Herpes simplex virus sometimes causes vesicular rashes on the finger tips of nurses and dentists following contact with an infected site, a condition called herpetic whitlow.

Varicella–zoster virus, a virus related to Herpesvirus, causes a mild form of childhood disease, chickenpox, presenting as a vesicular rash over the trunk and face. Vesicles may become pustular and crust followed by desquamation. The virus also causes shingles – a reactivation of herpes zoster virus along the sensory roots of nerves. It usually occurs in immunosuppressed patients and the elderly. The rash consists of very painful vesicular lesions along dermatomes, usually on one side of the body. The lesions eventually crust and heal.

Coxsackie virus A16, an enterovirus, causes hand, foot, and mouth disease, which is manifested by vesicular rashes on the hands and feet and very painful stomatitis. Other enteroviruses may produce macular rashes, including the echovirus, which causes a fleeting, non-specific rash.

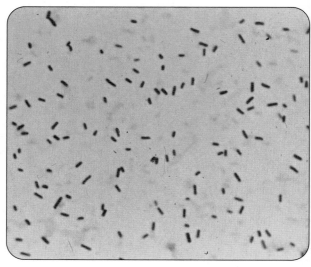

Figure 16.3 Gram stain of *Clostridium perfringens*. This is the organism that is responsible for gas gangrene.

Rubella (German measles) virus causes a macular rash over the face which then spreads to the trunk. Rubeola (measles) virus causes a more florid maculopapular rash over the face which spreads over the body. The rash fades in 10–14 days with large areas of desquamation.

Rare viral causes of skin afflictions include parvovirus, which produces the rash of erythema infectiosum (fifth disease), a red maculopapular rash (manifested as slapped-cheek appearance of bright red rash) that commonly occurs in children; papovavirus, which causes warts; and poxvirus; which manifests as molluscum contagiosum.

Bacterial Infections Causing Rashes

Bacterial infections may also manifest as rashes. *Neisseria meningitidis* causes severe septicaemic infection, with the release of large amounts of endotoxin. This elicits cytokine release from target cells such as the monocyte–macrophage cells (see Chapter 25). One of the effects of these cytokines is to evoke a moderate-to-severe haemorrhagic rash in the skin and internal organs.

Fungal Infections of Skin

Ringworm is caused by dermatophytes (e.g. *Microsporum canis*). There are various ringworm infections, such as common ringworm, ringworm of scalp, athlete's foot, body ringworm, and ringworm of nails; these are caused by a number of different dermatophytes. Fungal hyphae are visible in the skin scrapings from these sites and can be cultured on appropriate media (Figure 16.4).

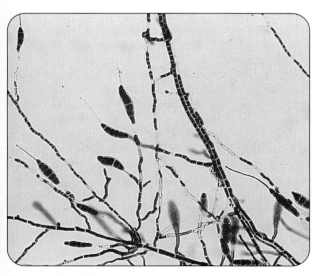

Figure 16.4 Microscopic appearance of skin fungi responsible for ringworm, *Microsporum canis*.

A number of major fungal infections of the skin are found in various tropical countries but are rarely seen in temperate areas such as the UK.

Candida albicans, a pathogenic yeast, has sometimes been found in mucocutaneous lesions or infections of the finger nails. This is more common in immunocompromised people (see Chapters 18 and 28).

INFECTIONS OF THE EYES

The eyes might seem to be rather vulnerable to infections from the environment because they are always moist and exposed. Fortunately, natural protective mechanisms, such as the presence of lysozyme in tears, prevent infections occurring readily. However, infections may be caused by highly virulent organisms that can survive within the protective barrier, or they may occur in the presence of damaged conjunctiva or when that protective barrier becomes compromised.

Gonococcal Infections of the Eyes

Ophthalmia neonatorum is a pyogenic (pus-producing) infection of the conjunctiva with extensive swelling of the eyelids in the newborn. It is caused by *Neisseria gonorrhoeae* and is usually acquired during passage through an infected birth canal. It manifests clinically within 1–2 days of birth. Gram staining of the exudate from the conjunctiva shows typical Gram-negative bean-shaped diplococci inside the pus cells as well as extracellularly. The causative organisms grow relatively easily when the exudate is cultured.

Ophthalmia neonatorum is highly contagious and extra care should be taken in delivery units and nurseries to prevent the spread of this infection by hand to other newborn babies during nursing care. The infection may be treated promptly with topical penicillin drops and systemic penicillin to prevent complications such as corneal ulceration and blindness. The mother should also be counselled to undergo investigation and treatment at a genitourinary medicine clinic, along with her sexual partner or partners.

Acute Pyogenic Conjunctivitis

Several pyogenic organisms, such as *Streptococcus pneumoniae*, *Haemophilus influenzae*, and *Staphylococcus aureus*, are often associated with pyogenic conjunctivitis. While pneumococcal and *Haemophilus* conjunctivitis is common in children, staphylococcal conjunctivitis occurs more often in older adults with defective tear production. Staphylococcal conjunctivitis has sometimes been associated with outbreaks of 'sticky eye' in nurseries.

In all these infections, there are acute inflammatory changes in the conjunctiva with redness and swelling. Topical treatment is the usual treatment. Chloramphenicol eye drops may be used for these infections in the elderly and are usually effective. Systemic treatment may be necessary in certain cases with more severe infection and acute swelling of the eyelids. Gram staining of a swab from the infected eye will confirm the presence of the organisms, which can be grown on common culture media. In nursery outbreaks caused by *Staphylococci*, special efforts should be made to control the outbreak by identifying the source of infection.

Chlamydia trachomatis Infection

Chlamydia trachomatis is an intracellular infection that affects the conjunctiva, producing follicular conjunctivitis. This is another example of an infection transmitted to newborn babies during birth through an infected birth canal. It is manifested by non-pyogenic inclusion conjunctivitis often leading to mild to severe keratoconjunctivitis or TRIC (trachoma inclusion conjunctivitis). Trachoma is prevalent in some endemic areas of Africa and the Middle East and is manifested by severe follicular conjunctivitis leading to fibrosis of the eyelids, secondary bacterial infections, and blindness. It is transmitted by hand and mechanically by flies. Erythromycin by oral route in neonates and tetracycline in adults are effective in the treatment of chlamydial infection.

Viral Infections of the Eye

Herpes simplex virus, varicella–zoster virus, and adenoviruses have been associated with eye infections. Viral infections of the eye often involve the cornea. Adenovirus type 8 has frequently been associated with epidemics of keratoconjunctivitis in ship-building yards. Herpes simplex virus and varicella–zoster virus often cause extremely painful keratitis. The rubella virus has been associated with congenital cataract; infection is usually transmitted *in utero*.

INFECTIONS OF THE UPPER RESPIRATORY TRACT AND EAR

The upper respiratory tract, including the ear and nose, is inhabited by a large number of commensal organisms, which usually provide an environment that prevents pathogenic organisms establishing an infection. However, in the face of overwhelming infection and a transient lowering of the host resistance, which may be caused by a number of factors, some pathogens may establish infection. Such infection may be manifested by acute or chronic disease process.

Infections of the Ear and Nose

The communication of the throat and nose to the middle ear by the eustachian tube makes it easy for throat infections to reach the ear. Common throat infections due to *Streptococcus pyogenes* are easily transmitted to the middle ear, precipitating an acute middle ear infection (otitis media). Organisms such as *Streptococcus pneumoniae* and *Haemophilus influenzae* (which are of little consequence as infecting organisms of the throat) may also be conveyed through the tube to the middle ear and can cause infections. Similarly, *Staphylococcus aureus* is present in the throat and nose of a large proportion of healthy people, but if it passes to the middle ear it may cause an infection.

Acute middle ear infections are common in children and are usually manifested by pain and fever. An examination of the ear may reveal a bulging and red tympanic membrane, owing to a collection of pus and exudate in the middle ear (see the Person-Centred Study in Chapter 28). This sometimes requires drainage to relieve the symptoms, as well as appropriate systemic antibiotic treatment.

Inadequately treated and neglected acute middle ear infections may lead to chronic discharging ear infection, often superinfected with Gram-negative organisms such as *Pseudomonas* species, *Proteus* species, and anaerobes such as *Bacteroides* species. This requires thorough surgical investigation and energetic treatment by an ear, nose, and throat (ENT) specialist, especially since most cases are associated with perforation of the tympanic membrane.

Virus infections of the upper respiratory tract constitute over half of all respiratory infections. There is inflammation and oedema of the lining membranes of the throat and the eustachian tube. This type of infection is often transmitted to the middle ear, where it may lead to a collection of exudate and give rise to similar manifestations to those described above for acute bacterial infection of the middle ear. Additionally, there may be added secondary bacterial infection complicating the viral infection, and this may require antibacterial therapy.

Bacterial infection of the nose is extremely rare. The nose may, however, be colonized with a number of opportunistic and pathogenic organisms, such as *Staphylococcus aureus* and *Streptococcus pneumoniae*. Virus infection of the nose is common; causative viruses include the rhinovirus, coronavirus, parainfluenza viruses, and adenoviruses.

Acute tonsillitis and sore throat

Streptococcus pyogenes group A is the most common cause of acute tonsillitis and sore throat, although a small proportion of cases can be due to group C or group G *Streptococci*. Some viral infections, including infections caused by adenoviruses, Epstein–Barr virus, and enteroviruses, may also give rise to sore throat and tonsillitis. In tonsillitis and sore throat there is an acute inflammatory response to the infection with the development of purulent patches over the tonsils and the posterior pharyngeal wall. There may be enlargement of the tonsils and pus formation in the tonsillar bed, which pushes the tonsils forwards and reduces the size of the air passage. The infection may also produce enlargement of the draining lymph nodes in the upper part of the neck. Patients usually have symptoms of systemic infection, with fever and malaise, and they are often highly infectious. Again, the infection may spread to the middle ear, sinuses, and lower respiratory tract.

Treatment of acute streptococcal tonsillitis should be started urgently. The usual treatment is with penicillin or erythromycin. Symptomatic treatment for sore throat and fever may also be urgent. Before commencing antibiotic therapy, a throat swab should be taken and sent to the microbiology laboratory for isolation and identification of the micro-organisms; antibiotic sensitivity is also determined by routine culture method (see Chapter 17). In the hospital environment, infection may spread to other patients and hence it is advisable to isolate the patient.

Diphtheria

Infection caused by *Corynebacterium diphtheriae* gives rise to acute sore throat and tonsillitis and often to severe respiratory distress owing to obstruction of the air passage. A highly infectious agent, *Corynebacterium diphtheriae* is a thin, Gram-positive organism that grows profusely in the throat with the production of a very powerful exotoxin, the diphtheria toxin. The infection leads to formation of a thick and tenacious pseudomembrane over the tonsils, causing partial or complete obstruction of the airway. There may be huge enlargement of the draining cervical lymph nodes, leading to an appearance called 'bull neck'. In advanced stages, toxins produced by the organism may cause myocardial damage, leading to cardiac failure. This toxin is also responsible for major tissue destruction at the site of the bacterial growth, leading to the pseudomembrane formation. Patients with diphtheria are usually treated with large doses of benzyl penicillin and diphtheria antitoxic serum (see Chapter 26).

Diphtheria is now a rare disease in the developed world, primarily because of improved hygiene but also because of the very successful immunization programme. Diphtheria toxoid, which is one of the most efficient immunogenic prophylactic agents, has helped to eradicate this infection almost completely in developed countries.

Whooping cough (pertussis)

Bordetella pertussis is a tiny, Gram-negative coccobacillus that has a major, damaging effect on the ciliated mucous membrane of the upper respiratory tract. The cause of this damage is not clear, but toxins produced during the growth of this organism may be responsible. The manifestation of the disease – severe bouts of paroxysmal cough – is usually preceded by infection with this organism several days earlier. Like diphtheria, the incidence of the disease has been considerably reduced owing to an immunization programme. Even so, cases are still seen and the infection tends to transmit to siblings and other children with close contact. (Some people are reluctant to have their children immunized because of some reports linking the vaccine with the development of neurological reactions). Unfortunately, patients are most infectious during the incubation period; attempted culture during the whoop stage usually fails to grow the organism.

Antibiotic treatment of infection due to *Bordetella pertussis* is unrewarding because the maximum damage occurs in the usually asymptomatic infectious period. Thus, when the patient is seen in whoop stage, the infection is already over and maximum damage to the ciliated membrane has occurred. Palliative treatment helps to alleviate distressing whooping cough, and a course of antibiotic treatment may help in the eradication of the carrier state. Unaffected children should be carefully observed and preventative antibiotic may be given to siblings and others in close contact.

Acute epiglottitis (croup)

This is a life-threatening condition in infants. It causes severe oedema of the epiglottis or upper part of the larynx, which obstructs the airway passage. It requires immediate intervention, with intubation or a tracheostomy. No attempt should be made to take a swab because this may precipitate severe stridor. The condition is generally caused by infection with certain types of *Haemophilus influenzae*, but other organisms, such as parainfluenza virus, respiratory syncytial virus, or *Corynebacterium diphtheriae* (diphtheria), may also precipitate epiglottitis (commonly known as 'croup' because of the crouping sound caused during respiratory effort in infected infants). Since *Haemophilus influenzae* is the most common cause, the usual antibiotic treatment is a third-generation cephalosporin or chloramphenicol.

INFECTIONS OF THE LOWER RESPIRATORY TRACT

The lower respiratory tract is normally sterile – the ciliated lining of tracheal and bronchial mucous membrane, the presence of a protective coat of immunoglobulin (secretory immunoglobulin A) on the membrane, and other protective mechanisms keep the lower respiratory tract germ free (see Chapters 23 and 24). However, when there is significant damage to these protective mechanisms (e.g. following virus infections, smoking, or inhalation of polluted air) microbes from the upper respiratory tract can spread downwards and cause infection.

Pneumococcal Pneumonia

Community-acquired pneumonia generally affects older adults and the debilitated, as well as chronic bronchitics and smokers. It also occurs in those with chronic conditions such as diabetes mellitus, cardiac and renal disease. Infection due to *Streptococcus pneumoniae* is the most common form of community-acquired pneumonia. Patients present with fever, shortness of breath, cough, and chest pain; they may also be toxic. They are often brought to an Accident and Emergency department. On chest X-ray, a major consolidation of one or both lung fields is usually found. Patients cough up copious amounts of rusty looking sputum and succumb rapidly if not treated promptly (see also Chapter 33).

Gram staining of the rusty, blood-stained sputum shows typical Gram-positive lanceolate diplococci in pairs and chains. Sputum culture yields typical pneumococcal colonies, and blood culture may also be positive. The organisms are sensitive to penicillin and erythromycin, but a small proportion of community isolates are now showing penicillin resistance. Patients with severe consolidation of both lungs may require positive pressure ventilation for maintenance of blood oxygen concentration.

Bronchopneumonia

Haemophilus influenzae and *Staphylococcus aureus* are often responsible for bronchopneumonia, especially in the elderly, producing acute exacerbation of chronic bronchitis. These micro-organisms are rare causes of primary acute pneumonia and may sometimes cause abscesses in the lung. Treatment is with antibacterial agents, such as ampicillin or amoxycillin–clavulanic acid (Augmentin) for *Haemophilus* infection, and flucloxacillin for staphylococcal infection.

Community-acquired atypical pneumonia

Mycoplasma pneumoniae is a significant cause of community-acquired pneumonia. It affects people of all ages but is more common in younger patients. It produces atypical manifestations of pneumonia, such as non-productive cough, fluctuating pyrexia, and general malaise. Chest X-ray shows patchy bronchopneumonic

changes. Mycoplasmal infection is generally susceptible to erythromycin.

Q fever (caused by *Coxiella burnetii*) and psittacosis (caused by *Chlamydia* species) are rare infections, and they are generally seen in the occupational groups involved in handling animals and birds. These infectious agents may also produce atypical pneumonia, and they are treated with tetracycline and erythromycin.

Legionella pneumophila is a small, Gram-negative, rod-shaped organism that causes moderate to severe atypical pulmonary manifestations. This infection is commonly thought to be associated with large modern buildings with centralized air conditioning systems, such as hotels, hospitals, and office blocks (see Chapter 15). It is also acquired from shower heads. Elderly patients with chronic bronchitis and smokers are more vulnerable to *Legionella pneumophila*. It causes patchy bronchopneumonia or lobar consolidation, and it can be rapidly fatal. Treatment is with erythromycin and tetracycline, but rifampicin and ciprofloxacin have also been found to be effective.

Viral Infections of the Respiratory Tract

Influenza still remains the major viral cause of respiratory infection. All three types of influenza viruses have been associated with human infection, but influenza A is the most common. The infection is transmitted from an infected person by droplets from the respiratory tract. After a short incubation period of 1–3 days, the disease manifests with sudden onset of chill, fever, headache, malaise, and aches and pains. This may be followed by bronchitis and tracheitis with non-productive cough and coryza. Secondary bacterial infection is common, particularly in children and the elderly, and this leads to a deterioration in the clinical condition. Severe primary infection may sometimes lead to pneumonitis and oedema of the lung with fatal consequences (see Chapter 33).

Treatment is generally palliative with bed rest and plenty of fluid to drink. If secondary bacterial infection arises, treatment with appropriate antibiotics is needed. Prophylactic vaccination is available and is usually offered to older adults, people with chronic bronchitis, and, in the face of epidemics, to some immunocompromised patients (see Chapter 28) and health care personnel.

Respiratory syncytial virus infections are common in children and can lead to severe manifestation such as acute bronchiolitis with respiratory distress. All four types of parainfluenza viruses have been associated with respiratory infection, but they are less severe and more likely to occur in children. Measles viruses, adenoviruses, and varicella–zoster virus have sometimes been associated with viral pneumonias.

Hospital-Acquired Pneumonias

Patients may develop chest infections while in hospital. These hospital-acquired chest infections arise because of stasis of lung secretions, which become secondarily infected with microbial agents found in the hospital environment, and also with patients' own commensal micro-organisms (see Box 16.2).

Patients' pulmonary function is compromised post-operatively because of anaesthetic-induced damage to the bronchial ciliated mucosa. This allows pathogens to migrate and establish infection in the lower respiratory tract. Furthermore, a number of interventions are used in patients requiring intensive therapy, such as intubation and ventilation, which also contribute to the establishment of infection. Patients with major immunocompromised states, such as haematological malignancies and HIV infection, often develop severe pulmonary infections (see Chapter 18).

It is essential that good physiotherapeutic manipulations are provided in order to minimize the accumulation of secretions during postoperative and recuperation periods. Patients with hospital-acquired pneumonia rapidly develop lobar pneumonia or broncho-pneumonia with consolidation. This is associated with high temperature, chest pain, and constitutional symptoms. Treatment with systemic antibiotics is usually necessary. Examples of such treatment are:

- flucloxacillin for *Staphylococci*;
- penicillin for pneumococci and *Streptococci*;
- cephalosporins for *Klebsiella* and *Haemophilus*;
- ciprofloxacin or ceftazidime (or both) for *Pseudomonas*; and
- erythromycin for *Legionella*.

If aspiration pneumonia is suspected, metronidazole is also given to prevent anaerobic infection. Infections in severely immunocompromised patients are often caused by *Pneumocystis carinii* or *Mycobacterium tuberculosis*. *Pneumocystis carinii* causes severe pneumonia in these patients and often requires the administration of oxygen. The infection is susceptible to trimethoprim–sulphamethoxazole (co-trimoxazole), but recurrence is common and prophylactic intermittent nebulized pentamidine is often recommended.

Tuberculosis

Mycobacterium tuberculosis causes a chronic course of infection of the lungs, leading to pulmonary tuberculosis. It can also cause infection in other parts of the body, but pulmonary infection predominates. The infection is transmitted by the air-borne route, and patients with active disease can disseminate a large number of organisms during coughing, sneezing, and even talking. The lung infection takes the form of single or multiple lesions –

BOX 16.2 COMMON CLINICAL PROBLEM: HOSPITAL ACQUIRED PNEUMONIA

Hospital-acquired pneumonia has become a major clinical and management issue involving sizeable resource implications.

Post-operative patients and immuno-compromised patients, particularly those requiring intensive therapy facilities, often develop pneumonia caused by common cross-infecting agents such as *Staphylococcus aureus*, *Klebsiella pneumoniae*, and *Pseudomonas aeruginosa* as well as the atypical microbes such as *Legionella pneumophila*, *Mycoplasma pneumoniae*, and *Pneumocystis carinii*.

Most of these agents are present in the hospital environments in large numbers and are transmitted via health-care workers and modern invasive and intensive therapy techniques. It is therefore extremely important for health-care workers to appreciate the problem both by the use of appropriate antimicrobial intervention, and in active nursing care.

---

the tubercles; multiple lesions often coalesce to form a large lesion. If the large lesions break down they may discharge their content into the bronchi or into a blood vessel. When the contents are discharged into a bronchus it is coughed up mixed with blood, and the patient may be highly infectious at this stage. However, if it is discharged into the bloodstream, the infection spreads throughout the body and causes miliary tuberculosis. A cavity may be formed, which may be clearly visible on X-ray. The tubercle lesions are visible as dense shadows on X-ray and help in the diagnosis.

Patients with tuberculosis present with low-grade, persistent fever, cough (which may be productive and blood-stained), pain in the chest, weakness, and night sweats. Patients lose weight rapidly and become anaemic. Chest examination and X-ray generally allow clinical diagnosis, which is confirmed by finding acid–alcohol-fast organisms in a stained sputum sample and by culturing these organisms on Löwenstein–Jensen medium after 4–8 weeks' incubation (see Chapters 17 and 33).

Tuberculosis of other parts of the body, such as bone and joints, kidneys, and meninges, are frequently seen and the diagnosis is confirmed by clinical evidence and by microscopy and culture of material from those sites. Patients with tuberculosis usually give a strong positive response to tuberculin injected intradermally into the forearm (see Chapter 26). Tuberculin is a purified protein produced from a liquid culture of *Mycobacterium tuberculosis*.

As mentioned above, tuberculosis is a highly infectious disease, killing more people world-wide than any other disease. On diagnosis, a patient should be treated in isolation until the sputum becomes negative on acid-fast stain. Regular treatment for 4–6 weeks may be necessary before the patient's sputum becomes negative. After this period, the patient may be managed as an out-patient, with regular follow up by clinical examination and X-ray. Therapy for tuberculosis generally involves 2 months' administration of combined isoniazid, rifampicin, ethambutol, and pyrazinamide followed by 4–6 months' treatment with isoniazid and rifampicin. This regimen, sometimes with minor modifications, is applied in most countries. Patients should be followed up regularly when the treatment regimen is completed, and household and other contacts should be examined.

INFECTIONS OF THE GASTROINTESTINAL TRACT

The gastrointestinal tract, which extends from the mouth to the anus, is inhabited by a large number of microbes, usually as commensals. These microbes are beneficial to the host in that they protect the intestinal tract against invasion by pathogenic organisms. The commensals that are generally found in the gastrointestinal tract include:

- Gram-negative aerobic bacteria, such as *Escherichia coli*, *Klebsiella aerogenes*, *Proteus* species, and *Pseudomonas* species;
- Gram-positive aerobic organisms, such as the *Streptococcus faecalis* group; and
- Gram-negative anaerobic bacteria, including *Bacteroides fragilis* as well as other species.

These organisms constitute the large bulk of faeces, but they do not cause any harm to the host under normal circumstances. However, some of these organisms are capable of a major pathogenic role when they are implanted elsewhere in the body. *Escherichia coli* is the most common cause of urinary tract infection when this organism enters the bladder as an ascending infection from the perineal region (see Chapter 36). Other gut organisms, such as *Streptococcus faecalis*, *Proteus* species, and *Pseudomonas* species, may also cause urinary tract infections. Most of these organisms, including the anaerobic *Bacteroides fragilis*, have been associated with postoperative blood-borne infections, producing bacteraemia, septicaemia, and wound infections.

Food Poisoning

Many infections of the gastrointestinal tract are acquired by consumption of contaminated food. These infections are usually manifested by symptoms of gastroenteritis, such as vomiting, diarrhoea and abdominal pain, and are collectively known as food-poisoning. Infections may also be transmitted by water contaminated with faecal materials. A number of highly pathogenic organisms are conveyed by this route, including the enteric fever agents, *Salmonella typhi* and *Salmonella paratyphi*; dysentery (caused by *Shigella* species), cholera (caused by *Vibrio* species), rotavirus, poliovirus, and the agents causing infectious hepatitis.

There are two types of food poisoning:
- toxic food poisoning; and
- infective food poisoning.

Toxic food poisoning

In toxic food poisoning, a ready-formed toxin in the food gives rise to severe bouts of vomiting and abdominal pain and may also cause diarrhoea. The symptoms are produced within a short period after consumption of the food, usually 2–4 hours. The toxin produces rapid action, predominantly affecting the stomach – hence the symptoms of severe vomiting and abdominal pain. Patients generally become dehydrated very rapidly and require urgent replenishment of electrolytes and fluid. The most common cause of this type of food poisoning is the ready-made toxin of *Staphylococcal aureus*, usually associated with dairy products, cold meat, and poultry. No specific treatment is required to treat this condition.

A rarer form of toxic food poisoning is caused by toxins of *Clostridium botulinum*. This organism, a strictly anaerobic spore-bearing organism, produces an extremely powerful exotoxin (botulinum toxin). This generally occurs in poorly canned foods and home-preserved fruit in which anaerobic conditions have been achieved and have allowed the germination of the spores of *Clostridium botulinum* and production of the toxin. When ingested, the toxin is rapidly absorbed from the stomach and transferred to the neuromuscular junctions of vital systems, particularly the respiratory muscles. The toxin prevents the transmission of impulses to the muscles, leading to paralysis. Some of the symptoms include diplopia (double vision) when eye muscles are affected, aphasia (inability to speak) when tongue muscles are affected, and often respiratory paralysis and death.

Bacillus cereus is sometimes responsible for toxic food poisoning. This organism can grow in cooked rice when it is left for a long time at room temperature. On rapid reheating, the toxin is not destroyed and profuse vomiting, abdominal pain, and diarrhoea can result.

Infective food poisoning

This is the most common type of food poisoning in the UK. There are several agents responsible.

Salmonella typhimurium and a number of other species of *Salmonella*, such as *Salmonella enteritides* and *Salmonella hadar*, are frequently involved. Several types of food have been responsible, including poultry and mince pies. Inadequate cooking of food, unsatisfactory storage of cooked food, and contamination of cooked food with raw food has often been implicated.

Symptoms usually begin several hours after consumption of the food; they include diarrhoea, abdominal pain, and sometimes vomiting. The infections are generally self-limiting and no antibiotic treatment is required. Fluid and electrolyte replacement is often necessary when diarrhoea is prolonged and results in dehydration. Patients with *Salmonella* food poisoning are often admitted to an infectious diseases unit, usually for rehydration. Special precautions must be taken to prevent the infection spreading to other patients and to the staff. *Salmonella* outbreaks have been reported from hospitals and other institutions such as prisons; careful epidemiological investigations are necessary to identify the source and contain the spread.

Campylobacter jejuni is one of the most common cause of gastroenteritis in the UK and Europe. This is a Gram-negative vibrio-shaped (comma-shaped) organism that is transmitted to humans from animals and poultry. Unpasteurized milk and milk products have been blamed for many outbreaks. After an incubation period of 1–3 days, the patient develops abdominal pain, which is often griping, diarrhoea, and sometimes blood-stained stool. The infection occasionally spreads to the bloodstream, leading to septicaemia. In moderate-to-severe cases, antibiotic treatment is needed. Erythromycin is the drug of choice and ciprofloxacin have been found to be very effective. These antibodies also help to eradicate the carrier state.

Enteric Fevers (Typhoid and Paratyphoid Fevers)

Salmonella typhi is responsible for most cases of enteric fevers. The infection is acquired by ingestion of unclean water, but it can also be transmitted by food contaminated during handling by a carrier excreting the organism. Normally, the acid content of the stomach kills the organisms, but some may survive when ingested in vast numbers. Furthermore, if the food is taken with a large amount of water, the stomach acid may be neutralized. Once in the small intestine, the organisms multiply and enter the intestinal mucosa, from where they are transported into the blood. This process takes about 7–10 days and constitutes the incubation period of the disease.

In the bloodstream, the organisms first cause a bacteraemia followed by multiplication both in the blood and in some internal organs such as spleen, liver, and bone marrow. Thus, a septicaemic state is established, with clinical manifestation such as headache, abdominal pain, fever (usually of the step-ladder type – i.e. gradually increasing), endotoxic shock with a fall in blood pressure, rashes (rose spots) over the body, confusion, and severe general malaise. Blood cultures taken during this stage usually give a positive result, and urine culture may also be positive. Specific treatment with an antibiotic such as ciprofloxacin or ampicillin plus appropriate supportive treatment is usually effective in curing the infection. (Chloramphenicol used to be the drug of choice for treatment of typhoid fever and is still regularly used in many endemic countries.)

If treatment is delayed, inadequate, or inappropriate, the organisms continue multiplying in the bloodstream and reappear in the gut in large numbers when they are excreted in the bile. In the small intestine, the organisms establish an ulcerating lesion in the lymphoid (Peyer's) patches, which may ultimately slough through the wall of the gut. This leads to perforation and spilling of the gut contents into the peritoneal cavity causing peritonitis, which is an acute abdominal emergency with a high fatality rate.

Relapse occurs in a small proportion of patients even after apparently adequate treatment. This more often happens in patients treated with chloramphenicol and trimethoprim–sulphamethoxazole (co-trimoxazole). Relapse is therefore more prevalent in endemic countries where these drugs still remain the choice of treatment. Some patients carry the organisms, usually in the gall bladder, for a long time, despite adequate treatment. These people continue excreting the organisms, and there is the risk that they will infect others by contamination of food and water, particularly if the person is a food-handler.

Typhoid fever remains a major communicable disease in some parts of the world. Therefore, people travelling to these areas should take protective vaccinations. Cases of this infection must be notified to the district Consultant for Communicable Diseases Control, who then initiates a contact-tracing investigation. A patient with typhoid fever should preferably be managed in an infectious diseases unit with appropriate isolation facilities

Salmonella paratyphi A, B, and C can cause similar infections of the gastrointestinal tract, but the disease is usually less severe. Treatment and general management follow the same pattern as the typhoid fever caused by *Salmonella typhi*.

Bacillary Dysentery

Shigella sonnei is the most common form of dysentery in the UK. It results in outbreaks of mild-to-moderate diarrhoea, especially in children and infants, but also in homes and institutions for people with special needs. Outbreaks of the infection also occur from time to time in other institutions such as hospitals and prisons. The infection is transmitted by the faeco-oral route and is frequently associated with poor hygienic standards and poor living conditions. It is common for this infection to be acquired in lavatories when inadequate hand-washing allows the infecting organisms to be carried on the hands. Poor personal hygiene is responsible for most outbreaks.

Shigella sonnei dysentery is generally a mild condition and does not require antibiotic treatment – palliative treatment is adequate in most cases. However, since the infection can cause a small outbreak or a large epidemic, it must be notified to the district Consultant for Communicable Disease Control, and community preventive measures are required to prevent spread of infections.

Shigella flexneri and other *Shigella* species (*Shigella dysentery* and *Shigella boydii*) produce severe dysentery in which invasion of the gut mucosa with inflammatory changes characteristically result in the presence of blood and large numbers of pus cells in the faeces. *Shigella dysentery* is the most severe form, and fulminating changes may be seen in the gut mucosa, with sloughing of large areas. There may be septicaemic episodes and evidence of neural involvement. Such infections are generally found in parts of the Indian subcontinent, the Middle East, South America, and parts of Africa. Again, poor personal and institutional hygiene is frequently the cause and the infection is transmitted faeco-orally.

Antibiotic treatment may be necessary for acute *Shigella* infections. Ampicillin, trimethoprim–sulphamethoxazole (co-trimoxazole), and ciprofloxacin are generally effective, along with treatment for symptomatic relief. Patients should be treated in an infectious diseases unit. Most of these infections in the UK are imported from overseas, although *Shigella flexneri* infection has occasionally been isolated in patients who have not been abroad recently.

Cholera

This is an acute enterocolitis caused by a small Gram-negative, comma-shaped organism, *Vibrio cholerae*, which had been a significant health problem in the countries of the Indian subcontinent and south-east Asia for hundreds of years. The incidence of cholera has fallen remarkably during the past 20–30 years, presumably because of public awareness, clean water supplies, improved sanitation, and health care facilities in endemic areas, as well as the efforts of national and international agencies such as the World Health Organization. Cholera is transmitted by the faeco-oral route and generally believed to be transferred via water contaminated with faecal material from infective people. The disease used to occur as major epidemics or even pandemics (affecting a number of countries), and it used to take a large toll of human life owing to the acute dehydration and irreversible shock that it causes.

The condition is manifested by acute persistent diarrhoea with the passage of large volumes of 'rice-water' stool. A milder form of the disease is due to a variant of the *Vibrio cholerae* strain; this is more common now than the classic *Vibrio cholerae* infection.

Treatment consists of replacement of electrolytes and fluid as soon as possible to prevent renal failure and other complications of acute dehydration. Antibiotic treatment may sometimes be necessary, in which case tetracyclines are generally used. This is a highly infectious disease; cases in the UK have usually been imported from an endemic part of the world by an infected patient. It is a notifiable disease in the UK, and in the event of a patient being received in a UK hospital, treatment is carried out in an infectious diseases unit.

Gastroenteritis in Infants and Children

In addition to the microbial agents described above, a number of other microbes have been associated with infantile gastroenteritis. *Escherichia coli*, a common intestinal commensal, has often been involved in acute gastroenteritis in infants, resulting in prolonged diarrhoea with consequent dehydration. A number of serotypes of *Escherichia coli* are recognized, based on the composition of the cell wall. Only certain serotypes have been found to be associated with infantile gastroenteritis (including serotypes O55, O111, and O126); these are the enteropathogenic strains of *Escherichia coli*.

Infantile gastroenteritis due to *Escherichia coli* often occurs as outbreaks in nurseries. It is associated with milk and other baby foods. No antibiotic treatment is necessary, but fluid and electrolyte replacement is required. In addition, strict infection-control procedures, including isolation of affected infants, are essential for management of the outbreak.

Some other serotypes have now been incriminated in acute manifestations, such as the *Escherichia coli* O157 serotype. This serotype has been associated with a haemolytic uraemic syndrome and haemorrhagic colitis characterized by bloody diarrhoea. The acute manifestations are caused by a powerful haemolytic exotoxin.

Rotavirus is a common viral cause of infantile gastroenteritis. This small RNA virus looks like a cart-wheel under electron microscopy. The infection is manifested by acute diarrhoea, often associated with vomiting. The infection generally occurs in maternity wards and nurseries. Where there is serious depletion of fluid and electrolytes, replacement therapy constitutes the main treatment of this infection. Rotavirus infection has also been involved in diarrhoea in older children and the elderly. Strict infection-control measures are required to prevent spreading of the infection.

Infections with other viruses (such as small round virus, adenovirus, and, more importantly, Norwalk agents) have been incriminated in a number of outbreaks of viral gastroenteritis. Electron microscopy of stool samples allows diagnosis of infection caused by these viruses.

Parasitic Infections of the Gastrointestinal Tract

Infections due to intestinal parasites are very widespread in parts of the world where a clean water supply is not easily available and the population is dependent on sources such as rivers, streams, and natural reservoirs for water. Unhygienic food habits may also be responsible for transmission of these infections. The two common types of intestinal infections are caused by amoebae (*Entamoeba histolytica*) and by *Giardia lamblia*.

Entamoeba histolytica produces infection of the lower bowel, with ulceration and bleeding from the intestinal wall. This gives rise to dysentery (amoebic dysentery) which is manifested by griping abdominal pain and passage of loose stool with mucus and blood. In severe cases there may be sloughing of the intestinal wall, leading to perforation and peritonitis. Satellite lesions may be formed in other parts of the body when the amoebae have been transmitted through blood from the primary intestinal ulcers. These sites include the liver, brain, and lung, and there may be single or multiple abscesses.

Mild and moderate cases may follow a chronic course with occasional acute exacerbations. Microscopic examination of a freshly voided stool specimen shows the presence of motile vegetative form of the parasites. Cysts of amoebae are found in chronic infections. Metronidazole is extremely effective in curing both colonic infections and visceral abscesses.

Giardia lamblia infection causes giardiasis. The organism is a flagellar parasite, which causes an acute infection usually of the small intestine, resulting in flatulent and frothy diarrhoea. Pear-shaped, flagellate, motile parasites are seen on microscopic examination of a fresh stool specimen. If the infection becomes chronic, cyst forms are more generally found. Chronic infection leads to malabsorption syndrome with white frothy faeces or steatorrhoea. The cystic forms are sometimes found in the jejunal aspirate in malabsorption syndrome. *Giardia* infection may be found both in children and adults. Treatment is with metronidazole. Special care should be taken to prevent outbreaks in nurseries and play schools when a child is infected.

INFECTIONS OF THE URINARY TRACT

The kidneys, the ureters, and the bladder can all become infected, usually with microbes from the intestinal tract. The perineum normally carries a large load of intestinal organisms, and these may be transmitted to the bladder through the urethra, as an ascending infection. This happens more frequently in females because the female urethra is shorter than the male urethra. Infection may develop in the kidneys when bacteria travelling in the bloodstream are seeded in there (e.g. *Staphylococcus aureus*). This causes pyogenic nephritis with small abscesses. *Mycobacterium tuberculosis* can also cause a blood-borne kidney infection (see Chapter 36).

Escherichia coli are the most common bacteria responsible for urinary tract infection (UTI) – 80 per cent of the cases of urinary tract infection treated in general practitioners' surgeries are caused by this organism. Sexually active females are often affected, as are the older adults, immunocompromised patients, and young children with anatomical abnormalities of the urinary tract. Other gastrointestinal organisms are occasionally associated with urinary tract infections, including enterococci, *Proteus* species, *Klebsiella* species, and *Pseudomonas* species. These organisms may be acquired in hospital, particularly if the patient has been catheterized or has had a minor urological investigation in which the instruments were not adequately sterilized.

Most urinary infections occur in the bladder, producing cystitis, which is manifested by urinary frequency, a burning sensation during the passing of urine, fever, and other systemic manifestations. On microscopy, infected urine specimens contain large numbers of pus cells (dead leukocytes) and often red blood cells. Culture on appropriate media may reveal the nature of bacterial growth if specific tests are used. Sensitivity tests are also performed to determine the most appropriate antibiotics against the causative organism. Oral antibiotics are usually prescribed for the treatment of urinary tract infections; these include nitrofurantoin, trimethoprim, and ampicillin. Hospital-acquired urinary tract infections may require systemic antibiotics. This is because many of the bacteria associated with these infections are resistant to common oral antibiotics.

Following repeated infections (often in association with anatomical abnormalities of the urinary tract), microbes may ascend upwards to the kidneys. This produces acute pyogenic nephritis and pyelonephritis, manifested by fever, loin pain, and systemic symptoms. Prompt treatment with systemic antibiotics is essential to prevent complications such as septicaemia and major damage to the kidneys. Staphylococcal metastatic lesions require active treatment with intravenous antibiotics to prevent the formation of large abscesses in the kidneys. Infections in the kidneys and ureters can also follow stone formations in these sites.

Tuberculosis of the kidneys is generally secondary to infection elsewhere, and is usually caused by blood-borne spread from pulmonary disease. Urine may contain large numbers of pus cells and red blood cells without any growth on common media. Symptoms of renal tuberculosis include persistent low-grade fever, loin pain, general weakness, and recurrent passage of red blood cells in the urine. Acid-fast stain of a centrifuged deposit of urine may show the presence of acid-fast bacilli, culture on an appropriate medium, such as Löwenstein–Jensen medium, allows the growth of *Mycobacteria*. Special tests are used to identify *Mycobacterium tuberculosis*.

Radiological investigation also helps in the diagnosis, both from local evidence and from evidence from other sites such as lungs.

Treatment consists of the usual antituberculous drug regimen consisting of rifampicin, isoniazid, ethambutol, and pyrazinamide for 8–10 months.

INFECTIONS OF THE BLOOD AND CARDIOVASCULAR SYSTEM
Bacteraemia and Septicaemia

The terms bacteraemia and septicaemia are frequently ascribed to blood-borne infections. Bacteraemia is generally a transient phenomenon that may occur in health, although it may be associated with diseases elsewhere in the body. Various amounts of bacteria may get into the bloodstream following simple everyday procedures like brushing of teeth and accidental lacerations as well as during surgical procedures. If the patient's defences are adequate and the microbes are not highly pathogenic, then they are eliminated with the help of phagocytes and other components of the host's immune systems such as complement (see Chapters 23 and 25). However, problems arise if the infecting dose of micro-organisms is high, the micro-organisms are virulent, and the host's immunological defence is relatively compromised. In this situation, the bacteria may continue to multiply in the bloodstream, which results in an acute infective state. Subsequently, the large numbers of organisms and their products accumulate in the bloodstream to give rise to various manifestations of severe blood-borne infections or septicaemia.

The Gram-negative organisms produce more acute manifestations owing to the release of cell-wall products such as lipopolysaccharide. Lipopolysaccharide, also known as endotoxin, causes activation of monocyte–macrophage cell lines which release a battery of cytokines (see Chapter 25). These cytokines activate a variety of pathophysiological events, leading to the establishment of symptoms of septic shock.

In its most severe form, septic shock can lead to:
• a fall in blood pressure, owing to peripheral vasodilatation;
• intravascular blood clotting, both in the peripheral capillaries and inside the internal viscera; and
• respiratory distress, owing to cellular consolidation of the lung fields.

Relatively mild manifestations of bacterial multiplication in the bloodstream are more regularly seen in clinical practice than severe septicaemia; these mild cases cause rigor, fever, and a feeling of being generally unwell.

The commonest organisms in Gram-negative septicaemia are *Escherichia coli* and other gut-derived organisms. *Escherichia coli* is mainly transmitted into the bloodstream from an infection of the urinary tract. Gram-negative organisms, including anaerobes such as *Bacteroides fragilis*, may also infect the bloodstream during both minor and major surgical procedures. Meningococcal septicaemia is a severe condition in which *Neisseria meningitidis* produces major septic shock with peripheral and central intravascular coagulation, caused by the release of a powerful endotoxin.

Gram-positive bacteria, notably *Streptococcus pyogenes* and *Staphylococcus aureus*, are still major causes of septicaemia. These organisms may enter the blood from sites such as skin and soft tissues, bone and joints, and other deeper sites. *Streptococcus pneumoniae* is the other major cause of Gram-positive septicaemia, especially in older adults with evidence of pneumonia and bronchitis. Blood-borne infection due to enterococci may be seen in patients with indwelling catheters and other urological manipulations.

Blood-borne infections require urgent investigation, preferably before antibiotic treatments are commenced. Ideally, blood cultures should be taken during febrile episodes and during an episode of chill and rigors in order to provide positive indication and adequate growth of the causative bacteria. Once blood has been drawn for culture, antibiotic therapy can be started. The result of antibiotic sensitivity tests on the cultured organisms determines whether the 'blind' antibiotic treatment, commenced earlier, should continue or requires modification. Mortality in severe blood-borne infections is high, and urgent action is necessary in terms of investigating the nature of the organism and starting antibiotic treatment and other supportive measures.

Endocarditis

Endocarditis is an infection of the endocardium (the inner smooth lining of the heart). Physically the endocardial surfaces are extremely smooth in texture and fail to allow adherence of most bacteria. However, infections occur in certain circumstances, even on healthy endocardium. This is sometimes seen with *Staphylococcus aureus* endocarditis, in which normal heart valve surfaces are affected, producing a large growth of the organism. This growth is known as a 'vegetation', and it may lead to destruction of the affected valves (see Chapter 32). This is an acute and severe condition requiring major antibiotic and often surgical intervention. Patients often have other foci of staphylococcal infection from where blood-borne infection of the valves has originated. Intravenous drug users are at increased risk of acute *Staphylococcus aureus* endocarditis.

Endocarditis is more often seen as a subacute-to-chronic infection, especially in people with previous damage to the endothelial lining of the valves (e.g. in congenital valve defects or following rheumatic heart disease). Patients with prosthetic valves are also more vulnerable to endocarditis. The endothelial surface in these conditions may be roughened and therefore allow small vegetations to form. Once a small fibrinous nidus is formed on the surface, the transient wandering microbes, generally non-pathogenic or only mildly pathogenic, may get lodged on the endocardial surfaces. When more fibrinous and cellular material is deposited, a small vegetation is formed within which the transient microbes start multiplying. The result is endocarditis.

The slow microbial multiplication results in a mild, subacute infection manifested by low-grade, persistent pyrexia, general malaise and weakness, anaemia, and, occasionally, splinter haemorrhages, which are characteristic haemorrhages under the nails.

The organisms most commonly involved in endocarditis include *Streptococcus viridans*, *Staphylococcus epidermidis*, and *Enterococcus faecalis*. On rarer occasions, organisms such as *Candida* species, *Coxiella* species, and some Gram-negative organisms have been involved. *Staphylococcus epidermidis* endocarditis has become very common, owing to the introduction of large numbers of new intravenous devices, such as the central intravenous lines used in the management of seriously ill patients. Undiagnosed or untreated endocarditis may result in serious haemodynamic complications caused by circulatory inadequacies. There may be thromboembolic complications owing to the discharge of small fragments of vegetations into vital sites such as the brain, lung, liver, and spleen. Bacterial thrombi may multiply in these new sites and cause abscesses.

Patients with endocarditis should be urgently investigated for the presence of the vegetations on their heart valves. Microbiological investigations include repeated blood cultures to identify the microbial cause and the appropriate antibiotics for its treatment. X-rays, echocardiograms, and other imaging techniques help to confirm the microbiological diagnosis.

Antibiotic treatment of endocarditis consists of a combination therapy including a penicillin, such as benzylpenicillin or amoxycillin (flucloxacillin for *Staphylococcus aureus*) and an aminoglycoside antibiotic, such as gentamicin. These two groups of antibiotics are bactericidal in their action (i.e. they actually kill the organisms rather than suppress their growth). They act synergistically (i.e. they help each other), resulting in rapid and complete killing. They are usually given intravenously for a relatively long period, about 4–6 weeks. Monitoring of drug levels to ensure that they are in the therapeutic but not the toxic range, particularly the aminoglycosides, is an essential aspect of prolonged treatment of endocarditis (see Chapters 11, 13 and 19).

Antibiotic treatment alone may not be adequate to cure the patient. Evaluation of the outcome of the antibiotic treatment is essential and, if necessary, surgical intervention may be required to rectify any valvular damage.

INFECTIONS OF THE CENTRAL NERVOUS SYSTEM

Both the meninges and the brain may be affected by a large variety of infections. These are transmitted predominantly via the bloodstream, but the central nervous system may also be directly infected (e.g. from an abscess in the middle ear or the sinuses, after a penetrating wound of the skull, or postoperatively). Most infections are caused by a variety of viruses and are generally mild, but bacterial infections can be extremely serious.

Meningitis

Meningeal infections are clinically manifested by severe headaches, fever, photophobia (sensitivity to light), irritability, neck stiffness, and drowsiness, which may progress to unconsciousness. Skin rashes, sometimes haemorrhagic, may be seen, especially in meningococcal meningitis (see Person-Centred Study). Usually in infection, both the meninges and the cerebrospinal fluid (CSF) show evidence of inflammatory changes. CSF taken by lumbar puncture (or from the fontanelles in newborn babies) shows an increased number of inflammatory cells. The inflammatory cells in acute infections are predominantly pus cells. In chronic infections and infections due to viruses, the inflammatory cells belong to lymphocytic series. There are other evidences of infection, mainly in the biochemical constituents of CSF; these include a reduction in glucose in bacterial infections and an increase in protein in tuberculous meningitis. Gram staining of CSF in untreated bacterial meningitis may show the presence of the causative bacterial agent.

Meningitis may be caused in newborn babies by aspiration of contaminated amniotic fluid into the respiratory tract during birth. Amniotic fluid may be contaminated by faecal material, especially in prolonged labour with ruptured membranes. The microbes involved are usually the maternal gut organisms such as *Escherichia coli* and group beta-haemolytic streptococci. Both these infections can rapidly establish a meningeal infection in which typical meningeal symptoms may not be evident. Mortality is very high in neonatal meningitis, and prompt diagnosis and rapid initiation of treatment is therefore vital.

Bacteria commonly involved in meningeal infections are *Haemophilus influenzae*, *Neisseria meningitidis* (the meningococcus), and *Streptococcus pneumoniae* (the pneumococcus). *Haemophilus influenzae* is a small, Gram-negative bacteria; it affects infants more frequently than older people. Meningococcus may cause the infection at any age but it is most common in adolescents and young adults. Pneumococcus is generally found in the very young and older adults.

All of these infections are transmitted by the airborne route; after a transient, often asymptomatic, pulmonary infection they are spread to the meninges via the bloodstream. The infection produces an acute inflammatory response in the meninges and the CSF, resulting in a pyogenic response.

Mortality is high in both meningococcal and pneumococcal meningitis, and it is therefore essential that antibiotic treatment is started as soon as meningitis is suspected. *Haemophilus meningitis* is relatively less severe, but should be treated with some vigour. A third generation cephalosporin such as cefotaxime is most appropriate for treatment. Incidence of *Haemophilus meningitis* has reduced significantly since the introduction of HiB vaccine (see Chapter 21). In most instances, patients will be first seen by their general practitioner, who should be aware of the gravity of the disease and commence treatment with either intravenous benzylpenicillin or intravenous ampicillin before arranging hospital admission. Benzylpenicillin is most effective against meningococcus and pneumococcus (although a small percentage of pneumococci are now resistant to penicillin). A broader spectrum antibiotic, such as a third-generation cephalosporin like cefotaxime or chloramphenicol, may be substituted. In hospital, a CSF specimen is normally taken by lumbar puncture, if safe, and this is rushed to the laboratory for microscopy, culture, and biochemical analysis. Blood for culture, taken at the same time as the CSF, may also be useful. Unfortunately, a lumbar puncture is contraindicated if there is raised intracranial pressure owing to an increased volume of CSF, and cultures may be negative if antibiotic treatment has been started before CSF and blood are taken. Meningitis is a notifiable disease. As far as possible it should be managed in isolation.

Tuberculous meningitis is a chronic infection of the meninges caused by *Mycobacterium tuberculosis*. It is usually secondary to pulmonary infection. This condition is rarely seen in children in the UK and is occasionally found in adults. It is often seen in patients with HIV infection and acquired immunodeficiency syndrome (AIDS). The disease causes a chronic persistent headache, low-grade pyrexia, and gradual weakness; it is often associated with behavioural changes and focal signs, owing to the involvement of several cranial nerves.

A CSF sample usually shows a moderate increase in lymphocytes with a large increase in protein. Treatment follows the same pattern as that of pulmonary tuberculosis, but the mortality is nevertheless rather high.

Viral meningitis, as mentioned earlier, is generally milder than bacterial meningitis, with symptoms of headache, irritability, and an influenza-like illness. The viruses commonly involved belong to the enterovirus group, including echovirus, Coxsackie virus, polioviruses, and also mumps virus and herpes simplex virus.

These infections may be transmitted to the central nervous system through the bloodstream. CSF microscopy shows a moderate increase in cell count, predominantly lymphocytes. Virological investigations, including tissue culture and electron microscopy, may help in the diagnosis. Viral meningitis is a self-limiting infection and no treatment is usually required, although herpes simplex meningitis is sometimes treated with acyclovir.

Encephalitis is inflammation of the brain which is caused predominantly by viruses. The viruses which cause meningitis are also associated with encephalitis, *Herpes simplex* being a common example. There are a number of other more virulent viruses, found in the tropical endemic areas that cause severe encephalitis. These usually belong to the group of arthropod-borne viruses.

Brain Abscess

Single or multiple abscesses in the brain are usually a consequence of infections elsewhere. These abscesses may be found in the brain tissue itself, between the brain and the dura mater (subdural region), or outside the dura mater (epidural region). Abscesses are the result of either blood-borne spread of pyaemic emboli (small clumps of pus that contain bacteria) from a primary source (e.g. a lung abscess or endocarditis).

Alternatively, a brain abscess may arise as a result of direct spread from an abscess in the middle ear or sinuses or from a dental abscess.

Patients present with symptoms of focal lesions in the brain, such as localized or generalized weakness or paralysis, fever, fits, and behavioural changes. Imaging investigations, including computerized tomography (CT) and magnetic resonance imaging (MRI) scan show the site and extent of the lesions.

Treatment consists of drainage of the abscess in a neurosurgical unit and antibiotic therapy. Since many of the abscesses are polymicrobial, it is usual to use a combination of antibiotics against anaerobic organisms, such as *Bacteroides fragilis*, and aerobic organisms such as *Streptococci*, *Staphylococci*, and pneumococci. Gram-negative organisms. such as *Pseudomonas* species and *Proteus* species, may sometimes be involved, especially if the abscess is a result of a middle ear infection. Antibiotics diffuse poorly into the brain tissue across the blood–brain barrier, and this needs to be taken into account during treatment.

SEXUALLY TRANSMITTED INFECTIONS

Neisseria gonorrhoeae and *Chlamydia trachomatis* are the two most common sexually transmitted infections, constituting over 80 per cent of these infections. HIV infection, which may be considered as a sexually transmitted infection, is clinically manifested with a wide involvement of multiple systems (see Chapters 18 and 28). A number of other agents are transmitted by the sexual route, such as *Gardnerella vaginalis*, *Candida albicans*, *Trichomonas vaginalis*, *Ureaplasma urealyticum*, and genital herpes.

Syphilis

Syphilis used to be an important sexually transmitted disease – it is still a serious infection, but the incidence has fallen significantly during the last 20–30 years. The infectious agent is a spirochaete, *Treponema pallidum,* which causes a primary lesion in the genitalia – a primary chancre. At a later stage the disease manifests systemically as secondary syphilis, during which patients develop systemic manifestations, rash, and oral ulcers. If the disease is untreated, it may either subside or present later as tertiary syphilis, when typical syphilitic granulomas, known as 'gummas', appear in the internal organs such as liver, brain, and bone. The organisms in the primary stage can be visualized in the exudates from the genital lesions using a dark ground microscope. In later stages, serology is usually indicative of infection, both of active disease and of past infection. Penicillin still remains the drug of choice, and the organism is exquisitely sensitive to it.

Gonorrhoea

Neisseria gonorrhoeae (gonococcus) is a Gram-negative, bean-shaped diplococcus. It is often found inside phagocytosed white blood cells (polymorphs) in the urethral discharge of infected patients. Patients may acquire the infection during sexual intercourse with an infected person. Within a short time, there is an acute inflammatory response, first involving the urethra and then other organs of the genital system. The patients present with dysuria (pain when passing urine), a burning sensation when passing urine, fever, and general malaise. If untreated, the infection may spread to the prostate, spermatic cord, and epididymis in the male, and to the cervix, endometrium, fallopian tubes, and ovaries in the female. Spread to deeper tissues may lead to pelvic inflammatory disease in females, in which there is a more generalized involvement of the pelvic organs, resulting in chronic low abdominal and back pain, fever, infertility, and other constitutional symptoms.

Gram staining of a urethral smear (from men) or an endocervical swab (from women) shows the presence of the red-stained diplococci both intracellularly and extracellularly (Figure 16.5). Swabs from other sites, such as rectum and throat, may also give positive results. The organisms can be cultured relatively easily on special culture media.

The infection is treated with penicillin, but because of the increased incidence of penicillin resistance, other antibiotics such as ciprofloxacin and spectinomycin are often used when immediate treatment is needed.

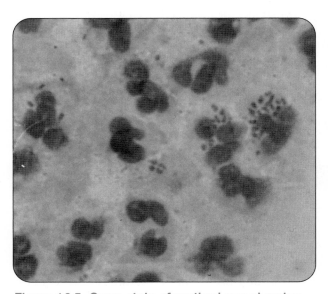

Figure 16.5 Gram stain of urethral pus showing *Neisseria gonorrhoeae* inside and outside pus cells.

Because of the possibility of re-infection, contact tracing and treatment of contacts is an important element in the long-term cure of the patient. Use of condoms also helps in the reduction of risk of infection.

Chlamydia trachomatis

Chlamydia trachomatis is an intracellular microbe. It is probably the most common cause of sexually transmitted disease. It produces clinical manifestations similar to those of gonorrhoea. The condition presents as a so-called non-specific urethritis or non-gonococcal urethritis in males, and as cervicitis in female. The urethral discharge produced is serous or mucoid, and special laboratory techniques are required to examine the specimen. A fluorescent antibody test can demonstrate the presence of the characteristic intracellular inclusion bodies. *Chlamydia trachomatis* may also be grown in tissue cultures, but the positive result is detected in less than half the cases. Tetracyclines are used to treat the infection and, as with gonorrhoea, contact tracing is extremely important to prevent re-infection.

KEY POINTS

- Some microbial agents are more virulent than others; some may even be completely harmless. Harmless microbes may occasionally cause disease, especially if the host is immunocompromised.
- Infecting microbes can be generally classified as bacterial, viral, fungal, or parasitic.
- Bacterial pathogens usually cause disease by releasing poisonous substances (toxins).
- *Streptococci* and *Staphylococci* are two major pyogenic organisms that cause superficial infection with production of pus.
- Many pathogenic bacteria – the anaerobes – cannot grow in the presence of oxygen.
- Many virus infections are manifested by skin rashes. The majority of the infections of the upper respiratory tract are caused by viruses.
- Diphtheria, which used to be a dreaded disease, is now virtually non-existent in developed countries, thanks primarily to the diphtheria toxoid vaccine.
- Pneumococcal pneumonia in older adults and influenza virus infection are two very common killer diseases.
- *Mycobacterium tuberculosis* infection is predominantly a lung disease that spreads by the air-borne route.
- *Campylobacter jejuni* is one of the most common cause of gastroenteritis in the UK. *Shigella sonnei* is the most frequent cause of dysentery in the UK, and the infection is spread by the faeco-oral route.
- Enteropathogenic *Escherichia coli* and rotavirus are the most common causes of infantile gastroenteritis. Strict infection-control measures are essential to prevent the spread of these infections.
- Eighty per cent of urinary tract infections are due to the bacteria *Escherichia coli*.
- Bacterial meningitis caused by *Neisseria meningitidis* is contagious and the contacts should be given prophylactic treatment. Viral meningitis is usually milder than bacterial meningitis.

FURTHER READING

Brooks GF, Butel JS, Ornston LN. Jawetz E, Melnick JL and Aldlberg EA (1995). Medical Microbiology, 12th edition. Prentice Hall International.

Elliott, Desselburger (1996) Lecture Notes on Medical Microbiology. Blackwell Science, Oxford.

Inglis TJJ (1998) Churchill's clinical microbiology pocket book. Churchill Livingstone, London.

Mims, PC (1998) Medical Microbiology, 2nd edition. Mosby, London.

Mims CA, Zuckerman M, Urwin G (1994) Case Studies in Medical Microbiology. Mosby, London.

Sleigh JD, Timbury MC (1998) Notes on Medical Microbiology. Churchill Livingstone, London.

Shanson DC (1998) Microbiology in Clinical Practice, 2nd edition. Wright, London.

INVESTIGATION OF THE INFECTED PATIENT

LEARNING OBJECTIVES

After studying this chapter you will have a clearer understanding of:
- the various ways of obtaining satisfactory clinical specimens for laboratory investigation and their safe transportation to the laboratory
- the clinical specimens that are used for the different microbiological investigations
- the microbiological investigations available to help in the diagnosis of infection
- the risks to health-care workers posed by clinical specimens

INTRODUCTION

Although many infections in patients who have been seen by their general practitioner or admitted to hospital can be provisionally diagnosed on clinical evaluation (see Person-Centred Study: Urinary Tract Infection), other infections require investigation by the laboratory, both for diagnosis of the nature of the infection and for confirmation of the provisional clinical diagnosis. Microbiology laboratories also advise on the antimicrobial agents that are most appropriate for the treatment of infections. An interactive laboratory service is therefore of great importance in the diagnosis and management of infected patients.

COLLECTION AND TRANSPORT OF MICROBIOLOGICAL SPECIMENS

In order to obtain the best service and advice from the laboratory, health care staff should be aware of the value of acquiring the appropriate specimens at the right time into the correct container. Most hospital laboratories in the UK provide guidance about safe practice in collection and transportation of clinical specimens from the wards and clinics to the laboratory. Health-care workers should be aware of these guidelines in order to maximize the usefulness of the pathology services available and to ensure the safety of the laboratory workers, the portering staff, their fellow health care workers, and themselves.

The quality of the results reported by the microbiology services are directly related to the quality of the clinical specimen sent for investigation. Dry sterile containers are used for the collection of many clinical specimens (e.g. blood, urine, sputum, cerebrospinal fluid, pus, and tissues). Specimens are obtained according to the direction given by the laboratory, properly secured by tightening the screw cap on the container, and adequately labelled with the name, date of birth, hospital number, and ward or clinic of the patient. Specimens must be transported in a sealed plastic bag and taken either via the hospital portering system or, in an emergency, by another health care professional. A laboratory request form must be enclosed (usually in a separate holder attached to the transport bag) to provide information about the patient, short clinical details, the nature of the specimen, the date and time of collection, and any other relevant clinical information, including drug therapies.

Prompt submission of microbiology specimens to the laboratory is particularly important to ensure that any microbes are viable for culturing. After all, if the microbes die because of a delay between the time that the specimen is collected and the time it arrives in the

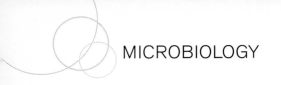

MICROBIOLOGY

laboratory, a second specimen for analysis will be needed and there will be a delay in obtaining a precise result. If it is an urgent out-of-hours request, the on-call laboratory technician should be bleeped so that he or she is alerted to the impending arrival of the specimen.

URINE SPECIMENS

A urinary tract infection is diagnosed and confirmed by the presence of organisms (see Figure 17.1) and possibly blood cells in the urine. Therefore, to prevent contamination with microbes from other tissues, patients are advised to collect a midstream urine specimen. The early part of the stream is voided, which flushes out the urethra, and the middle part of the urine is collected. In males, this is very straightforward; in females, it may be necessary to clean the vulva with clean tissue before the middle part of the stream is collected. In neonates and infants, it may be necessary to collect urine by suprapubic aspiration (i.e. introducing a long sterile needle into the bladder above the pubis and aspirating the urine directly into a plastic

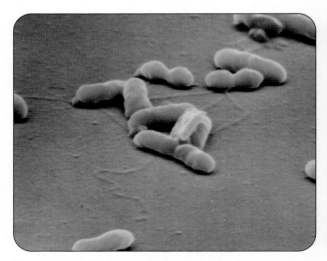

Figure 17.1 Electron micrograph of a *Proteus* species. This species normally inhabits the gastrointestinal tract, though if the organisms migrate into the genitourinary tract, they can cause a UTI.

pot). Alternatively, urine specimens are sometimes collected from newborn babies into a plastic bag, but this often gets contaminated with organisms from the perineum. A urine sample from a catheterized patient is not very helpful and is often found to be contaminated with commensal organisms from the urethra.

SPUTUM SPECIMENS

A satisfactory specimen of sputum is obtained by coughing up and collecting sputum; this can sometimes be helped by physiotherapy procedures. Salivary contamination should be avoided as far as possible. The patient should be advised to collect purulent, mucopurulent, or blood-stained sputum and avoid collecting mucoid sputum. If the patient is unable to produce sputum, particularly in cases of suspected tuberculosis or in children, a gastric aspirate may be obtained; these patients often swallow any phlegm that is produced. In adults, sputum production may be induced by spraying aerosol into the trachea. This evokes a strong cough reflex with production of sputum. Bronchoalveolar lavage is sometimes performed during bronchoscopy; this provides a satisfactory specimen for various microbiological investigations. Bronchoalveolar lavage involves introduction of physiological saline through the bronchoscopy tube; the fluid is then withdrawn carefully for cytological and microbiological examinations.

CEREBROSPINAL FLUID SPECIMENS

Cerebrospinal fluid (CSF) is collected by aspiration through an intervertebral space; in newborn babies CSF may be collected through the anterior fontanelle. Extreme care in the aseptic technique is necessary when performing a lumbar puncture to obtain CSF. In patients who have shunts for hydrocephalus, a CSF specimen may be collected from external reservoirs or shunt tubes. It is essential to transport this specimen to the laboratory as quickly as possible; urgent examinations are performed in the laboratory in order to provide the clinician with rapid preliminary results.

PUS AND TISSUE SPECIMENS

Pus and tissue specimens are collected aseptically and transported in sterile containers. Specimens of aspirated pus, in particular, need to be transported rapidly in order to retain the viability of the anaerobic microbes.

BLOOD CULTURES

Blood culture is an extremely important microbiological investigation. Samples of blood are collected, usually from veins but sometimes from arteries, and are used to inoculate blood culture bottles for aerobic and anaerobic organisms. The culture bottles are transported rapidly to the laboratory and are incubated as soon as possible, often in an automated blood culture system. Blood collected for culture out of ordinary laboratory hours should be taken in the blood culture bottles, and subsequently put in an accessible incubator available in most laboratories for this purpose. (A clotted blood may be required to evaluate antibody status (e.g. *Toxoplasma* or rubella antibodies) (see Chapter 24).)

FAECAL SPECIMENS

Faecal specimens are collected for examination for bacterial, viral, and parasitic infections. Specimens are generally received in special universal containers, which contain a spatula for obtaining the stool sample. It is advisable that the bladder is emptied before the specimen is produced to avoid contamination with urine. Faecal specimens are examined both by conventional methods, for the presence of bacteria and parasites, and by electron microscope, for viral agents. Freshly voided specimens ('hot stool' specimens) are sometimes sent rapidly to the laboratory for microscopic examination for parasites.

SWABS

A common investigation for infection involves taking swabs from the sites of infection, such as the throat, ear, and eye. Swabs may also be taken from a number of infected sites, such as wound or other lesions. The swabs are taken on wisps of cotton wool on a stick and are transported to the laboratory in a transport medium such as Stuart's transport medium. The medium contains thioglycolic acid, which uses up the oxygen and provides a reduced (oxygen-free) environment for any anaerobes to survive, and also allows the aerobic bacteria to be transported. There are various types of swabs available for viral, bacterial, chlamydial and special investigations, such as culture of *Bordetella pertussis*. It should be emphasized that if possible, the swab should be well loaded with the exudate specimen for a reasonable result to be obtained.

Swabs of the Genital Tract

High vaginal, cervical, and urethral swabs (from females) and penile and urethral swabs (from males) are transported in Stuart's transport medium for bacterial and fungal cultures. Special transport media for *Trichomonas* species and *Chlamydia* species are available.

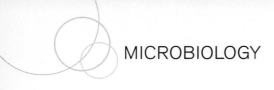

SERUM FOR ANTIBIOTIC LEVELS

For the determination of the serum levels of antibiotics in the patient's blood, clotted blood samples are collected in dry, sterile tubes. There are written protocols to provide guidance as to the scope and frequency of these tests. It is essential that these guidelines are available in the wards and are followed to obtain the best services from the laboratories.

SAMPLES FOR SEROLOGICAL TESTS

Clotted blood samples are collected for a variety of serological tests, for the diagnosis of viral infections, and to provide serological evidence of bacterial infections such as syphilis. Serological tests are also available for infections with organisms such as *Toxoplasma* and *Legionella* and for fungal and parasitic infections. Laboratories provide guidance to the availability and usefulness of these tests.

Virus Infections

A number of investigations are available for diagnosis of various virus infections. Some of these require specimens such as throat washings (for enteroviruses and influenza viruses), vesicular fluids (for herpes zoster virus and varicella–zoster virus), faeces (for enteroviruses, rotavirus, and other gut-derived viruses), nasopharyngeal aspirates (for respiratory syncytial viruses), and bronchoalveolar lavage fluid (for cytomegalovirus and measles virus).

Safety Precaution

It is extremely important to remember that specimens for laboratory investigations may contain highly pathogenic microbes. Therefore any such material should be handled with extreme care during collection and transfer to the laboratory. In particular, specimens obtained from patients who are likely to be at high risk [e.g. patients infected with hepatitis B or human immunodeficiency virus (HIV)] must be clearly labelled with identification stickers so that the portering and laboratory staff are aware. Hospitals have written guidelines for collection and transportation of high-risk specimens and for dealing with spillage or other accidents involving these specimens. It must be emphasized that all specimens for laboratory investigation should be considered as hazardous and therefore should be handled with due care and precaution.

PROCESSING CLINICAL SPECIMENS IN THE LABORATORY

MICROSCOPY

CSF Specimens

Some specimens for microbiological investigations require microscopic examination for an urgent provisional diagnosis on which immediate treatment could be based. For example, CSF specimens are examined by microscopy to ascertain whether there has been an increase in the cell count in the CSF and, if so, to what extent; the type of cell can also be identified at this early examination. A count of fewer than 5 white cells (usually lymphocytes) is normally found in uninfected CSF. A count of more than 5 white cells that consists predominantly of polymorphs (neutrophils) indicates an acute bacterial infection (e.g. pyogenic meningitis). Infections due to *Haemophilus influenzae*, meningococcus, or pneumococcus may give rise to a large increase in these cells.

In viral infections, a moderate increase in lymphocytes is usually seen, and this is also true for tuberculous meningitis. Microscopy therefore serves as a good indicator and the results are usually telephoned to the clinician for immediate attention.

A Gram stain is performed at the same time as these examinations, and this provides an indication of the nature of the organisms involved. For instance, a Gram-positive diplococcus indicates the pneumococcus whereas a Gram-negative diplococcus suggests the meningococcus; and a Gram-negative thin, rod-shaped bacteria points to *Haemophilus influenzae*. Occasionally, a meningeal infection may be caused by a fungus (e.g. *Candida* species or *Cryptococcus* species). Gram staining will often allow these organisms to be visualized. A special stain, such as India ink negative stain, is sometimes required to detect *Cryptococcus neoformans* in the CSF.

Urine Specimens

Microscopic examination of urine specimens is generally performed before the sample is cultured. This often gives valuable information about the nature and extent of urinary infection and helps in decision making about early treatment. The following information is obtainable from microscopy of urine:
- the presence or absence of white or red blood cells;
- the presence or absence of epithelial cells;
- the presence or absence of crystals;
- the presence or absence of casts; and
- results of dipstick tests.

White or Red Blood Cells in the Urine

Normal urine has no more than 10 white cells (pus cells) or red cells per ml. An increase in the white blood cell count indicates a possible urinary tract infection either in the bladder (cystitis) or in the kidneys and ureters (pyelonephritis). An increase in the red blood cell count could be due to bleeding (haematuria) either in the kidneys or the ureters; this is commonly caused by the trauma that renal stones produce. Chronic infection such as tuberculosis of the kidneys may also cause haematuria. Red blood cells may also be present in the urine of patients with bacterial endocarditis, chronic kidney diseases, and a variety of non-infective conditions (Figure 17.2).

Epithelial Cells in the Urine

Epithelial cells are sometimes found in the urine. A small number of squamous epithelial cells are normally found in a properly taken midstream specimen of urine. The early part of the urine stream will flush out any loose epithelial cells that are normally found in the urethra. A preponderance of epithelial cells in the urine indicates that the specimen has not been collected properly or that there has been concentration of urine, possibly because of dehydration.

Crystals in the Urine

Crystals of different shapes and sizes are sometimes found during microscopy. These have very little microbiological significance but are often reported by the laboratory. They may indicate various metabolic abnormalities and may provide clues to the clinician about other underlying diseases (e.g. uric acid may point to a diagnosis of gout).

Casts in the Urine

Casts of various morphologies may occasionally be found during microscopy. The basic matrix of a cast consists of a hyaline deposit of protein in the renal tubules, the hyaline casts. These occur when damage to the renal tubules allows the colloidal protein to leak out of the blood vessels into the tubules. The presence of the casts is, therefore, an indication of renal damage and is often seen in association with infections (e.g. pyelonephritis). Pus cells or red blood cells may be found embedded on hyaline matrix, forming the pus or white blood cell casts and red blood cell casts.

Dipstick tests

Rapid tests are available for immediate detection of protein, sugar, nitrite, blood or haemoglobin, and white cells in the urine. These can be performed at the patient's bedside, in out-patient clinics, or general practitioners' surgeries. The tests are based on a series of dried reagents on the dipsticks which, when immersed in freshly voided urine, results in a change of colour of the reagents. These can be read within minutes by comparing the change in colour of the dipsticks or segments of the dipsticks with standards. Many laboratories are now introducing the dipsticks for rapid results and for screening urine specimens, to enable them to culture only the specimens that give positive results.

Faecal Specimens

Faecal specimens are examined microscopically for the presence of ova and cysts of parasites and for mature parasites, particularly in people who have been travelling in areas where infection with these organisms is endemic.

Other Specimens

Various other clinical specimens are also examined by microscopy for early indication of infection. One of the most common examples of this is the acid-fast stained smears of sputum for tuberculosis. In pulmonary tuberculosis, patients often cough up blood-stained sputum (haemoptysis), which requires urgent investigation. If the sputum contains large numbers of acid-fast stained organisms, the patient requires immediate isolation to prevent the spread of the infection to others. Aspirates from other sites (e.g. the pleural, pericardial or peritoneal cavities) are often stained for acid-fast bacilli and other infective organisms.

Throat swab are taken where there is the suspicion of diphtheria, or when rusty coloured or purulent sputum is produced in pneumonia. Any abscess pus may be examined by staining and microscopy for rapid diagnosis.

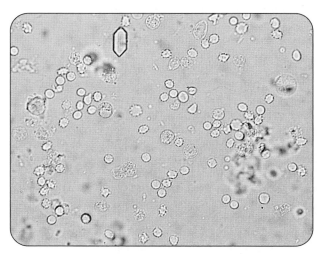

Figure 17.2 Pus cell, red blood cells, and crystals in urine infected with *Escherichia coli*.

Fluorescence microscopic examinations are sometimes used for visualizing a number of pathogenic organisms – after smears of specimens are stained with a fluorescent dye, they are examined under ultraviolet light. Acid-fast bacilli are often examined after staining with a fluorescent stain such as auramine–rhodamine, and a number of viruses may be examined by staining with antisera labelled with fluorescent dye such as the respiratory syncytial virus, influenza virus, parainfluenza virus, and other respiratory viruses. When stained, the fluorescing organisms appear brightly stained in a dark background (see Chapter 24).

CULTURE

Microbiological investigation of clinical specimens is dependent on culturing them to isolate the offending pathogens on various artificial media and then identify these pathogens by various tests. There are a number of artificial media that are routinely used for culturing common bacteria and fungus. More fastidious pathogens require selective media (which will allow selective growth of some organisms while inhibiting others). An enriched media allows enhanced growth of some organisms. Most common media contain a semi-solid base made of agar (a variety of Chinese seaweed).

Clinical specimens are usually cultured on a number of media, including:

- a blood agar medium (agar plus 4–5 per cent blood); this supports the growth of most common organisms;
- a chocolate agar (a blood agar that has been heat-treated to destroy some natural inhibitory products); this allows growth of some fastidious organisms such as *Haemophilus* species and *Neisseria* species; and
- a medium for the growth of anaerobic organisms, which is sometimes used.

Many clinical specimens may contain organisms derived from the gut. These organisms grow better in the presence of bile salts, and therefore a bile salt containing-medium such as McConkey's medium or CLED is often routinely used. Most pathogenic *Mycobacteria* require an egg-based medium (Löwenstein–Jensen) for their growth and preliminary identification.

Culture plates are inoculated on their surface with the clinical specimens and incubated, generally at 37°C. Some specimens that are being investigated for a fungal infection may require incubation at lower temperatures (e.g. 30°C). Between 24 and 48 hours' incubation is adequate for most common pathogenic organisms, but some organisms, such as pathogenic *Mycobacteria*,

require several weeks (usually between 3 and 8 weeks). Most pathogenic bacteria grow in an ordinary incubator in aerobic conditions, but some organisms require an anaerobic environment and others require a small amount of carbon dioxide for optimal growth.

The organisms grow on the surface of these media as small colonies. The appearance of these colonies sometimes gives an indication of the identity of the organism, such as golden yellow colour of the colonies of *Staphylococcus aureus* (Figure 17.3), the beta-haemolytic colonies of *Streptococci*, or the swarming colonies of *Proteus mirabilis*.

IDENTIFICATION
Staining

Staining of a smear of the isolate shows the characteristic morphology of the organisms, which aids in the identification of the type of infection. Gram stain allows preliminary identification of a large number of bacterial agents. For example, it may reveal such bacteria as cocci (spherical organisms) or bacilli (rod-shaped organisms), and it will show if the microbe stains dark violet (Gram positive) or red (Gram negative).

Special stains such as the acid-fast (Ziehl–Neelsen) stain for *Mycobacteria*, the Albert stain for *Corynebacterium*, and the Leishman or Giesma stain for malarial parasites are other stains that are commonly used. Fungal cultures are often stained by lactophenol cotton blue and other special stains.

Corynebacterium diphtheria, the causative organism of diphtheria, is identified by its characteristic black colonial growth on media containing potassium telurite or the typical halo that is seen around the black

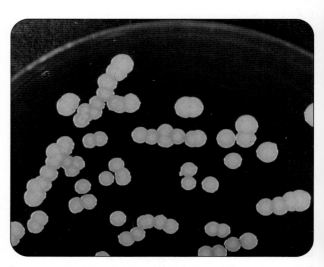

Figure 17.3 Blood agar plate of colonies of *Staphylococcus aureus*.

colonies on Tinsdale medium. Tiny transparent colonies with large areas of clear haemolysis are characteristically produced by beta-haemolytic *Streptococci*. Similarly, pink colonies formed on McConkey's medium or yellow colonies on CLED medium by *Escherichia coli* aids a presumptive diagnosis. There are special media containing antibiotics that selectively inhibit some organisms and allow growth of others, such as Thayer–Martin medium, which allows the growth of *Neisseria gonorrhoeae*. Characteristic growth and pigment production on special fungal media allows identification of many pathogenic fungi.

Biochemical Tests

Various other tests, including a battery of biochemical and serological tests, are also used to identify the organisms.

Simple tests are routinely used in clinical laboratories (such as the coagulase test to differentiate between coagulase-positive *Staphylococcus aureus* and coagulase-negative *Staphylococcus epidermidis*, and the optochin sensitivity test to differentiate between optochin-sensitive *Streptococcus pneumonia* and optochin-resistant *Streptococcus viridans*).

Many biochemical tests that help identify bacteria are based on the ability of the microbe to ferment a number of sugars (e.g. glucose, sucrose, mannitol, lactose, maltose). When a broth containing a small amount of these sugars is fermented by these bacteria, acid is produced, which, in the presence of an indicator, results in a colour change of the broth. Different bacteria produce their own characteristic patterns of fermentation, which allows the pathologist to distinguish between the types of organisms. This, along with a number of other special tests, forms the basis of most biochemical identification of bacteria. Certain commercial biochemical kits are available which allow precise identification of many bacterial isolates.

Serological Tests

Commercially available antibodies are used in the serological identification of isolated strains. These may be used as a primary identification test or to confirm the identity determined by other biochemical tests. These serological tests are based on a simple agglutination (clumping) test, in which a panel of known antibodies are used to visualize the agglutination of a saline emulsion of the isolate on a microscopic slide. Cultures of *Salmonella* species and *Shigella* species from cases of intestinal infections are often identified by this method.

Special serological tests are available for the diagnosis of virus infections. These include:

- examination of fluorescent antibody-stained clinical specimens under a light microscope in ultraviolet light;
- culture of viruses in cell cultures;
- examination of clinical specimens under an electron microscope; and
- serological tests for the presence of specific antibodies.

Direct examination of clinical specimens, such as nasopharyngeal aspirates, under a light microscope in ultraviolet light relies on the fact that fluorescing spots will be seen on the cells in the aspirate when antibodies made against certain viruses (e.g. respiratory syncytial virus) are stained with fluorescent dye (see Chapter 24).

Viruses may be identified by culturing them in cell cultures; some viruses have characteristic damaging effects on the cells (cytopathic effect or CPE) or alter the cells' ability to adsorb to red blood cells (the haemadsorption test). Occasionally it may be necessary to identify the type of the virus further by using a neutralization test.

Direct examination using an electron microscope may be used to demonstrate the presence of rotavirus and other enteric viruses in faecal specimens (Figure 17.4), herpesvirus in vesicle fluid, or the presence of viruses in CSF responsible for meningoencephalitis.

Serological tests are used to detect the presence of specific antibodies in patients' blood; tests used include complement fixation (see Chapter 25), agglutination test, enzyme-linked immunosorbent assays (ELISA), and fluorescence antibody tests (see Chapter 24).

In most microbial infections, especially those that invade the bloodstream and deeper tissues, the host immune system reacts by producing antibodies. These antibodies are produced against the many components of the microbial agent, such as proteins, glycoproteins

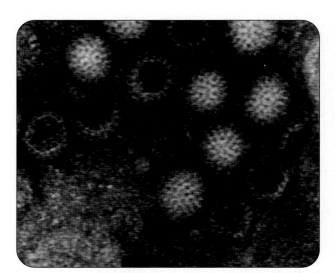

Figure 17.4 Electron micrograph of rotavirus.

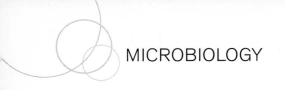
and polysaccharides. In the early stages of the disease, most antibodies belong to the immunoglobulin M (IgM) class; later, IgG is the predominant antibody (see Chapters 23 and 24). The antibodies are detected within a few days after the initiation of infection and are therefore of less value in the early diagnosis of infection. However, it often affords a confirmation of the early diagnosis and also helps in the follow-up of the progress of the disease process. Serological evidence of infection is also of value in the epidemiological investigation of diseases especially virus infections.

A large number of serological tests are available for bacterial and viral infections. These test for the presence of antibodies in body fluid. Laboratories require about 5–10 ml of clotted blood in a sterile tube for these tests. For most virus infections, a sample is taken during the acute stage of the infection, and a second sample should be sent during the next 7–14 days. Laboratories usually provide a list of the serological tests that are available for clinical use (Box 17.1).

Detection of microbial antigens by specific antibodies

A large number of tests are now available to detect the presence of microbial infections by detection of microbial products with the help of known positive specific antibodies. This is particularly important when the patient has been partially treated, as in meningitis, when the culture is likely to be negative. When specific antibody-coated latex particles are mixed on a microscope slide with the CSF from a patient with meningitis, clumping (agglutination) of these coated particles may be seen if the whole organism or components of these organisms are present in the CSF. Antibodies against *Neisseria meningitidis*, *Haemophilus influenzae*, or *Streptococcus pneumoniae* are useful for this particular detection method. It is an extremely rapid test, and a diagnosis can be made within minutes of receiving the specimen in the laboratory. A

variety of other antibody-coated reagents are now available for the rapid diagnosis of a number of microbial infections (e.g. syphilis, *Toxoplasma*, *Chlamydia*).

Good-quality monoclonal antibodies are available against a large number of common viruses and chlamydia. These are used to detect the presence of viral and chlamydial antigens in a variety of clinical specimens. Viral antigens detected by these methods include respiratory viruses such as influenza virus and parainfluenza virus; mumps virus; measles virus; respiratory syncytial virus from throat washing, nasopharyngeal aspirate, or bronchoalveolar lavage; cytomegalovirus in buffy coat (white blood cell fraction of blood products), urine, and tissues; herpes simplex virus and varicella zoster virus in vesicle fluids and skin scrapings; and herpes simplex virus in CSF.

Antibiotic Sensitivity Tests

When a bacterial isolate is thought to be responsible for initiating an infection, these are tested to determine their sensitivity to a variety of different antibiotics. Most microbiology laboratories have a written protocol indicating appropriate antibiotics for different isolates. For example, aminoglycosides (e.g. gentamicin) and cephalosporins are predominantly used for Gram-negative infections, whereas penicillins and macrolides (e.g. erythromycin) are often used to treat Gram-positive infections. Some of these are routinely tested; others are reserved for extended sensitivity in cases when the isolate is resistant to the first set of antibiotics. In acute infections, antibiotic treatment needs to be started urgently, and the choice of antibiotic will therefore depend on clinical judgement. Once the sensitivity result is available from the laboratory, usually after about 36–40 hours, the treatment plan may require modification.

Antibiotic sensitivity tests are performed using the disc diffusion test, in which small filter paper discs containing a fixed amount of antibiotic are placed on the surface of a uniformly inoculated plate. After the appropriate incubation time, the plate is examined for zones where growth has been inhibited by the different antibiotics. A standard organism with known antibiotic sensitivity is included as a control on the same plate to allow comparison of the zones and to give a satisfactory indication of the sensitivity of the isolate (Figure 17.5).

Minimal inhibitory and minimal bactericidal concentrations

In certain clinical situations, it may be necessary to determine the minimum concentration of antibiotic that will inhibit or kill the microbe. The minimum concentration of antibiotic that will inhibit microbial growth is the minimal inhibitory concentration (MIC); the minimum concentration of antibiotic that will kill the microbe is the minimal bactericidal concentration (MBC).

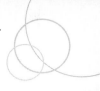

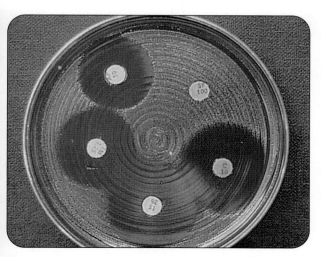

Figure 17.5 Antibiotic sensitivity testing. The plate shows the effect of a number of different antibiotics on the growth of a microbe, and is compared with a known control organism. Test microbe: central area; control microbe: outside colonies.

The MIC is determined by the addition of known concentrations of an antibiotic into different culture test tubes, then adding broth culture medium containing the offending microbes. After the appropriate time period of incubation, the minimal amount of the antibiotic that has resulted in inhibition of growth is determined by lack of turbidity (cloudiness) in the test tube.

Taking samples for culture from each of the negative tubes and culturing the samples on agar plates will show if there were any viable organisms remaining. The lowest concentration of antibiotic which shows no growth is considered as the MBC of the antibiotic to that isolated microbe.

Antibiotic Assays

Antibiotic assays in clinical specimens are particularly necessary when relatively toxic drugs are used for the treatment of a patient. Antibiotic assays are usually performed in the local laboratory or a reference laboratory using automated systems.

A common example of regular assays includes evaluation of the serum level of gentamicin. Prolonged use and high levels of serum gentamicin causes kidney damage, resulting in renal failure; there is also the risk of damage to the eighth cranial nerve, leading to ototoxity and deafness. In view of these potential hazards, the serum level of gentamicin is regularly monitored during treatment with this drug, and the dosage adjusted to the appropriate therapeutic but non-toxic level.

Other drugs that require monitoring include vancomycin, which also has both renal and ototoxic effects, streptomycin, which has ototoxic effects, other aminoglycosides (e.g. amikacin, amphotericin B, netilmicin for nephrotoxicity, and sometimes rifampicin for its hepatotoxic effects).

Epidemiological Investigations

Hospitals are a major site of small and large outbreaks of infection. A large concentration of microbial pathogens is regularly found in hospital environments. Some of these microbes have circulated in the hospital environment and developed multiple drug resistance owing to intense antibiotic pressure. In combination with the fact that many in-patients are to a greater or lesser extent immunocompromised during their hospital stay, these multiple-resistant organisms could create major clinical and management problems. Multiple-resistant *Staphylococcus aureus* (MRSA) inhabits and causes major outbreaks of infection, especially in high-activity areas such as intensive therapy units. These issues will be discussed in more detail in Chapter 20.

KEY POINTS

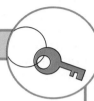

- The laboratory service is of great importance in the diagnosis and management of patients with infection.
- Collection of appropriate specimen and rapid transportation is vital for obtaining satisfactory and useful laboratory results.
- All specimens for laboratory investigations should be considered potentially hazardous and should therefore be handled with the utmost care.
- Initial microscopy result of specimens such as CSF and urine may help in the early diagnosis and treatment of infection.
- Guidelines provided by the laboratories are extremely valuable for the optimal use of the laboratory facilities.

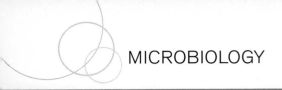

MICROBIOLOGY

FURTHER READING

Collee JG, Fraser AG, Marmion BP, Simmons A (1996) Mackie and McCartney's Practical Medical Microbiology. Churchill Livingstone, London.

Cooke EM, Taylor L (1991) Nursing Advisor. Hare's Bacteriology and Immunity for Nurses, 4th edition. Churchill Livingstone, London.

Greenwood D, Slack R, Peutherer JF (1997) Medical Microbiology. A Guide to Microbial Infections, Pathogenesis, Immunity, Laboratory Diagnosis and Control, 15th edition. Churchill Livingstone, London.

Hart CA (1996) Medical Microbiology. Mosby-Wolfe, London.

Pattison JR (1995) A Practical Guide to Clinical Bacteriology. John Wiley and Sons, Chichester.

Sleigh JD, Timbury MC (1998) Notes on Medical Bacteriology. Churchill Livingstone, London.

Stokes T (1997) Screening for chlamydia in general practice: a literature review and summary of the evidence. J Pub Health Med 19(2):222–32.

INFECTIONS IN IMMUNOCOMPROMISED PATIENTS

INTRODUCTION

There are many complexities associated with suppression of the immune response, as demonstrated in the Person-Centred Study. In this case, the suppression was initiated by medical intervention in order to prevent rejection of the kidney graft (see Chapter 29). As a result of the immunosuppressive drugs, the patient became vulnerable to a number of infections. The associated infections are usually caused by microbial agents of low virulence such as *Pneumocystis* species and *Candida* species.

THE IMMUNOCOMPROMISED HOST

Immunity against infection is associated with the ability of a host to counter the effect of the infecting agents and get rid of the infection. This is achieved by the competent response of the host with the aid of different components of the body's defence system (see Chapter 22).

These components include:
- the phagocytic and innate defence mechanisms;
- the humoral (antibody-dependent) immune system; and
- the cellular immune system.

The host may lose its ability to protect itself due to a variety of reasons. Congenital deficiencies in the immune mechanisms are rare but they do occur, exposing the host to subversion by infecting agents. An example is chronic granulomatous disease, in which defects in the phagocytic cells allow repeated and chronic infections by such organisms as *Staphylococcus aureus*. Defects in the humoral immune system in which immunoglobulins are not produced in adequate amounts may lead to recurrent bacterial and viral infections. Congenital defects of the cellular immune system often lead to a variety of opportunistic infections with microbes of low pathogenicity, including *Pneumocystis carinii*.

Acquired defects of the immune system can result from a number of different factors. Some of these arise in normal health and are associated with physiological states, such as occurs in premature and newborn infants, pregnancy, and old age. The immune system may be suboptimal during these periods and may therefore allow infection with mild-to-moderate pathogens.

IMMUNE STATUS *IN UTERO* AND IN THE NEWBORN

Preterm and newborn babies possess the components of the immune system, such as functional B lymphocytes and T lymphocytes, but they have not been assaulted by a wide variety of antigens (i.e. the cells

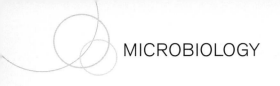

are naïve). It takes time for mature B lymphocytes to become established and, as a result, immunoglobulin production is reduced in neonates. This applies especially to immunoglobulin G (IgG) but also, to some extent, to IgM. This makes these babies vulnerable to many serious infections (e.g. Gram-negative septicaemia and infections due to *Staphylococci* and *Streptococci*).

Antibodies from the mother, especially IgG, against a number of viruses and bacteria cross the placental barrier and are transferred to the fetus *in utero*. Therefore, the fetus is normally protected against infections. This is specially true if the mother has significant quantities of antibodies in her bloodstream. Examples of maternal antibodies providing protection in the newborn includes, amongst others, rubella, polio, tetanus and diphtheria.

There are, however, some infections that may be transmitted from the mother to the fetus. These may have serious consequences, often leading to congenital deformities. Rubella virus, cytomegalovirus, and *Toxoplasma* are the three common culprits that have been associated with various congenital malformations in the fetus. If these infections have been confirmed by laboratory tests, the patients need to be counselled about the risk of the malformations and the possible course of actions, including termination of the pregnancy. Some other infections, such as syphilis, herpes simplex, hepatitis B, and human immunodeficiency virus (HIV), have also been associated with intrauterine infections.

T-lymphocyte-dependent immunity is not transferred from mother to child. In neonatal infection due to *Listeria monocytogenes*, in which early septicaemic or late meningitic manifestations are common and lead to high mortality, general immunodeficiency has been thought to be present. Both macrophage-dependent and T-lymphocyte-associated immunodeficiency has been described. Transmission of *Toxoplasma gondii* to the fetus occurs in a number of cases of early pregnancies, but it is not clear whether this is associated with immune status (see Chapter 24).

IMMUNE STATUS IN PREGNANCY

In pregnancy, immunity against infections appears to be slightly diminished. Rapid development of miliary tuberculosis and tuberculous meningitis during the third trimester of pregnancy has been reported. This was thought to be associated with decline in the cell-mediated immune function. Similarly, varicella pneumonitis has also been ascribed to waning cellular response in late pregnancy. Herpes simplex infection during pregnancy could result in disseminated disease, probably as a result of relative depression of T-lymphocyte immunity (see Box 18.1).

BOX 18.1 SOFT CHEESE, PREGNANT WOMEN AND LISTERIOSIS

Considerable confusion occurred recently surrounding publicity of infection in pregnant women caused by opportunistic bacteria such as *Listeria monocytogenes*. It was reported that soft, ripened cheeses such as brie, camembert, and blue vein, and all types of pâté were involved in the transmission of this infection to pregnant women (who are potentially immunodeficient), as well as to older adults and other relatively immunocompromised people. After investigation it was confirmed that these foods contain significantly increased numbers of *Listeria monocytogenes*. Further evidence suggested this bacterium could also be transmitted in cook-chilled meals prepared from farm animal products (including poultry) unless served piping hot. These foods should be avoided by pregnant women as well as by the older adults and other vulnerable groups. They should also avoid contact with these animals.

IMMUNOSUPPRESSION AS A CONSEQUENCE OF OLD AGE AND DEBILITATING DISEASES

Chronic debilitating diseases such as malignancy, diabetes mellitus, and malnutrition reduce the ability of the host to respond immunologically to many infections. Neutropenic patients, whether the neutropenia is caused by primary disease such as acute leukaemia or whether it follows cytotoxic treatment, are also at increased risk of infections, mainly with bacteria and fungi.

Similarly, many older adults are less able to defend themselves against many infections presumably due to sub-optimal immune mechanisms. People recovering from major surgical interventions are also likely to be more vulnerable to infection, including persistent wound infection (see Chapters 23 and 28).

DRUG-INDUCED IMMUNOSUPPRESSION

Prolonged use of certain antibiotics can induce significant immunosuppression, as can corticosteroids used for the treatment of inflammatory connective tissue and joint disorders. In particular, patients taking systemic corticosteroids are at higher risk of developing severe infection with varicella–zoster virus.

Chemotherapeutic agents used for the treatment of malignancies, particularly haematological malignancies (e.g. leukaemia, lymphoma), induce a major suppressive effect on the immune system (see below).

Immunosuppressive agents are regularly used after organ transplantation to suppress the immune system in order to prevent rejection of the transplanted organ (see Person–Centred Study). These agents include azathioprine, cyclosporin A, and prednisolone. Drug-induced immunosuppression makes a patient vulnerable to infection by a number of opportunistic pathogens (see Chapter 29).

Clinical Problem: Increased Risk of Infection with Chemotherapy

Patients with haematological malignancies (e.g. leukaemia) are aggressively treated with antineoplastic chemotherapy. This has resulted in a greatly improved prognosis, including an improvement in the quality of life. Unfortunately, it has also been associated with an increased risk of infection, including common infections associated with central venous catheters (e.g. coagulase-negative *Staphylococcus*, *Staphylococcus aureus*, and Gram-negative septicaemia with *Escherichia coli*, *Pseudomonas* species, *Klebsiella* species). Fungal infections are also an increasing cause of mortality, especially those due to *Candida* species and *Aspergillus* species. It is therefore extremely important that an effective antibiotic programme to deal with these infections is planned before chemotherapy is initiated and that appropriate surveillance is maintained during the course of treatment.

IMMUNOSUPPRESSION ASSOCIATED WITH INFECTIONS

The most significant example of immunosuppression associated with infections is found in patients infected with HIV. The virus is transmitted by homosexual and heterosexual activities, via shared needles among intravenous drug misusers, via blood and blood product transfusions, and by vertical transmission from an infected mother to her fetus.

The virus selectively infects cells of the immune system – T helper lymphocytes (also known as CD4+ cells), macrophages, and other mononuclear phagocytic cells. As a consequence, the defence system is compromised, leaving the patient vulnerable to infections. Both the cellular and antibody immune functions are affected as a result. As the HIV infection progresses, the patient becomes progressively more immunodeficient, with reductions in the numbers of CD4+ cells. Other virus infections co-exist, such as cytomegalovirus, herpes simplex virus, and Epstein–Barr virus.

Chronic infections, such as malaria, leishmaniasis, leprosy, and tuberculosis can also cause significant suppression of the immune system, making the patient susceptible to a number of microbial agents, most of which are generally of low pathogenicity – the so-called 'opportunistic pathogens' (e.g. opportunistic *Mycobacteria*, *Pneumocystis carinii* infection of the lung, *Toxoplasma gondii* and cytomegalovirus) (Figure 18.1).

MAJOR OPPORTUNISTIC INFECTIONS

BACTERIAL INFECTIONS

There are a number of common bacterial infections that may be associated with the immunocompromised state. *Staphylococcus aureus*, *Pseudomonas aeruginosa*, *Klebsiella pneumoniae*, and *Streptococcus pneumoniae* are examples of the infections often found in these patients. Pneumococcal bacteraemia occurs in a significantly high proportion of HIV-infected patients, and staphylococcal endocarditis and multiple abscesses are also being more frequently reported. These infections often arise in patients in whom there is a defect in antibody production. Antibodies are required for coating many of these microbes before they can be engulfed by the phagocytes for killing, a process known as 'opsonization'. If there is a defect in antibody production or a defect in the killing mechanism of the phagocytes (as occurs in chronic granulomatous

disease), the pathogens will survive, multiply, and cause disease (see Chapters 23 and 28).

Mycobacterial Infections

Chronic infections due to *Mycobacteria*, especially *Mycobacterium avium intracellulare* and *Mycobacterium tuberculosis*, cause considerable concern in the management of HIV infections. These infections occur when the CD4+ cell count is very low (often as low as 100 cells/ml). In particular, infection due to *Mycobacterium tuberculosis*, which occurs early in the course of HIV infection, has been of great concern because of its rapid progression to active and infectious disease in HIV-infected persons, and because of its potential for developing multiple drug resistance (multiple drug resistant tuberculosis – MDRTB). The rapid progression of tuberculosis in HIV patients is due to the inability of their immune system to ward off the infectious focus by forming a granuloma; this leads to extensive necrosis with numerous acid-fast bacilli. Granuloma formation occurs with the recruitment of large numbers of activated macrophages and sensitized lymphocytes. These normally help to contain multiplication of mycobacteria and consequent tissue damage (see Chapters 17 and 26).

In recent years, HIV-infected patients in the USA have been reported to be involved in institutional outbreaks of tuberculosis, caused by both drug-sensitive and drug-resistant strains of *Mycobacterium tuberculosis*; some of these infections have been fatal. Of

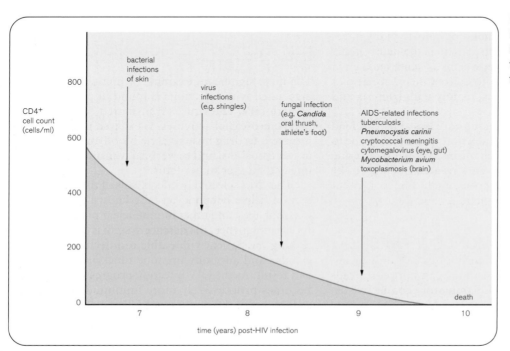

Figure 18.1 Typical infections that occur in HIV infection as the CD4+ cell count falls.

particular concern has been the transmission of infections to health care professionals from these infected patients. This had presumably resulted from the fact that health care professionals are not routinely protected by BCG vaccination in the USA (see Chapter 21). Special precautionary measures have resulted in the containment of transmission of tuberculosis, and particularly MDRTB, amongst the health care workers in the USA. In the UK, everyone is vaccinated with the Bacillus Calmette–Guérin (BCG) vaccine under the national immunization programme. This vaccine provides protection against tuberculosis and maintains a level of general resistance to this infection for a long period of time. Health care professionals in the UK, particularly those who are directly involved in patient care, are generally tested for delayed hypersensitivity to tuberculin antigen using the Mantoux test (see Chapter 27) when they begin work in the health service, and they are offered BCG vaccination if they are not immune to tuberculosis. Incidence of MDRTB remains low in the UK. Consequently, transmission of MDRTB infection has not yet posed any serious threat in the UK.

Most patients with tuberculosis are treated as outpatients, especially once their sputum has become negative on smears for acid-fast bacilli; treatment usually continues for 6–8 months. This is the normal procedure for both HIV-positive and HIV-negative patients. During the early stage of the disease, when the sputum shows the presence of acid-fast bacilli on smear tests, the patients are usually isolated in special facilities, such as in single rooms in an infectious diseases unit. Patients with MDRTB require special facilities, such as negative-pressure isolation units, from which the air is extracted several times an hour so that it does not pass to other areas of the hospital. Special precautions are required in the care and management of these patients (see Chapter 20).

Infections due to *Mycobacterium avium intracellulare* (MAI) has often been associated with significant debilitation in patients with HIV infection who have a very low CD4+ cell count. MAI is an organism of low virulence and rarely causes infection in people with a competent immune system. MAI infections that do occur in these people are generally mild and affect only the lymph nodes. In HIV-infected people, however, MAI behaves as an opportunistic infection and multiplies in various deeper tissues, including the blood. Patients with CD4+ cell counts of less than 50 cells/ml may rapidly develop disseminated MAI infection, in which the organisms may be found in the blood, lung, bone marrow, spleen, liver, lymph nodes, and gut wall. This leads to significant clinical manifestations of fever, night sweats, cough, and sometimes abdominal pain and diarrhoea. Severe anaemia may develop owing to the involvement

of bone marrow; this is a negative predictor for survival.

Treatment of MAI infection is particularly difficult because of the innate resistance of these organisms to most common antimycobacterial agents. A combination of second-line antimycobacterial agents, including rifabutin, amikacin, and the recently introduced drug, clarithromycin, have been used for the treatment of MAI infection with varying success.

Opportunistic infections caused by other non-pathogenic *Mycobacteria*, such as *Mycobacterium kansasii*, *Mycobacterium gordonae*, have been reported, but often these are really terminal colonizations rather than infections.

HIV infection and syphilis (caused by infection with *Treponema pallidum*) may occur simultaneously. Neurological involvement is often the main effect of syphilis in HIV-infected patients. The infection frequently fails to respond to standard treatment. In addition, routine laboratory investigations often demonstrate that the patient has not raised antibodies against *Treponema pallidum* in the blood or the cerebrospinal fluid (CSF). This is particularly common in patients whose CD4+ cell count is less than 200/μl. Severity of treponemal disease increases as the HIV infection progressively depletes the body of CD4+ cells.

FUNGAL AND PARASITIC INFECTIONS
Infection with *Pneumocystis carinii*

A major cause of morbidity (and mortality) in HIV-infected patients is infection with the opportunistic pathogen *Pneumocystis carinii*. It is usually associated with a low CD4+ cell count. Other immunocompromised patients (e.g. those on chemotherapy for malignancy and those actively immunosuppressed by drugs) are also susceptible to infection with this organism.

The parasite is found in the environment as tiny airborne particles, which, when inhaled by an immunocompromised host, may initiate a major pulmonary infection. Diagnosis of the infection is dependent on the demonstration of the parasites in induced sputum or bronchoalveolar lavage fluid. The parasites are stained with fluorescent-labelled antibody or silver stain for microscopy (see Chapter 24 for details of these techniques).

The X-ray of patients with *Pneumocystis carinii* infection reveals patchy bronchopneumonic consolidations throughout both lung fields, and this consolidation leads to disturbance in oxygen intake with oxygen starvation and consequent shortness of breath, which may be severe. Patients have a dry cough, fever, and severe malaise, and they require immediate attention to relieve oxygen deprivation. Therefore, oxygen supplementation is necessary. Treatment with trimethoprim–sulphamethoxazole (co-trimoxazole) is effective against the infection (see Chapter

19). Pentamidine (given intravenously) is also effective but it is very toxic. Pentamidine is also frequently given in an aerosol preparation as a preventive measure against the infection. Dapsone and trimethoprim combination has also been used effectively to treat infection due to *Pneumocystis carinii*.

Infection with *Toxoplasma gondii*

Toxoplasma gondii is a protozoal parasite, which, like *Pneumocystis carinii*, is found in the environment. This parasite, when inhaled, may initiate a mild asymptomatic pulmonary infection in health (Figure 18.2). It has been demonstrated that a substantial number of healthy people have antibodies against the parasite; this number increases with age, which indicates a subclinical, latent existence of this parasite in the normal healthy population. However, suppression of the immune system can mobilize these dormant parasites to produce an active infection. This has been demonstrated on occasions in patients who have been actively immunosuppressed as a requirement for their treatment for organ transplantation, or who are immunosuppressed as a result of chemotherapy for malignant conditions.

In HIV-infected people and patients with acquired immunodeficiency syndrome (AIDS), progressive immune suppression is associated with gradual reduction in the CD4+ T lymphocyte count, often to about 100 cells/ml. At these levels of CD4+ cells, dormant pathogens such as *Toxoplasma gondii* can then establish an infection involving various parts of the body, predominantly the brain and the eyes. Definitive diagnosis may be provided by brain or needle biopsies in conjunction with a polymerase chain reaction test (see Chapter 7). The presence of antibody may aid in the diagnosis.

Pyrimethamine plus sulfadiazine is an effective treatment regimen. Other drugs such as trimethoprim plus sulphamethoxazole and dapsone plus pyrimethamine have also been useful in the treatment.

Gastrointestinal Infections

Diarrhoea and abdominal pain and other vague abdominal discomforts are frequent signs in many immunocompromised patients. Infections of the upper and lower intestinal tract with a number of bacterial pathogens are common in HIV-infected patients and occur throughout the various stages of the disease. Infections due to *Salmonella* species are the most common form of bacterial gut infections. The diarrhoea can be severe and may lead to fulminant disease; the severity depends on the invasiveness of the *Salmonella* species and the severity of the immune dysfunction. Patients with HIV infection are also at increased risk of infection with other *Shigella* species and *Campylobacter* species. They

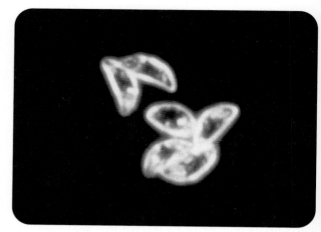

Figure 18.2 The appearance of *Toxoplasma gondii* under dark-ground microscope.

often suffer from protracted diarrhoea, colitis, and abdominal pain and they may develop malnutrition, weakness, and anaemia.

Protozoal parasites, including *Giardia lamblia* (Figure 18.3) and *Entamoeba histolytica*, two common pathogenic gut parasites, have also been involved.

Cryptosporidia species, *Isospora* species, and *Microsporidia* species, which are occasionally implicated in self-limiting gut infestations and diarrhoea in healthy people, have been associated with persistent diarrhoea in patients with HIV. The diarrhoea resembles the acute manifestation of cholera – voluminous stools with or without abdominal pain, often continuing until the death of the patient. The prevalence of these infections varies geographically and involves 3–10 per cent of HIV infected patients. Laboratory diagnosis is dependent on the demonstration of the parasites in the faeces by Ziehl–Neelsen stain, which stains the parasite red, or by staining with fluorochrome dye such as auramine–rhodamine. Treatment of these infections has so far not been very successful.

Candidal Infections

Candida albicans is an opportunistic pathogen that commonly causes infection in immunocompromised patients. Predisposing factors included active immunosuppression, prolonged use of corticosteroids or antibiotics, diabetes mellitus, and other forms of debilitating disease. Candidal infection is considered to be a forerunner of the chain of opportunistic infections in HIV-infected individuals.

One of the earliest manifestations of this infection is significant oral thrush. In more advanced stages, *Candida albicans* causes a severe oesophagitis with ulcerations and diffuse cheesy plaques. Patients

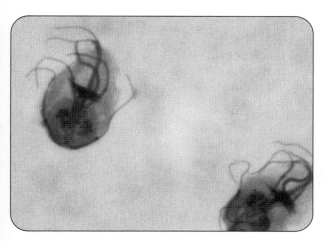

Figure 18.3 Microscopic appearance of a protozoan parasite, *Giardia lamblia*.

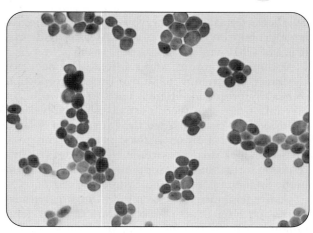

Figure 18.4 Microscopic appearance of the opportunistic fungal infection, *Candida albicans*.

experience retrosternal pain and discomfort, pain on swallowing, anorexia, and loss of weight. Endoscopic examination of the oesophagus shows the extent of the disease. Biopsy taken during endoscopy shows the presence of invasive fungal hyphae, which is a diagnostic feature of the infection. Differential diagnosis from cytomegalovirus can be made from the biopsy picture as well as the clinical appearance of the lesions. *Candida albicans* may cause disease elsewhere, including visceral dissemination, blood-borne infection, and neurological involvement. It grows easily on laboratory culture media and can be identified by simple tests. *Candida* species other that *Candida albicans* have sometimes been found to cause infection in HIV patients (Figure 18.4).

Local infections can be treated with topical application of nystatin. Deeper infections require oral fluconazole or ketoconazole. The length of treatment depends on the extent and severity of infection. On rare occasions, especially when there is a deep seated infection such as candidal septicaemia, systemic treatment with amphotericin B may be required, either alone or in combination with flucytosine.

Infection with *Cryptococcus neoformans*
Central nervous system infection in immunocompromised patients is predominantly due to *Cryptococcus neoformans*. This is a yeast-like organism with a large capsule. It is acquired from the environment, and has been shown that co-infection with HIV enhances the replication of the virus. Indeed, the incidence of infection with *Cryptococcus neoformans* was very low until the onset of HIV disease. A large proportion of HIV-infected patients have been found to develop cryptococcal meningitis. *Cryptococcus neoformans* causes

chronic progressive meningitis and a number of other clinical infections, including pulmonary infection. The presence of capsulated organisms in the CSF confirms the diagnosis. Sometimes the organism cannot be seen in the CSF, but the degraded products from the organism (antigen) may be detected by other methods. Cryptococcal meningitis is treated by intravenous administration of amphotericin B plus flucytosine or fluconazole. Long-term treatment is usually required to prevent recurrence.

Invasive Aspergillosis
Invasive aspergillosis has often been reported in patients with HIV infection, the major sites of involvement being the lung and the central nervous system. The condition is often a terminal event and is usually associated with treatment with other toxic drugs that have aggravated the immunosuppressive effects of HIV infection.

VIRAL INFECTIONS
Cytomegalovirus
Concurrent infections with HIV and other viruses may lead to a molecular interaction between the viruses, amplifying the infecting process of either one or both viruses. As a result of the boost in the activity of the two viruses, there may be considerable multiplication of both viruses within the same cell. This has been shown when a patients is infected with cytomegalovirus (CMV) and HIV. CMV infection is associated with significant morbidity and mortality in HIV infection. Infections of the eye, lungs, gastrointestinal tract, and nervous system are frequently observed and lead to progressive and symptomatic disease. Evidence of co-infection with the two viruses have been found in the

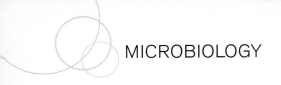
cells of the retina, central nervous system, and lung. A large proportion of patients with AIDS provide evidence of CMV viraemia.

CMV is ubiquitous, and serological evidence of subclinical infection is found in a varying proportion of healthy people in different parts of the world. In HIV-infected people, there is usually a high prevalence of antibody to the virus, and the virus can be isolated from a large proportion of these patients. The presence of a large load of the virus in HIV-infected patients results in further immunosuppression and a reduction in the total numbers of circulating $CD4^+$ cells.

Active immunosuppression following organ transplantation often leads to reactivation of CMV (and probably also to new infection), resulting in clinical manifestation of the disease. It is therefore a common practice to test for the CMV antibody status of the organ recipient and, if possible, the organ donor before transplantation (see Chapter 29).

Epstein–Barr Virus

Epstein–Barr virus (EBV) is ubiquitous with a worldwide distribution. It causes a variety of clinical disease complexes, primarily involving the lymphatic system. The most common clinical manifestation is glandular fever, often seen in young adults, with symptoms of fever, malaise, swelling of the neck lymph nodes, sore throat, and tonsillitis. There is a typical haematological picture consisting of mononuclear leukocytosis with atypical lymphocytes. In immunocompetent patients, the disease is generally of mild-to-moderate severity and self-limiting, lasting 2–3 weeks.

Other forms of EBV infections have been documented in association with Burkitt's lymphoma, other lymphomas, and nasopharyngeal cancer (see Chapter 31). Serological evidence of the association with the EBV virus and the presence of virus genomic material have been regularly found in these conditions. However, the actual role of the virus in the disease process has not yet been clearly established.

In immunocompromised patients, including HIV-infected patients and those with AIDS, the virus has been regularly found in association with lymphoproliferative conditions, including non-Hodgkin's lymphoma. It has been shown that during HIV infection, even in the early stages, there is reactivation of latent EBV.

Herpes Simplex Virus

Herpes simplex virus (HSV) is an extremely common virus found in association with a wide variety of clinical diseases (Figure 18.5). In immunocompetent people, the severity of HSV infection ranges from very mild to moderate. Manifestations in children include oral infections (gingivostomatitis), pharyngeal infections,

and ocular infections (caused by HSV-1); manifestations in adolescents and young adults include genital infections (caused by HSV-2). Recurrent infection is not uncommon and often occurs in the sites where primary infections occurs [e.g. the mouth (herpes labialis), the eyes (keratoconjunctivitis and keratitis), and the genitals].

HSV infection in a compromised host may result in a more severe manifestation, including disseminated disease, and it may present in atypical sites, including the central nervous system. Other herpes viruses, such as human herpes virus 6 (HHV-6) have also been found in association with HIV infection.

ANTIBIOTIC THERAPY IN THE IMMUNOSUPPRESSED HOST

As described above, a variety of conditions may result in immunosuppression. Immunodeficiency may be due to physiological factors (e.g. it is seen in newborn babies and the older adults). It may be due to drug therapy. Some common viral infections, such as influenza, measles, and EBV infection, make patients particularly susceptible to bacterial infections. It is well known that following a major influenza epidemic, staphylococcal infection may take a large toll of lives. Chickenpox and measles in the children are often complicated by septicaemia. Therefore, immunosuppressed people require protection with antibiotics against secondary bacterial infections as well as other appropriate therapy.

Bacterial infections that are often found during investigations of these patients include those due to

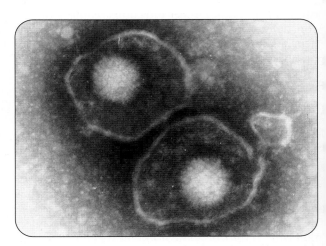

Figure 18.5 Electron micrograph of herpesvirus. Note the typical large envelope around the virus particle.

Staphylococcus species, the pneumococcus, *Streptococcus* species, and the meningococcus. These bacterial infections may rapidly develop into severe invasive disease and lead to septicaemia, meningitis, cellulitis, and pneumonia in immunodeficient patients; hence, prompt and adequate treatment with appropriate antibiotics is required.

Empirical and prophylactic antibiotic treatment is sometimes needed in patients with other forms of immunosuppression, such as post-splenectomy or in lymphoma, leukaemia, and other types of malignancy. Multivalent pneumococcal vaccine and long-term prophylaxis by penicillin is often used to prevent pneumococcal infection in splenectomized patients. Prophylactic co-trimoxazole is now regularly used to prevent *Pneumocystis carinii* pneumonia in HIV-infected people.

KEY POINTS

- The number of patients with compromised immune mechanisms has increased significantly in the recent past.
- Immunosuppression caused by infection such as HIV accounts to a large extent for this increase.
- There has been a large increase in active immunosuppression treatment, in both oncology and transplantation services.
- Many infections in immunocompromised patients are due to agents that are usually less pathogenic in normal health.
- Infections in immunocompromised patients are often due to endogenous microbes (i.e. microbes derived from patients' own flora).
- Antibiotic treatment of these infections is often difficult owing to the absence of help from the host defence system, which normally complements the antibiotic-induced suppression of infection.
- Antibiotic treatment of infection in immunocompromised patients is often required for longer periods than in immunocompetent patients.

FURTHER READING

Bolton CF (1996) Infections. Baillieres Clin Neur 5:599–626.

Bogstedt AK, Nava S, Wadstrom T, Hammarstrom L (1996) *Helicobacter pylori* infections in IgA deficiency: lack of role for the secretory immune system. Clin Exp Immunol 105:202–4.

Chaignaud BE, Vacanti JP (1995) Opportunistic infections in immunocompromised patients. Semin Pediatr Surg 4:245–51.

Corbett EL, De Cock KM (1996) Tuberculosis in the HIV-positive patient. Br J Hosp Med 56:200–4.

Davis CL, Gretch DR, Carithers RL Jr (1995) Hepatitis B and transplantation. Infect Dis Clin North Am 9:925–41.

Fleisher TA (1996) Evaluation of the potentially immunodeficient patient. Adv Intern Med 41:1–30.

Hadley S, Karchmer AW (1995) Fungal infections in solid organ transplant recipients. Infect Dis Clin North Am 9:1045–74.

Horsburgh CR Jr, Schoenfelder JR, Gordin FM, Cohn DL, Sullam PM, Wynne BA (1997) Geographic and seasonal variation in *Mycobacterium avium* bacteremia among North American patients with AIDS. Am J Med Sci 313:341–5.

Hughes I, Jenney ME, Newton RW, Morris DJ, Klapper PE (1993) Measles encephalitis during immunosuppressive treatment for acute lymphoblastic leukaemia. Arch Dis Child 68:775–8.

Jacobson MA (1997) Treatment of cytomegalovirus retinitis in patients with the acquired immunodeficiency syndrome. N Engl J Med 337:105–14.

Kontoyiannis DP, Rubin RH (1995) Infection in the organ transplant recipient. An overview. Infect Dis Clin North Am 9:811–22.

Maes HH, Causse JE, Maes RF (1996) Mycobacterial infections: are the observed enigmas and paradoxes explained by immunosuppression and immunodeficiency? Med Hypotheses 46:163–71.

Manez R, Breinig MC, Linden P, *et al.* (1997) Posttransplant lymphoproliferative disease in primary Epstein–Barr virus infection after liver transplantation: the role of cytomegalovirus disease. J Infect Dis 176:1462–7.

Marshall BG, Shaw RJ (1996) New technology in the diagnosis of tuberculosis. Br J Hosp Med 55:491–534.

Miller ML, Szer I, Yogev R, Bernstein B (1995) Fever of unknown origin. Pediatr Clin North Am 42:999–1015.

Nehring WM, Larson B, Boyer SG (1997) Caring for the child with HIV infection or AIDS. Key points for community care. Adv Nurs Pract 5:37–8.

Ormerod P (1996) Tuberculosis and immigration. Br J Hosp Med 56:209–12.

Patel R, Paya CV (1997) Infections in solid-organ transplant recipients. Clin Microbiol Rev 10:86–124.

Ryan KJ (ed) (1994) Sherris Medical Microbiology. An Introduction to Infectious Diseases. Prentice-Hall International.

Smith S, Sweetser MT, Wilson CB (1996) The immunocompromised host. Pediatr Rev 17:435–40.

Wheeler JG (1996) Evaluating the child with recurrent infections. Am Fam Physician 54:2276–82,2285–6.

Wood CGA, Whittet S, Bradbeer CS (1997) ABC of palliative care: HIV infecton and AIDS. BMJ 315:1433–6.

ANTIMICROBIAL THERAPY

LEARNING OBJECTIVES

After studying this chapter you will have a clearer understanding of:
- the nature and mechanisms by which antimicrobial drugs exert their action on microbes
- the strategies developed by the microbe to bypass the damaging effects of antibiotics
- the mechanisms by which microbes develop resistance to antibiotics
- the possible adverse side-effects of antimicrobial drugs on the patient
- the rationale for using distinct groups of antibiotics on different types of infections

AN HISTORICAL PERSPECTIVE

Since time immemorial infectious diseases have taken their toll both in terms of mortality and morbidity. Major infectious illnesses such as cholera, plague, pneumonia and scarlet fever have been responsible for the death of large numbers of people, and there was virtually no remedy to combat these apocalyptic devastations. This continued for centuries until chemists, microbiologists, and pharmacists came up with a major breakthrough in the fight against infectious diseases in the 1930s – sulphonamide.

Sulphonamide provided the first successes against such contagious diseases as scarlet fever, septicaemia, urinary infections, and dysentery. However, there was a price to pay. Early sulphonamides were too toxic and induced a number of serious side-effects. Other antimicrobial agents (e.g. quinine for malaria; arsenic preparations for syphilis, trypanosomiasis and leishmaniasis) were also introduced but the attempt to develop antimicrobials against common infections were not rewarded with success until the early 1940s.

Although penicillin had been discovered in 1929 by Alexander Fleming at St Mary's Hospital in London, it was not until early 1940s that the exceptional antimicrobial effect of penicillin on *Streptococcus* species, the pneumococcus, and the gonococcus became evident. This revolutionary discovery formed the basis of modern antimicrobial therapy. Today, a large number of antibiotics (both natural and synthetic) have been developed, with significant effect on most major microbial pathogens.

Meanwhile, the sulphonamide molecule was modified and improved to develop less toxic and more effective products. By the mid-1940s a large number of sulphonamide derivatives had been produced. These had remarkable effects on *Streptococcus* and *Pneumococcus*. A number of other chemotherapeutic agents against infectious agents have been developed since then, which are by definition, not antibiotics. These chemotherapeutic agents are chemically well-defined compounds that could be synthesized in the laboratory. Antibiotics, on the other hand, are substances that are synthesized during the process of a biological activity, such as the growth of microbial organisms. (Both chemotherapeutic drugs and antibiotics are collectively antimicrobial drugs.) However, with the progress of technology, it is now possible to synthesize many of these compounds in the laboratory on a large scale – a prerequisite for commercial exploitation.

HOW DO ANTIMICROBIAL DRUGS WORK?

BACTERICIDAL ACTIONS VERSUS BACTERIOSTATIC ACTIONS

Penicillins and other beta-lactam antibiotics damage the cell wall of growing bacteria, leading to weak spots in the wall. Bacterial cells have high internal osmotic pressure owing to the presence of large concentrations of electrolytes and other nutrients. With the weakened wall, this leads to rapid fluid absorption and swelling of the damaged cells until they burst. Other antibiotics act by other modes, such as restriction of vital protein synthesis (e.g. aminoglycosides) and nucleic acid metabolism (e.g. rifampicin) to cause cell death.

Bactericidal antibiotics cause bacterial death; they are more powerful in the containment of infection than bacteriostatic antibiotics, which generally prevent the replication of bacteria by inhibiting the synthesis of non-vital proteins (e.g. tetracyclines) or metabolites (e.g. sulphonamides). This leads to maiming but not killing of the affected bacteria. These disabled bacteria are then normally wiped out by the body's immune mechanisms. However, if the infection is overwhelming and the host's resistance is inadequate, such bacteria may persist for a long time and, when the antibiotic treatment is stopped, they multiply again causing relapse of the infection. It is therefore imperative that severe infections such as meningitis, endocarditis, and septicaemia are treated with bactericidal drugs.

THE SULPHONAMIDES – THE FIRST MODERN ANTIMICROBIAL AGENTS

The sulphonamides are generally easy to manufacture and are available in both oral and parenteral forms. They are well absorbed and uniformly distributed in the body, attaining a useful concentration in most tissue compartments, including the cerebrospinal fluid (CSF). Most drugs fail to achieve a significant concentration in the CSF due the barrier created by a partition between blood and the CSF – the so-called blood–brain barrier. The sulphonamides are able to achieve therapeutic concentration in the brain tissue because their small molecular weight enables them to cross this barrier more readily than other drugs. They were therefore a major antimicrobial treatment for infection of the brain and the meninges before the advent of new antibiotics.

Unfortunately, the sulphonamides suffered from two major disadvantages. These drugs, being bacteriostatic in action (inhibiting but not killing the microbes), were unable to create a major impact in the treatment of major infectious diseases, whereas active bactericidal drugs had more significant effects. Secondly, the sulphonamides were toxic to many tissues, especially the kidneys during their excretion through this organ. Some of the earlier sulphonamides accumulated substantially in the kidneys, leading to crystallization. A major adverse side-effect is hypersensitivity (allergy) to the compound, which may manifest as moderate-

to-severe skin rash (see Chapters 13 and 26). These drugs may also depress bone marrow function (see Chapter 31).

Sulphonamides exert their antimicrobial effect by interfering with folic acid synthesis in the bacterium. This is an essential nutrient for nucleic acid production, and without an adequate supply of deoxyribonucleic acid (DNA) and ribonucleic acid (RNA), bacterial replication is inhibited. However, some bacteria have found a way to subvert this mechanism so that the sulphonamides fail to disrupt the folic acid synthetic pathway.

Synergy

Trimethoprim, like the sulphonamides, interferes with folate synthesis, which is essential to a cell for its nucleic acid and its protein requirement (see Chapter 1). Moreover, when trimethoprim is given in combination with sulphonamide, the two act together on the folic acid synthesis pathway. Accordingly, each drug helps the other to inhibit the nucleic acid synthesis of the bacterium even more effectively. This phenomenon – synergy – is exploited in development of drug combinations.

For instance, sulphamethoxazole (a sulphonamide drug) and trimethoprim are, individually, bacteriostatic agents that inhibit the growth and replication of bacteria but do not completely prevent it. However, sulphamethoxazole and trimethoprim given together in the optimum dose are extremely effective and bactericidal against a number of Gram-positive and Gram-negative bacteria. This combination, co-trimoxazole, has for many years been used as the most effective treatment of urinary tract infections. (Trimethoprim by its own right is also a very effective drug for the treatment of urinary tract infections, especially those caused by common agents like *Escherichia coli*.) Co-trimoxazole has also been very useful in respiratory tract infections, having activity against infection with *Streptococcus* and *Haemophilus* species and the pneumococcus. Likewise, *Neisseria gonorrhoeae* is highly sensitive to co-trimoxazole, which has potential as a major antibacterial drug for penicillin-resistant *Neisseria*. A significant proportion of co-trimoxazole is able to diffuse into the CSF and it is therefore a major candidate for the treatment of infections of the central nervous system.

THE PENICILLINS – A NEW ERA OF ANTIMICROBIAL THERAPY

The pharmaceutical industry has taken great interest in penicillin since its discovery by Alexander Fleming and the demonstration of its antibacterial activity by Florey and Chain. Its enormous potential was evident during the Second World War, when penicillin saved many lives. The first penicillin, penicillin G or benzylpenicillin, was developed as a parenteral antibiotic and was effective against Gram-positive bacteria. This preparation was found to be unsuitable for oral use because of its instability in gastric acid.

The discovery of the chemical nature of the penicillin molecule (it is a beta-lactam molecule) led to the development of newer penicillins. Ampicillin, an aminopenicillin, was one of these; it could be given orally and by parenteral route (Figure 19.1). However, it became apparent that many bacteria produced an enzyme (penicillinase or beta-lactamase) that could metabolize the penicillin molecule and render it ineffective. Therefore, a unique penicillin was developed, the penicillinase-resistant flucloxacillin or oxacillin. It was a significant breakthrough because of the rapid evolution of penicillin-resistance in *Staphylococcus* species, especially in the hospital environment. Subsequently other more complex penicillins have been synthesized that are active against both Gram-positive and Gram-negative bacteria (broader-spectrum penicillins). These penicillins include carbenicillin, piperacillin, and azlocillin, which have remarkable effects against *Pseudomonas* species and a number of other difficult-to-treat Gram-negative bacteria.

The penicillins act by interfering with the formation of the bacterial cell wall. The cell wall is a vital structure for maintaining the structural integrity of the bacterial cell. The cell is therefore protected from adverse interference caused by changes in osmotic pressure. But the cell wall also has an active role, to allow inflow and outflow of electrolytes and other nutrients essential for growth and survival. The bacterial cell wall is composed of layers of complex sugars interlinked by amino-sugars. Some penicillins interfere with the interlinking of these compounds, which results in gaps within the cell wall. The cytoplasmic sap may protrude through these gaps and take in a large amount of water, so the cells may burst by osmotic lysis.

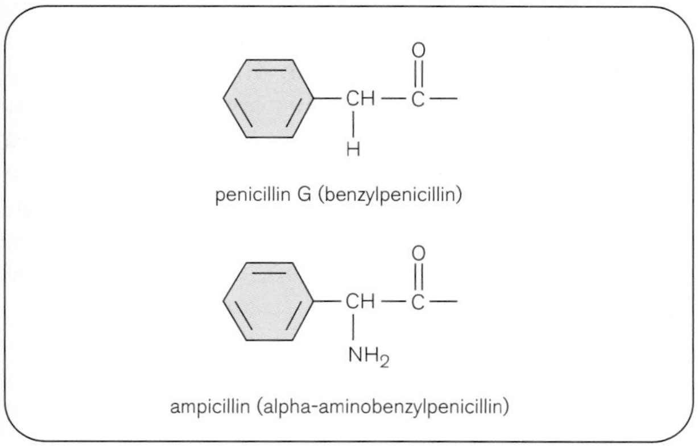

THE CEPHALOSPORINS AND OTHER ANTIBIOTICS THAT ACT AGAINST THE CELL WALL

As the search continued for more effective and wider-spectrum antibiotics, a new group of antibiotics that acted against cell walls was discovered. These were cephalosporins, a biologically active product derived from a fungus. The cephalosporins have similar molecular structures to the penicillins, but have a much broader spectrum of activity and are relatively more resistant to the inhibitory effects of beta-lactamases. Many of the cephalosporins are particularly effective against a wide range of Gram-negative bacteria. Although several of these antibiotics are available for systemic use only, some can be given by the oral route. Other antimicrobial drugs, such as teicoplanin and vancomycin, also exert their effect by inhibiting cell wall synthesis.

Allergies and Adverse Reactions to Penicillins and Cephalosporins

The cell-wall active antibiotics are generally less toxic than others to the patient's tissues. In fact, penicillin is probably the least toxic of any antibacterial drug; however, they may produce allergic manifestations. A small proportion of people are naturally allergic to penicillin, and penicillin administered to such a patient could result in a mild-to-moderate local reaction or even in severe systemic anaphylactic reactions, which are occasionally fatal (see Chapters 13 and 26). It is therefore useful to remember to ask the patient about any past history of penicillin allergy before penicillin is administered. Secondly, as far as possible, a skin test should be performed before the drug is injected. Some cephalosporins can also induce allergic manifestations and are cross-allergic penicillins. These therefore should not be prescribed to a patient with a history of penicillin allergy.

Other toxic effects due to penicillins are rare; they include haemolytic anaemia, thrombocytopenic purpura, and other haemorrhagic disorders (see Chapter 31). However, cephalosporins can give rise to more serious side effects, including renal toxicity and haematological disturbances.

POLYPEPTIDE ANTIBIOTICS

Polypeptide antibiotics exert their antimicrobial influence by interfering with the bacterial cell membrane,

Figure 19.1 Chemical structures of penicillin G and ampicillin. Both drugs are active against Gram-negative bacterial infections, and both are destroyed by the enzyme, beta-lactamase.

which is found beneath the cell wall. They affect many of the biochemical reactions of the cell. Examples of such drugs are colistin and polymyxin B, which are effective against Gram-negative bacteria (e.g. *Pseudomonas* species) and used in topical preparations for ear, eye, and skin infections (Figure 19.2).

THE AMINOGLYCOSIDES

The second important group of antibiotics, apart from the penicillins, that have proved extremely useful for the treatment of serious infections are the aminoglycosides. One of the first aminoglycosides to be introduced was streptomycin, which was discovered by Waksman in 1948. It was the first effective drug for the treatment of tuberculosis.

Subsequently, a number of other similar compounds have been developed that exert a significant effect against a wide range of organisms. Gentamicin is a notable example with strong bactericidal effect against many Gram-negative and some Gram-positive bacteria. Gentamicin is the mainstay of treatment of acute Gram-negative septicaemia and other major infections involving Gram-negative organisms. It is also used in combination with a cell-wall antibiotic such as ampicillin or cephalosporin to maximize the bactericidal effect – in combination, these drugs act synergistically, which results in enhanced killing of the pathogens. A combination of these drugs is probably one of the best antimicrobial strategies and is regularly applied in clinical situations. Gentamicin plus ampicillin or a

cephalosporin is the most frequently used antibiotic combination for the treatment of both major Gram-negative systemic infections and infections such as endocarditis.

The aminoglycosides interfere with protein synthesis at the cellular level. During the process of cell replication, proteins are manufactured in the ribosomes located in the cytoplasm (see Chapter 1). Some of these proteins are essential for the survival and growth of bacteria, and thus inhibition of protein synthesis results in stunted growth and other damage.

In common with other antibacterial drugs, this predominantly affects the bacterial cells, with very little adverse effect on the patient's cells. Nevertheless, the aminoglycosides do have toxic side-effects that need to be taken into consideration during treatment with these agents. The common sites affected include the kidneys and the eighth cranial nerve. The effect is more remarkable in the kidneys, where the drug accumulates in the renal cortex and causes toxic necrosis. Fortunately, the aminoglycoside-induced renal damage is reversible with the cessation of treatment. However, the effect on the eighth cranial nerve is more prolonged, and both the hearing (auditory) and balancing (vestibular) functions are affected, and damage may be permanent. Therefore it is imperative that a safe serum level is maintained by adjusting the dosage of the drug (see Chapters 9 and 12). Monitoring the serum levels throughout the course of treatment with these drugs allows for these adjustments to be made (Box 19.1). A number of other aminoglycosides are available, some of which were claimed to have similar activity but with lesser toxicity. The side-effects of the different aminoglycosides vary; whereas gentamicin is more likely to cause adverse effects, netilmicin is relatively less toxic.

THE TETRACYCLINES

The tetracycline group of antibiotics was developed several decades ago and became popular for treatment of infections in children. The drug was cheap and could be given orally, although systemic preparations were also available. However, several problems were encountered during treatment with these antibiotics, the major one being the effect on teeth and bone in fetuses and children.

Tetracyclines deposit in deciduous teeth and cause yellow discoloration. To prevent discoloration of teeth caused by tetracycline treatment, it is advised that the drug should be avoided:

• during pregnancy, particularly in the last 2 months so as not to affect the fetus; some even suggest that from 14 weeks' gestation the drug should not be prescribed; and

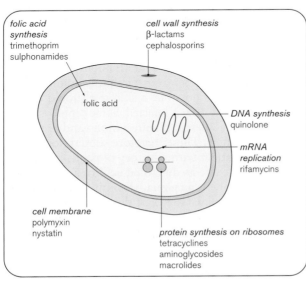

folic acid synthesis
trimethoprim
sulphonamides

cell wall synthesis
β-lactams
cephalosporins

folic acid

DNA synthesis
quinolone

mRNA replication
rifamycins

cell membrane
polymyxin
nystatin

protein synthesis on ribosomes
tetracyclines
aminoglycosides
macrolides

Figure 19.2 Sites where antimicrobial drugs act to destroy bacterial cells. Examples of the drugs that act at these sites are given.

BOX 19.1 ROUTINE MONITORING OF GENTAMICIN

Monitoring of aminoglycoside concentrations is performed by taking blood samples:
- half-an-hour before a parenteral dose is injected (trough level)
- 1 hour after the dose (peak level)

For gentamicin, plasma levels are generally considered to be safe when:
- the trough concentration is below 2 mg/l and peak level is about 10 mg/l.

- If the levels are significantly different from these levels, the dosages are adjusted, taking into account the concentrations measured, the body weight of the patient, and the serum creatinine and urea levels, which are used in assessing renal function (see Chapter 6).
- The microbiology laboratory (where this investigation is performed) needs to be closely involved in monitoring and determining the appropriate dosage of these antibiotics.

- in childhood up to the age of 12 years, so that both deciduous and second teeth are not adversely affected.

The tetracyclines are also deposited in growing bones, leading to calcium depletion in the skeleton. Furthermore, they may induce major gastrointestinal disturbances and skin rash, and resistance can develop rapidly to these drugs. These days the tetracycline group of antibiotics are not generally used except in the treatment of particular infections.

Tetracyclines act by inhibiting protein synthesis in the bacterial ribosomes. They are active against a number of Gram-positive organisms such as *Streptococcus* and *Staphylococcus* species. Although the tetracyclines have some activity against Gram-negative bacteria, they are rarely used for these infections except for the treatment of respiratory infections due to *Haemophilus influenzae*. Tetracyclines are effective against atypical pulmonary infections (e.g. infections with *Mycoplasma pneumoniae* and *Chlamydia trachomatis*, and Q fever, which is due to *Coxiella burnetii*). Tetracyclines such as doxycycline have been valuable for the treatment of sexually transmitted diseases particularly chlamydial infection and pelvic inflammatory disease. Although they are usually active against *Neisseria gonorrhoeae*, tetracyclines are not commonly used for the treatment of this infection, because they are only bacteriostatic and they can cause adverse side-effects.

THE MACROLIDES

The macrolides are another important group of antibiotics. Their primary activity is against Gram-positive bacteria, but they are also extremely effective against organisms such as *Mycoplasma pneumoniae*, *Legionella pneumophila*, *Chlamydia trachomatis*, and

Chlamydia psittaci. The macrolides are also active against Gram-negative bacteria, including *Haemophilus influenzae* and *Campylobacter jejuni*. Erythromycin, an early macrolide, has been very extensively used in Gram-positive infections, especially in patients who are allergic to penicillins. It is available in both oral and systemic forms but it is associated with significant side-effects, predominantly gastrointestinal effects and skin rash.

Newer derivatives of macrolides have recently been introduced (e.g. clarithromycin and azithromycin); these are more active and less toxic and have a wider spectrum of activity. Clarithromycin is active against a number of opportunistic *Mycobacterium* species (e.g. *Mycobacterium avium intracellulare* and *Mycobacterium leprae*); azithromycin has been shown to have significant effects against chlamydial infection.

The mode of action of the macrolides is very similar to other antibiotics that affect bacterial protein synthesis by binding to the ribosomes in the cytoplasm.

FUSIDIC ACID

Fusidic acid is an antibiotic with a very narrow spectrum of activity. It is a fairly non-toxic preparation, and its clinical use is restricted to the treatment of *Staphylococcus aureus* infection. It is highly effective against both penicillin-resistant and penicillin-sensitive strains. Because fusidic acid concentrates in the bony tissues it is particularly useful for staphylococcal bone infections, including osteomyelitis.

Fusidic acid and penicillins act synergistically against staphylococcal infections. The main disadvantage of fusidic acid is that bacteria rapidly develop resistance if treated with it alone. Fusidic acid inhibits protein synthesis leading to cell death.

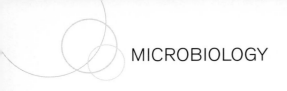

However, it does not penetrate the cell wall of Gram-negative bacteria, so it is not an effective treatment against such organisms.

CHLORAMPHENICOL

Chloramphenicol is another antimicrobial agent that inhibits protein synthesis, and although it is chiefly a bacteriostatic drug, it can have bactericidal activity against *Neisseria meningitidis* and *Haemophilus influenzae*. It is rarely used because it can cause bone marrow suppression, leading to a diminished blood cell production; this effect is dose-dependent, and although it is reversible in most patients, some patients develop aplastic anaemia after prolonged treatment, which may be fatal.

THE RIFAMYCINS AND THE QUINOLONES

This group of antibiotics have their site of action on nucleic acid. Rifampicin, a rifamycin, is an extremely powerful bactericidal drug against a number of *Mycobacterium* species, especially *Mycobacterium tuberculosis* and *Mycobacterium leprae*. Rifampicin is also highly active against *Staphylococcus* species and is often used for the treatment of deep-seated multiple-resistant *Staphylococcus aureus* (MRSA) infections (see Chapter 16), particularly when there is involvement of the central nervous system and lungs. The rifamycins act by inhibiting an enzyme that transcribes RNA from the DNA template (see Chapter 7).

Quinolones are a group of synthetic antibiotics with powerful activity against a wide variety of Gram-negative and some Gram-positive bacteria. They act on DNA gyrase, an enzyme that is responsible for packaging and configuring large amounts of nucleic acid in the cell cytoplasm. Inhibition of this enzyme causes rapid death of the bacterial cell. Ciprofloxacin is a major quinolone antibiotic; it has remarkable effects on most clinically significant Gram-negative infections. It is widely used either alone (as monotherapy) or in combination with other antibiotics such as gentamicin.

METRONIDAZOLE

Metronidazole is another compound with damaging effects on the DNA of bacterial cells, although its nature of action is not clear. Metronidazole acts only in an anaerobic environment and therefore anaerobes are the main target of its action. Most anaerobic bacteria, including *Bacteroides* and *Clostridium* species are susceptible to this antibiotic. Some protozoal parasites are also sensitive to metronidazole (e.g. *Giardia lamblia*, *Entamoeba histolytica*, and *Trichomonas vaginalis*).

MICROBIAL RESISTANCE TO ANTIBIOTICS

Microbes are endowed with rather complex and clever mechanisms by which they can bypass the damaging effects of various antibiotics.

Innate Resistance

A microbe may be innately or naturally resistant to an antibiotic, either because:
- the antibiotic does not penetrate the bacterial cell wall and therefore fails to cause damaging effects; or
- the bacteria releases substances (e.g. enzymes) that destroy the antibiotic.

For instance, tetracyclines do not penetrate the cell wall of many Gram-negative bacteria and are therefore ineffective against these organisms. *Bacteroides fragilis* produce beta-lactamase, an enzyme that destroys penicillins, and hence penicillins have no action against this bacteria.

Primary Resistance

Organisms often become resistant to a drug while a patient is being treated. If a resistant organism subsequently infects another patient, then the original antibiotic will not be able to be used for the treatment of this infection. This phenomenon is known as primary resistance. A large number of *Staphylococcus aureus* in hospitals are resistant to penicillin when first isolated (before treatment is even started). These are therefore primary resistant organisms.

Secondary Resistance

When an organism becomes resistant to a drug while the infected patient is being treated with that drug, the organism is said to have secondary (or acquired) resistance. This is the most frequent form of antibiotic resistance found both in the hospitals and in the community. There are various ways it can be induced, and is more likely to occur if the patient either:
- does not complete the full course of antibiotics; or
- does not take the doses as prescribed.

HOW DO MICROBES BECOME RESISTANT TO ANTIBIOTICS?

There are a number of mechanisms by which microbes may become resistant to antibiotics.

Development of Antibiotic-Destroying Enzymes

A microbe may start to produce antibiotic-destroying enzymes after the patient has commenced treatment with the drug. The mere presence of the antibiotic in the environment of the organism may induce this enzyme production. Alternatively, the organisms may procure tiny amounts of genetic material (plasmids) that are enzyme-inducing genes; these genes may be acquired, for example, from the environment or from other microbes. These plasmids prompt the production of large amounts of enzymes that modify the antibiotics, rendering them ineffective. Beta-lactamase production is often induced during treatment with a beta-lactam or a cephalosporin antibiotic. Gram-negative enteric organisms (e.g. *Pseudomonas* species) often acquire resistance to aminoglycoside antibiotics (e.g. gentamicin) by way of plasmids during treatment with this antibiotic.

Spontaneous Bacterial Mutation

During an infection a large number of organisms are harboured in the patient's body. If the organism is susceptible to the particular antibiotic used in treatment, all the bacterial cells barring a few are likely to be eliminated during treatment. The few unaffected bacteria are called spontaneous mutants. The proportion of spontaneous mutants vary depending on:
• the nature of the organism itself; and
• the type of antibiotic used as therapy.

Normally, the small number of spontaneous mutants that remain are eliminated by the body's immune defence mechanism. However, if there are too many mutants, or if the immune defence mechanism is compromised, these antibiotic-resistant mutant microbes may multiply to significant numbers.

A major manifestation of mutation is the alteration of the target site of the action of antibiotics. To elicit an effect, an antibiotic such as penicillin must bind to a site located on the microbes which possess characteristic penicillin-binding proteins (PBPs). These proteins are situated between the cell wall and the cell membrane, the so-called periplasmic space. A microbial mutation that results in the PBP being modified may lead to the development of a site that the antibiotic cannot readily adhere to. Accordingly, if the drug's active target is a PBP, it will be unable to effect damage on the cell because it is unable to adhere to it. Resistance to various beta-lactams and cephalosporins are caused by this mechanism.

Mutations that lead to alterations in the protein manufacturing sites at the ribosomes are responsible for resistance to macrolides like erythromycin. As a result, the antibiotics fail to bind to the attachment sites on the microbial ribosomes and are therefore ineffective. Rifampicin resistance in *Mycobacterium tuberculosis* and quinolone resistance in *Escherichia coli* may occur because of mutations in the bacterial genes that modify theses target sites of action.

Alteration of Antibiotic Penetration

Penetration into the bacterial cell is essential for many antibiotics to exert their therapeutic effect, particularly those that act intracellularly on nucleic acid and ribosomes. The cell wall of most bacteria possess porin channels, special structures that allow the passage of drugs into the cell. (Although this is not the main function of porin channels, drug companies have exploited this 'design fault' for the delivery of antimicrobial agents.) Antibiotic resistance in many Gram-negative enteric organisms is associated with the interference in transport through these channels owing to a reduction in size or other changes in porins. Some antibiotics are actively pumped out of the cell by an efflux system, which repel the drug from entering into the cell; this occurs in tetracycline resistance.

Development of Bypass Mechanisms

Resistance to sulphonamides and trimethoprim is associated with the development of a bypass mechanism, which allows the microbe to evade the inhibitory mechanism of these drugs. These drugs act by obstructing the bacterial synthesis of folic acid by binding to and inhibiting an essential enzyme in this metabolic pathway. However, some bacteria have evolved a way of resisting these drugs by making a 'bogus enzyme' as a decoy to which the drugs attach. Consequently, folic acid synthesis continues unaffected because the 'true' enzymes are available for action (Figure 19.3).

CHOICE OF ANTIBIOTIC

The list of antimicrobials increases every week. As described before, the nature and the type of microbes against which they are effective is distinct for the various groups of antibiotics. Similarly, their mode of action against the infection and the mechanisms by which the microbes develop a resistance to the drugs differs. Most hospitals develop a local antibiotic policy for general use. These policies are prepared in discussion with microbiologists, pharmacists, and clinicians and are regularly updated to keep pace with new developments and to take account of adverse side-effects and cost. There is also a list of special preparations that are dispensed only at the discretion of microbiologists and special users; this list is likely to include new and expensive antibiotics.

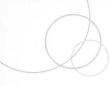

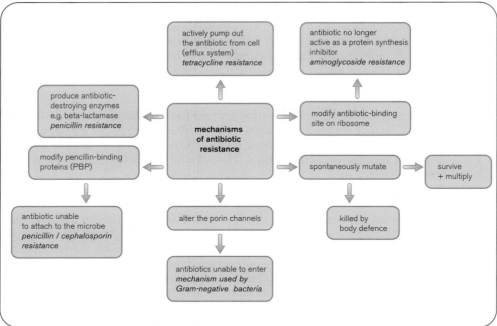

Figure 19.3 Mechanisms of antibiotic resistance used by microbes.

When infection is suspected, a clinical specimen is usually sent to the microbiology laboratory for isolation of the offending pathogen and the determination of the antibiotic sensitivity. A laboratory normally selects a number of antibiotics for sensitivity test based on the nature of the specimen, the clinical information provided with the specimen, and the history of the patient's antibiotic therapy. Once the antimicrobial drugs have been tested against an isolated organism, the microbiologist indicates the choice of appropriate antibiotics to be used for the treatment of the infection. In so doing, the microbiologist takes into account the spectrum of activity of the antibiotic, its relative toxicity, and the patient's ability to deal with excretion products of the drug. For example, rifampicin is a hepatotoxic drug, and therefore its use needs to be carefully assessed in a patient with liver damage. The age of the patient is another important consideration in deciding about the use of an antibiotic. Some antibiotics must be prescribed with care in older adult patients because their hepatic and renal systems are less efficient at dealing with drugs. For example, aminoglycosides are more efficiently cleared from the bloodstream in young adults than in older adults (see Chapters 9 and 12).

Whether an oral or systemic preparation is more appropriate also needs to be evaluated, depending on the urgency of action, the ease of administration, and the cost. In acute life-threatening infections, intravenous administration is preferred to other routes because of the need for rapid delivery of the drug to the site of infection. When the patient's condition has been stabilized, a suitable oral preparation may be used as maintenance therapy (Table 19.1)

CHOOSING THE APPROPRIATE DOSE

Dose is an important factor in treatment with any drug. The adequate dose depends on distribution and metabolism of the drug within the body and its elimination and possible toxic effects (see Chapter 9). If a suboptimal concentration of the drug is obtained, it may fail to achieve its therapeutic activity and result in the emergence of resistance to the antibiotic. Conversely, if the dose is excessive, toxic damage to the tissues (especially in the kidneys and liver) may be precipitated. For instance, aminoglycosides may cause damage to nerves if given in excess.

It is therefore essential that accurate dosage of the drug is determined by taking into consideration the minimal inhibitory concentration of the drug. This is established in the laboratory by testing concentrations of drugs against an organism and determining the minimum level (and therefore the dose) that will inhibit the growth of the organism. It is also necessary to consider whether that concentration (in practice, between four and eight times that concentration) can be achieved without resulting in toxic effect on the patient.

It is essential that the concentration of some drugs (e.g. the aminoglycosides) is monitored regularly in

Summary of Common Infections and Treatment (part I)

Site or type of infection	Causative agent	Treatment
Sore throat and tonsillitis	*Streptococcus pyogenes*	benzyl penicillin/erythromycin
Ear infections	*Streptococcus pyogenes* *Streptococcus pneumoniae* *Haemophilus influenzae*	benzyl penicillin/erythromycin benzyl penicillin/erythromycin, also amoxycillin benzyl penicillin/erythromycin, also augmentin
Eye infections	*Streptococcus pneumoniae* *Haemophilus influenzae* *Moraxella* *Neisseria gonorrhoeae* (neonatal infection)	benzyl penicillin, ampicillin or amoxycillin, erythromycin + topical chloramphenicol benzyl penicillin
Pyogenic infections (superficial or deep)	*Staphylococcus aureus*	flucloxacillin (benzyl penicillin if the isolate is sensitive to it), fusidic acid, erythromycin
Bacterial pneumonia	*Streptococcus pneumoniae* *Haemophilus influenzae* *Staphylococcus aureus*	benzyl penicillin, amoxycillin cephalosporin flucloxacillin
Atypical pneumonia	*Legionella pneumophila* *Mycoplasma pneumoniae* *Chlamydia pneumoniae* *Chlamydia psittaci*	erythromycin, ciprofloxacin erythromycin, tetracycline tetracycline, erythromycin azithromycin, tetracycline
Viral pneumonia	Influenza A Respiratory syncytial virus Parainfluenza viruses Adenovirus Measles virus Varicella	role of antiviral treatment is limited; in severe influenza infection amantadine is given; respiratory syncytial virus may need to be treated with ribavirin derivatives; severe varicella pneumonia may need treatment with acyclovir
Bacterial meningitis	*Neisseria meningitidis* *Streptococcus pneumoniae* *Haemophilus influenzae* Group B *Streptococcus* (in neonates) *Escherichia coli* *Listeria*	benzyl penicillin, cephalosporin benzyl penicillin, chloramphenicol amoxycillin, cephalosporin, chloramphenicol benzyl penicillin cephalosporin + gentamicin ampicillin + gentamicin
Viral meningitis	ECHOvirus Coxsackie virus Poliovirus Mumps virus Herpesvirus	mild and self-limiting; usually no treatment is required; herpesvirus infection is occasionally treated with acyclovir
Cryptococcal meningitis	*Cryptococcus neoformans* (commonly associated with immunocompromised state)	amphotericin B
Brain abscess	polymicrobial cause	metronidazole/chloramphenicol, benzyl penicillin
Anaerobic infections	*Bacteroides fragilis* *Clostridium* spp. anaerobic *Streptococcus*	metronidazole clindamycin benzyl penicillin ± trimethoprim
Septicaemia	Gram-negative organisms	gentamicin/cephalosporin or meropenem/ciprofloxacin

Table 19.1 Summary of common infections and treatments. (continued overleaf)

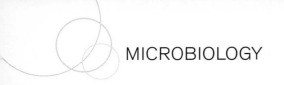

Summary of Common Infections and Treatment (part II)

Site or type of infection	Causative agent	Treatment

Endocarditis	*Streptococcus viridans*
	Enterococcus faecalis
	Coagulase-negative
	  Staphylococcus
	Staphylococcus aureus
	methicillin-resistant
	  Staphylococcus aureus
		benzyl penicillin + gentamicin
		penicillin/ampicillin + gentamicin
		vancomycin + gentamicin
		
		flucloxacillin + gentamicin
		vancomycin or teicoplanin + gentamicin/rifampicin

Gonorrhoea	*Neisseria gonorrhoeae*	benzyl penicillin/ciprofloxacin/septrin/spectinomycin
Non-specific urethritis	*Chlamydia trachomatis*	tetracycline/doxycycline/erythromycin/azithromycin
Pelvic inflammatory disease	*Neisseria gonorrhoeae* *Chlamydia trachomatis* anaerobes	benzyl penicillin doxycycline metronidazole
Vaginal discharge	*Candida albicans* *Trichomonas vaginalis* anaerobic vaginosis (*Gardnerella vaginalis*) *Neisseria gonorrhoeae*	nystatin, co-trimoxazole metronidazole penicillin/metronidazole penicillin (see above)
Gastroenteritis, enterocolitis	*Campylobacter jejuni* *Clostridium difficile* *Giardia lamblia* *Entamoeba histolytica* *Shigella sonnei,* *Salmonella enteritidis*	erythromycin/ciprofloxacin metronidazole/vancomycin metronidazole metronidazole no antibiotic treatment no antibiotic treatment

Table 19.1 Summary of common infections and treatments. (continued)

BOX 19.2 A HOSPITAL IN COURT - THE ADVERSE SIDE-EFFECTS OF ANTIMICROBIAL THERAPY

A patient with endocarditis was prescribed long-term therapy with intravenous penicillin and gentamicin. After 10 days' treatment the patient complained of difficulty in hearing. Blood samples for gentamicin levels were sent to the microbiology laboratory, and the level was found to be extremely high, indeed much above the acceptable level. Gentamicin was discontinued, but the patient's hearing deteriorated further. It was discovered that during the first 10 days of treatment, no blood samples had been sent to the laboratory. A mix-up in the instructions to other medical staff was given as the cause.

The patient was, subsequently, successfully treated for his endocarditis but lost his hearing completely. The hospital was sued for negligence and the case was settled out of court with considerable financial compensation to the patient.

This case highlights the importance of routine monitoring of toxic drugs. Hospitals have written policies regarding monitoring of these drugs. If these are not followed appropriately, a situation such as that described above may develop. The medical and nursing staff should be aware of these hazards and take necessary and timely action to prevent them happening.

the patient's blood during treatment (Box 19.2). On the other hand, some drugs (e.g. benzylpenicillin) are very safe and non-toxic and monitoring the concentration is therefore not required. However, benzylpenicillin may give rise to serious allergic reactions in hypersensitive patients. It is therefore essential that the absence of history of previous allergic reaction is confirmed or a skin test performed before penicillin is prescribed.

CHOOSING THE APPROPRIATE ROUTE OF ADMINISTRATION

Infections acquired in the community are often treated with oral antibiotics prescribed by general practitioners. Severe infections that require hospitalization and infections acquired in hospital often need to be treated with systemic antibiotics. In general, patients with these infections are more seriously ill, are unable to take oral medications, and often require long-term treatment with different combinations of antibiotics and other drugs. Many of these patients may have infusion lines inserted in their circulatory system. Antibiotics may therefore be given by this route for rapid distribution through the body to attain high concentration at the site of infection; in life-threatening infection, this is the preferred route. Furthermore, absorption of drugs from the gut is not always satisfactory, and in unconscious patients the oral route is inappropriate. On very rare occasions an antibiotic may be given by the intrathecal route, in which the drug is injected directly into the CSF; this may be done, for example, in shunt infections. Topical or local application of antibiotics is often required in eye and ear, nose, and throat infections as well as in skin infections (see Chapter 9).

TREATMENT WITH DRUG COMBINATIONS

For severe life-threatening infections, a combination of antibiotics is often used. This is particularly seen in therapy for endocarditis, meningitis, brain abscess, and septicaemia. Similarly, a combination of antibiotics may be used when there is a possibility of polymicrobial infection (more than one type of microbe involved), such as in a brain abscess or an intra-abdominal abscess. In this situation, drug combinations are expected to deal with many different pathogens, as in the case of brain abscess treated with metronidazole for anaerobes and penicillin for *Streptococcus* species. More importantly, combined antibiotics are used to achieve synergy between two antibiotics, in which one antibiotic improves the activity of the other. This is the case when a penicillin and an aminoglycoside are given together to treat endocarditis. Similar effects are obtained by treating Gram-negative septicaemia with a combination of an aminoglycoside and a beta-lactam antibiotic (preferably a cephalosporin).

The use of combination treatment allows the clinician to prescribe a lower, less toxic dose of antibiotics. For example, subtherapeutic doses of amphotericin B in combination with fluconazole are given to treat deep fungal infections. This regimen is as effective as full dosage of amphotericin B plus fluconazole, but it is less toxic. Similarly, the treatment of tuberculosis and leprosy both require prolonged antibiotic therapy in which a number of drugs are prescribed together. The reason for a multiple-drug regimen is to prevent the emergence of drug resistance. Both these infections have a considerable bacterial load and because long-term therapy is needed, spontaneous resistant mutants may be selected out. The second and the third drug used in the therapeutic management are expected to deal with the mutants that might emerge to the first drug.

ANTIMICROBIAL PROPHYLAXIS

Antibiotics are sometimes prescribed to prevent an infection. This is particularly important in the prevention of postoperative infections. Many patients undergoing surgical procedures are vulnerable to infection, either from their own commensal micro-organisms or from the environment. As discussed before, humans carry a very large number of commensal organisms in their internal environment, notably in the gut, the vagina, and the respiratory tract. These microbes are also present on the body surfaces (e.g. on the skin and mucous membranes). An infection may be established if these organisms settle on the operation site during surgery or on the wound postoperatively. Some of these infections may be superficial, but major systemic infections may result which require active medical intervention.

Postoperative infections more frequently occur following abdominal surgery, especially when there is a risk of spillage of bowel contents (e.g. in resection of the gut due to malignancy or operation for the removal of an infected appendix). The gastrointestinal tract (especially the large bowel) harbours a large number of different bacteria which are generally non-pathogenic for the gut. However, if these organisms find their way into the blood stream or operations site, they can establish major systemic or local infections (see also Chapter 23). Bowel organisms that are often involved in these infections include *Bacteroides fragilis* and a number of other Gram-negative organisms; Gram-positive bacteria are sometimes involved.

Because of this potential hazard, it is a common practice to:

- remove as much as possible of the faecal content by mechanical emptying of the gut pre-operatively with an enema (e.g. Fletcher's phosphate enema, which is a commercially prepared solution and delivery system for this purpose); and
- give antibiotic cover during operation (metronidazole is the antibiotic used most frequently as prophylaxis for bowel operation; other antibiotics effective against Gram-negative organisms are sometimes used – e.g. cephalosporins or aminoglycosides).

Patients with congenital heart defects and those with damaged or scarred heart valves or endocardium are vulnerable to infections of the endocardium, which lead to endocarditis (see Chapter 32). They require antibiotic prophylaxis during any surgical procedure including minor procedures such as tooth extraction. Such antibiotic prophylaxis is also necessary for those older patients in the UK who suffered rheumatic fever in the pre-antibiotic era.

People who have been in contact with patients with highly contagious infections are often given prophylactic antibiotics (e.g. a short course of rifampicin given to people who have come into contact with meningococcal meningitis). This includes siblings of infected children occupying the same household as well as classmates. Children in contact with a patient of pulmonary tuberculosis are often given isoniazid as prophylaxis.

ANTIVIRAL DRUGS

So far, progress of antiviral chemotherapy has been rather slow. This is partly because most common viral infections are self-limiting illnesses of short duration and are managed relatively easily. The main disincentive, however, is that the action of the antiviral agents may also have a toxic effect on the patient's own cells. As has been described in Chapter 16, viruses multiply inside the host cells and any attempt to interfere with the viral nucleic acid synthesis is likely to affect the host nucleic acid, resulting in damage to the tissues. However, with the advent of major virus infections such as human immunodeficiency virus (HIV) and the increased exacerbation of many latent virus infections in immunocompromised patients, there has been renewed interest in research and development of antiviral agents. A number of antiviral agents have now been developed; some of these are already in clinical use; others are undergoing clinical trials. Some of these are described briefly below.

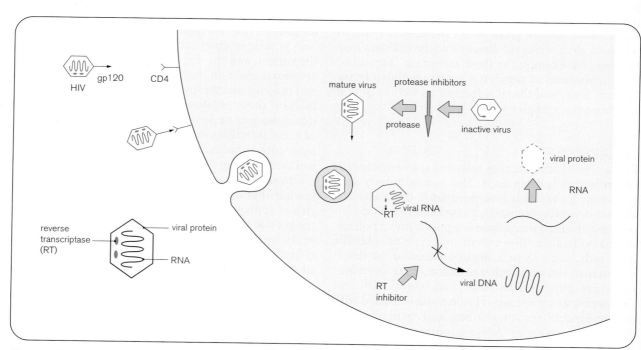

Figure 19.4 Mechanisms by which antiviral drugs inhibit viral infections. The mechanisms shown here are inhibition of reverse transcriptase (RT) (e.g. zidovudine) and inhibition of protease (e.g. saquinavir).

Amantadine and Rimantadine

Amantadine and rimantadine are synthetic primary amines that inhibit replication of influenza A virus but have no effect on influenza B. Rimantadine is as effective as amantadine but less toxic and is often used for prophylaxis in older adults who are unable to tolerate influenza vaccine owing to hypersensitivity to egg protein (influenza vaccine is prepared from egg-grown virus).

Acyclovir, Ganciclovir, and Fanciclovir

Acyclovir and ganciclovir are nucleoside analogues (guanine analogues) and are active against a range of herpes simplex virus (HSV) infections. Acyclovir is relatively non-toxic and is used against HSV infection of both superficial and deep sites. Superficial sites include skin and mucous membrane and corneal infections. Deeper infections usually affect immunocompromised hosts, and include HSV encephalitis and neonatal herpes.

Ganciclovir has been prescribed for cytomegalovirus infection, particularly severe infections associated with immunocompromised states (e.g. in transplant patients).

Fanciclovir is often used for the treatment of herpes zoster and genital herpes. Idoxuridine is another nucleoside analogue with activity against HSV. This preparation is too toxic and has now been superseded by acyclovir.

Ribavirin

Ribavirin is a synthetic nucleoside with activity against a wide range of experimental virus infections. It is a well-recognized treatment for severe respiratory syncytial virus (RSV) infection in children and is given as an inhaled aerosol.

Zidovudine

Zidovudine (AZT) is a synthetic nucleoside analogue that inhibits the replication of HIV in experimental tissue cultures. It is used for the treatment of HIV in both late infections (e.g. advanced acquired immunodeficiency syndrome) and in the early stages of HIV infection. It also reduces the transmission of maternal infection to the fetus. Zidovudine has also been used in HIV-positive asymptomatic children.

It is a toxic drug, especially with its effects on bone marrow; it may lead to an increased risk of anaemia, poor clotting activity, and exacerbation of the immunocompromised state. Therefore, the effect of the drug should be regularly monitored by blood tests (see Chapter 28). Zidovudine has been found to synergize with other agents, and clinical trials are now progressing with various combinations including interferons, acyclovir, and proteinase inhibitors.

Ritonavir and Saquinavir

Ritonavir and saquinavir are two of the more recent antiviral agents used in the treatment of HIV infection. They act as protease inhibitors and affect the assembly of new virus particles inside the host cell, and so retard the progress of the viral infection (Figure 19.4).

KEY POINTS

- Antibiotics have different target sites of action on bacteria, such as the cell wall, cell membrane, ribosomes, and nucleic acids. They cause disruption of function at those sites.
- Bacteria become resistant to antibiotics, often rapidly, unless treatment is appropriately regulated.
- The mechanism of resistance varies from antibiotic to antibiotic and often develops during the course of treatment.
- The therapeutic range of some antibiotics is narrow and regular monitoring is essential to determine if the blood levels are therapeutic and to avert toxicity to the patient.
- Treatment with combinations of drugs may be more effective in serious infections and often has a synergistic effect.
- For treatment of infections, the appropriate antibiotic, correct dose, and proper route of administration are extremely important for optimum effect.
- Antiviral chemotherapy is still in its early stage of development.

FURTHER READING

Anon (1997) Drugs for HIV infection. Med Lett Drugs Ther 39:111–16.

Corey L, Holmes KK (1996) Therapy for human immunodeficiency virus infection – what have we learned? N Engl J Med 335:1142–4.

Crumpacker CS (1996) Ganciclovir. N Engl J Med 335:721–9.

Dawson A, Newell R (1994) The extent of parental compliance with timing of administration of their children's antibiotics. J Adv Nurs 20:483–90.

Del Mar C, Glasziou P, Hayem M (1997) Are antibiotics indicated as initial treatment for children with acute otitis media? A meta-analysis. BMJ 314:1526–9.

Drake-Lee A (1996) Sinusitis. Br J Hosp Med 55:674–8.

Eaglstein WH, Falanga V (1997) Chronic wounds. Surg Clin North Am 77:689–700.

Edwards J Sr, Cook E, Shearer R, Davidhizer R (1997) What the licensed practical/vocational nurse should know about pharmacological therapy for AIDS sufferers. J Pract Nurs 47:48–57.

Foxworth J (1997) Recognizing and preventing antibiotic-associated complications in the critical care setting. Crit Care Nurs Q 20:1–11.

Karlowicz KA (1997) Pharmacologic therapy for acute cystitis in adults: a review of treatment options. Urol Nurs 17:106–14.

Kramer MS, Shapiro ED (1997) Management of the young febrile child: a commentary on recent practice guidelines. Pediatrics 100(1):128–34.

Kroner BA (1995) Rational antibiotic selection. J Am Acad Nurse Pract 7:557–64.

Lipsky JJ (1996) Antiretroviral drugs for AIDS. Lancet 348:800–3.

Little P, Williamson I, Warner G, Gould C, Gantley M, Kinmonth AL (1997) Open randomised trial of prescribing strategies in managing sore throat. BMJ 314:722–7.

Macfarlane J, Prewett J, Rose D, et al. Prospective case-control study of role of infection in patients who reconsult after initial antibiotic treatment for lower respiratory tract infection in primary care. BMJ 315:1206–10.

Misson J, Clark W, Kendall MJ (1997) Therapeutic advances: protease inhibitors for the treatment of HIV-1 infection. J Clin Pharm Ther 22:109–17.

Musch DC, Martin DF, Gordon JF, Davis MD, Kuppermann BD (1997) Treatment of cytomegalovirus retinitis with a sustained-release anciclovir implant. The Ganciclovir Implant Study Group. N Engl J Med 337:83–90.

Nathwani D, Davey P (1996) Intravenous antimicrobial therapy in the community: underused, inadequately resourced, or irrelevant to health care in Britain? BMJ 313:1541–3.

Payne D, McKenzie SA (1996) Oral antibiotics for common infections in children: for and against. Br J Hosp Med 56:481–5.

Quinn JP (1997) Rational antibiotic therapy for intra-abdominal infections. Lancet 349:517–18.

CONTROL OF HOSPITAL INFECTION

20

LEARNING OBJECTIVES

After studying this chapter you will have a clearer understanding of:
- the various ways by which hospital cross-infections occur and the common pathogenic microbes involved
- the role of hospital staff in inadvertently facilitating cross-infection
- the methods of preventing hospital infections, including the isolation of infected patients
- the development of appropriate guidelines and protocols for preventing hospital infection, and monitoring by regular surveillance
- the establishment of a management structure for hospital infection control

INTRODUCTION

The Person-Centred Study (see below) demonstrates the action taken to control the spread of methicillin-resistant *Staphylococcus aureus* (MRSA) within a hospital unit with high-intensity activity. Intensive therapy units (ITUs) receive patients from across the whole hospital as well as patients referred from other hospitals and the community. Patients have often developed infection with MRSA in the referral unit, and this is then transmitted to other patients in ITU, leading both to infection and transient colonization. Hospitalized patients in general, and ITU patients in particular, are more prone to become secondarily infected or colonized, because:
- their body defence against infections is generally reduced; and
- they are in close geographical proximity to other patients.

The effects of these infections, the so-called cross-infections, are often multiple and may result in serious illness with prolonged periods of hospitalization and often death. Extended hospital stay increases the cost of treatment and results in beds being blocked, as well as economic loss and hardship to the family. Cross-infected patients often require expensive antibiotics, with the

attendant risks of toxicity and development of drug resistance. Regrettably, health care professionals, including doctors and nursing staff, are often unaware of the extent of the problem in the early stages and further assist in spread if infection control practices are relaxed.

By definition, the nature of the illness suffered by patients in ITUs is serious. Consequently they often undergo invasive procedures, such as the insertion of intravenous lines, catheters of various descriptions, intubation and ventilation, and nasogastric or total parenteral nutrition. These are all potential sources and sites of colonization by pathogenic organisms and opportunistic commensals. Thus organisms can gain access to deeper tissues and blood, resulting in infection.

COMMON CROSS-INFECTING ORGANISMS AND THEIR MECHANISMS OF SPREAD

Large numbers of pathogenic and opportunistic microbes lurk in the hospital environment and become established on the surface of patients who are vulnerable to infection owing to reduced physiological and immune resistance. Often the microbes survive and multiply as commensal organisms on the body surfaces

265

PERSON-CENTRED STUDY: METHICILLIN-RESISTANT *STAPHYLOCOCCUS AUREUS*

An Intensive Therapy Unit (ITU) recorded eight cases of infection caused by methicillin-resistant *Staphylococcus aureus* (MRSA) within a period of 6 weeks. The Infection Control Team of the hospital initiated a major outbreak investigation in conjunction with the ITU Team. All ITU patients were screened for the presence of MRSA in nasal, axillary, and perineal swabs. Several patients were found to carry the organism. A strict isolation and decontamination procedure was instituted and the medical and nursing staff on the ITU were targeted to follow a rigid protocol. The Infection Control Team met the ITU Team

every day to take stock of the control measures. It took several weeks to clear all patients known to be carrying MRSA, some being transferred back to isolation rooms in the referral wards. The infected patients were treated aggressively with the appropriate antibiotics. Two patients died of septicaemia and five patient gradually gave negative results following microbiological examination over the following few weeks. One patient continued to have positive wound swabs for over 2 months, but this patient was not deemed to be infected and was discharged.

(e.g. the skin) without harming the host, but sometimes they enter deeper tissues and cause infection.

Common sources of these cross-infecting organisms include the skin and nose, superficial wounds and ulcers, and infected hands of the patients. Spread may also occur during coughing, sneezing, and blowing the nose, as well as during bed-making (Figure 20.1).

STAPHYLOCOCCUS AND *STREPTOCOCCUS* SPECIES

Staphylococcus species are skin organisms that are dispersed regularly with desquamated skin flakes. *Staphylococcus aureus* is pathogenic and is frequently found as the responsible cross-infecting organism. Although *Staphylococcus epidermidis* is found more often on the skin surface, it is rarely involved in hospital infection. A large proportion of healthy people carry *Staphylococcus* species in their nose. Many health care workers carry the organisms in their nose, hands, axillae, and perineal region, presumably having acquired them during the course of their work. In the hospital, organisms shed by infected and colonized patients disperse in large numbers. Once these are scattered through the air they settle on other patients. *Streptococci*, which are less robust but more infectious, are transmitted by the same method as *Staphylococci*. *Streptococci* belonging to groups A, C, and G are most often associated with most hospital infections.

Hospital cross-infections due to pneumococci have also been reported in which the infection has been transmitted to patients occupying adjacent beds. These and the other cocci described above can be inhaled by

debilitated patients, precipitating acute respiratory infections such as staphylococcal, streptococcal, or pneumococcal pneumonia.

The *Staphylococcus aureus* that become resistant to many antibiotics, including methicillin (MRSA), are especially important because they are refractory to most common anti-staphylococcal antibiotics; vancomycin remains the mainstay of treatment of these infections. MRSA have been found superficially colonizing wounds and ulcers, but they can also produce more difficult-to-treat infections in deeper sites, such as septicaemia and respiratory infections.

ENTEROCOCCI

Enterococci, particularly the vancomycin-resistant enterococci (VRE), have recently been encountered in many hospital cross-infection outbreaks. These are extremely difficult organisms to eliminate because they are resistant to most common antibiotics (see Chapter 19).

AIR-BORNE INFECTIONS

Respiratory infections caused by air-borne viruses (e.g. influenza) are generally transmitted in hospital as cross-infections in the same way as in the community, though with increased communicability owing to close living conditions.

Meningococcal meningitis infection, which is acquired by inhalation, has the potential to cause cross-infection in hospital. Health care staff who are closely involved in the management of these patients are especially at risk, particularly where mouth-to-mouth

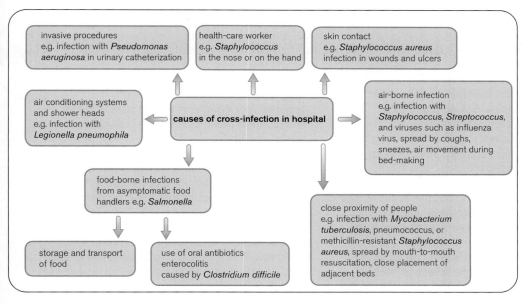

Figure 20.1 Causes of cross-infection in hospital.

invasive procedures e.g. infection with *Pseudomonas aeruginosa* in urinary catheterization

health-care worker e.g. *Staphylococcus* in the nose or on the hand

skin contact e.g. *Staphylococcus aureus* infection in wounds and ulcers

air conditioning systems and shower heads e.g. infection with *Legionella pneumophila*

causes of cross-infection in hospital

air-borne infection e.g. infection with *Staphylococcus*, *Streptococcus*, and viruses such as influenza virus, spread by coughs, sneezes, air movement during bed-making

food-borne infections from asymptomatic food handlers e.g. *Salmonella*

storage and transport of food

use of oral antibiotics enterocolitis caused by *Clostridium difficile*

close proximity of people e.g. infection with *Mycobacterium tuberculosis*, pneumococcus, or methicillin-resistant *Staphylococcus aureus*, spread by mouth-to-mouth resuscitation, close placement of adjacent beds

resuscitation may be required, so prophylactic antibiotics are essential for these staff. Meningitis is commonly associated with community transmission, especially in children and adolescents in institutions such as schools and colleges.

Tuberculosis is transmitted by the air-borne route and is therefore a cross-infection problem. Necessary protective action is therefore needed. In particular, multiple-drug-resistant tuberculosis requires very stringent isolation facilities to prevent dispersion of these organisms in the hospital environment (see Person-Centred Study: Rapid Spread of Multiple-Drug-Resistant Tuberculosis in a Large Hospital).

The hospital environment allows various other infections to be communicated with relative ease. Legionnaires' disease, an acute bronchopneumonia, is caused by environmental bacteria, *Legionella pneumophila*, often found in association with air-cooling systems in hospitals. The organisms are transmitted via air-conditioning ducting and shower heads and may affect patients with relative immunosuppression. Outbreaks of legionnaires' disease have been reported from many hospitals around the world.

THE COLIFORMS

A large number of Gram-negative organisms may be detectable in infected wounds and ulcers. Although they are capable of spreading via the air-borne route, these organisms are more commonly spread by hand, both the hands of patients and the hands of health care workers. *Pseudomonas aeruginosa* is the most common of these Gram-negative organisms; it may

infect patients whose normal defence mechanisms are compromised (e.g. during chemotherapy or tissue injury of the skin and mucous membranes). *Pseudomonas aeruginosa* may be responsible for precipitating septic shock, disseminated intravascular coagulation, and adult respiratory distress syndrome in these patients (see Chapters 25, 31 and 33).

Other bacteria such as resistant coliforms are also sometimes responsible for cross-infection. Coliform infections associated with urinary catheters occur regularly in hospital patients; these often involve multiple-resistant Gram-negative bacteria.

GASTROINTESTINAL INFECTIONS

Gastrointestinal infections leading to symptoms of diarrhoea and vomiting are a frequent complication in hospitalized patients, especially the more vulnerable groups. Many of these are cross-infections caused by rotavirus and other similar viruses, transmitted in these patients owing to poor hygiene.

The hospital environment also permits the spread of enteric infections caused by *Clostridium difficile* in patients with a history of antibiotic use, especially oral antibiotics. Oral antibiotics tend to suppress the commensal gut flora, which allows selective multiplication of *Clostridium difficile*. A toxin released by this organism produces acute enterocolitis – the so called antibiotic-associated colitis.

Hospital catering facilities have often been associated with outbreaks of food-borne infections caused by *Salmonella* and *Shigella* species; these are often due to inadequate storage facility or poor personal hygiene

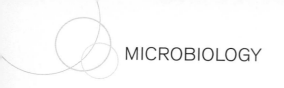
PERSON-CENTRED STUDY: RAPID SPREAD OF MULTIPLE-DRUG-RESISTANT TUBERCULOSIS IN A LARGE HOSPITAL

A female patient with multiple-drug resistant pulmonary tuberculosis was admitted to an isolation unit of a large teaching hospital. She was human immunodeficiency virus (HIV) antibody negative. The isolation unit had several other patients with advanced HIV infection. None of these patients had tuberculosis. However, within a few weeks, three of the HIV-positive patients had developed pulmonary tuberculosis, and one of them soon died. It was then established that the HIV-negative index case was occupying an isolation room that did not have a negative-pressure isolation facility. Her infection had probably spread through the unit and infected the HIV-positive patients. She was therefore transferred to another hospital with facilities for negative-pressure isolation. The HIV-positive patients were also relocated to other hospitals with this facility.

The *Mycobacterium tuberculosis* isolates from each of these four patients were found to be identical by genetic fingerprint studies (see Chapter 7), indicating that the infection had spread from the index case to the other patients. Lack of appropriate negative-pressure isolation facility was the most likely cause of this outbreak. The episode also shows how a slow chronic infection can spread very rapidly in the right environment to immunosuppressed patients.

on the part of staff. An additional factor in these infections is the person who is an asymptomatic carrier (sometimes referred to as a secreter), with detectable levels of the organism in the body fluids (e.g. nasal secretions, saliva, urine, and stools). Such a person as a member of the catering staff would represent a significant reservoir of infection.

HOST FACTORS ASSOCIATED WITH CROSS-INFECTION

Compromised Host Defence Mechanisms and Prolonged Hospitalization

Patients with serious and protracted illness become debilitated, and their non-immune and immune defence mechanisms become weakened. This makes these patients vulnerable to infection with various microbial agents in the environment of the hospital (Figure 20.2).

Patients undergoing prolonged hospitalization are subjected to various minor and major procedures, and consequently they are more exposed to environmental organisms.

Effects of Drugs

The use of antibiotics, immunosuppressive and cytotoxic drugs, and many other medications suppress the host's ability to mount an active reaction to environmental micro-organisms. Some of these actually suppress the functions of immune cells, which are particularly important in providing protection against infections. Cyclosporin A is a very effective immunosuppressive agent used for prevention of rejection of transplants; it suppresses the activity of T lymphocytes, which are the immune cells that protect against many intracellular infections (see Chapter 29).

Extent and Duration of Surgical Procedures

Patients undergoing major surgical procedures and prolonged operative manipulations are more prone to developing hospital infections, both locally, owing to stasis of the blood, as well as generally, owing to devitalization of tissues.

Inadequate Physical Movement

Inadequate physical movement delays wound healing and allows stasis of pulmonary secretions. Secretions in the lung act as a good nidus for bacterial growth. Inadequate physical movement also allows pressure sores to develop, which become a common site for superadded hospital infection. Nursing care and physiotherapy aimed at those deemed to be a high risk are essential in the prevention of pulmonary infection and pressure sores in long-term hospitalized patients (see Chapter 4).

ATTRIBUTES OF INFECTIOUS AGENTS INVOLVED IN HOSPITAL INFECTIONS

The microbial agents that are usually involved in hospital cross-infections are probably no more pathogenic than common microbes. It is merely the increased

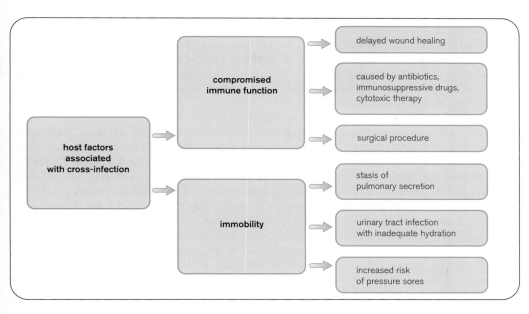

Figure 20.2 Host factors assocated with cross-infection.

opportunity for them to establish a focus of infection that allows disease to occur. Hence the cross-infecting organisms are often called 'opportunistic infections'; these include infections with *Escherichia coli*, *Staphylococcus epidermidis*, and *Klebsiella* species. Many of these microbial agents are now found in increasing numbers in the hospital environments.

The increased use of antibiotics can lead to an alteration of the commensal flora of the host. For instance, the prolonged use of broad-spectrum antibiotics eliminates the protective gut flora, allowing organisms that are more resistant to colonize the gut. An infection established by these resistant organisms may be difficult to treat. In addition, the organisms often create an altered environment which is beneficial for their survival, so they may be found within or on the surface of equipment that is now commonplace in modern medical practice.

One microbial strain may be more communicable than another, for instance, the epidemic strain of MRSA (E-MRSA). E-MRSA has been found to persist in the hospital environment for longer periods than other strains of MRSA. Multiple-resistant strains of some other bacteria, such as *Pseudomonas* and *Klebsiella* species, have sometimes been associated with major hospital cross-infections. It is not clear whether the antibiotic-resistant microbes are more communicable than their more sensitive counterparts but the lack of susceptibility of these strains to commonly available antibiotics make them more difficult to treat.

It is interesting to note that the multiple-resistant organisms generally dilute out or disappear fairly rapidly when a colonized patient returns to the community. Therefore it is advisable that a patient colonized with a multiple-resistant organism without evidence of active infection should be discharged from hospital as soon as practicable and nursed by community nurses. This strategy not only releases hard-pressed hospital beds, but also removes patients from the hospital environment, where they are a potential source of infection to other in-patients. It also relieves pressure on the nursing staff because these patients require special care, such as barrier nursing and strict isolation.

PREVENTION OF HOSPITAL CROSS-INFECTION

As discussed above, the hospital environment and other in-patients are the major sources of hospital cross-infection. It is therefore extremely important to identify the immediate sources of organisms so that all necessary measures can be taken to contain the spread. The preventive methods and their implementation, described below, are developed and based on good practices and are now standard procedures in most hospitals. Each hospital has its own written policies, which are co-ordinated by its Infection Control Committee.

PREVENTION OF CROSS-INFECTION IN THE WARDS
Hand-washing

Good nursing and medical care is one of the most important prerequisites for the prevention of hospital cross-infection. Health care workers should understand and appreciate the general principle regarding the intrinsic and extrinsic factors involved in the causation of infections. They should take extra caution when examining and managing an infected patient. Careful hand-washing is the vital precautionary measure. Nursing and medical staff should understand that infected hands are the most common route of transmission of infection from patient to patient.

Thorough soap and water washing is often adequate for removal of most infectious agents from the hands. Periodically, it may be expedient to use an alcohol-based detergent solution between patients when there are several to be examined in rapid succession. Water-based detergent soaps are now generally available in most hospital wards. These are mild and user-friendly and come in convenient containers for hands-free operation.

Isolation of Infected Patients

One of the main principles for the prevention of hospital infection is to break the chain of transmissibility. Infected patients in a large ward are significant sources of infection to other patients. It is therefore appropriate that they are separated from others by isolating them.

It is advisable that staff entering isolation rooms should wear protective clothing (e.g. disposable aprons and gloves). Visitors should not be allowed to enter the isolation facilities without the permission of the medical and senior nursing staff, and they must also be advised on the appropriate protective clothing. The rooms should have a minimal amount of equipment and furniture. The disposal of body fluids, clinical waste, and bed linen is carried out according to local guidelines. The entrance to the rooms should have appropriate signs and instructions for all staff.

Standard isolation

There are several levels of isolation. The simplest level is standard isolation, in which the patient is moved to a single room equipped with the necessary facilities. This may engender some apprehension and distress, and the patient must be reassured about the need for isolation. The medical and nursing staff should be made aware and the domestic staff should be advised of appropriate precautions. Common infections like staphylococcal (usually MRSA) and streptococcal wound infections, burns, and gastroenteritis are treated in standard isolation.

Respiratory isolation

Infections transmitted by the respiratory route require a slightly more elaborate isolation procedure, in which the isolation room door must be kept closed at all times and the staff attending the patient should wear face masks. Many virus infections (including chickenpox), bacterial infections (such as tuberculosis, staphylococcal and streptococcal respiratory infections), and meningeal infection due to *Meningococcus* are managed by respiratory isolation.

Strict isolation

Infections due to some highly virulent pathogens require strict isolation, which necessitates the establishment of a high-level containment area. The isolation rooms are fitted with their own facilities, including nursing care trolleys. The isolation rooms must have negative-pressure ventilation, and staff should wear special masks, such as high efficiency particulate air filter masks. Infections such as viral haemorrhagic fevers, Lassa fever, plague, and anthrax require this level of isolation. Similar facilities are also appropriate for the management of multiple-drug-resistant tuberculosis. Health care professionals working in these units are specially trained and are aware of the basic disciplines that are required to be followed in these units. These rooms have their own independent ventilation and, when required, they can be decontaminated by formalin gas without affecting other areas.

Protective isolation

This isolation facility is required to protect patients susceptible to common infections. Such patients include immunodeficient patients, those with bone marrow aplasia, and bone marrow transplantation patients, who are susceptible to a large number of opportunistic infections from the environment. Burns patients are isolated because they are particularly vulnerable to airborne infections (owing to the large areas of raw and devitalized skin surface), not because they are possible sources of infection. Hence they are isolated to prevent them becoming infected, not because they are a possible source of infection. The isolation rooms are fitted with a positive pressure filtered air supply.

PREVENTION OF INFECTION IN THE LABORATORIES

Hospital laboratories handle a very large volume of infected material derived from patients. Strict precautions are necessary, both by the requesting medical teams and by the laboratory workers, to prevent transmission of infection from patients to the laboratory workers. Hospitals provide guidance regarding the best practices in the collection and transportation of specimens and the transmission of information regarding infected patients.

Medical and nursing staff are responsible for making sure that clinical specimens being sent to the laboratory are safe to handle. All specimens collected from patients must be tightly stoppered and sent in sealable plastic bags. If leaking, a specimen could pose serious hazard to the laboratory workers. Highly hazardous specimens must be clearly indicated by special tags or warning stickers, and they are often transported wrapped in double bags. Information about possible infection should be provided so that necessary precautions may be taken. This includes specimens from a patient suspected or confirmed to be suffering from infection with human immunodeficiency virus (HIV), multiple-drug-resistant tuberculosis, hepatitis B, and a number of other bacterial and viral infections.

Laboratory staff should consider all clinical specimens as hazardous and deal with them accordingly. Good laboratory technique is essential for safe handling of the specimens. The specimen bottles should be taken out of the bags by trained staff after ensuring that the specimen has not leaked. If there is any doubt, the laboratory staff should take advice from senior staff. Specimen containers from some infections may need to be handled with gloves. Thorough washing of hands after handling clinical specimens must be rigorously followed.

Portering staff should be adequately advised and trained about handling clinical specimens. Some hospitals have dedicated laboratory portering staff and provide written guidance for portering of clinical specimens. These should be strictly observed. The staff should seek advice from the Occupational Health Department or senior laboratory staff if they have any cause for concern about any specimen (e.g. contamination with blood known to be infected with hepatitis B) (see Chapter 23).

Ancillary and domestic staff should be given adequate advice and training regarding infection control measures for the prevention of infection. If in doubt they should contact the senior laboratory and ward administrative staff.

SAFE DISPOSAL OF CLINICAL WASTE

Disposal of clinical and domestic waste presents important health and environmental risks. Hospital management and health care workers should be aware of their statutory obligations with regard to safe disposal of hospital waste and the protection of the environment. Safe and effective storage and disposal of waste is the responsibility of the hospital, whether carried out by hospital staff or by contractors. Hospitals are legally required to have local guidelines and policies based on good practice and national guidelines.

Disposable materials are discarded in strong plastic that are colour-coded to denote the type of waste (e.g. paper waste, clinical waste). These are collected by hospital porters and incinerated locally or transported to commercial incinerator facilities.

No sharp items must be included in these bags. Sharp items and glass are disposed of in special impenetrable leak-proof containers, usually made of plastic. These boxes should never be filled to the limit. Once the box is ready to be disposed of, the lid should be secured with tape. It is also advisable to write the name of the ward or department that has used the box. These boxes are transported in the same way as other disposables for incineration. Sharp and needle-stick injuries can occur before, during, and after use of these items. It is therefore essential that staff are trained in the disposal of sharps. Users of hypodermic needles should be strongly advised against re-sheathing the needles after use.

Contaminated bed linen and patient clothing are put in water-soluble bags with dissolvable stitches for laundering in a washing machine with a hot wash cycle (90°C).

Excreta and body fluids can be disposed of directly into a bedpan washer or macerator. Spillage of blood and body fluid or other infected material can be dealt with by covering the spillage with chlorine granules or hypochlorite, removing them with disposable paper towels, and then cleaning the area with detergent and water. Laboratory waste should, where appropriate, be autoclaved to be made safe before disposal.

DECONTAMINATION, STERILIZATION AND DISINFECTION

Hospitals generate a large volume of contaminated materials, some of which are disposed of as clinical waste. However, a considerable amount of material is re-used after cleansing or sterilization. Such re-used material includes surgical instruments, delicate and electronic equipment, patient clothing, bed linen, and a variety of other items of daily use.

Sturdy surgical equipment is decontaminated by autoclaving. This involves the application of steam under pressure, which is the most effective sterilising procedure, and destroys most pathogenic microbes, including spores. The surgical instruments are decontaminated by thorough cleansing with a detergent and water to remove blood and tissue contamination, then they are repackaged for sterilization by autoclaving. This process is usually carried out in a central sterile supply department (CSSD) under strict guidelines. A number of other items are also sterilized by autoclaving, such as wound dressing material. Heat is also used for disinfecting patient clothing and bed linen, using a conventional household washing machine with a hot wash cycle.

Delicate equipment, like endoscopes and other electronic equipment, are disinfected by immersing in glutaraldehyde solution. They are then cleansed by washing with water and sterilized again by immersing in glutaraldehyde. Before re-use, they are washed in sterile water to remove the glutaraldehyde.

Sterile disposable ventilator and intubation equipment is now available, as are a number of other disposable items which are available ready sterilized (e.g. a variety of intravascular catheters). A large number of sterile disposable items are also available for routine health care use (e.g. disposable syringes and needles). These items are generally sterilized with ionizing (gamma) radiation by commercial suppliers.

CONTINUOUS SURVEILLANCE

The hospital Infection Control Team maintain regular surveillance mechanisms in close collaboration with the microbiology laboratory. In particular, surveillance of infection by drug-resistant organisms such as MRSA and vancomycin-resistant enterococcus (VRE) can serve as a marker for efficient functioning of the infection control programme of a hospital.

MRSA has, in recent years, attracted a considerable interest, both within the medical establishment and from the public. The purchasers of health care have been particularly concerned about the cost involved in the treatment and surveillance of MRSA. The Infection Control Team has a major role in the prevention of hospital infection by these and other organisms, which puts cost pressures on hospital treatment. National and local MRSA policies have been established relating to:

- the admission and discharge of patients who are infected or colonized with MRSA; and
- the isolation and treatment of these patients.

Adherence to these policies by the medical establishment and the hospital managers is absolutely essential for the prevention of the spread of these infections within the hospital.

Policies and guidelines relating to the prevention of other infections have also been produced, at both the national and the local level. These include policy and guidelines for the prevention of:

- hepatitis B infection, including the management of needle-stick injuries to health care workers;
- infections caused by pyogenic *Streptococcus* species, VRE, and *Clostridium difficile*; and
- other hospital-associated intestinal infections, tuberculosis, and *Legionella* infection.

Hospitals are also expected, through their Infection Control Team, to monitor the provision of clean air supply, especially in the operation theatres and ITU, safe water supply, and hygienic and safe food distribution to patients. In addition, they maintain strict surveillance and implement policies for the prevention of infection from blood and blood products. The Infection Control Team also maintain a close surveillance to ensure that their policies on procedures in the hospital are adhered to (e.g. policies to prevent infection from arterial and venous lines, including those used for total parenteral nutrition).

DEALING WITH NEEDLE-STICK AND SHARP INSTRUMENTS

Despite training, education and protective measures, cases of needle-stick and sharps injuries often occur in health care workers. Hospitals usually have a policy to deal with these accidents. After a sharps injury, the victim should:

- try to squeeze out as much blood as possible from the injury site;
- wash the site thoroughly in tap water;
- seek help from the occupational health department, or out of hours from the microbiologist on call or the infectious diseases unit;
- try to identify the sharp, if this is possible and safe;
- try to identify the previous user of a hypodermic needle (Figure 20.3).

The major concern about needle stick is the risk of acquiring hepatitis B from a carrier or an infected person and, to a lesser extent, HIV (HIV is less infectious than the hepatitis B virus – less than 0.3 per cent of people who suffer needle-stick injuries with HIV-infected blood become HIV positive).

If a risk is identified and the injured worker has not been immunized against hepatitis B, hepatitis B immunoglobulin and hepatitis B vaccine are given, if possible within 24 hours. Blood samples are also collected from the patient who was the potential source of the infection to test for the presence of hepatitis B markers. In addition, blood is taken from the member of staff who suffered the injury, and the serum is stored for future reference.

If there is suspicion that the patient may have been HIV positive, the occupational health department should arrange testing, prophylaxis, and counselling according to the guidelines provided by the Department of Health, General Medical Council, and the Hospital Infection Control Committee.

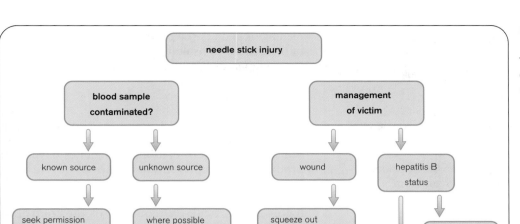

ANTIBIOTIC POLICIES

The use of antibiotics for the treatment of infections is a major factor in the development of hospital cross-infection. Prolonged use of antibiotics often leads to the selection of drug-resistant organisms. Appropriate and prudent use of antibiotics is therefore an important requirement in the prevention of the development and spread of resistant organisms, such as multiple-resistant enteric organisms. Many hospitals have developed their own antibiotic policies for both prophylaxis and treatment. Microbiologists and the pharmacy department co-ordinate these policies and monitor their strict observance. The infection control doctor has often been involved in the development of antibiotic policies in the hospital through the Drugs and Therapeutics Committee. This has enabled them to contain major infection problems with resistant organisms and has also allowed a considerable saving in antibiotic costs to these hospitals.

ORGANIZATION OF HOSPITAL INFECTION CONTROL

Hospital infection control is best managed by an infection control committee that includes specialists from different medical areas of the hospital with a consultant microbiologist heading the group (Box 20.1). The head of the Infection Control Committee also performs the function of the infection control doctor. The infection control doctor would normally be supported by a team of infection control nurses, who are responsible for day-to-day surveillance of infection control in the hospital. The infection control budget should ideally be separate from the microbiology budget and managed directly by the hospital. It is therefore expedient for the Infection Control Committee to have representation from the hospital management as well as the nursing establishment. The Consultant for Communicable Disease Control (or the proper officer) of the district and the Director of Public Health are also generally involved with the Infection Control Committee because of their role in the containment of infectious diseases in the community.

The Infection Control Committee:
- considers all aspects of infection control and advises the hospital management with regard to the development of policies and guidelines for the hospital;
- offers advice regarding new building development, operation theatre structure, hospital catering, and maintenance of safe hospital environment, including disposal of clinical waste; and
- meets at regular intervals to review the effectiveness

BOX 20.1 MEMBERSHIP OF AN INFECTION CONTROL COMMITTEE

- the infection control doctor (consultant medical microbiologist), who acts as chairman
- a consultant infectious diseases physician or general physician
- two or three consultant members (including perhaps a paediatrician and a general surgeon)
- a senior infection control nurse
- a consultant microbiologist
- a pharmacist
- a senior nursing manager (chief nurse's representative)
- a management representative (chief executive's representative)
- the District Consultant for Communicable Disease Control
- the Director of Public Health
- a consultant in occupational health
- other invited members, such as site services manager and the catering manager, for discussion of specific issues involving their areas

of the infection control programme and to bring new issues for discussion.

The chairman of the committee is responsible for presenting the infection control issues to the medical advisory mechanism of the hospital (e.g. the Medical Advisory Committee). In effect, the chairman is authorized by, and administratively responsible to, the chief executive of the hospital for the implementation of the infection control policies. In the event of an outbreak of infection, the infection control doctor in consultation with the medical director and the chief executive take management responsibility for dealing with any major hospital infection.

Hospital cross-infection problems do sometimes spill over to the community such as issues relating to meningitis and gastrointestinal infections. Involvement of the District Consultant for Communicable Diseases Control and the Director of Public Health is therefore essential.

Guidelines and Protocols

The Infection Control Committee should develop local guidelines and protocols for the control of infection in the hospital. National guidelines have been produced for the prevention of various infections in hospitals. These often serve as the basis on which local guidelines are developed. Infection control protocols are particularly required for the control of MRSA infection, infections caused by blood-borne virus diseases such as hepatitis B and HIV, and general infectious outbreaks such as gastroenteritis and respiratory infections especially tuberculosis. The Infection Control Committee also provides guidelines for the prevention of urinary tract infections in patients with long-term urinary catheters. Besides the guidelines for the prevention of specific infections, the Infection Control Committee should provide advice on cleaning, disinfection, and terminal disinfection of the hospital wards. Written guidelines should also be provided for catering, domestic, portering and mortuary staff. The Infection Control Committee should also be responsible for providing guidance to all staff regarding maintenance of a safe hospital environment.

Training and Education

An understanding of the mechanisms of hospital cross-infections and the principles and practice of preventing these infections are major contributing factors in their control. The infection control nurses should conduct a continuous updating programme for the nursing staff, who are the cornerstone of the infection control programme of a hospital. A continuous training and education programme also needs to be provided by the Infection Control Team for all staff in a hospital. The hospital management should make available necessary resources for such programmes.

KEY POINTS

- Hospital cross-infection is a major contributory factor to longer hospital stays and increased cost of treatment.
- Some of the major causes of hospital cross-infection are the MRSA, VRE, and a number of difficult-to-treat Gram-negative organisms. Infected patients are the main source of these hospital infections.
- Spread of hospital infections occurs primarily through air-borne transmission and by hand.
- Transmission can occur due to incomplete and unsatisfactory cleaning and sterilization of medical and surgical equipment, bed linen, and other inanimate objects.
- Transmission can occur because of careless disposal of clinical waste.
- Health care workers, especially nurses and doctors, are mainly responsible for transmission of hospital infections.
- Thorough hand washing with water-based or alcohol-based anti-infective detergent solutions by medical and nursing staff considerably reduces the incidence of hospital cross-infection.
- Isolation of an infected patient into a separate self-contained room reduces the risk of environmental spread of the infection.
- Good infection control guidelines and protocols, developed under the guidance of a hospital Infection Control Committee, are essential for the control of hospital infections.
- The infection control and surveillance service should be adequately resourced.

FURTHER READING

Association of Medical Microbiologists, Hospital Infection Society, Infection Control Nurses Association and Public Health Laboratory Service (1993) Standards in Infection Control in Hospitals.

Casewell M, Philpot-Howard J (1994) Hospital Infection Control – Policies and Practical Procedures. WB Saunders, London.

Finn L (1997) Nurses' documentation of infection control precautions: 1 [Review]. Br J Nurs 6:607–11.

Finn L (1997) Nurses' documentation of infection control precautions: 2. Br J Nurs 6:678–84.

Gould D, Chamberlain A (1997) The use of a ward-based educational teaching package to enhance nurses' compliance with infection control procedures. J Clin Nurs 6:55–67.

Guidelines on post-exposure prophylaxis for health-care workers exposed to HIV (1997) UK Health Department, June.

Kinoshita M, Sawabe E, Okamura N (1997) Concept of segmentation in nosocomial epidemiology:epidemiological relation among antimicrobial-resistant isolates of *Pseudomonas aeruginosa*. J Infect 35:269–76.

Marshall BG, Shaw RJ (1996) New technology in the diagnosis of tuberculosis. Br J Hosp Med 55:491–*534.

Mayall B, Martin R, Keenan AM, Irving L, Leeson P, Lamb K (1996) Blanket use of intranasal mupirocin for outbreak control and long-term prophylaxis of endemic methicillin-resistant *Staphylococcus aureus* in an open ward. J Hosp Infect 32:257–66.

Meredith S, Watson JM, Citron KM, Cockcroft A, Darbyshire JH (1996) Are healthcare workers in England and Wales at increased risk of tuberculosis? BMJ 313:522–5.

Wilson J (1995) Infection Control in Clinical Practice. Baillière Tindall, London.

VACCINES: ONE OF MEDICINE'S SUCCESS STORIES

LEARNING OBJECTIVES

After studying this chapter you will have a clearer understanding of:
- historical perspectives to the development of current vaccines for the prevention of infectious diseases
- the background to the mechanisms of natural immune protection against infectious diseases
- the methods used in the development of different vaccines – bacterial, viral, subunit, live, and dead vaccines
- the mechanisms of action of different vaccines by the involvement of antibody and cellular immune responses
- the routes of administration and complications associated with vaccinations
- the current guidelines for childhood vaccination in the UK
- the recommended immunization protocols for overseas travellers

INTRODUCTION – AN HISTORICAL PERSPECTIVE

With the discovery of the causes of various infectious diseases, it became necessary to find ways to control and eradicate those infections that used to take large tolls on human lives. Historically, major epidemics of communicable diseases such as smallpox, plague, tuberculosis, cholera, and diphtheria affected large areas of the world and devastated the economic and social life of the people living in those areas. Vaccination and immunization against some of these infections became established, and this was followed by the discovery of effective antimicrobial agents (see Chapter 19).

Smallpox vaccine is one of the success stories and it gave a major boost in the development of other more recent vaccines. By 1980, the World Health Organization (WHO) had officially declared that smallpox had finally been eradicated from the world. This was an outstanding achievement and demonstrated that infectious diseases could be conquered. Smallpox used to cause devastating epidemics affecting very large numbers of people. In the late 18th century, smallpox was rampant in England, and it was Edward Jenner who found that milkmaids who were regularly in contact with cowpox-infected cattle were resistant to infection by smallpox. This led Jenner, in 1796, to the development of a vaccine taken from infected cattle, which proved to be effective in protecting against smallpox infection. The vaccine against smallpox was one of the early discoveries in the fight against infectious diseases. With the improvement of the socioeconomic condition of the developed world and the implementation of large-scale vaccination programmes, the disease virtually disappeared from the Western world, but it remained a dreaded scourge for the developing and underdeveloped world. Concerted and multidisciplinary action taken jointly by the WHO and national Governments of the affected countries finally resulted in this great achievement.

Later, with the discovery of various viruses that caused major epidemics (e.g. measles, rubella and polio), meant that methods were devised for their cultivation, and vaccines against these agents became available (Figure 21.1).

Today, a large number of vaccines are used in immunization programmes for the prevention of infectious diseases. The national immunization programmes are generally very effective in most developed countries.

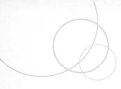

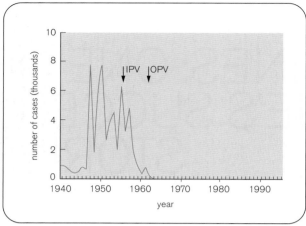

Figure 21.1 Notified cases of paralytic poliomyelitis, England and Wales (1940–1995). Note the dramatic decline in the incidence of poliomyelitis following the introduction of mass immunizations. [Data from Department of Health, Welsh Office, Scottish Office Department of Health and DHSS (Northern Ireland). *Immunisation against infection* 1996; by permission of Her Majesty's Stationery Office.] (IPV, injectable polio (Salk) vaccine; OPV, oral polio (Sabin) vaccine.)

However, the major economic and logistic problems in many developing countries have resulted in uneven and inadequate protection against these infectious agents.

The social and economic achievements of the developed world have also helped in the control and eradication of many infectious diseases. Thus, major infectious diseases such as measles, rubella and diphtheria have been virtually eradicated from these countries. Moreover, a sustained surveillance programme, as is practised in countries like the UK, is another major factor that has helped to keep these infections at bay.

WHAT IS A VACCINE?

The word 'vaccine' is derived from 'vaccinia', the name of a virus that causes cowpox and was used by Edward Jenner to immunize humans against smallpox. Today, the word 'vaccination' is used to mean immunization against infectious diseases. The term 'vaccine' is also used synonymously with 'antigen' or 'immunogen' to mean a substance or agent that, when given to a person, can evoke specific response by the body's immune system. The activation of the immune system may result in enhanced resistance to an infecting agent containing that antigen (see Chapter 23).

An antigen may be a component of an infectious agent – a protein, an amino-sugar, or a lipoprotein actively secreted during growth, or a substance released as a breakdown product. An antigen may also be a whole organism. Most bacterial, fungal, and parasitic antigens used as vaccines are non-living, whereas viral antigens are generally live but altered in virulence (attenuated).

An example of a viral vaccine is the polio vaccine. Between 6000 and 8000 cases of paralytic poliomyelitis were notified in England and Wales each year in the period 1945–1955. The killed polio vaccine (Salk vaccine) was introduced in 1956; this was replaced by the inactivated oral polio vaccine (Sabin vaccine) in 1962. This has reduced the notification rate to 28 during the period 1985–1995, of which 19 cases were associated with vaccination. This exemplifies the tremendous impact of vaccination against infectious diseases (see Figure 21.1).

HOW DO VACCINES WORK?

A vaccine (often known as an antigen) is given as a synthetic mimic of an infectious agent. On introduction into the host, whether it is given by injection or by mouth, the vaccine is perceived as foreign or dangerous by the immune cells, and so it should elicit a reaction. A number of different cell types are involved in this reaction, including the lymphocytes and the phagocytic cells (e.g. macrophages). The phagocytic cells engulf and process the vaccine, which may be the whole micro-organism or a broken down and altered product of a microbe such as a toxoid (e.g. tetanus toxoid). Subsequently, the host cells are able to display fragments of the vaccine antigen on their outer surface to signal the presence of danger to other immune cells – the T and B lymphocytes. Once the lymphocytes have recognized that the phagocytes have engulfed and processed a 'foreigner', they become activated and respond. The B lymphocytes, which are responsible for antibody production, release antibodies into the circulation.

The immune response to the first exposure of an antigen is called the primary immune response. This is generally short and does not result in much protection to the host. However, the immune system has its own strategy for remembering the first encounter with the vaccine. Therefore, if either the vaccine is encountered again, or the disease it has mimicked is encountered, then an enhanced response is raised – the secondary immune response. This is much faster and greater than the primary immune response. These activities are generally responsible for the immune status of the host (see Chapter 23).

Multiple doses of vaccine are frequently required for an adequate immune response. Immunity to many bacterial, viral, and other infections is dependent on B-lymphocyte-derived immunity – the humoral immune response. Several different types of antibody [e.g. immunoglobulin G (IgG)] are produced in varying amounts in response to immunization to different antigens (see Chapter 24).

The immune status of a vaccinated person can often be ascertained by examining his or her serum antibody levels against a particular infective agent or a fraction of the agent. This is exemplified by the presence of adequate levels of the rubella antibody, which is obligatory for all nursing and medical staff employed to work in a hospital. Similarly, all health-care workers involved in invasive surgical procedures must be immunized against hepatitis B, and their antibody level tested to confirm a satisfactory immune response before they are involved in those procedures. Some antibodies may not persist in the blood stream indefinitely because the immunological memory does not last for ever, so it may need an occasional boost.

Immunity in the form of the long-persisting IgG antibodies, that are small enough to pass across the placental barrier to reach the fetus, forms the basis of immunity in the newborn, often known as maternal immunity. This lasts for about 12–18 months after birth. During this period, the baby is considered to be immune to a number of infectious diseases (see Chapter 23).

Some infections that persist inside cells may not be as readily detected by the antibody arm of the immune system. Hence, the T lymphocytes are designed to recognize and respond to intracellular organisms (e.g. viruses) by a mechanism called the cell mediated immune response. This is essential for the elimination of pathogenic organisms such as *Mycobacterium tuberculosis*. Bacillus Calmette–Guérin (BCG) vaccination, given to protect against tuberculosis, activates the T lymphocytes, which then circulate in the bloodstream as memory cells. If these memory cells come into contact with the tubercle bacilli (e.g. as may happen when a health-care worker is caring for a patient with active tuberculosis), the cells will actively proliferate and implement cytotoxic mechanisms to kill the infected cell as well as the microbe. In the UK, the BCG vaccination is offered to school children; likewise many health authorities in the UK expect their staff to be protected against tuberculosis. It is routine practice for health-care workers directly involved in patient care to have the Mantoux test (see Chapter 26) to ascertain their immune status against tuberculosis, and for the BCG vaccination to be offered if the skin test is negative (see Figure 21.2).

BCG vaccination is not available in the USA as part of a national programme. As a result, health care workers there are vulnerable to infection by tuberculosis if they are exposed to the disease while caring for a patient. This was demonstrated during the outbreak of acquired immunodeficiency syndrome (AIDS) in the late 1980s and early 1990s. There were several reports of the spread of both drug-sensitive and multiple-drug-resistant tuberculosis amongst health care workers looking after AIDS patients, and several died of tuberculosis. Since then all health-care workers in the USA who will be working with immunocompromised patients are offered vaccination with BCG and their skin test reaction tested before they are allowed to work with these patients.

Many virus infections render the patient immune to that virus for a very long time. This is because a persistent minimal infection state is established, which means the level of immunity against the infection is maintained. On re-exposure to the same virus, an enhanced immune response occurs, which prevents further infection. Active immunization against virus infection with a live vaccine follows the same pattern, and the immunity conferred persists for a very long time, like the natural infection. Killed viral vaccines, such as the influenza vaccine, provide only short-lived immunity, however, and revaccination at intervals is required. The cellular immune response is involved in protection against virus infection and is generally associated with live vaccines. Vaccination against viruses also activates cytotoxic T lymphocytes and natural killer cells, which kill virus-infected cells (see Chapter 24).

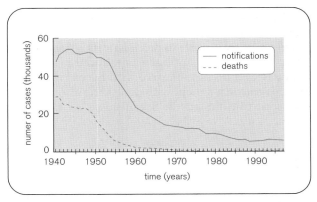

Figure 21.2 Notified cases of tuberculosis and deaths from tuberculosis, England (1940–1995). Note the impact of BCG vaccination on the notification rate of tuberculosis to the Office of National Statistics following the introduction of a mass vaccination programme after 1950. [Data from Department of Health, Welsh Office, Scottish Office Department of Health and DHSS (Northern Ireland). *Immunisation against infection* 1996; by permission of Her Majesty's Stationery Office.]

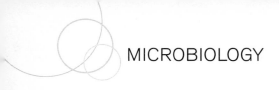

MICROBIOLOGY

TYPES OF VACCINES

WHOLE ORGANISM

Many bacterial vaccines contain whole killed organisms (e.g. whooping cough, cholera, and typhoid vaccines). The bacterial cultures are grown in liquid or solid media, washed thoroughly with saline. The microbes are then killed either by moderate heat or by the application of alcohol, acetone, or other similar substances. The killed organisms retain their ability to activate the immune system. The whole organism suspensions are standardized against known standards before being used as immunogens. On injection, these vaccines evoke antibody (humoral) responses to the bacteria and afford protection to the vaccinated person.

TOXOIDS

Some pathogenic bacteria actively produce very powerful exotoxins, which are proteinaceous in nature and can be isolated in purified form (e.g. tetanus and diphtheria toxins). They are highly toxic in this form but are made harmless, or detoxified, when combined with formalin solution (formolization). Their immunogenicity is, however, retained when formolized. These formolized toxins are called toxoids, and these are regularly used for immunization against tetanus (caused by *Clostridium tetani*) and diphtheria (caused by *Corynebacterium diphtheriae*). Toxoids are often combined with an adjuvant such as aluminium phosphate or aluminium hydroxide, which acts to boost the immune response (see Chapter 24). The antibody produced in response to injection of a toxoid neutralizes the toxin, so it is unable to precipitate its adverse symptoms. However, the antibodies produced in response to the toxoid do not interfere with bacterial growth. For this reason a patient with diphtheria also needs an antibiotic to eliminate the organisms.

ATTENUATED AGENTS

Attenuated agents are living organisms with reduced virulence but unaffected immunogenicity. Attenuation is achieved by repeatedly subculturing (or passaging) through artificial media or an unnatural host (or host tissue cultures). The BCG vaccine, for example, which is used to protect against tuberculosis, is a live attenuated bovine strain of the tuberculosis organism that has been subcultured over 100 times in artificial media. The BCG vaccine gives immunity for 10 years or longer. The rubella virus vaccine and measles virus vaccine are also attenuated by passaging through tissue cultures that are not normal hosts for these viruses. As already mentioned, a large number of virus vaccines are live

attenuated vaccines. These give long-lasting immunity in comparison to the dead vaccine.

The poliovirus vaccine is available in both a live attenuated form as well as a formalin-killed form (see above). The live attenuated form (known as the Sabin vaccine) gives long-term protection ,whereas the dead vaccine provides short-term protection. Although the live vaccine has various advantages it suffers from the risk of mutation of the attenuated strains to a virulent form; some vaccinated people have developed polio in the past. Killed polio vaccine (Salk vaccine) is safe but is logistically inconvenient as it is given by injection and requires regular boosting.

SUBUNIT VACCINES

A whole micro-organism contains a mixture of a large number of different antigens. Some of these antigens may be irrelevant while others may be harmful to the host. Attempts are therefore being made to produce vaccines that contain relevant targets to stimulate the immune response but are free from toxic or harmful components of the micro-organisms.

New subunit vaccines have recently been produced from a number of bacteria. *Haemophilus influenzae* type b is a highly pathogenic bacteria that causes life-threatening infections such as meningitis and acute epiglottitis. A subunit vaccine containing capsular polysaccharide, conjugated with large protein molecules, is now being routinely used in the UK with excellent results. The introduction of *Haemophilus influenzae* type b vaccine in 1992 resulted in a rapid reduction in the notification of infection caused by this organism, from about 200 notifications a year down to notifications in single figures during the past 2–3 years (Figure 21.3). The incidence of childhood meningitis due to *Haemophilus influenzae* type b has also been drastically reduced in other countries where this vaccine has been introduced.

Meningococcal subunit vaccines have also been developed against types A and C, and these are now used to protect contacts and to eradicate the carriage of *Neisseria meningitidis* in the pharynx during convalescence. Likewise, a pneumococcal polyvalent vaccine has been introduced; this contains polysaccharide capsular material from a number of prevalent pneumococcal types. Attempts to develop an acellular whooping cough vaccine are currently being actively pursued. A number of components of *Bordetella pertussis* are being examined as possible candidates for synthesis as the whooping cough vaccine.

A subunit vaccine used to be prepared from hepatitis B surface antigen (HBsAg), which contained small glycoprotein particles separated from the plasma of

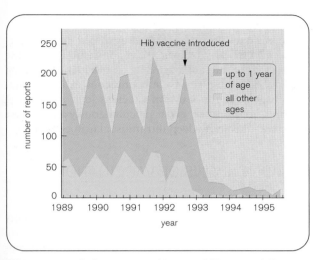

Figure 21.3 Laboratory reports of Haemophilus influenzae type b by age, England and Wales (1989–1995). The introduction of *Haemophilus influenzae* type b (Hib) vaccine in 1993 caused a rapid decline in the rate of *Haemophilus influenzae* type b infection. [Data from Department of Health, Welsh Office, Scottish Office Department of Health and DHSS (Northern Ireland). *Immunisation against infection* 1996; by permission of Her Majesty's Stationery Office.]

hepatitis B carriers. However it was deemed unsafe because some people who received the vaccine became infected with hepatitis B virus. It has now been superseded by a safer recombinant vaccine.

RECOMBINANT VACCINES

The advances in molecular biology techniques has allowed sites on the microbe to be selected and synthesized as recombinant proteins (see Chapter 7). The progress in biotechnology methods has enabled such proteins to be prepared 'in bulk', exploiting the intracellular machinery of other cell types. Therefore it is now possible to develop new vaccines, with specially targeted components of microbial cells, that do not have the potential risk of infection.

This field of work has been particularly productive in the field of viral vaccines (e.g. hepatitis B virus). Many viruses have protein capsids and glycoprotein cell envelops, which have been recognized as the major antigenic components. Once the gene sequence and its control mechanism for constructing these proteins are identified, it is relatively straightforward to synthesize the genes and insert them into a bacteria, virus, or yeast – an example of genetic cloning.

Such microbes in themselves are innocuous; they are merely exploited for their intracellular machinery to decode and produce recombinant proteins from the newly acquired genetic constructs. The microbes are grown in large volumes of media and synthesize the recombinant proteins. These may be isolated and purified for use as vaccines. Such proteins can activate the immune system to afford protection against the infectious organism that naturally expresses them on the outer surface.

Recombinant vaccines are expected to be safer. But if they are to be of use, it is essential that the proteins that are selected and cloned are a precise mimic of the sites on the infectious agent. If this is so, the immune cell should recognize and respond to them if they encountered the infection. HBsAg gene has been successfully cloned in yeast and the recombinant vaccine is now being used effectively and widely against hepatitis B. A recombinant rabies virus vaccine has also been produced in vaccinia virus. This expresses the rabies glycoprotein.

More recently the gene cloning of the surface glycoprotein gp120 of HIV virus has been investigated as a potential vaccine against developing AIDS (see also Chapter 28). Vaccinia virus, which is virtually avirulent, has now been used as a host for encoding genes from hepatitis B, the influenza virus, and the herpes virus, either singly or for inserting multiple genes to produce polyvalent vaccines.

FUTURE DEVELOPMENTS

Recently, the emphasis has further advanced to identify the small areas on a pathogenic microbe (peptide epitopes), which the immune system can recognize. The amino acid sequence in the peptide chain is then established, which allows the determination of the genetic constitution of these epitopes (see Chapter 24). Once this is known, these epitopes can be synthesized and used for protection. This synthetic product may be attached to a carrier molecule or introduced into a carrier micro-organism, such as vaccinia, for expression. Considerable research in the biotechnology industry is now being done to develop synthetic vaccines. Another area of development in vaccine research is to directly introduce genes responsible for protection to the host – the so-called deoxyribonucleic acid (DNA) vaccine. This is in the very early stage of development, and several candidate vaccines are now under investigation (see Chapter 30 for a discussion of vaccines against cancer).

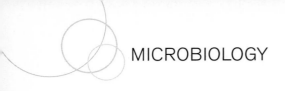

MICROBIOLOGY

STORAGE OF VACCINES

On receipt of a vaccine, the manufacturer's recommendation should be noted with regard to the storage, dilution, distribution, and shelf life (expiry date). Most vaccines are stored at 0–4°C. Vaccines should never be frozen because freezing causes deterioration of the vaccine and consequent loss of activity. Storage facilities should be regularly checked to ensure that the optimum conditions are maintained, and these data recorded. For transportation of vaccines, special cool boxes should be used to preserve the vaccines; storage during transit to rural areas in developing countries can pose real problems. Unused open ampoules and empty vials should be safely disposed of based on written guidelines.

ROUTE OF ADMINISTRATION OF VACCINES

ORAL VACCINES

Live attenuated polio virus vaccine, a combination of all three types of polio virus, is administered orally in syrup form or added to a lump of sugar. The vaccine, on entering the intestine, evokes a mild gut infection. This allows the development of local immunity in the gut, where IgA antibodies are produced. The vaccine viruses then enter the blood stream and elicit an initial IgM response followed by an IgG response. Research in the development of oral cholera and typhoid vaccines is still continuing, and an oral typhoid vaccine is now available.

INJECTABLE VACCINES

Most other vaccines in general use are injected into the host by intradermal, subcutaneous, or intramuscular injection.

Intradermal Injection

BCG, a live attenuated vaccine against tuberculosis, is given by intradermal injection (or percutaneously in infants by the multiple puncture technique). A fine 26 G needle is inserted under the skin, more or less horizontally to the surface, for about 2 mm with the bevel of the needle upwards. The bevel should be just visible under the skin surface. Resistance is felt during injection and a small blanched bleb is produced. A small local ulceration may follow during the next 2–3 weeks, which usually heals with a scar. The presence of a scar indicates a successful BCG vaccination. Typhoid and rabies vaccines are also given by the intradermal route.

Subcutaneous and Intramuscular Injection

Most immunizations are effected by these routes. Freeze-dried and dried vaccines are reconstituted with the appropriate diluents according to the manufacturers' instructions and given by subcutaneous or deep intramuscular injection. Several vaccines (e.g. hepatitis A vaccine) are routinely given subcutaneously and are less effective if given by deep intramuscular injection.

COMPLICATIONS OF VACCINATION

MINOR COMPLICATIONS

Being foreign substances, vaccines can give rise to many constitutional side-effects, such as mild-to-moderate fever, pain and redness at the site of injection, and generalized malaise, headache, and shivering. These side-effects are often associated with killed whole bacterial vaccines and some viral vaccines produced in tissue cultures. Most of these side-effects do not require any treatment, but occasionally analgesic and antipyretic treatment may be necessary.

MORE SEVERE COMPLICATIONS

Moderate vaccine reactions are often associated with live attenuated viral vaccines. They are caused by active virus multiplication in the body with consequent manifestation of the disease that the virus produces, albeit in a milder form. This can occur with rubella and measles vaccines, for example. Live attenuated BCG vaccine often produces localized ulceration at the site of injection, which may take a long time to heal.

Severe anaphylactic reactions may follow certain vaccines including those live virus vaccines that are produced in embryonated eggs (e.g. measles vaccine). Sometimes common vaccines like diphtheria, tetanus, and pertussis (DTP vaccine) have given rise to severe anaphylactic reactions.

MAJOR COMPLICATIONS

These usually occur in people who are immunologically compromised. BCG vaccination in immunodeficient and immunocompromised patients can give rise to major generalized BCG infection. Similarly, any live viral vaccines may give rise to complications that may result in generalized manifestations. Convulsions, encephalitis, and other serious neurological reactions have occasionally been reported, but the evidence is not strong enough to relate these to particular vaccines. Vaccine-associated major infections have arisen in the past with live oral polio vaccine owing to the conversion of the attenuated virus into its virulent form.

CONTRAINDICATIONS TO VACCINATION

Some vaccines are unsuitable for certain situations and should be avoided. These include:

- patients with febrile illnesses, especially in children, when vaccination should be delayed until recovery;
- patients on immunosuppressive therapy (e.g. corticosteroids and other immunosuppressive substances for organ transplantations; or bone marrow transplantation)
- patients on cytotoxic drugs for the treatment of malignancy;
- patients with evidence of allergic manifestations (e.g. vaccines containing traces of egg or antibiotic, which may be used in their preparation, are often contraindicated in children with a medical history of anaphylaxis;
- patients with immunosuppressive diseases such as HIV infection and deficiencies of T lymphocytes;
- pregnancy (some live vaccines, like rubella and polio, are to be avoided).

Live vaccines are particularly contraindicated in most of the above conditions. Killed vaccines are not contraindicated as such (except in allergic patients) but they are unlikely to evoke strong immune response in these patients.

PREGNANCY AND VACCINATION

As a general rule all forms of vaccination should be avoided in pregnancy. Live viral vaccines are particularly contraindicated. These include live polio, measles, and rubella vaccines (Figure 21.4), and yellow fever vaccine. However, there may be compelling reasons for vaccinating during pregnancy; if so, a decision must be taken depending on the relative risk of infection to the mother. An example of this might be yellow fever vaccination for a pregnant woman travelling to an area where yellow fever is endemic. Inactivated vaccines, such as influenza, injectable polio vaccine, and hepatitis A, should not be given during pregnancy unless there is a definite risk.

THE VACCINATION PROGRAMME IN THE UK

NEWBORN BABIES

Most newborn babies have maternal antibodies against a variety of infectious agents. Protection from the maternal antibodies persists for up to about 18 months of age. Therefore, the vaccination programme is initiated within 3 months of birth as the maternal immunity starts waning. However, immunization against

tuberculosis is usually started within a few weeks of birth in those newborn babies who have come into contact with cases of tuberculosis. Similarly, babies of immigrants from endemic areas are given BCG vaccination within a few weeks of birth.

INFANTS

Conjugate *Haemophilus influenzae* type b vaccine is recommended at the age of 2 months, with three doses at monthly intervals. Unimmunized children up to 13 months of age are at high risk and should be given this vaccine simultaneously with other childhood vaccines. *Haemophilus* infection in infants gives rise to meningitis and epiglottitis. These manifestations are rarely seen in older children, and hence vaccination against this infection is more appropriate for infants.

Infants are also more likely to acquire infections leading to diphtheria, pertussis, and tetanus, and hence immunization against these infections is recommended in early infancy. A combination of diphtheria, pertussis, and tetanus (DPT) vaccines are given, starting from the age of 2 months. Three doses, with an interval of 1 month between each dose, completes the primary vaccination. Oral polio vaccine (OPV) is included in this schedule at the same time.

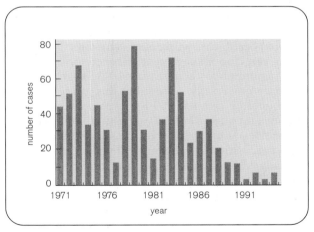

Figure 21.4 Confirmed cases of congenital rubella syndrome and congenital rubella infection, England and Wales (1971–1994). The effect of vaccination on the incidence of congenital rubella infection shows a continued reduction in cases recorded in England and Wales. [Data from Department of Health, Welsh Office, Scottish Office Department of Health and DHSS (Northern Ireland). *Immunisation against infection* 1996; by permission of Her Majesty's Stationery Office.]

Booster doses are necessary to maintain adequate immunity. These are given at the school-starting age, and again at about 13 or 14 years of age.

A combined measles, mumps, and rubella (MMR) vaccine is now available to be given to all children in two doses; shortly after the first birthday (about 12–15 months of age) and before school entry. The MMR vaccine comes in a freeze-dried formulation containing attenuated measles, mumps, and rubella viruses. It is administered by deep subcutaneous or intramuscular injection. Attenuation is achieved by repeated subculturing of the viruses in tissue culture. Immunization provides more than 90 per cent protection against the three viruses and persists for a long time – as long as 18 years against the rubella virus. MMR vaccine should be given to all children who missed the measles vaccination, to non-immune adults in institutional care, and to students in higher and further education who have not received measles or MMR vaccine.

AT SCHOOL ENTRY

All children should have a booster diphtheria and tetanus toxoid as well as a further dose of oral polio vaccine. In addition, the second dose of MMR is given simultaneously.

MIDDLE SCHOOL AGE AND ADULTS

Children between the ages of 12 and 15 years should receive BCG vaccination. Immunity persists for a long time but health-care workers who are directly involved in the care and management of tuberculosis patients may require a booster dose after 10–15 years. This has not been universally agreed, but this group of workers should be skin tested 10–15 years after the BCG vaccine and offered repeat vaccination if the skin test is negative or only weakly positive. As discussed above, BCG vaccination is frequently offered to infants from specially vulnerable groups, such as communities where tuberculosis is widespread.

Until recently, rubella vaccination was given to school girls at about the age of 12 or 13 years. Since the introduction of the MMR vaccine, rubella vaccination is no longer necessary. However, rubella vaccine is still recommended for women who are seronegative for rubella (i.e. those with no detectable anti-rubella antibodies), because the infection during pregnancy could harm the unborn child. Women wishing to conceive and who are not immune to rubella should be offered the vaccine, then advised on the use of adequate contraception so they do not become pregnant in the first 3 months of being immunized. However, rubella vaccine may be safely given to women in the postpartum period.

Adults without a history of tetanus, diphtheria, and polio vaccination are also advised to have the full course of these vaccines. Tetanus and a low-dose diphtheria vaccine (Td) is now available and is generally given as a booster at school leaving age. Table 21.1 summarizes the UK Immunization Schedule recommended by the Department of Health.

VACCINATION FOR HIGH-RISK GROUPS

Dead bacterial vaccines and toxoids do not normally pose any problem to immunocompromised and high risk patients. However, live bacterial vaccine such as BCG should be avoided in these people because of the risk of their developing disseminated infection. Similarly, many viral vaccines are also avoided in immunodeficient and immunocompromised people.

Vaccines against hepatitis A, hepatitis B, influenza, and the pneumococcus are often recommended for high-risk patients. Asplenic patients (i.e. those whose spleens have been removed), either as a consequence of accidental damage or following elective removal because of disease, are more prone to infection by capsulated bacteria such as pneumococci. It is advocated that asplenic people, whether children or adults, should be vaccinated with a single dose of these vaccines, preferably pre-operatively, especially in elective cases (see the Person-Centred Study in Chapter 31). *Meningococcus*, also a capsulated organism, can also cause severe infection in asplenic people. A single dose of meningococcus vaccine containing types A and C antigens is particularly advised for asplenic people travelling to endemic areas.

It is recommended that patients with chronic bronchopulmonary and cardiac diseases should have an influenza vaccine every year during the winter months.

VACCINATION FOR TRAVELLERS

International travelling has expanded and with it there is an increased risk of acquiring communicable diseases from endemic parts of the world. In the past, the World Health Organization recommended that a number of measures be taken to protect people travelling to the endemic countries. These measures included vaccination against smallpox, cholera, and yellow fever. However, smallpox has now been eradicated and cholera is no longer a major threat as long as sensible precautions are taken.

Therefore, yellow fever vaccination remains the one mandatory vaccine requirement for travellers to yellow fever endemic countries. Nevertheless, travellers are advised to take adequate protection against a number of infections while travelling in countries where

Immunization Schedule in the UK

Vaccine	Age at vaccination	Comments
diphtheria, pertussis, tetanus, polio, haemophilus B	first dose at 2 months second dose at 3 months third dose at 4 months	all children should have this primary course by 6 months; there are very few adverse reactions; satisfactory antibody levels are achieved
measles, mumps, rubella (MMR)	12–15 months	children who are missed can be vaccinated at any time after 12 months
diphtheria, polio, tetanus booster and second MMR	3–5 years	school entry
BCG	10–14 years	infants born in families with higher risk of tuberculosis can be vaccinated at birth or as early as possible after birth
tetanus, diphtheria, polio booster	13–18 years	school-leaving age

Table 21.1 Immunization schedule in the UK.

these are prevalent. Travellers from the UK are advised to have vaccination against typhoid and hepatitis A and have booster doses against polio and tetanus when travelling to countries in south-east Asia and other parts of eastern Asia, some parts of Africa, and South America.

Meningococcal vaccine is recommended for some parts of the world (e.g. sub-Saharan Africa, India, and Nepal) where Group A meningococcal infection occurs in small and large outbreaks). Group B meningococcal infection predominates in the UK, but no vaccine has yet been developed for this infection.

Prophylactic rabies vaccine is advised for those people who are occupationally exposed to the disease whilst working or travelling in endemic countries.

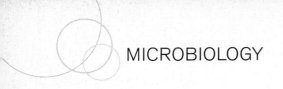

KEY POINTS

- A vaccine is given as the synthetic mimic of an infectious disease. On introduction into the host, whether it is given by injection (subcutaneous, intradermal, or intramuscularly) or by mouth, the vaccine is perceived as foreign or dangerous by the immune cells, it should elicit a reaction.
- Bacterial vaccines contain whole killed organisms (e.g. whooping cough, cholera, and typhoid vaccines), which have been grown in liquid or solid media, washed with saline, then killed (e.g. using moderate heat or the application of alcohol or acetone). The killed organisms retain their ability to activate the immune system.
- Toxoid vaccines are prepared by isolating the toxin released from the microbes and then rendering them harmless by treatment with formalin solution.
- Attenuated vaccines are living organisms with reduced virulence; this is achieved by repeatedly subculturing (or passaging) them through artificial media or an unnatural host (or host tissue cultures) (e.g. BCG vaccine).
- On receipt of a vaccine, the manufacturer's recommendation should be noted with regard to the storage, dilution, distribution, and shelf life (expiry date). Storage facilities should be regularly checked so that the optimum conditions are maintained. Unused open ampoules and empty vials should be safely disposed of based on written guidelines.
- The more severe complications following vaccine administration are associated with live attenuated vaccines, where the virus replicates in the body and may cause the manifestation of the disease.
- Vaccine therapy may be contraindicated in people who are immunocompromised, have a febrile illness, or are pregnant.

FURTHER READING

Anonymous (1996) Randomised controlled trial of single BCG, repeated BCG, or combined BCG and killed *Mycobacterium leprae* vaccine for prevention of leprosy and tuberculosis in Malawi. Karonga Prevention Trial Group. Lancet 348:17–24.

Beverley PC (1997) Vaccine immunity. Immunol Today 18:413–15.

Brewer TF, Wilson ME, Nardell EA (1995) BCG immunization: review of past experience, current use, and future prospects. Curr Clin Top Infect Dis 15:253–70.

Davies F, Luke LC, Burdett-Smith P (1996) Patients' understanding of tetanus immunization. J Accid Emerg Med 13:272–3.

Department of Health, Welsh Office, Scottish Office Department of Health, and the DHSS (Northern Ireland) (1996) Immunisation against Infectious Diseases. Her Majesty's Stationery Office, London.

Gangarosa EJ, Galazka AM, Wolfe CR, et al. (1998) Impact of anti-vaccine movements on pertussis control: the untold story. Lancet 351:356–61.

Greco D, Salmaso S, Mastrantonio P, et al. (1996) A controlled trial of two acellular vaccines and one whole-cell vaccine against pertussis. Progetto Pertosse Working Group. N Eng J Med 334:341–8.

Hayward C (1996) The legacy of Jenner: vaccination past, present and future. J R Coll Physicians 30: (6) 571–8.

Jeremijenko A, Kelly H, Sibthorpe B, Attewell R (1996) Improving vaccine storage in general practice refrigerators. BMJ 312:1651–2.

Loomis SC (1997) Varicella vaccination. An overview for the occupational health nurse. AAOHNJ 45:592–5.

McDonald P, Friedman EH, Banks A, Anderson R, Carman V (1997) Pneumococcal vaccine campaign based in general practice. BMJ 314:1094–8.

Mims C, Stephen J, Dimmock N, Nash A (1995) Mims' Pathogenesis of Infectious Diseases, 4th edition. Academic Press, London.

Salisbury D, Begg N (1996) Immunisation against infectious disease. Her Majesty's Stationery Office, London.

Schneerson R, Robbins JB, Taranger J, Lagergard T, Trollfors B (1996) A toxoid vaccine for pertussis as well as diphtheria? Lessons to be relearned. Lancet 348:1289–92.

Tingle AJ, Mitchell LA, Grace M, et al. (1997) Randomised double-blind placebo-controlled study on adverse effects of rubella immunisation in seronegative women. Lancet 349:1277–81.

Trollfors B, Taranger J, Lagergard T, et al. (1995) A placebo-controlled trial of a pertussis-toxoid vaccine. N Engl J Med 333:1045–50.

Wirsing von Konig CH, Postels-Multani S, Bock HL, Schmitt HJ (1995) Pertussis in adults: frequency of transmission after household exposure. Lancet 346:1326–9.

Immunology

TISSUES AND CELLS OF THE IMMUNE SYSTEM

LEARNING OBJECTIVES

After studying this chapter you will have a clearer understanding of:
- the historical perspective of immunity
- the tissues and cells of the immune system and their differing functions in defence
- the mechanism of phagocytosis to eliminate antigens
- the recirculation of immune cells throughout the different compartments of the body for its protection

INTRODUCTION – AN HISTORICAL PERSPECTIVE

Information about infection and the immune system has been around for centuries, although it may not have been expressed in those terms. Descriptions of epidemics led to realization that affected people were protected from further infections with the same disease. Similarly, it became known that an infection could be prevented by prophylactic activities or quarantine.

As far back as the fifth century BC, the Chinese reported a crude attempt at immunization against smallpox by a technique called variolation. This involved drying the crusts from skin lesions to a powder and then either inserting them into a small cut in the skin or, more often, inhaling them into the nostrils. Crusts were obtained from people with milder disease and people who were at the recovery stages of the disease, because these were considered less virulent and therefore more efficacious.

For centuries this method was about the only formal method of immunization that was practised. In the 18th century, the wife of a British ambassador to Constantinople, Lady Mary Wortley Montagau, having witnessed the preventative effects of variolation, allowed her own children to be immunized against smallpox. So impressed was Lady Mary that she set up what can only be described as a 'clinical trial'. She persuaded many of her socialite friends, the Royal

household, and some condemned prisoners (encouraged by the offer of a Royal pardon) to agree to variolation. Although the medical records for this era are incomplete, it was clear that smallpox was partly controlled – yet variolation was made illegal in 1840 because it could have the serious side effect of causing active smallpox.

Edward Jenner, a general practitioner from Gloucestershire, was also interested in this disfiguring disease, and attempted to understand the reasoning behind the folklore that milkmaids who had contracted cowpox became immune to smallpox. His records were safely documented; therefore it is known that Jenner's first patient to be immunized was a young boy, James Phipps, who received the cowpox inoculation from the lesions of a milkmaid called Sarah Nelmes on 14 May 1796. Jenner is one of the better known early immunologists in the battle against smallpox, a disease that was finally declared by the World Health Organization to be eradicated on 8 May 1980. The hide of Edward Jenner's cow, affectionately known as Blossom, is displayed in the medical library of St George's Hospital Medical School, London, his own medical school

These early immunologists recognized the significance of their results to public health, but did not understand the mechanisms by which they were brought about. For example, Louis Pasteur discovered the concept of attenuated vaccination by serendipity, as has happened in many medical

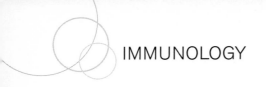

discoveries. He was interested in a fowl cholera bacillus, which he grew in culture. One summer he left his cultures out on the laboratory bench while he went on holiday. When he returned to work, Pasteur injected these bacteria into chickens only to find that they did not give the usual fatal outcome. He concluded that the bacteria must have been less virulent or dead because they were 'old'. It would seem research funds were as scarce in those days as they are today, because, to save money, he used the same birds again with a fresh virulent culture, but they still failed to contract the disease. Only then did Pasteur realize that the injection with the first batch of bacteria must have offered some protection to the birds. Having discovered a way of inducing immunity that was not life-threatening, he went on to use the same technique and produced attenuated vaccines for anthrax and rabies. A boy called Joseph Meister was the first of Pasteur's patients to receive the vaccine against rabies, which was given as an emergency because he had been repeatedly bitten by a rabid dog. The treatment saved his life, and in later years Joseph became a custodian for the Pasteur Institute in Paris (see Person-Centred Study: Immunization for Travel).

In 1901, Emil von Behring won a Nobel Prize for demonstrating that immunity in one animal could be transferred in the serum to another (see Chapter 23). The active component was given many names, including antitoxin, precipitin, and bacteriolysin. It was not until the 1930s that the name 'antibody' was finally coined and ascribed to the abilities to neutralize toxins and either lyse (burst) or agglutinate (clump) bacteria.

Elie Metchnikoff, a Russian zoologist, first saw motile cells surrounding a thorn in a starfish and went on to observe white blood cells engulfing microbes and named this process 'phagocytosis'. He also found that the phagocytic cells in the immunized animals were more active, and so concluded that it was cells rather than antibodies that were the real tool in the immune system. The question as to which was the essential part of the immune system (cells or antibodies) became the subject of lively discussion for many years. We now know that both are needed to give adequate protection. Only much later was it realized that there were different antibodies in the plasma to bind specific bacteria. Any material that could be bound to an antibody and immobilized by it was named an 'antigen'. It is now accepted that an antigen can be just about anything – a living organism that causes an infection, or bee venom or house dust that might provoke an allergic reaction. Whether living or dead, synthetic or chemical, anything that produces a specific reaction by the immune system is called an antigen.

In the whole living world, both plant and animal, mechanisms have evolved as a means of protection against a potentially hostile environment. In lower animals, like the earthworm, there is a phagocytic cell called a coelomocyte. Humans and other mammals have a more complex defence network, which forms the immune system. It would seem a perfect solution to have a system available for any assault, whether it was alive, dead, or synthetic.

However, as with all mechanisms, it can become defective or hyperactive. Our immune system is also highly educated, for generally we do not mount a persistent immunological attack against our own tissues and cells, only against foreign or dangerous antigens. Occasionally, though, this education is incomplete owing to some self-reacting immune cells escaping into the circulation rather than being killed. When this happens, the immune cells may make an active attack on the patient's own body tissues, resulting in a state called autoimmunity. For example, in patients with insulin-dependent diabetes mellitus their lymphocytes have attacked the beta-cells in the islets of Langerhans, so there is a progressive immunological destruction of these insulin-producing cells. Any remaining cells valiantly synthesize and supply the hormone until they are all finally killed. Hence, the onset of the disease is somewhat abrupt, for when no cells remain, the only hope of survival is an alternative source of insulin (see Chapters 27 and 35).

The immune system is both aggressive and specific – immunity against one disease (e.g. polio) does not automatically protect the individual from another (e.g. cholera). The system can even detect differences between different peoples' cells and tissues, which is evident in patients undergoing organ or tissue transplantation. In this instance, an immunologically foreign tissue is donated as a replacement for a diseased or defective structure; without a constant supply of immunosuppressive drugs (which are required for the rest of the patient's life), the body considers the transplant as foreign and rejects it. The hostile damage is not entirely surprising; after all, transplantation is a surgical intervention, not a normal physiological process, and however clinically worthwhile the graft might be, it is still a foreign tissue (see Chapter 29).

We should be grateful that in normal events our active immune system will attack foreign antigens. The topical nature and media coverage of the epidemic of the acquired immunodeficiency syndrome (AIDS) bears witness to the suffering and affliction that results when a fundamental part of immunity is inactive or missing. The ultimate effect is that a patient with AIDS is vulnerable and less able to eliminate infections, so the microbes multiply unchecked (see Chapter 28).

Another peculiarity in our defence system is that it occasionally mounts an allergic reaction, which is an abnormally vicious response to what might be considered a harmless substance. Very unpleasant symptoms may arise as a result of an allergy to grass pollen or the nickel of a watch strap. These are examples of hypersensitivity reactions that may be life-threatening if the patient suffers anaphylactic shock (see Chapter 26).

WHAT IS THE IMMUNE SYSTEM?

To protect against disease, the immune system is distributed throughout the body as a highly regulated net-

work of different cells, tissues, and soluble molecules. It has three major objectives:
- to identify foreign organisms and substances;
- to dispose of them; and
- to communicate between other cells and tissues to try to ensure an adequate response while minimizing the damage to surrounding healthy tissue.

The major organs of the immune system are sometimes referred to as the lymphoid organs, which may be subdivided into primary and secondary lymphoid organs (Figure 22.1).

The primary lymphoid organs are where the immune cells are produced and matured. These include the bone marrow and thymus in adults, but the liver during fetal life. Secondary lymphoid organs are the sites where the immune cells circulate and respond to antigens. These are the spleen, the lymphatic system

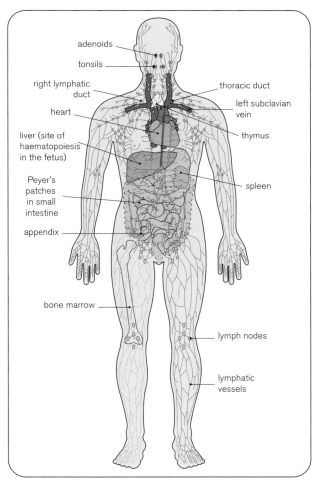

Figure 22.1 The primary and secondary lymphoid organs of the immune system.

with its lymph nodes, and the mucosal-associated lymphoid tissue (MALT). At first glance, the lymph nodes, spleen, and MALT appear to be distinct tissues with their own unique anatomy. However, on closer inspection, they have certain structural similarities in that they possess discrete areas in which immune cells interact with one another. This arrangement is critical for the immune response to be effective in the recognition and disposal of antigens.

CELLS OF THE IMMUNE SYSTEM

Mature immune cells are readily transported in the blood and lymphatic systems to areas where their defence activities are required. The white blood cells include the monocytes and lymphocytes as well as the granulocytes (neutrophils, basophils, and eosinophils) (Figure 22.2). Although the platelets and red blood cells have other physiological functions and are not strictly part of the immune system, they do offer some assistance. The haemostatic properties of platelets cordon off an area of infection by the formation of a platelet and fibrin plug. The red blood cells may be used to 'shepherd' antibody–antigen complexes (also known as immune complexes) from the periphery to the spleen for their disposal. This is an essential process, because immune complexes that lodge in tissues can provoke the inflammatory processes seen in diseases such as glomerulonephritis (see Chapters 25 & 27).

LYMPHOCYTES

Lymphocytes represent up to 20 per cent of the white blood cells circulating in the peripheral blood of healthy adults. There are two main populations of lymphocytes – T lymphocytes and B lymphocytes. They are manufactured by the bone marrow but migrate into the blood stream and lymphatic system to be matured in other lymphoid tissues for their part in the immune response. These cells endow us with the ability to be immune to specific diseases by virtue of the antigen receptors in their cell surface. Although B and T lymphocytes look the same when viewed down the microscope, they have some distinguishing features other than their antigen receptors, the cell surface markers. However, these are only detectable when the cells are subjected to specific histological examination.

B Lymphocytes

In humans, B lymphocytes mature in the liver during fetal life and in the bone marrow in adults. In birds, B lymphocytes mature in a sac at the end of the gut called the bursa of Fabricius (see Chapter 24); humans do

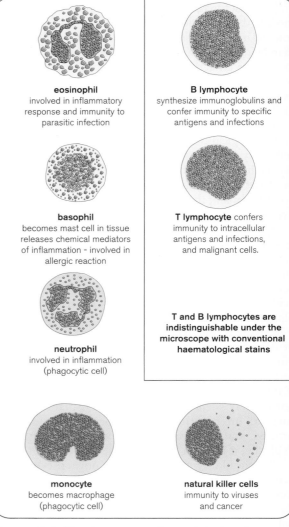

eosinophil
involved in inflammatory response and immunity to parasitic infection

B lymphocyte
synthesize immunoglobulins and confer immunity to specific antigens and infections

basophil
becomes mast cell in tissue releases chemical mediators of inflammation - involved in allergic reaction

T lymphocyte confers immunity to intracellular antigens and infections, and malignant cells.

neutrophil
involved in inflammation (phagocytic cell)

T and B lymphocytes are indistinguishable under the microscope with conventional haematological stains

monocyte
becomes macrophage (phagocytic cell)

natural killer cells
immunity to viruses and cancer

Figure 22.2 The immune cells and their roles.

not have this organ. B lymphocytes are the immune cell type that produce immunoglobulins, which is another name for antibodies. These molecules are the antigen receptors of the B lymphocytes, which are displayed on their cell surface. Immunoglobulin production generally takes place in discrete and defined areas of the bone marrow, spleen and the lymph nodes.

The reason why immunoglobulins are detected in body fluids is because they are secreted after the B lymphocytes has encountered the antigen. The cells that subsequently become 'antibody secreters' are referred to as plasma cells. The immunoglobulins bind to their specific infectious or foreign antigen to form an immune complex, thereby limiting infections and neutralizing toxins. In fact, it is essential that B lymphocytes meet their specific antigen in order to survive; otherwise they die within a few days. Unfortunately, immunoglobulins are also responsible for adverse effects suffered in hypersensitivity reactions such as hay fever and haemolytic disease of the newborn (see Chapter 26).

There are five main classes of immunoglobulins, immunoglobulin G (IgG), IgM, IgA, IgD, and IgE (see Chapter 24). They are predominantly found in specific areas of the body, and at various stages of the immune response.

T Lymphocytes

There are three types of T lymphocytes – cytotoxic T lymphocytes, T helper cells, and T suppressor cells. Each performs a different task, and their names give a reasonable clue to their role in immunity. They displace antigen receptors, known as T-cell receptors. Unlike the immunoglobulins, these remain bound to the cell surface and are not secreted into body fluids.

Cytotoxic T lymphocytes

Cytotoxic T lymphocytes kill cells that are infected with a virus, cells that are malignant, and cells that are considered to be a foreign tissue (e.g. a transplanted organ). Their attack follows the recognition of the foreign antigen (see Chapter 24) using their antigen receptors. Upon successful binding, they lyse and kill their target by releasing enzymes and substances called perforins that *perforate* the cell membrane. The attachment of the lymphocyte is aided by a specialised cell surface marker with adhesive properties called CD8. In fact, CD8+ cells is a name often used when referring to cytotoxic T lymphocytes.

T helper cells

These cells assist other immune cells so that:
- the cytotoxic T cells can kill defective or infected cells;
- B lymphocytes can produce immunoglobulins; and
- inflammatory cells and phagocytes take part in the immune response.

T helper cells also possess receptors for binding to cell surface antigens; this is aided by another adhesive molecule, CD4, hence T helper cells are also referred to as CD4+ cells.

Reduced numbers of T helper cells are a significant reason for the impaired immune response found in patients infected with the human immunodeficiency virus (HIV). The virus enters the T helper cells and, once infected, their ability to work as immune cells is severely impaired and they are ultimately eliminated. Hence, patients who develop full-blown AIDS do not die from the HIV infection as such; rather,

they die because of an inability to limit infections that an active immune system could more effective control. HIV-infected patients essentially have an infection-induced immunodeficiency because the cell type with the ability to stimulate other immune cells is in short supply – rather like having a car without its starter motor.

T suppressor cells

The T suppressor cells are somewhat of an enigma, because the nature of their part in immunity is not fully understood. They are considered to have the task of tempering potentially aggressive activities since they inhibit other immune cells. T suppressor cells become stimulated during the immune response in order to act as one of the controllers.

NATURAL KILLER CELLS

The knowledge about natural killer cells is somewhat limited in comparison with other immune cells. In fact, they have been confused or mistaken for lymphocytes. Certainly the two cell types look similar when viewed down the microscope – hence the other name for natural killer cells, large granular lymphocytes.

Natural killer cells are produced by the bone marrow and fulfil a vital surveillance operation, namely to kill virus-infected and malignant cells. It might be considered that this is unimportant since these functions have also been attributed to T lymphocytes. However, the cytotoxic T lymphocytes are only useful in the assault on a specific antigen that they have previously encountered. Natural killer cells are more indiscriminate and will rapidly destroy just about any virus-infected cells and tumour cells that they confront. A testimony to their essential role in immunity is found in Chediak–Higashi syndrome, in which patients have inadequate natural killer cell function and are therefore more prone to developing malignancies such as lymphomas (see also Chapters 30 & 31).

GRANULOCYTES

Three of the immune cell types, the eosinophils, basophils, and neutrophils, are collectively referred to as granulocytes. They are so-named because of the granules in their cytoplasm, which are visible under a light microscope.

Eosinophils

Eosinophils make up between 1 and 3 per cent of the total leukocyte count in peripheral blood. In order to see them microscopically, they are stained with the acidic histological stain called eosin, which gives their cytoplasmic granules a red–orange appearance. They congregate at the site of allergic reactions and parasitic infections; hence their numbers may be raised in patients suffering from such disorders. Eosinophils display receptors for IgE antibodies on the cell surface and release a toxin called major basic protein. Both of these substances act against parasitic infections, which is highly advantageous because certain parasites have outer coats that resist the enzymes produced by macrophages and neutrophils. Although eosinophils are capable of phagocytosis, they are not particularly successful at it. However, they do produce cytokines (e.g. transforming growth factor-beta) to act as an antidote to the substances that would cause inflammation and so reduce the inflammatory response of the basophils and mast cells.

Basophils

Basophils are not phagocytic, and they make up the smallest individual mature population of white blood cells in the peripheral circulation – less than 1 per cent of the total white blood cell count. Their granules appear blue–black with conventional histological stains, and contain chemical mediators of inflammation (e.g. histamine) which promote vasodilatation and vascular permeability, and the anticoagulant, heparin. Basophils are the circulatory counterparts of the mast cells that reside in tissues. These cells display receptors on the cell surface that bind to free IgE antibodies. They also actively release the contents of their cytoplasmic granules (degranulation), which stimulate the adverse symptoms experienced in allergic reactions (see Chapter 26).

Neutrophils

Neutrophils make up to about 70 per cent of the white blood cells in normal healthy adults. Viewed down the microscope they have multilobed nuclei. Within their cytoplasm are granules that hold enzymes such as lysozyme and myeloperoxidase, used to destroy and degrade bacteria in phagocytosis. In the response to a stressor (e.g. surgery), the number of neutrophils in peripheral blood is often raised. Many of these cells would have left the bone marrow in haste and so might be slightly immature. Consequently, their nuclei look different in that the lobes are not so well developed; hence they are known as band forms.

Upon leaving the bone marrow, the neutrophils reside in the blood for just a few hours before migrating into the tissues, and have a comparatively short life span, dying within about 2 days. Neutrophils capture iron within an iron-binding protein called lactoferrin. An antimicrobial effect is thus produced because iron, which is an essential nutrient for microbes to grow and colonize, is bound to lactoferrin and not available to the microbes.

Neutrophils are also known as the inflammatory cells. They respond to factors that chemically attract them to the area of infection or injury. Some of the substances that neutrophils secrete provoke the vascular permeability and vasodilatation found at the site of inflammation. In particular, neutrophils are partly responsible for the formation of pus. Hence, the ability of neutrophils to be anaerobic is significant (i.e. not require oxygen) since they are commonly found in the interior of an abscess.

MONONUCLEAR PHAGOCYTIC CELLS
Monocytes and Macrophages

Monocytes are cells with a large single nucleus and a non-granular cytoplasm. They make up about 8–10 per cent of the white blood cell count in healthy adults. As they mature and enter different tissues of the body they are known as macrophages and are ascribed different names according to where they reside. For instance, a monocyte that ends up in the lung is called an alveolar macrophage; in the liver it becomes a Kupffer cell; in the brain a microglial cell. They form part of the mononuclear phagocyte system and have a major role in phagocytosis. Essentially they are scavengers; they engulf cellular debris to prevent inflammation, and to this end they produce enzymes and free radicals. However, they also fulfil another, highly significant, role – macrophages, from whatever tissue source, display the material they have previously phagocytosed on their cell surface to act as a 'flag' or 'sign board'. In so doing, they act as antigen-presenting cells to alert other parts of the immune system to the presence of the antigens they have engulfed.

Macrophages are a major cell type found at the site of injury and inflammation. Similarly, in the medically controlled Mantoux test for tuberculosis, aggregated macrophages and T lymphocytes are the cause of the raised and inflamed lumps at the site of the injection that are found in a positive result. The inflamed lesion persists for about 1 week and is an example of a granuloma (see Chapter 26). Active macrophages also respond by producing immunological factors, such as the complement proteins, which stimulate inflammatory reactions, and the cytokines involved in regulation of immune cell activities (see Chapter 25).

Another distinct property of macrophages is their role in healing – they recruit other immune cells to a specific area where there is tissue injury. They synthesize growth factors required for healing and repair, and even some coagulation factors to limit infections by means of the blood clotting mechanism.

Dendritic Cells

Dendritic cells, another type of mononuclear phagocytic cells, are produced by the bone marrow. They are so-named because they have long processes that look similar to the dendrites found on nerve cells. Once they have dispersed throughout the body, the dendritic cells engulf antigens, then migrate to the nearest lymphoid organ to display antigens to lymphocytes. Dendritic cells are found in most organs, where they can gather up unwanted antigens so that they can be disposed of (e.g. follicular dendritic cells are phagocytes operating in the lymph nodes).

PHAGOCYTOSIS

The original observations by Elie Metchnikoff, in which he studied the engulfing of bacteria by phagocytes, were accurate. As a general rule, at areas of infection or inflammation neutrophils phagocytose smaller particles and bacteria, whereas macrophages are the scavengers of larger particles and cell debris. However, these cells must be attracted into the vicinity, a process known as chemotaxis. Some of the activated complement proteins are responsible for enticing and recruiting immune cells to where they are required. Phagocytosis commences when the phagocyte puts out pseudopodia to surround and enclose the particle or organism. This type of intracellular vacuole is called a phagosome; it limits the offender but does no more. For the demise of the offender, the phagosome must fuse with the cell lysosomes ('suicide bags'), which possess powerful digestive enzymes. A key characteristic of a microbe, which governs whether or not it survives, is its ability to resist phagocytosis; some bacteria have an anti-phagocytic capsule (e.g. encapsulated pneumococci).

Digestion goes hand-in-hand with an increase in energy production in the form of glycolysis (see Chapters 1 and 2). The metabolism of the phagocyte changes, with an increased oxygen consumption for the manufacture of hydrogen peroxide, which is an effective toxic agent within the phagosome (Figure 22.3). The cytoplasmic granules of neutrophils contain enzymes, such as myeloperoxidase, that require a good supply of hydrogen peroxide. Macrophages do not have this enzyme and so are not so efficient at killing certain pathogens (e.g. *Candida albicans*).

Although most organisms are killed with the discharge of the enzymes into the phagosome, there are some that are not. In fact some microbes have evolved survival strategies whereby they resist phagocytosis and multiply within the phagosome (see Chapter 16).

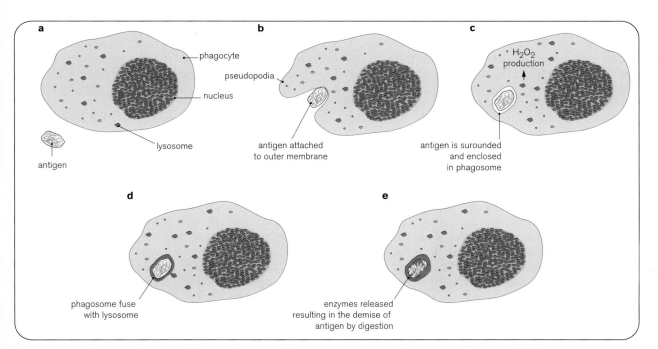

Figure 22.3 Phagocytosis. (a) The antigen and the phagocyte come into close proximity. (b) The phagocyte puts out pseudopodia and the antigen becomes attached to the surface of the phagocyte. (c) The antigen becomes enclosed in the phagosome, energy changes occur in the phagocyte, and hydrogen peroxide is produced. (d) The lysosome fuses with the phagosome. (e) Enzymes are released from the lysosome to digest the antigen.

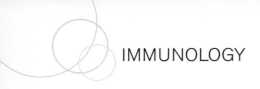

IMMUNOLOGY

THE LYMPHOID ORGANS AND TISSUES

THE BONE MARROW

At birth, the bone marrow occupies all the bones, but it is gradually replaced by fatty marrow. In adults, haematopoiesis (production of blood cells) predominantly occurs in the bone marrow of a select set of bones – the sternum, the iliac crest, and the vertebrae from 10th thoracic vertebra (T10) to the fourth lumbar vertebra (L4). The bone marrow contains the haematopoietic stem cells, the immature cells that are required for blood formation. These cells are called pluripotent stem cells because they have the capacity of differentiating (developing) into all the various cell types circulating in the peripheral blood (i.e. white blood cells, red blood cells, and platelets). The supply of stem cells in the bone marrow is maintained by a process known as self-renewal, so that blood cells may be replenished when they die or get used up in immunological activities. Generally, the development of the stem cells are influenced by the microenvironment of the bone marrow.

The production of the different blood cell types is dependent on the provision of different stimuli in the form of colony-stimulating factors and cytokines, that are specific soluble factors sometimes referred to as the immunological hormones. Various factors act on these immature precursor cells to direct their line of development. The immature cells then become committed into being one or other of the blood cell types (see Chapters 1 and 31). Homeostatic mechanisms operate to regulate the daily production of blood cells in order to ensure that the numbers of different cells types are maintained. Hence, normal ranges of these cells have been established, and variations identified according to the age and sex of the person (see Appendix 2).

THE THYMUS

The thymus is made up of two lobes and is located just below the thyroid gland. It is a primary lymphoid organ, and it provides the appropriate environment for the development of active T lymphocytes. Lymphocytes migrate from the bone marrow and those committed to becoming T lymphocytes enter and mature within the thymus. Here they acquire their T-cell receptors and their cell surface markers, and here they are educated about 'self' or non-dangerous antigens.

The thymus has an outer cortex and inner medulla; the immature T lymphocytes are found in the cortex and are sometimes referred to as thymocytes, as the cells mature they progress to the medulla. In the thymus, T lymphocytes are, for the first time, exposed to the tissue-type antigens called human leukocyte anti-

gens (HLA). (The HLA are the tissue-type antigens that are tested and matched between the donor and recipient of a transplant graft, in order to reduce the risk of rejection). Lymphocytes that would react against self-antigens or HLA are eliminated by a process of programmed cell death, known as apoptosis (see Chapter 4). In fact it has been estimated that over 95 per cent of lymphocytes entering the thymus are deleted without ever maturing into active immune cells.

The thymus develops during fetal life and reaches its maximum size by puberty, after which it starts to regress. By about the age of 30 years the thymus has atrophied, and although there is still some thymic activity in old age, it is by no means as effective as it was at puberty. The increased incidence of infections, malignant, and autoimmune diseases with advancing age has partly been attributed to reduced thymic activity. Thymic atrophy has also been associated with an acute rise in steroid levels in response to stress, malnutrition, or pregnancy (see Chapters 23 & 28).

THE SPLEEN

The spleen is a secondary lymphoid organ located behind the stomach and near the diaphragm, high in the abdominal cavity. It acts as a blood reservoir (particularly for platelets, granulocytes, and red blood cells) and operates a blood filtering system. Blood-borne antigens are therefore trapped and phagocytosed by the resident macrophages to help prevent systemic infections. There are two main tissue types within the spleen, the red pulp and white pulp (Figure 22.4).

The Red Pulp

The red pulp is the site where old and defective red blood cells are destroyed. In diseases in which the red blood cells have a reduced life span (e.g. sickle cell disease and beta-thalassaemia) patients often develop splenomegaly because the red pulp had to 'work overtime'. Therefore a splenectomy may be performed in order to slow down the rate at which the cells are destroyed. But this can result in patients having a greater risk of blood-borne bacterial infections. In particular, young children who have had a splenectomy have an increased incidence of infections with the pneumococcus and *Haemophilus influenza* (see Person-Centred Study in Chapter 31). Therefore, these patients should be immunized against these organisms before surgery and prescribed long-term prophylactic antimicrobial drugs.

The White Pulp

White pulp is a lymphoid tissue in which there are designated areas for the activities of T lymphocytes and

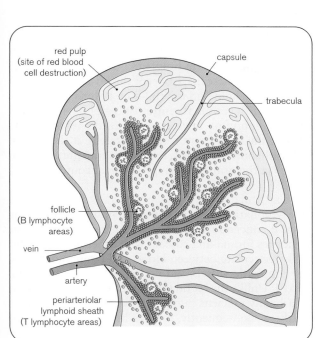

red pulp
(site of red blood
cell destruction)

capsule

trabecula

follicle
(B lymphocyte
areas)

vein

artery

periarteriolar
lymphoid sheath
(T lymphocyte areas)

Figure 22.4 Structure of the spleen. Note the periarterial lymphatic sheaths (T-lymphocyte areas) in close proximity to the follicles (B-lymphocyte areas). The red pulp areas are the site of red blood cell destruction.

B lymphocytes. For T lymphocytes to take part in active immunity they must see antigens exhibited by antigen-presenting cells. In the white pulp of the spleen, the phagocytic cells from the periphery (e.g. follicular dendritic cells and macrophages) display their engulfed foreign antigens to T helper cells. The T lymphocyte areas are found surrounding the arterioles supplying the spleen, called the periarteriolar lymphoid sheath (PALS). As previously mentioned, B lymphocytes need the 'help' of T lymphocytes to produce immunoglobulins. Accordingly, the internal structures and geography of the spleen allows the T and B lymphocytes areas to be in close proximity. The follicles where the B lymphocytes reside are found interspersed between the PALS. Upon antigen stimulation the follicles develop germinal centres. It is here that the B lymphocytes rapidly divide and become plasma cells, which secrete immunoglobulins for subsequent immobilisation and elimination of antigens.

LYMPHATIC VESSELS AND LYMPH NODES

Lymphatic vessels and lymph nodes are dispersed more or less throughout the whole body; however, there are few areas that are not served by this system. Within the lymphatic vessels is lymph, fluid that was originally in the capillary network but has subsequently passed into the extracellular space. As the fluid is collected and drained into the lymphatic vessels, the lymph delivers antigens from the many different epithelial surfaces, and the organs nearby to be displayed to the immune cells residing in the lymph nodes. The lymph then returns to the blood via the thoracic duct, which pours into the left subclavian vein. Thus, the same fluid circulates from blood to extracellular fluid to lymph and then back to blood.

Lymphocyte Activities in the Lymphatic System

Lymphocytes that have not come into contact with an antigen are said to be naïve. As they progress from the bone marrow and thymus they enter the lymphatic system. Once a B lymphocyte has recognized and responded to its specific antigen it is no longer naïve, and it may then return to the bone marrow to secrete immunoglobulins. Alternatively the lymph nodes are sites where B lymphocytes produce immunoglobulins with great affinity for antigen with the assistance of the T helper cells.

The lymph nodes are encapsulated by connective tissue, with discrete areas crammed with lymphocytes, macrophages, and other phagocytic cells. Groups of lymph nodes are strategically located in chains at junctions of the lymphatic vessels in the neck, groin, and other parts of the body such as the skin. The cells make contact and react with the antigens as they are filtered through and sampled by the lymph node. Thus the lymph drains through nodes that contain the immune cells that provide a 'guard' for most organs and connective tissues.

As with the spleen, lymph nodes contain discrete areas called follicles, which develop into germinal centres as B lymphocytes divide and change into immunoglobulin-secreting plasma cells; the necessary T helper cells reside in connecting areas. B lymphocytes come into the lymph nodes and must pass through areas where the T lymphocytes reside in order to enter the follicles. As a result, B and T lymphocytes are obliged to make contact with each another and with other immune cells (e.g. follicular dendritic cells), which in turn maximizes the potential for their mutual co-operation.

Lymph nodes are by no means fixed and static, since they alter their size with the progress of the immune response. Therefore, some patients present with enlarged lymph nodes (lymphadenopathy). For example, large lymph nodes, which may be palpable where the lymph has drained from a malignant tissue, or from the site of entry of a foreign antigen (e.g. as in a throat infection). If they are enlarged it is because they are packed with

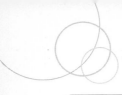

IMMUNOLOGY

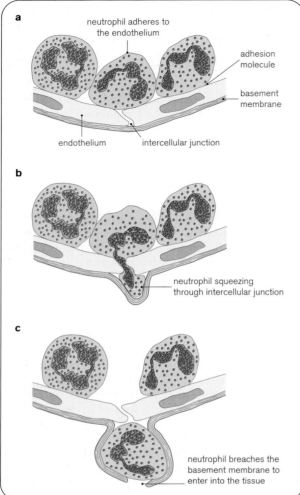

Figure 22.5 Sequence of events in diapedesis of an immune cell. (a) The immune cell adheres to the surface of the endothelium. (b) The immune cell squeezes between the cells of the intercellular junction. (c) The immune cell breaches the basement membrane and enters the tissue.

active immune cells dealing with the antigens that have been swept in. But once the antigen has been eliminated, the lymph node activities subside and so it shrinks back to a smaller size.

Mucosal-Associated Lymphoid Tissues

The mucosal-associated lymphoid tissues (MALTs) are specialized lymphoid tissues at the interface between the body and the external environment. MALT includes the mucosal surfaces of the gut, respiratory tract, and genitourinary tract. MALT acts as a guard by trapping foreign antigens before they are allowed to penetrate

these surfaces. Hence, there are vast numbers of immune cells in MALT for this purpose. In addition, immunoglobulins (mainly IgA) are detectable (see Chapter 24); these help prevent the invading microbes from taking hold and multiplying. Peyer's patches are nodules with germinal centres of lymphocyte activity; they are found on the outer wall of the intestine and protect the body from foreign antigens at the intestinal epithelium. Similarly, the tonsils trap antigens that enter via the oral and nasopharyngeal routes.

Cellular Trafficking in the Lymphatic System

The lymphatic system has an efficient way of gathering up and concentrating antigens into areas that are the ideal sites for making contact with other immune cells. Cells recirculate between blood and lymphoid tissues, i.e. lymphatic vessels and nodes, spleen, thymus, and MALT. Unlike the blood that rapidly circulates because of a highly efficient pump, the lymph merely agitates (shakes). Consequently, it takes hours for an immune cell to pass around the entire lymphatic system, whereas blood is pumped around the body in a matter of minutes. Because of this continuous movement of lymph and blood, the whole body is protected. For example, tetanus toxoid is normally given as an injection in the deltoid muscle of the arm. However, this does not mean that only the injection site is protected. The immune cells that react against the tetanus toxoid do not remain static but recirculate in the cardiovascular and lymphatic systems. When the immunized person comes into contact with tetanus again, the immune cells are attracted and driven to congregate at sites where they are most needed to respond to and eliminate infection.

Many antigens could potentially enter the body at the epithelial surfaces (skin, gut, respiratory tract, and genitourinary tract), for it is at these sites that they are in direct contact with the external environment. However, there appears to be an inner circulatory process within MALT, and therefore all areas can be protected against antigens.

White blood cells detected in the blood are generally in transit to other parts of the body, and this movement is described as trafficking or migration. Their destination depends on whether they are naïve cells or actively employed in an immune response. The majority of these cells migrate out of the blood and into the lymphatic system by first sticking to endothelial cells lining specialized areas called high endothelial venules (HEVs) – so-named because they are lined with tall cells. The HEVs have molecules on the surface that promote the adherence of immune cells, allowing them to attach. Then they squeeze between the endothelial cells and into the tissues and lymphatic vessels – a process called diapedesis (Figure 22.5).

In the figure labels:
- neutrophil adheres to the endothelium
- adhesion molecule
- basement membrane
- endothelium
- intercellular junction
- neutrophil squeezing through intercellular junction
- neutrophil breaches the basement membrane to enter into the tissue

Cells tend to be 'programmed' to proceed to special areas. The directing of cellular traffic is known as 'homing', and this process is by no means random. Lymphocytes and other immune cells possess homing receptors on the cell surface for binding to molecules on the endothelium of HEV and other capillary walls. These receptors are responsible for cellular adherence and are particularly important in the initial stages of the migration process. There are a number of different adhesion molecules, and if they are either absent or defective, immune cells do not move efficiently into an infected tissue. This is the problem for certain patients who have a rare inherited condition called leukocyte adhesion deficiency (see also Chapter 28). As a result, these patients are more prone to bacterial infections and impaired wound healing because the cells are not readily available at the sites where they are needed.

KEY POINTS

- Both immune cells and antibodies are needed to give adequate protection.
- Any material that can be bound to and immobilized by an antibody may be termed an antigen
- Neutrophils are phagocytic cells that make up around 70 per cent of the white blood cells in the blood, but these numbers may be increased in response to stress (e.g. surgery).
- Macrophages are monocytes that mature in different tissues of the body and take part in phagocytosis and antigen presentation in order to alert T helper cells to foreign antigens.
- B lymphocytes differentiate into plasma cells, which secrete immunoglobulins into the soluble medium of body fluids to limit bacterial infections and neutralize toxins.
- There are three known types of T lymphocyte – cytotoxic T lymphocytes kill other cells that are infected with virus, malignant, or considered to be foreign tissue (e.g. transplanted tissue); T helper cells assist other immune cells in their activities; and T suppressor cells control the potentially aggressive immune response by inhibiting other T and B lymphocytes.
- Natural killer cells fulfil a vital surveillance operation by seeking out and destroying many virus-infected cells and tumour cells.
- Eosinophil numbers are raised in response to allergic reactions and parasitic infections.
- Basophils are the circulatory counterparts of mast cells; they reside in tissues and produce histamine, which stimulates the adverse symptoms experienced in allergic reactions.
- The primary lymphoid organs are areas of immune cell production and activities; these areas are the bone marrow and thymus in the adult, and the liver in the fetus.
- Secondary lymphoid organs are the sites where the immune cells circulate; these include the spleen and the lymphatic system with its lymph nodes and mucosal-associated lymphoid tissue (MALT).
- Secondary lymphoid organs possess discrete areas for the immune cells to interact with one another and to make contact with the antigens.
- The body is defended because the active immune cells that have reacted against foreign antigens re-circulate around in the blood and lymph.
- The majority of the lymphocytes migrate from the blood into the lymphatic system by sticking to the endothelial cells lining the capillary wall at specialized areas called high endothelial venules. They then squeeze between the endothelial cells and into the tissues and lymphatic system.

FURTHER READING

Dudgeon JA (1980) Immunisation in times ancient and modern. J R Soc Med 73: 581–6.
Kuby J (1997) Immunology, 3rd edition. WH Freeman, New York.

Parish CR (1996) Immune deviation: a historical perspective. Immunol Cell Biol 74:449–56.
Roitt I, Brostoff J, Male D (1997) Immunology, 5th edition. Mosby, London.

THE IMMUNE RESPONSE

LEARNING OBJECTIVES

After studying this chapter you will have a clearer understanding of:
- how the individual components of the immune system interact and deal with unwanted antigens and infections
- the events following antigen recognition by the lymphocyte
- the ways that internal and external factors such as age, sex, nutrition, and stress influence the efficiency of immunity

INTRODUCTION

The immune response is the action and reaction of the tissues, cells, and soluble factors of the immune system united in combat against a hostile invader. It is able to mobilize the appropriate cell types to the area of infection. These cells in turn destroy the intruder, while aiming to minimize the damage to the surrounding cells.

In addition to warding off external invaders, the immune system co-ordinates a surveillance network – it detects and destroys abnormal cells that have the potential to develop into malignant cells, and it scavenges dead cells that could cause internal damage. It would be a misconception to consider that the immune response only operates when a patient was ill. On the contrary, the immune system is in a constant battle with both the internal and external environment. Only when the immune response has been overpowered are the clinical symptoms of a disease presented. Thus, the outcome of an infection is a balancing act between the persistence of the microbe and the fighting efficiency of the immune system.

Healthy people have two eliminating strategies that work 'in concert' with each other – the natural immune system and the specific immune system. The natural immune system is around all the time, being activated by contact with antigens, tackling them at the same rate, and never increasing the pace. It would seem a perfect arrangement to have an immune system that is ready and waiting. However, it can be easily 'used up', moreover some bacteria and viruses have learnt deceptive ways of evading this system. Therefore, once the natural immunity has been either overwhelmed or eluded, the specific immune system responds. Specific immunity is exactly that: specific. Once stimulated, its attack increases as a result of contact with a distinct antigen.

Nonetheless, separation of the two types of immunity is really done for academic convenience, because they assist one another and neither is inferior. For example, the Anthony Nolan Bone Marrow Trust is a charity set up in memory of a boy who lived in the sterile environment of a bubble as he waited in vain for a bone marrow transplant. He had chronic granulomatous disease, a genetic defect in the neutrophils (natural immunity). On the other hand, patients with acquired immunodeficiency syndrome have a virus-induced defect of their lymphocytes (specific immunity). Either way, these diseases evoke an immunodeficiency that has disastrous consequences.

NATURAL IMMUNITY

The natural immune system is the first line of defence and includes the physical barriers of the skin and

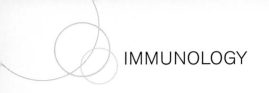

mucosal surfaces, the cells (e.g. natural killer cells and phagocytes), and a number of soluble factors found in body fluids (Table 23.1).

PHYSICAL AND CHEMICAL BARRIERS

The interface between the individual and the external environment includes the skin and the mucosal surfaces of the gastrointestinal, respiratory, reproductive, and urinary tracts. Bacteria do not generally penetrate

an intact skin, and the acidic secretions of the sweat glands limit their growth. But skin may be disrupted accidentally by a cut or burn, deliberately in surgery, or by the invading activities of a micro-organism. The other surfaces can be breached by microbes in food, air, or water. The gastric secretions in the stomach offer some defence in that their acid pH is bactericidal. In the respiratory tract, with the mechanical assistance of the coughing and sneezing reflexes, the cilia sweep organisms up and out, enabling the air in contact with

Natural and Specific Immunity: Immune Resistance, Barriers, Cells, and Soluble Factors

	Natural	Specific
immune resistance	first line of defence; does not discriminate antigens and infections	can specifically discriminate antigens and infections
barriers	mucous membranes skin	antibodies secreted into the mucus
cells	neutrophils, basophils eosinophils monocytes, macrophages natural killer cells	T lymphocytes B lymphocytes
regulating molecules	cytokines produced by cells of natural immunity	cytokines produced by lymphocytes
important molecules	lysozyme, complement, acute-phase proteins	antibodies

Table 23.1 Components of natural and specific immunity.

PERSON-CENTRED STUDY: IMMUNITY TO RUBELLA

Fifteen-year-old Jenny had been absent from school for 3 days because she had symptoms that were remarkably like influenza (fever, headache, malaise). Then she developed lymphadenopathy and a rash. Her general practitioner made a provisional diagnosis of rubella, which was confirmed with a number of blood tests. The full blood count revealed an increased number of lymphocytes, which looked reactive, and her erythrocyte sedimentation rate was raised at 29 mm/hr (normal range: 1–10 mm/hr). These results indicated the presence of an infection, which was probably viral. The haemagglutination inhibition test was positive for rubella, and serum rubella

antibodies test was also positive. The advised treatment was palliative – non-steroidal anti-inflammatory drugs for the fever and discomfort, and camomile lotion to reduce the itching caused by the rash. Jenny remembered that she had been away from school when the rest of her class were immunized against rubella. Moreover, although Jenny had received the MMR vaccine in infancy (see also Chapter 21), rubella immunity had not been sustained, because immunological memory does not necessarily last indefinitely. But her general practitioner verified that having suffered the disease and raised anti-rubella antibodies, Jenny did not need to received the vaccine.

the alveoli to be sterile (see the Person-Centred Study: Immunity to Rubella, in which the rubella virus could have been transmitted to Jenny through the respiratory tract via infectious air-borne droplets).

Lysozyme is an enzyme that is found in all the body fluids (including tears, nasal secretions, saliva, and breast milk). It is secreted mainly by the macrophages and it is an important chemical defence against certain types of bacteria that have a cell wall but no protective outer capsule (see Chapters 15 and 16). Lysozyme selectively digests peptidoglycan, a substance within the bacterial wall made of protein and sugar, thereby killing the bacterium by osmotic lysis. The surrounding human cells are safe from the attack because peptidoglycan of this type is not found in human tissues.

Despite their antibacterial attempts, the physical barriers are by no means sterile. They are colonized by harmless bacterial, usually called the commensal bacteria, whose mere existence crowds out potentially harmful microbes. But commensal bacteria can be killed by a change in the pH of the barrier secretions (e.g. by the use of douches or medicated or alkaline soaps). Antibiotics and radiotherapy can also wipe out the commensal organisms, allowing other harmful organisms to grow (see Chapter 18). For example, candidal (thrush) infections are a frequent problem for patients prescribed antibiotics. Although it is a benign fungus living in the gut and reproductive tract, the resulting invasive damage can cause considerable discomfort if allowed to multiply out of control (see Person-Centred Study: *Candida albicans* Infection).

CELLS AND SOLUBLE FACTORS

The cells that work as part of the natural immune system include the natural killer cells and the phagocytes (see Chapter 22).

Natural Killer Cells

Natural killer cells are one of the least studied features of the natural immune system, yet they fulfil two critical roles:
- they are the first line of defence against viruses; and
- they cause the lysis of abnormal cancerous cells.

Jenny's natural killer cells (see Person-Centred Study: Immunity to Rubella) would have tried to limit her viral infection, but they failed.

Neutrophils and Macrophages

The neutrophils and macrophages are the phagocytes that meander around in amoeboid fashion and phagocytose (eat) all manner of waste (e.g. dead cells, microbes, tissue debris, immune complexes). They are able to squeeze in between cells by diapedesis and roam throughout the circulation. They may be recruited to an infected area by a process of chemical attraction (i.e. chemotaxis). Efficient phagocytosis requires more than just chemotaxis, and hence opsonization has evolved to aid the process.

Opsonization

Some soluble factors found in body fluids can adhere to the outer bacterial surface like a chemical 'badge', and they are collectively referred to as opsonins. Receptors for the 'badges' are present on the surface of the phagocytes. Microbes covered in opsonins that then come into close proximity with a phagocyte bearing an opsonin receptor have 'signed their own death warrant' – the opsonins bind with their receptor on the phagocyte, thereby allowing the bacterium to move so close to the phagocyte that engulfing is inevitable. This process is called opsonization; another way of putting it is that opsonins 'make "bugs" tastier to the phagocytes' (Figure 23.1).

There are several different molecules that can act as opsonins to aid phagocytosis; these include:

PERSON-CENTRED STUDY: *CANDIDA ALBICANS* INFECTION

A woman with a urinary tract infection was prescribed antibiotics and recommended to drink plenty of fluids, and take particular care in personal hygiene. Within about 3 days of commencing treatment, she complained of pruritus with an offensive white vaginal discharge. This was diagnosed as the fungal infection Candida albicans (thrush). Candida albicans is present in the mouth, skin, and female reproductive tract, but numbers are normally maintained at a low level in healthy people because the fungus is crowded out by the commensal bacteria. However, these commensal bacteria had been destroyed by the antibiotic therapy, allowing room for the Candida to multiply. The infection was treated with vaginal pessaries and cream containing an antifungal agent.

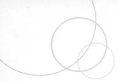

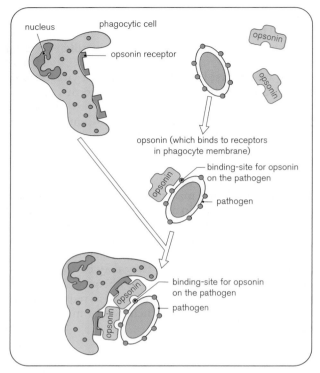

Figure 23.1 Opsonization as an aid to phagocytosis. Opsonins bind to the outer surface of bacterial cells and to opsonin receptors on the cell membrane of phagocytes, thereby aiding the process of phagocytosis.

- the acute-phase reactant proteins,
- the immunoglobulins (or antibodies; see Chapter 24), and
- activated complement fragments (see Chapter 25).

In times of stress, such as during infection, acute-phase reactant proteins are produced by the liver at a phenomenal rate, thereby promoting and assisting phagocytosis just when it is needed. Jenny's raised erythrocyte sedimentation rate (see Chapters 6 and 31) reported in the Person-Centred Study: Immunity to Rubella was the result of the increased level of serum acute-phase reactant proteins in response to her infection. Similarly, when bound to their antigen, immunoglobulins also act as opsonins, and this is an example of the natural and specific immune systems working together.

Complement fragments act just as their name suggests, to enhance the immune response. Some microbes have substantial amounts of sugar on their outer surface that can stick to tissues like heart valves, as well as the artificial invasive devices used in clinical practice. Thus, opsonization serves to aid phagocytosis and reduce the extent of microbial growth in and around the body, and to help prevent a focus of infection at the site of an indwelling catheter or intravenous line.

Cytokines

All of the immunologically active cells, whether they are part of the natural or the specific immune system, secrete cytokines (immunological hormones), soluble factors that regulate the immune response (see Chapter 25). Cytokines have a key role in the 'cross-talk' between the natural and specific immune systems – macrophage-derived cytokines can activate the lymphocytes (cells of specific immunity), and lymphocyte-derived cytokines can activate and modulate the functions of the macrophages (cells of natural immunity). Some cytokines (e.g. interleukin-1 (IL-1) stimulate the temperature-regulatory system in the hypothalamus of the brain to induce fever and a change in sleep patterns. Other cytokines may stimulate an inflammatory reaction around the site of infection. The antibacterial effects of the inflammatory and fever responses are an integral part of natural immunity. Jenny's fever and rash (see Person-Centred Study: Immunity to Rubella) were some of the uncomfortable symptoms provoked by the cytokines and complement proteins, products of her many active immune cells fighting the infection. Clinicians have exploited the use of genetically engineered cytokines as therapy for disease states in which it is efficacious to stimulate the patient's immune system (e.g. recombinant IL-2 has been used to treat cancer) (see Chapters 25 and 30).

SPECIFIC IMMUNITY

The specific immune response is orchestrated by the lymphocytes – T lymphocytes and B lymphocytes. The secretory products of these cells include immunoglobulins and cytokines, which assist in the immune response (see Table 23.1). The various components of this system are present before infection strikes (like natural immunity), but they must wait to make contact and adapt to the antigen before mounting an attack. As a general rule, the B lymphocytes combat extracellular infections (outside the body's cells) and the cytotoxic T lymphocytes deal with intracellular infections (inside the body's cells).

CELLS AND SOLUBLE FACTORS

Specific immunity has two special properties that are not exhibited by the natural immune system:
- the ability to discriminate between different antigens; and

- the ability to remember these antigens in the case of subsequent encounters.

Viruses are really intracellular parasites. Thus, immunoglobulins produced by the B lymphocytes can neutralize viruses only if they burst out of the cell. Immunoglobulins are detectable in all body fluids, where they act as an internal defence, and externally on the outer mucosal surfaces of the physical barriers. The defence conferred by the immunoglobulins is known as humoral immunity. Antibodies raised in response to the rubella virus would have been detectable in Jenny's body fluids during and after her infection (see Person-Centred Study: Immunity to Rubella).

Human Leukocyte Antigens

Since cytotoxic T lymphocytes deal with intracellular infections, one might well ask how the cytotoxic T lymphocyte knows if a cell is infected when the infection is hidden inside the cell. This task has been assigned to the tissue receptors found on every nucleated cell in the body known as the human leukocyte antigens (HLA) class I (see Chapter 24). The HLA class I fulfil a positive role in the immune response by alerting the cytotoxic T lymphocytes to the presence of a viral infection. HLA class I are synthesized in the same way as all other proteins (see Chapter 2), but if the cell is infected with a virus they pick up small pieces of the virus (viral peptides) on their pathway to the exterior surface of the cell, and they display these viral peptides like a 'sign board'. A cytotoxic T lymphocyte will recognize and respond to an antigen only if it is bound to HLA class I (Figure 23.2a). In Jenny's infection (see Person-Centred Study: Immunity to Rubella), the rubella viral peptides would have been displayed with the HLA class I on the outer surface of infected cells, which

the cytotoxic T lymphocyte would have recognized and killed.

Other immune cells, such as macrophages, engulf foreign antigens and are able to use another type of HLA, the HLA class II, to 'advertise' that an extracellular antigen has invaded the body. In this instance, the digested antigen is also gathered up on its way through the cell, but it is displayed with the HLA class II on the surface. Cells that process and display antigens in this manner are called antigen-presenting cells. T lymphocytes can sense the difference between antigens bound to HLA class I and antigens bound to HLA class II. An antigen bound to HLA class II attracts the attention of another type of T lymphocyte, the T helper cells (Figure 23.2b). The T helper cells in turn may alert the B lymphocytes to start producing immunoglobulins (to act as opsonins) for efficient phagocytosis of the antigen. Here again, the cells of natural immunity (antigen-presenting cells) have assisted the cells of specific immunity (lymphocytes) to discard an extracellular antigen. The communication and activities of the different immune cells to remove a foreign antigen is called cell-mediated immunity. Jenny's infection (see Person-Centred Study: Immunity to Rubella) required both humoral and cell-mediated immunity (i.e. antibodies and cells) to efficiently eliminate the rubella virus.

THE LYMPH NODES

The lymph nodes are a filtering network for the body as well as being one of the areas where the lymphocytes (and macrophages) multiply and perform their various functions. In viral infections (such as rubella), there are vast numbers of energetic lymphocytes, so that the lymph nodes expand to accommodate the working cells. Jenny's raised lymphocyte count (see

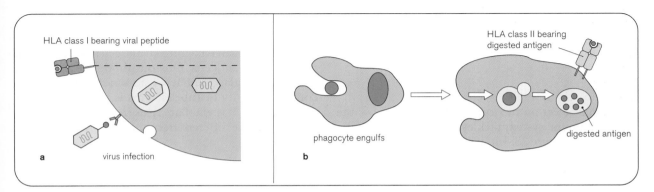

Figure 23.2 HLA class I and HLA class II systems. This cartoon explains the usefulness of HLA class I and HLA class II specific immune systems. (a) A virus infects a cell and it displayed with HLA class I. (b) A phagocytic cell engulfs a bacterium and it is displayed to the immune system with HLA class II.

Person-Centred Study: Immunity to Rubella) was a response to the viral infection, which induced the expansion of her lymph nodes (i.e. lymphadenopathy).

WHAT HAPPENS WHEN A LYMPHOCYTE AND ANTIGEN MEET?

A lymphocyte can only 'see' the outer surface of an antigen that has many different recognizable shapes and protrusions known as epitopes. There are receptors on the outer surface of the lymphocytes that recognize antigenic epitopes. Once the antigenic epitope has bound to one of these receptors on the surface of the lymphocyte, it sets off a chain reaction within the cell (signal transduction), which leads to its activation. The activated lymphocyte is remarkably energetic – it multiplies (proliferates) to make thousands of identical copies of itself at a rate several orders of magnitude faster than a tumour cell. At about the same time the cell changes (differentiates) to actively take part in the immune response.

Consequently, if the cell is:
- a T helper cell, it starts alerting and assisting defence activities of other immune cells;
- a cytotoxic T lymphocyte, it lyses its target (i.e. an infected or abnormal cell);
- a B lymphocyte, its antigen receptor (which is an immunoglobulin molecule) is modified so it can be secreted into body fluids. Thus, from being anchored in the cell membrane, the immunoglobulins are released at a remarkable rate, and the immunoglobulin-secreting B lymphocyte is subsequently referred to as a plasma cell.

The simultaneous release of cytokines regulates the cellular activities and provokes some of the unpleasant clinical symptoms that occur in infection, such as fever. Once the antigen has been fought and defeated, the lymphocytes may die. Alternatively, they become memory cells, which remain dormant but are still potentially active and able to respond rapidly and effectively if the antigen is encountered again (Figure 23.3).

CLONAL SELECTION THEORY

The clonal selection theory aims to explain how the specific immune system tackles a multitude of different antigens (Figure 23.4.). Perhaps the most intriguing aspect of the specific immune system is that it has the capacity to recognize and respond to an almost infinite number of different antigens and infections. The specific immune system is so perceptive that the most subtle differences (e.g. between species of *Salmonella*) can be distinguished one from another. It all comes down to the central role of the antigen receptors on the surface of the T and B lymphocytes in the immune response.

It is a strange concept, but as each lymphocyte leaves the bone marrow or thymus it has many antigen receptors on its surface, all of which are identical to one another, but different from those found on any other lymphocyte – just like snowflakes, each lymphocyte is unique. Thus, at any one time, a person has millions of individual lymphocytes with receptors, each with a differently shaped and specific for different antigenic epitopes. As an antigen makes random contact with the circulatory lymphocytes, the receptor will bind to the epitope with the best fit, urging the cell to multiply. The identical daughter cells created from the cell divisions of one activated lymphocyte are called clones. All the clones derived from one original cell will react to the same part of the antigen because they have identical receptors.

The clonal selection theory is an invaluable scheme, which allows the immune system to be ready and waiting for any eventuality. With time, microbes change their genetic make-up, so the immune system must adapt accordingly if it is to be a fighting force. It has taken centuries for humans to evolve and change genetically, since our lifespan is generally for around 70 years. In contrast, microbes live for only a few days, so they alter at a much faster rate. Hence, in order to accommodate these changes, the lymphocyte population provides a wide variety of receptors ready for many microbes, some of which have not yet evolved. The mechanism for the production of such diversity in the lymphocyte receptors is explained in Chapter 24.

PROPERTIES OF THE SPECIFIC IMMUNE RESPONSE

The behaviour of the lymphocyte in the specific immune response has four basic properties – it can recognize, respond to, be regulated by, and remember an antigen.

Recognizing an antigen

A lymphocyte can recognize an antigen and distinguish it from other antigens. Obvious though it may seem, immunity to glandular fever does not automatically confer immunity to rubella. This is because the cells that recognize Epstein–Barr virus (responsible for glandular fever) are different from those that recognize the rubella virus.

Responding to an antigen

A lymphocyte can respond to and destroy a foreign invader by means of its antigen receptors while recognizing the surrounding tissues as not being dangerous and so leaving it alone. When a tissue or cell in the body becomes a direct and persistent target for an

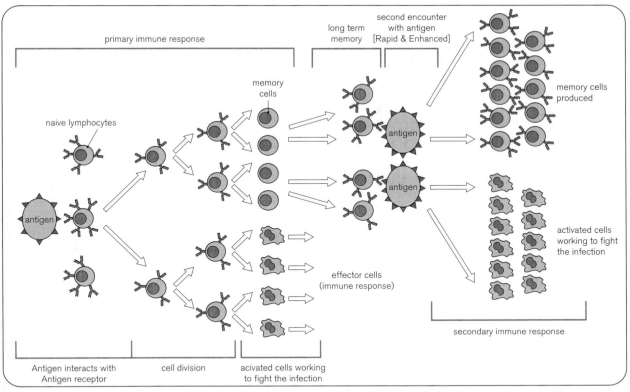

Figure 23.3 Meeting of a lymphocyte and an antigen. The lymphocyte recognizes the antigen by means of the cell surface receptors. The rapid chain of events that follows this contact includes cell division, activity to eliminate the infection, release of cytokines, and formation of memory cells in case of subsequent encounters.

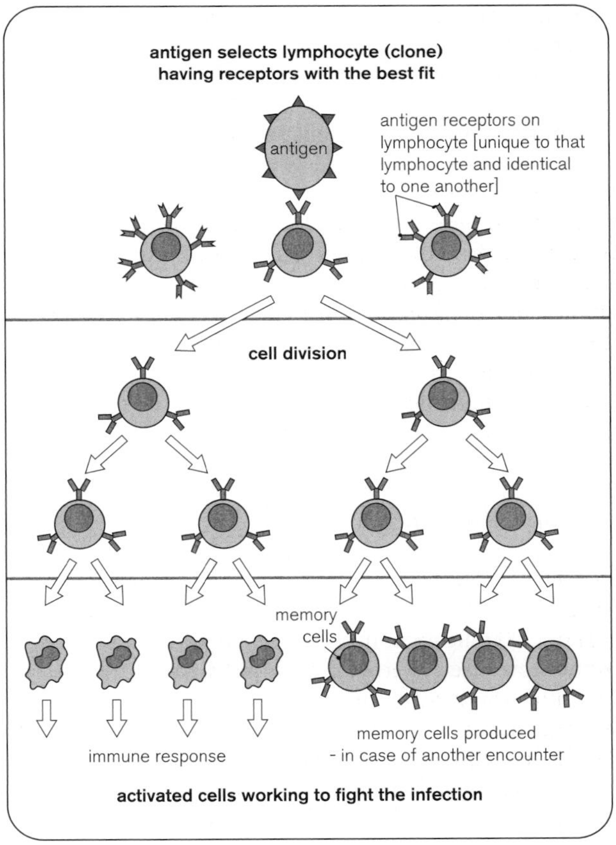

Figure 23.4 The clonal selection theory. Each lymphocyte that leaves the bone marrow has unique antigen receptors on its cell surface – all the receptors on the one cell are identical, but they are different from the receptors on other lymphocytes leaving the bone marrow. Rapid cell division when a lymphocyte encounters an antigen allows many identical lymphocytes to be produced, thereby limiting the antigen and its effects on the patient's well-being.

immunological attack, an autoimmune disease is precipitated. Rheumatoid arthritis is a well known example of a disorder that is the consequence of a breakdown in the immunological tolerance to 'self' tissues. Although the disfigured joints are the more obvious physical signs of disease, other tissues are also affected, since rheumatoid arthritis is a systemic disorder (see Chapters 27 and 39).

Regulation by an antigen

A lymphocyte can regulate the rather aggressive immune response, which declines with time, thus serving to help protect the surrounding tissues. Lymphocytes remain active for a relatively short time before they die or become dormant as memory cells. As the antigens are progressively eliminated, the reason for more lymphocytes to be activated is removed. The reduced cytokine levels and the diminished cellular activities 'turn down' the response still further.

Remembering an antigen

A lymphocyte can remember (if it is a memory cell). The first time the immune system mounts an attack against a particular antigen is the primary immune response, which has rather a slow onset, taking around 12 days to reach peak activity (Figure 23.5). The memory cells generated in this process remember the antigen and 'wait in the wings'. The probability of meeting the infectious agent again is high, and if contact is made again, the memory cells will respond (the secondary immune response). This time, the cells react with a response that is significantly faster and greater than the primary immune response (e.g. a rapid release of many immunoglobulins molecules by the B lymphocytes). Therefore, provided the antigen is efficiently eliminated, there should be no clinical symptoms. Now that Jenny's immune system (see Person-Centred Study: Immunity to Rubella) has mounted an attack on the rubella infection, she should not present with the clinical symptoms again.

The immunological memory does not necessarily last for ever, and second attacks of infections are known to occur. Hence regular immunizations are required for infections like polio to sustain immunity because memory cells do not survive indefinitely.

TYPES OF SPECIFIC IMMUNITY

Specific immunity can be conveyed by either:
- the activities of the individual's immune system (active immunity); or
- the administration of antibodies from another person whose immune system has previously responded to the antigen (passive immunity).

Active immunity relies on the immunological memory

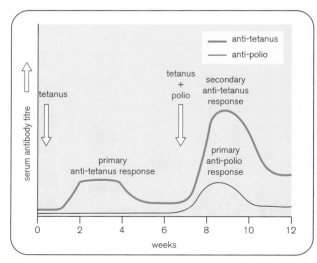

Figure 23.5 Primary and secondary immune response.

and may be acquired by one of two ways, either by suffering the infection or by contact with a 'man-made mimic' (i.e. a vaccine). For instance, a patient may acquire immunity to cholera by contracting the potentially life-threatening disease, or may be immunized with the commercially prepared cholera toxin (see Chapter 21). Passive immunity bestows temporary protection without having to wait for the immune system to become active. The transfer of maternal immunoglobulins to the fetus is one example of this, in which immunity is the result of activity on the part of the mother's immune system (see also Box 23.1).

INTERNAL AND EXTERNAL FACTORS AFFECTING THE IMMUNE RESPONSE

The immune system is just one of the body's many physiological systems, all of which are influenced by the personal characteristics of the individual as well as by external factors. For example, the immune response is less active in infants and older adults than it is in healthy young adults. Likewise, genetic and environmental elements can also have an influence on immune function and susceptibility to disease.

INTERNAL FACTORS AND THE IMMUNE RESPONSE

The Fetus and the Infant

The immune system, along with all the other physiological systems, develops and declines throughout the life cycle. The fundamental difference between the

BOX 23.1 PASSIVE IMMUNITY

Passive immunity is regularly exploited in occupational health, where the serum of an immune person may be given to a non-immune person for immediate protection against a disease. For example, an intramuscular injection of immunoglobulins (antibodies) against hepatitis B surface antigen may be given to a non-immune health care professional who has been in contact with the body fluids of a patient known to be a carrier of the hepatitis B virus. Accordingly, the injected immunoglobulins soak up any viral particles before they are allowed to multiply and cause hepatitis.

immune system of the neonate and that of the mother is the 'antigenic inexperience' of the neonatal immune system – the neonate has been in contact with few antigens. A fetus lives and bathes in the sterile environment of the uterus, so that the only infections (e.g. rubella) or harmful agents (e.g. thalidomide) that it encounters are those that cross the placenta. The components of the immune system are formed in fetal life – lymphocytes and complement proteins are detected as early as the sixth week of gestation, and neutrophils are apparent by the second trimester of pregnancy.

The transfer of significant amounts of immunoglobulins from mother to the fetus happens at around 32 weeks' gestation (see Chapter 24). Therefore, a preterm baby would have proportionally fewer immunoglobulins. Fortunately, all the components of the immune system are formed and immediately begin to mature, irrespective of gestational age, once in contact with the outside world. Inadequate placental transfer of immunoglobulins is a problem for neonates who are small-for-dates (intrauterine growth retardation) and for infants born to mothers with pre-eclampsia (toxaemia) – a defective placenta is a consistent pathological feature of both these conditions. Intravenous immunoglobulins can be given to assist, but these babies still have an increased risk of infection. Statistically, these children are more likely to be hospitalized in the first 5 years of life because of a compromised and immature immune system.

It is noteworthy that passive immunity is not always efficacious, since a mother with an autoimmune disease could transfer harmful antibodies across the placenta to the growing fetus. For example, a neonate born to a mother with Grave's disease may present with a secondary hyperthyroidism, precipitated by the placental transfer of the mother's anti-thyroid antibodies (see Chapter 27). Haemolytic disease of the newborn is another example of this, in which the transfer of maternal-derived antibodies *in utero* harms the baby (see Chapter 26).

The onset of labour and delivery are vulnerable times for the neonate. The raw surfaces of the uterus and umbilical cord can permit the transmission of infectious agents that did not cross the placenta. Tetanus has been known to be a significant cause of neonatal mortality in developing countries; this could be prevented by the aseptic management of the umbilical cord. Nonetheless, a dramatic decline in its incidence has occurred in areas where the mothers have been immunized against tetanus, because the maternal antitetanus antibodies pass across the placenta to the baby whilst *in utero* and confer passive immunity.

The rapid colonization of the infant's skin and mucosal surfaces with commensal bacteria takes place almost immediately after its first contact with people. Many natural killer cells are available as defence against viruses. The number of circulating neutrophils in the fetus increases dramatically with the onset of labour, but their phagocytic ability is suboptimal, so an infection may be exaggerated in a neonate. Soluble opsonin levels are low in the neonate (complement proteins are about two-thirds adult levels), putting phagocytes in danger of being damaged by the micro-organisms they are trying to kill.

Contact with other people brings about an assault on the infant's immune system by many different antigens. It would be folly to deliberately expose a child to someone with a raging infection, but cosseting may also put a child in jeopardy by delaying the maturing process of the immune system. Lymphocytes are available, but their responsiveness is rather slow at first because of their 'antigenic innocence' Their consequent inefficiency at secreting cytokines influences the cells of natural immunity – a young child has an increased risk of infections such as salmonellosis, tuberculosis, and listeriosis, since the causative organisms of these infections are killed by macrophages, which require cytokines derived from active lymphocytes.

Breast-feeding is undeniably a good back-up for the infant's immunity. Breast-fed infants are less prone to diarrhoea than bottle-fed infants because their gastrointestinal tracts become colonized with bacteria that produce large quantities of lactic acid and acetic acid, which lower the pH and inhibit the growth of organisms that cause diarrhoea such as *Shigella* species and *Escherichia coli*. Weaning promotes further changes in the commensal organisms occupying the gut. The immunoglobulins in breast milk have always been considered an added bonus of breast-feeding. However, these are trivial in comparison to the maternal white blood cells donated each day, which approximately equal the numbers in the infant circulation. As a result, the infant has added protection from bacterial invasion of the mucosal surfaces.

A young child is vulnerable to infections such as meningitis and pneumonia in the first 2 years of life. The reason for this lies in the non-recognition of the microbial outer coat, which has large quantities of sugar displayed on it. A child's immune system does not readily produce immunoglobulins in response to these sugars, consequently the organisms can multiply unchecked. Immunization with a modified vaccine against such infections is therefore essential to prevent these fatal childhood diseases (see Chapter 21).

The Older Adult

Ageing is a multifaceted phenomenon that occurs at different rates – some people are healthy, active, and independent at 80 years of age; others have chronic illness and are disabled. It is generally accepted that older patients seem to be more vulnerable to infection, which is often attributed to the increased social stresses and a 'tired immune system'. The physical barriers of the skin and mucosal surfaces are affected by dietary changes, drugs, changes in endocrine hormones (particularly in women), and simply by their 'years of service'. Older adults do not perspire as efficiently, allowing the colonization of bacteria that cause pruritus (see also Chapter 16). The gut may become overgrown with infectious antigens because of reduced gastric acidity (achlorhydria) and motility. Breathing can be shallower, so secretions may stagnate in the lungs, increasing the opportunity for microbes to grow. In addition, old people are often less agile and more prone to accidents and are therefore at risk of injury and subsequent infections.

Neutrophils of older adults may be able to phagocytose antigens, but they do not arrive at the site of infection as quickly because the chemotactic effects are suboptimal. Natural killer cell activity is also reduced, which may partially explain the increased incidence of cancer in old age. As cytokine levels are lower, the fever response, which is often one of the first signs of an infection, is blunted in older patients, so diseases may progress undetected.

Lymphocyte numbers do not alter significantly but their functional capacity to combat new infections wanes. It is well established that the thymus degenerates with age; consequently the area responsible for maintaining an adequate and mature T lymphocyte population is compromised. An older person at least has the advantage of an immunological memory, which an infant does not have. Therefore, provided they are assaulted with antigens that they have previously met,

the memory cells should respond accordingly; it is new antigens that possibly could give them problems. The low levels of serum cytokines, particularly interleukin-2, which promotes T lymphocyte activity, put older people at risk of viral infections (see Chapter 25). Antibody production to infections by B lymphocytes that require T helper cell activity is also impaired, yet older people still produce antibodies, for the incidence of autoimmune diseases like rheumatoid arthritis increases with age. In such disorders, it is thought that antibodies are made against the debris created by tissue damage stirred up with recurrent infections.

Genetics

The activities and interactions of the individual components of the immune system are affected by the genes that control them. Minor variations in these genes can either lead to an increased susceptibility to infection or promote immunity. For instance, patients with an inherited deficiency of one of the complement proteins have recurrent pyogenic infections (see Chapter 25). Genes have also been described that can confer resistance to viral infections. Their influence is thought to be conveyed by altering the release of specific cytokines that inhibit the viral multiplication (e.g. interferon). The HLA molecules are inherited, and studies have linked certain molecular types with disease states such as ankylosing spondylitis and insulin-dependent diabetes mellitus (see also Chapter 24).

Ethnic Origin

Ethnic differences could be viewed as an outward indicator of genetic variation. However, in evaluating the effects of ethnic origin on resistance to infections, socioeconomic variables must also be considered. Clearly, the risk posed by diseases encountered by people in their country of domicile (where the antigens are likely to have been encountered before) are different from diseases encountered by people in a country that they are just visiting (where the antigens are likely to be a novel challenge to the immune system). African immigrants in the UK who visit their country of origin on holiday will be at risk of malaria if they do not take prophylactic quinine, even though they may not have required the antimalaria therapy when they lived in Africa. However, because they will have lost their immunity, the prophylaxis is essential. It has also been suggested that black people are more susceptible to tuberculosis than white people but that they have a greater resistance to influenza and diphtheria. Doubtless, ethnic variation in the susceptibility to specific infections could be estimated in people who share the same environment (e.g. people in prisons and members of the armed services). However, racial discrimination should also be considered, since this may create other tensions that affect immunity (see below).

Sex

As far as the influence of sex hormones on the immune response is concerned, information remains both incoherent and scanty and may be confused further if social and economic conditions are also included. A sex-linkage has been clearly illustrated in autoimmune diseases. For example, in systemic lupus erythematosus a female:male ratio of 10:1 is observed; this is attributed (in part) to an abnormal metabolism of sex hormones (see Chapter 27). Receptors for oestrogens and androgens have been identified on some immune cells, but the hormone binding to them appears to have opposite effects. Oestrogens have been shown to up-regulate immunity in females, yet it would seem that the androgens have a down-regulatory effect in males. This disparity might account for the ability of females to mount a greater antibody response to diseases like rubella and hepatitis than males do.

EXTERNAL FACTORS AFFECTING THE IMMUNE RESPONSE

The media are constantly promoting lifestyles for longevity, wealth, and success. Diet, stress levels, and exercise may interact and influence one another. The net effect of one or more of these factors may subsequently modify a person's sensitivity to his or her environment by way of the immune system.

Nutrition

The physical and mental welfare of a person are affected by changes in nutritional status, and the immune system is equally susceptible. In developing countries, chronic infections arising from contaminated food and drinking water and poor sanitation may complicate the delicate balance of host and environment. Yet malnutrition is not unique to poverty and deprivation, for it may be precipitated by malabsorption syndromes such as coeliac disease (gluten-sensitive enteropathy), malignancy, and bizarre diets, in which the resulting nutritional inadequacies ultimately produce a sub-optimal immune response.

At 15 years of age, Jenny was near the end of her adolescent growth spurt, and at the peak age (statistically) for contracting rubella (see Person-Centred Study: Immunity to Rubella). An inadequate diet compounded by infection may have affected her growth and development at this crucial time. Teenagers are particularly conscious about their image and this can result in eating disorders and erratic changes in dietary habits that could lead to malnutrition.

The skin and mucosal surfaces are susceptible to dietary changes (e.g. in vitamin A status). Changes may affect their integrity and permit microbes to breach them. Vitamins and trace elements, although present in minute concentrations in the body fluids, are essential cofactors for the enzymes that drive the metabolic reactions (see Appendix 1).

The activated immune cells have a high metabolic rate since they rapidly multiply in response to antigen stimulation, and therefore their activities can be affected by vitamin and mineral deficiencies.

The thymus gland requires an adequate supply of dietary zinc and vitamin B6 to function as the site of lymphocyte maturation. Poor nutrition, and protein–energy malnutrition in particular, influences the ability of the immune cells to kill pathogens and secrete regulatory cytokines. However, despite being malnourished, people with a gut infection invariably have high levels of immunoglobulins in the mucosal surface – a valiant attempt by the immune system to limit the infection within the gut.

Vitamin and mineral supplements should be used with caution. Although excess water-soluble vitamins (vitamin B complex and vitamin C) are excreted in the urine, the fat-soluble vitamins (vitamins A, D, E and K) are stored and accumulate in the adipose tissue. Although short-term supplements of the micronutrients may facilitate recovery in time of stress, such as after surgery or burns, a vast overindulgence may diminish the immune response. Supplements of vitamins A and D that are surplus to requirements are known to promote infections that cause septicaemia in malnourished people. Many of the multivitamin pills contain iron, an essential nutrient for phagocytosis, but microbes also need it – some pathogens will go as far as lysing red blood cells to acquire iron if a suitable form is not freely available in the patient's body fluids (e.g. beta-haemolytic *Streptococcus*). A child with protein–energy malnutrition should never be given iron supplements because this would encourage the growth of microbes, particularly those responsible for infections such as meningitis and cholera.

Overnutrition may also exert an adverse effect on the immune system. Overnourished people consume enough energy to store as fat, but their choice of foods may limit the vitamin and mineral intake required for an adequate immune response. Postoperative sepsis is a more frequent occurrence in obese patients than in lean ones. Moreover, the macrophages of obese people are diverted to phagocytose excess lipid in the circulation, resulting in fewer cells at hand to clear pathogens. Nevertheless, the macrophages are activated whatever they phagocytose and secrete cytokines and highly reactive substances such as free radicals,

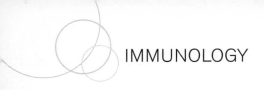

which are known to damage cell membranes and deoxyribonucleic acid (see Chapter 4). The injury to blood vessel walls caused by free radicals, compounded by the excess circulatory lipids, is proposed as a cause for the onset of atherosclerosis.

Selenium and vitamin E supplementation appears to increase natural killer cell activity in older adult patients. The anti-oxidant effects of these nutrients scavenge the free radicals that have been implicated in the ageing process. Dietary intervention has also been utilized to treat certain diseases, such as cancer and rheumatoid arthritis, and circumstantial evidence suggests that symptoms are improved.

Stress

Stressors affect people in different ways – some thrive on it while others may become oppressed. Stress may be induced by various stimuli (e.g. mental anguish, injury, pain, hospitalization, academic examinations). The subsequent communication of the central nervous system with the adrenal gland stimulates the release of cortisol and adrenaline (the 'fight-or-flight' hormone). Their effects, although still open to debate, seem to be a reduction in the activities of the immune cells, thereby increasing susceptibility to infection. The adrenal hormones also promote excess mucus secretion, thus inducing the symptoms of an infection without the presence of a microbe. Mental stress can cause changes in behaviour, sleep patterns, and dietary habits, and encourage the use of drugs such as nicotine and narcotics; all these factors may depress the immune response. In addition, poorer hygiene and certain sexual behaviour may increase the chances of exposure to unwanted antigens. Natural killer cell activities are lower during stress, which may explain the increased frequency of viral infections during stress and, possibly, the occurrence of stress-induced cancer (see Chapter 30).

Clinicians are aware that surgery has an effect on the immune system – a patient's recovery period is in proportion to the time spent in theatre and the trauma that the surgery has produced. Some anaesthetics and the blood transfusions that accompany major operations may inhibit immune cell function. Although the stress-induced depression of immunity may increase the propensity to postoperative infection, it may also be seen as a safeguard, since an aggressive immune reaction produced at the same time as the postoperative catabolic response might be incompatible with survival. A good clinical gauge of recovery is a return to normal immune activity.

Exercise

Light exercise has long been advocated for good aerobic respiration and neuromuscular control and a sense of general well-being. Regular exercise is upheld to maintain a competent immune system, especially in older adults. However, exercise in sports training and the mental anguish of competing are stressful. Cortisol and adrenaline have depressive effects on the immune system, irrespective of the stresses that stimulated their release. A significant minority of the top athletes did not compete in the 1988 and 1992 Olympic Games owing to illness – many of them contracted upper respiratory tract infections, thought to be due to a disturbance in antiviral activity (natural killer cells) caused by the stress of training. Strenuous exercise, even in the finest athletes, causes muscular damage and local inflammation. The migration of immune cells to promote repair and scavenge the dead cells sometimes produces a transient reduction in circulatory numbers of white blood cells. It is possible that the cells were so intent on repairing the muscular damage that other surfaces were therefore put at risk of infection.

KEY POINTS

- The immune system acts not only when the symptoms of an infection are present; it is in a constant battle with both the internal and external environments.
- Healthy people have two eliminating strategies – the natural immune system and the specific immune system, which are equally important and assist one another.
- The natural immune system is the first line of defence; it does not discriminate between infections and is activated on contact with an antigen.
- The specific immune system has the ability to discriminate between different antigens, and the attack increases as a result of contact with antigen.
- Features of specific immunity include: recognition of the antigen by way of cell surface receptors on lymphocytes, response by rapid cellular division to produce many identical cells for eradicating the infection, the ability to regulate by way of cytokines that control the response so that the response waxes and wanes as the antigen is eliminated, and an ability to remember the antigen in case of subsequent encounters.
- The immune system develops and declines throughout the human life cycle: the neonate's immune system is intact but naïve because it has been assaulted by relatively few antigens while in the sterile environment of the uterus. In older people the functional capacity has become suboptimal, compounded by the ageing physical barriers (e.g. the skin and mucosal surfaces).
- Immunity is affected by sex, ethnicity, stressors that stimulate the release of adrenaline, and the individual genetic make-up.
- Dietary excess and deficiencies can affect the functional efficiency of immune cells and tissues.

FURTHER READING

Asadullah K, Woiciechowsky C, Döcke WD, Liebenthal C, *et al.* (1995) Immunodepression following neurosurgical procedures. Crit Care Med 23(12): 1976–83.

Bambang Oetomo S, Bos AF, de Lei L, *et al.* (1993) Immune response after surfactant treatment of newborn infants with respiratory distress syndrome. Biol Neonate 64:341–5.

Chandra RK (1993) Nutrition and the immune system. Proc Nutr Soc 52:77–84.

Crockett M (1995) Physiology of the neonatal immune system. J Obstet Gynecol Neonatal Nurs 24:627–34.

Grant HW, Chuturgoon AA, Kenoyer DG, Doorasamy T (1997) The adaptive immune response to major surgery in the neonate. Pediatr Surg Int 12(7):490–3.

Hoffman-Goetz L, Pedersen BK (1994) Exercise and the immune system: a model of the stress response? Immunol Today 15:382–7.

Hsu LC, Lin SR, Hsu HM, *et al.* (1996) Ethnic differences in immune responses to hepatitis B vaccine. Am J Epidemiol 143:718–24.

Kuby J (1997) Immunology, 3rd edition. WH Freeman, New York.

Mannick E, Udall JN Jr (1996) Neonatal gastrointestinal mucosal immunity. Clin Perinatol 23:287–304.

Meydani SN, Meydani M, Blumberg JB, *et al.* (1997) Vitamin E supplementation and *in vivo* immune response in healthy elderly subjects. A randomized controlled trial. JAMA 277:1380–6.

Nelson RJ, Demas GE (1996) Seasonal changes in immune function. Q Rev Biol 71:511–48.

Newman J (1995) How breast milk protects newborns. Sci Am 273:76–9.

Roitt I, Brostoff J, Male D (eds) (1997) Immunology, 5th edition. Mosby, London.

Rumore MM (1993) Vitamin A as an immunomodulating agent. Clin Pharmacol 12:506–14.

Salo M (1992) Effects of anaesthesia and surgery on the immune response. Acta Anaesthesiol Scand 36:3201–20.

Shahid NS, Steinhoff MC, Hoque SS *et al.* (1995) Serum, breast milk, and infant antibody after maternal immunisation with pneumococcal vaccine. Lancet 346:1252–7.

Shephard RJ, Rhind S, Shek PN (1994)Exercise and the immune system. Natural killer cells, interleukins and related responses. Sports Med 18:340–69.

Shinkai S, Konishi M, Shephard RJ (1997) Aging, exercise, training, and the immune system. Exerc Immunol Rev 3: 68–95.

Stoll BJ, Lee FK, Hale E, Schwartz D, *et al.* (1993) Immunoglobulin secretion by the normal and the infected newborn infant. J Pediatr 122:780–6.

Westwood OMR (1997) Nutrition in practice. Nutrition and immune function part I. Nursing Times 93:(15) insert 1–6.

RECOGNITION OF AND RESPONSE TO ANTIGENS

INTRODUCTION

The success of immunization in the control of infections is testimony to the persistent vigilance of the immune system against foreign antigens. However, vaccines simply exploit the normal functions of specific immunity. Furthermore, personal experience and epidemiological data have provided enough evidence to support the general belief and expectation that suffering from an infection is one way of developing an immune resistance. This effect does not arise because one never comes into contact with the same infection again but because lymphocytes (as memory cells) remember and react rapidly when the infection is encountered, so that the unpleasant symptoms are not experienced a second time. For instance, hepatitis B vaccine offered to health care professionals (and others likely to be exposed to the hepatitis B virus) dramatically reduces the risk of an infection and a potentially fatal outcome.

The 20th century has witnessed great strides in immunology. It is now known that specific immunity is conferred by the T and B lymphocytes, for they are able to discriminate very minute differences between antigens. For example, it is known that there is more than one type of viral hepatitis (see also Chapter 34). People can be immunized against hepatitis A or hepatitis B as appropriate. Although the pathological effect of the diseases are similar, the lymphocytes perceive the difference between the two infectious agents.

CELLULAR ACTIVITIES THAT CONFER IMMUNITY TO SPECIFIC ANTIGENS

Once the outer body surfaces have been breached, some antigens remain in the body fluids whereas others enter cells and infect them. The phagocytes (neutrophils and macrophages) are indiscriminate in their disposal of unwanted antigens – they endocytose just about anything. Conversely, the antigen receptors on lymphocytes bestow them with the ability to recognize a discrete and specific facet of the outer surface of the antigen (see Chapter 23). B lymphocytes secrete immunoglobulins (a soluble form of the antigen receptors) into the extracellular fluids to limit antigens directly before they attach or enter a cell.

T lymphocytes respond to antigens via T-cell receptors, which remain membrane-bound, and the consequences of these actions are perceived by their effects on other cells. For instance, the activities of immune cells may be assisted by T helper cells or restrained by T suppressor cells. Alternatively, cytotoxic T lymphocytes recognize an infected or abnormal cell and proceed to kill the cell or to prompt the distressed cell to kill itself by a programmed cell death (apoptosis) (see Chapter 4).

Two of the fundamental questions about lymphocytes that this chapter seeks to address are:
- what exactly it is that the lymphocytes 'see' or detect; and
- how they discriminate between foreign antigens.

B LYMPHOCYTES AND IMMUNOGLOBULINS

WHAT DOES THE B LYMPHOCYTE RECOGNIZE ON AN ANTIGEN?

All antigens have a highly complex structure, so it would be virtually impossible for lymphocytes to bind to them as a whole. Instead, lymphocytes recognize a small, distinct part of the antigen, the epitope. An antigen is made up of many parts, or epitopes, so one lymphocyte may recognize one epitope of the antigen, whereas other lymphocytes may recognize different epitopes. B and T lymphocytes recognize different features, and this has decided advantages in ensuring that foreign or dangerous antigens will be detected and eliminated.

Immunoglobulins can be raised against just about any type of antigenic molecule, provided it is located outside a cell. Proteins and carbohydrates are the most likely candidates, but immunoglobulins can also be raised against fats or even nucleic acids such as DNA. For instance, the presence of antinuclear antibodies in plasma are a diagnostic indicator of systemic lupus erythematosus, an autoimmune disease (see Chapter 27). An in-depth knowledge of antigen structure is an essential part of vaccine design. Making the right choice of epitope is critical because it must mimic exactly what the immune system is able to detect when it encounters the causative agent of the disease. As all antigens are intricately folded, the immunoglobulin molecule can only bind the exposed parts on the outer surface of the folds; the inner parts are not detectable. If an antigen is likened to an unpeeled orange, immunoglobulins recognize and bind to the outer peel, not the inner fleshy segments.

The twists and turns of the molecular folds create the overall three-dimensional configuration of the antigen. The antigen's folds are like a ball of string, in that sections far distant from one another on the unravelled strand may be brought much closer together in the ball. Immunoglobulins may bind a small, continuous section of the 'string' (a linear epitope) or 'straddle' two stretches of the 'string' (a discontinuous epitope). The size of the epitope is largely determined by the capacity of the antigen-binding site on the

lymphocyte receptor (this is true for both T and B lymphocytes) and hence the epitope with the best fit binds to the immunoglobulin.

One of the intriguing features of immunoglobulins is their ability to recognize a shape of the antigenic epitope rather than its chemical content. This has certain pathological implications – if an immunoglobulin recognizes a shape on a foreign antigen that happens to be also found on the surface of a tissue or cell in the body, it is likely to bind. Then an immunological attack may be provoked on the patient's own body (i.e. an autoimmune disorder) (see Chapter 27). If you liken the antibody–antigen interaction to a key and lock, it is like having two keys for one lock, one made of brass and the other of steel – both open the lock!

IMMUNOGLOBULINS – THE ANTIGEN RECEPTORS OF THE B LYMPHOCYTES

Immunoglobulins have been given a variety of names since they were first described. The term most often used is 'antibodies', which in many ways describes their function in disposing of unwanted antigens. However, after they were isolated from serum and plasma, by a technique called electrophoresis, the name 'gamma-globulins' was used because they were found to be abundant in the third band of globulins (gamma is the third letter of the Greek alphabet). The name immunoglobulins was finally adopted because they were the gamma-globulins that offered immunity.

Immunoglobulins bind extracellular pathogens and toxins via their specific antigen-binding site. Once the pathogens and toxins are bound, their target is neutralized – microbes are prevented from replicating and toxins are precluded from binding to cellular components when captured in an immune complex. For example, antibodies against cholera toxin block its binding to gut epithelium so that the undesirable symptom of diarrhoea is avoided. Similarly, an antiviral antibody thwarts the entry of the virus into cells and therefore prevents the cells becoming infected with the virus. The antibody may do this by inhibiting the virus from attachment, or fusing with host cell membrane (as with influenza virus), or uncoating the virus for deposition of its genetic material into the host cell (as with polio).

Besides acting as a harness to neutralize their specific antigen, immunoglobulins facilitate the activities of other immune cells. However, they rely on other immune cells displaying antibody receptors onto which they can bind. Therefore, to fulfil both these roles, immunoglobulin molecules need two distinct recognition areas:
- unique binding site for a specific antigen; and
- a relatively common point of attachment that is easily recognizable by other immune cells bearing an antibody receptor.

Rodney Porter was one of the first scientists to separate the two working sections of the immunoglobulin molecule, and it earned him a Nobel Prize. He showed that immunoglobulins had well-defined functional areas and proved it by 'cutting' them with enzymes and separating them into fragments. He labelled the part of the immunoglobulin that bound to antigens as the Fab region, and the remaining section he called the Fc region (Figure 24.1).

THE STRUCTURE OF THE IMMUNOGLOBULIN MOLECULE

The basic structure of the immunoglobulins is one of two long proteins and two short proteins, known as the heavy chains and the light chains, respectively. These four proteins associate in a distinctive arrangement to form a 'Y' shape. There are two major types of light chains, kappa and lambda. Immunoglobulins are constructed from either kappa or lambda chains in B lymphocytes arising from the bone marrow, for the type of light chain they produce is governed by which genes are switched on in the cell (see Chapter 7). The 'arms of the 'Y' are formed when the light chains (whether kappa or lambda chains) attach to the heavy chains. At the top of these arms are the two identical antigen-binding sites, which are unique to the new B lymphocyte (and part of the Fab region isolated by Rodney Porter).

The Fc region is the area where the two heavy chains are in parallel. A number of different binding sites are contained on this part of the molecule; these sites are required for immunoglobulins to fulfil their various functions in the immune response. There are binding sites for complement proteins, to assist the humoral arm of immunity. There is also a recognition site for their attachment to antibody receptors on other immune cells (hence antibody receptors are often referred to as Fc receptors). The ends of the two heavy chains are integrated into the plasma membrane to anchor the immunoglobulin in the cell. However, following an encounter with an antigen, new immunoglobulins are synthesized with a minor structural change so that they can be released into the body fluids rather than be anchored in the outer cell membrane (Figure 24.2).

Generation of a Vast Number of Different Lymphocytes

The immunoglobulins are encoded by a number of genes within the human genome, and these genes are transcribed and translated on the ribosomes for synthesis, as with any other protein (see Chapters 1 and 7). Nevertheless, a special mechanism has evolved so that a vast array of different immunoglobulins can be produced to neutralize the multitude of dangerous antigens in our environment. How then does our genome,

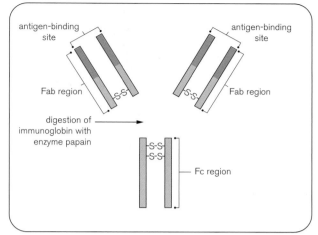

Figure 24.1 Digestion of immunoglobulin G molecule with papain. The enzyme papain cuts the molecule to produce two functional regions: Fab (the unique site for binding to specific antigen) and Fc (the common point of attachment, which is easily recognized by other immune cells).

which has a finite amount of DNA, have the capacity to hold enough genes to synthesize such a vast number of different immunoglobulins?

Many of the amino acid sequences and the overall shape of all immunoglobulins are very similar – two heavy chains and two light chains. Moreover, it is essential that certain parts of this working molecule are uniform (like the Fc region for instance), so it can be operate 'in concert' with immune cells involved in defence. These uniform sections of the immunoglobulin molecule are known as the constant region. Only a few genes are needed for the construction of the constant regions of immunoglobulins, since they have a fixed amino acid sequence.

However, the region containing the antigen-binding sites needs to be unique to the specific B lymphocyte (diverse and variable in shape), so it can 'fit' one of the many different shapes of antigens. Therefore, there is a hypervariable region within the immunoglobulin molecule for it to cope with one of the many potentially dangerous antigens that may invade the body. Thus, a greater number of genes are required to make the vast number of different antigen binding sites than are required to make the constant regions (Figure 24.3).

The hypervariable regions of the heavy chains are encoded on three different sets of genes – the variable (V), diversity (D), and joining (J) genes. Although the human genome is protected from damage by being bound up as chromosomes, special DNA enzymes move in and act on the V, D, and J genes to separate them.

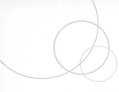

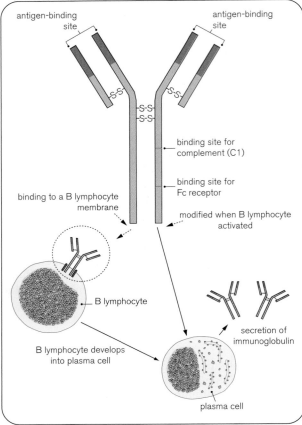

Figure 24.2 A closer look at the immunoglobulin molecule. The functional areas are the sites for binding to antigen (arms of the' Y'); the sites for binding to complement and Fc receptors (e.g. on phagocytic cells); the site for integration into the membrane of the B lymphocyte, which is modified so that immunoglobulin can be secreted when the B lymphocyte develops into a plasma cell.

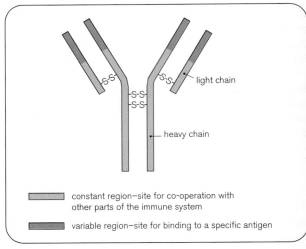

Figure 24.3 Constant and variable regions of an immunoglobulin molecule. These regions are encoded by different sets of genes.

sections where the V, D or J genes, and constant regions genes combine together. They are then decoded, using the intracellular machinery, so that the B lymphocyte synthesizes its own unique immunoglobulin molecule.

Another unusual feature of the immunoglobulins occurs as the B lymphocyte matures with the progress of the immune response. There is a mild mutation of the genes that code for the antigen-binding site. This happens so that antibody molecules emerge to bind their antigen more avidly – the mutation to the 'hot spot area' of the molecule is known as somatic hypermutation. In reality, the genetic rearrangement results in some cells producing antibodies whose antigen binding is improved, whereas with others, the antigen-binding is diminished (see also Box 24.1).

IMMUNOGLOBULIN ISOTYPES

Up to now, the discussion of the immunoglobulin molecules has concentrated on their overall structure and how the diversity in their antigen-binding sites is created. However, immunoglobulins can be subdivided into five smaller classes, or isotypes – immunoglobulin G (IgG), IgM, IgD, IgA, and IgE. The isotypes differ by virtue of their structure, their predominant location in the body (e.g. blood, mucosal surfaces), and their timing in the immune response (first encounter or second encounter with the antigen). Ultimately, the isotype of immunoglobulin produced is governed by the route by which the antigen entered the body and whether or not it has been previously encountered by the immune system (Figure 24.4).

Then, in a random manner, one of each type of gene (one V gene, one D gene, and one J gene) is selected and combined to form the gene sequence that will make one antigen-binding site. It is rather like shuffling a pack of cards, in which the chances of them recombining in the same order are almost infinite. The same mechanism applies to the hypervariable regions of the light chains, with differences created by 'shuffling' the genetic code of the two set of genes (i.e. V and J genes) for the manufacture of light chains.

The genes used to construct the constant regions, and the random selection of genes of the antigen-binding site (hypervariable regions), are spliced (stuck) together Further sequence diversity is achieved by the addition or deletion of short base sequences at the

The structures of the different immunoglobulin isotypes are slight modifications on the general theme. All are made up of the 'main building blocks', two heavy and two light chains, with some isotypes being single units and others being multiple units. The IgD, IgE, and IgG molecules are single units (monomeric), whereas the secreted form of IgA is made up of two identical immunoglobulin molecules (dimeric) joined together by a J chain (joining chain). IgM is assembled from five immunoglobulin molecules (pentameric), also linked together by a J chain.

Immunoglobulin G

This is by far the most abundant immunoglobulin and accounts for about 75 per cent of the immunoglobulin in the serum of healthy adults. In turn there are four sub-classes of IgG (IgG1, IgG2, IgG3, and IgG4). Each of these has a very similar structure but fulfils only slightly different functions and is found in different proportions in body fluids. These antibodies are released at the 'tail end' of the primary immune response and predominantly in the secondary immune response. Once they are caught up in an immune complex, they can activate the cascade of complement proteins, a phenomenon sometimes referred to as complement fixation (see Chapter 25). IgG molecules are also particularly good as opsonins and assist phagocytic cells bearing the appropriate Fc receptor. Likewise, the passive immunization of IgG from the mother to the fetus is facilitated by unique Fc receptors on the placenta.

Immunoglobulin M and immunoglobulin D

IgM is the initial isotype secreted in response to the first encounter with an antigen. It is very effective at binding and activating the complement proteins once it is part of an immune complex. IgM makes up about 10 per cent of the immunoglobulin found in normal serum. This figure includes the naturally occurring blood group antibodies (the anti-A and anti-B antibodies) (see Chapter 31). Maternal IgM is not conveyed to the growing fetus because these large molecules do not generally cross an intact placenta.

Interestingly, a rather obscure immunoglobulin, which does not seem to be secreted, is co-represented on B lymphocytes that display cell surface IgM – the IgD antibodies. These antibodies are thought to function as part of the mechanism that triggers the cell to secrete IgM molecules, for once active secretion of IgM has got underway, IgD is no longer detectable.

Immunoglobulin A

IgA is the predominant immunoglobulin found in body secretions (e.g. mucus, sweat, tears, saliva). Therefore as might be expected, serum levels of IgA are relatively low,

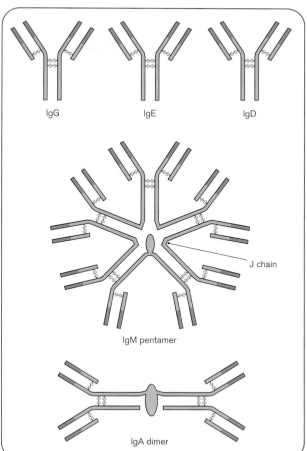

Figure 24.4 Overall structure of the immunoglobulin isotypes.

about 10–15 per cent of total serum immunoglobulin. B lymphocytes and plasma cells that secrete IgA are located mainly at the external surfaces of the gut, respiratory tract, and genitourinary system. Thus, pathogens that would otherwise breach the mucosal surfaces and provoke an infection are rapidly neutralized by being trapped in an immune complex. The transfer of IgA through the mucosal epithelial cells and into the external secretions is facilitated by their J chain or secretory piece. To a more limited extent, IgM antibodies can be transported into the mucosal secretions by virtue of their J chain. Since immunoglobulins are proteins, it might be expected that they would be destroyed by the proteolytic enzymes in the gut. Here the J chain fulfils another role in offering some protection from digestion.

Immunoglobulin E

These antibodies evoke allergic reactions when they are manufactured in response to certain antigens (e.g.

pollen, peanuts). Once bound, with a mast cell on one side and the antigen on the other (mast cell–IgE–antigen), IgE stimulates the release of the chemical mediators of inflammation by the mast cell, and this precipitates adverse symptoms (e.g. urticaria; rhinitis, as in hay fever; and, in extreme cases, anaphylaxis) (see Chapters 13 and 26). Although IgE levels are relatively low in body fluids, raised levels are a recognized feature in people who are predisposed to allergic diseases. However, IgE also has a protective role against parasites that penetrate the external surfaces. The parasite–IgE immune complexes bind on the mast cell surface via specific Fc receptors, with the result that an inflammatory reaction is provoked and other immune cells are recruited. The outer surface of parasites cannot be effectively digested by phagocytes, but eosinophils together with IgE antibodies can limit the infection by extracellular digestion (see Chapter 25).

B LYMPHOCYTES CAN SWITCH FROM ONE ISOTYPE OF IMMUNOGLOBULIN TO ANOTHER

One of the more intriguing aspects of B lymphocytes is their ability to change the isotype of immunoglobulin they produce while retaining the ability to bind the same antigen. For instance, IgM antibodies are the isotype released in response to the first encounter with an antigen. However, with the second encounter, another isotype is secreted (IgG, IgA, or IgE, depending on the route by which the antigen entered the body). *How does the B lymphocyte perform this switch in the type of isotype it produces?*

The various isotypes utilize different heavy chain constant region genes for their manufacture. So in effect the B lymphocyte selects and decodes the heavy chain genes required to make IgG, IgA, or IgE. Consequently the switch mechanism generates a distinctive change in the overall immunoglobulin structure, but the highly specialized area of the antigen-binding site remains the same. Some cytokines are involved as the signal to stimulate the B lymphocyte to switch isotype.

For example, an antitetanus B lymphocyte secretes IgM in response to its first encounter with the tetanus toxoid. These antibody molecules were manufactured from a set of IgM constant region genes, and the B lymphocyte's unique selection of variable region genes which, when decoded, produced an antigen-binding site with specificity for the tetanus toxoid. By the time of the second assault, the B lymphocyte rapidly produced IgG antibodies. The same variable region genes are required to construct the antitetanus binding site, but the switch is made so that the IgG constant region genes are used instead of the IgM constant region genes.

BOX 24.1 WHAT ARE MONOCLONAL ANTIBODIES?

- The immunoglobulins in body fluids, whether IgG, IgM, IgA, or IgE, bind one of a variety of targets.

  In the response to antigen, the B lymphocyte changes into an immunoglobulin-secreting plasma cell and is triggered to start rapidly dividing.

  Many identical copies of the original B lymphocyte are made, and these copies are often referred to as clones.

  The immunoglobulins detectable in body fluids are polyclonal antibodies because they were made by a multitude of different B lymphocyte clones that were specific for their own distinct target antigens.

- Conventional monoclonal antibodies were first made in 1976 by a genetic biotechnology technique devised by two immunologists, Kohler and Milstein, and it earned them a Nobel prize.

They manipulated cells to produce and secrete immunoglobulin molecules, all of which were identical. There is nothing very special about that. Any one B lymphocyte produces immunoglobulins that are all the same – but here was the stroke of genius. The engineered cells were immortalized so the immunoglobulin genes would never mutate (i.e. there would be no somatic hypermutation).

This is analogous to taking one B lymphocyte out of the body and 'locking it in time'. As a result, the monoclonal antibody molecules bind the same epitope with the identical binding ability (or affinity) and they never switch isotype.

- Monoclonal antibody production is one of many examples of genetic engineering being beneficial in clinical diagnosis and treatment. Monoclonal antibodies are used as innovative therapies for cancers and autoimmune diseases and for the prevention of transplant rejection.

IMMUNOGLOBULINS ASSIST OTHER IMMUNE CELL ACTIVITIES

The structure of immunoglobulin molecules is complex, and the antigen-binding sites are often seen as the most significant part of the molecule. However, the constant regions are an equally exquisite part of the immune system, for cells bearing Fc receptors (antibody receptors) can use them to potentiate their own defence activities (see Figure 24.2). Some immune cells bind the free immunoglobulin molecule, whereas other cells bind immunoglobulin only after it has harnessed its antigen. Fc receptors on natural killer cells are used in their antiviral and anti-tumour activities for a mechanism called antibody-dependent cell mediated cytotoxicity. IgG molecules form a bridge for the natural killer cell to be drawn closer and kill its antibody-bound target using toxic granules.

Two or more immunoglobulin-bound antigens within close proximity in body fluids tend to aggregate (clump) and form an immune complex. If they lodge in other tissues they stimulate inflammation. However, macrophages can clear immune complexes since their Fc receptors allow the phagocytic mechanism to be more efficient. Nonetheless, the inflammatory response can prove useful by promoting the migration of cells into an area of infection (e.g. neutrophils found in the centre of an abscess; platelet aggregation in wound healing). Neutrophils are assisted in two ways by antigen-bound immunoglobulins, which can act as an opsonin, and can precipitate the degranulation of the neutrophil to kill the pathogen by a cytotoxic process. Unfortunately, adverse reactions may also be precipitated by immunoglobulin–Fc receptor binding – IgE molecules trigger an allergic reaction if they are bound to their allergen (see Chapters 13 and 26).

The secretion of immunoglobulins must be controlled; thus in addition to the influence by the cytokine network, B lymphocytes have another mechanism which involves Fc receptors to control immunoglobulin output. Fc receptors on the surface of immunoglobulin-secreting cells are able to bind the excess molecules in the immediate area. This signal initiates a feedback mechanism that inhibits the immunoglobulin production.

LABORATORY DETECTION AND USES OF ANTIBODIES

One obvious way to find out if a patient has been in contact with an antigen or infectious agent is to analyse body fluids for the presence of specific antibodies. A prime example is the test for human immunodeficiency virus (HIV), which detects IgG antibodies against the virus. Laboratory testing is also useful to confirm the response of a patient's immune system to a vaccine. Women of child-bearing age are often investigated for immunity against rubella virus and *Toxoplasma gondii* because of the possible fetal abnormalities caused by these micro-organisms (see Person-Centred Study: Toxoplasmosis IgM and IgG Antibodies and Pregnancy).

A simple agglutination (clumping together) of cells or latex particles has been exploited to detect the presence of antibodies in a number of diagnostic tests (e.g. titres of rheumatoid factor in autoimmune diseases). The results of the test are easily visualized on a microscope slide or in a test tube. The serum immunoglobulins of healthy people are polyclonal antibodies. However, in some diseases, a large amount of one or two distinct immunoglobulin molecules is produced by one or two malignant cells (see Box 24.2).

One of the routine investigations performed in the day-to-day management of patients and blood donors is blood grouping and rhesus status. The presence of naturally occurring serum anti-A and anti-B antibodies, and other atypical antibodies are evaluated by the blood transfusion laboratory (see Chapter 31).

Estimation of the serum levels for the different isotypes (IgG, IgM, IgA, and IgE) may be requested and the results compared with the established normal range. Isotype measurements are a useful clinical parameter when investigating a patient for a possible immunodeficiency disorder (e.g. selective IgA deficiency) or monitoring treatments such as immunoglobulin replacement therapy (see Person-Centred Study in Chapter 28, and the Appendix 2).

Immunohistochemical Techniques

Clinical laboratories use commercially prepared antibodies to detect and measure antigens on cells and in body fluids. Thus, antibodies raised against specific cellular antigens may be used in immunohistochemical techniques to visualize the cells by microscopy. The procedure is relatively straightforward – a dye is chemically cross-linked with the antibody whose target is one of the cellular components of interest (see Chapter 6).

Immunoassay is a modification of this technique performed in a test tube to measure the precise level of a biological molecule (e.g. a hormone or vitamin) in a body fluid. Some immunoassays incorporate the use of a radioactive isotope as a means of detection (e.g. a radioimmunoassay to estimate the levels of luteinizing hormone in the urine). An enzyme-linked immunosorbent assay (ELISA) uses an enzyme, and a precise result is determined by the intensity of a colour change. ELISA is extremely sensitive for detecting the presence of antigens and antibodies (see Box 24.3).

Body fluids other than serum are taken for antibody analysis; one of the diagnostic tests for multiple sclero-

IMMUNOLOGY

sis is the presence of oligoclonal bands (which are immunoglobulins derived from just a few cells). Mucus is another example, for couples with problems conceiving may be tested for the presence of antisperm antibodies in the genital tract of both partners. Unfortunately, natural conception is unlikely if they are found because the antibodies stop sperm swimming up the female reproductive tract to fertilize an oocyte.

T LYMPHOCYTES AND HUMAN LEUKOCYTE ANTIGENS

DISCOVERY OF T LYMPHOCYTES

Phagocytosis and antibodies were some of the first defence strategies to be characterized. The fact that lymphocytes were the immune cell type that conveyed specific immunity to a precise antigen was not realized until much later.

By the late 1960s it was acknowledged that there were two major types of lymphocyte (i.e. T lymphocytes and B lymphocytes). Intriguingly, cellular immunity conveyed by T lymphocytes was discovered accidentally by two PhD students in Ohio. One of the students, Bruce Glick, was fascinated by the small sac at the end of the gut in chickens, bursa of Fabricius, and wanted to discover more about its function. Therefore, he did the obvious experiment of taking the organ out of chickens at various stages of their development and then observing them. No striking differences were found between the birds with the organ and those without it. Furthermore, the lack of the bursa of Fabricius did not seem to do the chickens any harm. Having lost interest in the project, he did not sacrifice

---

BOX 24.3 HIV TEST

The initial screening test for HIV status uses the ELISA technique, but it can give false-positive results. Therefore, if the result is positive, a Western blot test is used to verify the positive result.

- In this test, the HIV antibodies in the patient's serum bind to surface antigens on the outer coat of the HIV molecule. These antigens have been isolated and standardized for pathology laboratories to use in the Western blot analysis.
- The HIV antigens are applied to a solid phase, called a gel, and separated by electrophoresis, a technique that uses an electric current.

- The gel is delicate and breaks easily, so once separated, the HIV antigens are transferred or 'blotted' on to sturdy nitrocellular paper, which is less fragile.
- The blot is incubated with the patient's serum to assess whether it has antibodies that could bind to the HIV antigens.
- The result is visualized using a similar autoradiographic technique to that used in Southern blotting (see also Chapter 7).

---

the chickens but simply let them scratch about and lay eggs! Another student, Tony Chang, needed some birds to demonstrate the production of antibodies to a class of students and, to be economical, he used his colleague's chickens. Imagine his embarrassment when the chickens failed to synthesize antibodies! Rather than simply putting the experience down to a 'bad day at the laboratory', Chang worked with Glick to do a few more experiments. They went on to show that the bursa of Fabricius was the site of antibody production in birds.

A further, very significant observation was made by Glick, who found that, although chickens without the bursa of Fabricius did not make antibodies, they were still able to combat viral infections and reject skin grafts. T lymphocytes, which are responsible for these immunological activities, were finally discovered, and, later still, the existence of the different subtypes of T lymphocyte were confirmed (i.e. T helper lymphocytes, T suppressor lymphocytes, and cytotoxic T lymphocytes).

WHAT DO T LYMPHOCYTES SEE

T lymphocytes only recognize and respond to antigens if they have been processed inside a cell. Foreign antigens enter cells by one of two routes, by either:

- infecting the cell (e.g. viruses, intracellular bacteria); or
- being engulfed and internalized by phagocytosis or endocytosis.

For example, viruses must invade other cells to survive – a virus replicates by discharging its nucleic acids into the cell and this subsequently becomes incorporated into the host cell's genome. Thus, every time the cell replicates, so does the viral DNA. Moreover, this virus-derived genetic material may be decoded to synthesize proteins on the intracellular machinery (see Chapters 1 and 7). However, the resultant proteins are still foreign because they were not a product of the host cell's DNA. Consequently, despite their concealed location, viruses do not go undetected by the immune system because of a mechanism whereby the foreign viral proteins are displayed by the immunological sign boards – the human leukocyte antigen system (HLA).

Viral proteins must be an appropriate size for 'slotting' into the peptide groove of HLA class I molecules. Therefore, intracellular enzymes cut the viral peptides into smaller fragments. The whole idea of the processing is to generate peptides that will fit into this groove – rather like holding a cricket ball (peptide) in the gloved hand (HLA). Peptides exhibited by HLA are the antigenic epitopes which are recognized by T lymphocytes. Thus, cells with antigen receptors of a complimentary shape bind these epitopes. Cytotoxic T lymphocytes are equipped to kill abnormal or infected cells because they recognize antigenic epitopes slotted into HLA class I. All nucleated cells and platelets have HLA class I on the cell surface (red blood cells do not), so, theoretically, when any of these cells become infected, the infection should be detected and eliminated (Figure 24.5a).

The other major type of immunological sign board, HLA class II molecules, are not found on every cell in the body, only on a few selected immune cell types that are capable of displaying to other immune cells that foreign antigens and danger are around (Figure 24.6b). These cells are the antigen-presenting cells, and they belong to the mononuclear phagocytic system (e.g. macrophages, dendritic cells). A foreign anti-

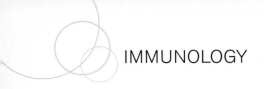

gen in the extracellular fluids is phagocytosed by a macrophage. Once engulfed, the antigen is digested into smaller peptide fragments by lysosomal enzymes. Accordingly, these peptides may be slotted into the groove of HLA class II, but they are recognized by another type of T lymphocyte, the T helper cell. In effect, by being an antigen-presenting cell, the

macrophage fulfils at least two vital functions in immune defence:

- it kills the antigen; and
- it alerts other immune cells to the presence of a foreign antigen by activating the T helper cells, which are the cells that 'kick start' the rest of the immune system.

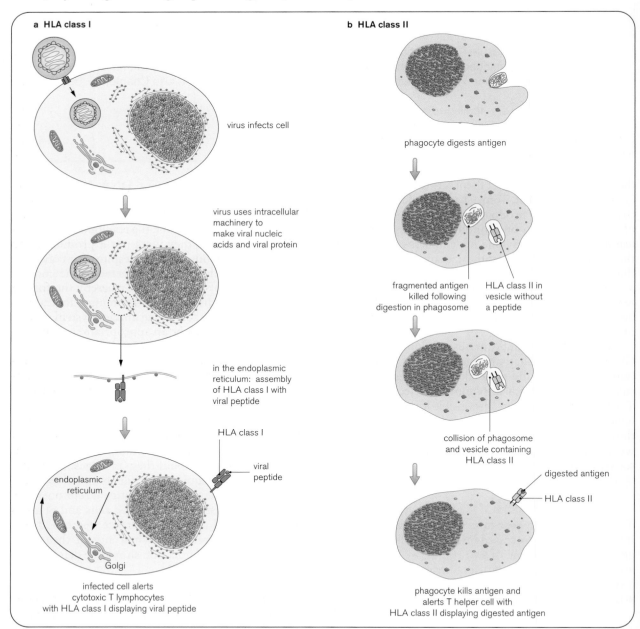

Figure 24.5 Peptides acquired by HLA. (a) HLA class I acquires viral peptides in the endoplasmic reticulum for display on the cell surface. (b) HLA class II acquires its peptides from phagocytosed fragments, and so alerts the immune system to extracellular antigens.

The Immune Response to a Virus Infection in the Skin Surface

Consider the case of a virus that has infected a skin cell and must be eliminated. However, most of the lymphocytes reside in the lymphatic organs (i.e. the lymph nodes and spleen), so they must be alerted to the presence of the skin infection. One of the essential roles of the antigen-presenting cells is to warn other immune cells of an unwanted antigen. Hence, they engulf and process the virus, then migrate to the nearest lymph node to display it to the lymphocytes. If they did not do this, the lymphocytes would be oblivious of the infection, which would mean that the natural immune system (phagocytes, natural killer cells, and complement) was the only line of defence.

The antigen-presenting cells guard the surfaces at the interface between the internal and external environment, since this is where a foreign or dangerous antigen is most likely to penetrate. Langerhans' cells are the chief antigen-presenting cells in the skin. They engulf the virus, then travel to the lymph nodes, where the T and B lymphocytes are located. The T helper lymphocytes are some of the first cells to recognize and respond to the Langerhans' cells, which display the antigen on HLA class II (the type of HLA that T helper lymphocytes are programmed to recognize). Accordingly, the T helper lymphocytes alert and encourage the cytotoxic T lymphocytes to migrate out of the node and kill the infected cells. When B lymphocytes are also stimulated, virus-specific immunoglobulins are released – this is called T-lymphocyte-dependent antibody production.

An intriguing function of the B lymphocytes has been identified in laboratory experiments – they are able to endocytose the antigen captured on the membrane-bound immunoglobulin. Once the antigen is internalized, the B lymphocyte can process it for display on HLA class II, like any other antigen-presenting cell in lymphatic organs and tissues. B lymphocytes therefore manufacture antibodies to neutralize the infection and alert other immune cells about the danger.

Antigens Differ in the Magnitude of the Immune Response They Induce

Many factors influence whether an antigen will be identified as sufficiently foreign to provoke an immune response. To a certain extent, a person's genetic make-up has an influence, amply demonstrated by the fact that some people succumb to infections more easily than others. Similarly, in the more controlled conditions of a vaccine trial, there is significant variation in the results when evaluating the serum levels (titres) of antibody. The hepatitis B vaccine is a classic example of an antigen that stimulates a massive response in some subjects, whereas others completely fail to respond.

For an antigen to be detected, it should ideally be unfamiliar. This is because antigens are more antigenic if they are foreign. Early in fetal life, lymphocytes are educated to tolerate and not respond to the body's own cells and physiological molecules, since they are not dangerous. Once out of the sterile uterus, the neonate's immune system rapidly responds to the foreign antigenic stimulation of their immediate environment. The chemical structure and composition of the antigen are deciding factors – antigens easily phagocytosed by antigen-presenting cells are more likely to be effectively displayed to the rest of the immune system. Size is another feature – small antigens are less easily detected than large ones.

The route of entry into the body determines the organs and lymph nodes, and thus type of immune cells, that the antigen encounters (see Chapter 21). Antigens penetrating by the oral route evoke an immune response in the mucosal surfaces and cause the production of IgA or IgE. The spleen is the target organ for blood-borne antigens (e.g. infection following the non-sterile preparation or administration of an intravenous drug). Conversely, antigens given by subcutaneous injection (e.g. rubella vaccine) are directed to the nearest lymph node and are ultimately likely to stimulate the production of IgG.

Devising the dosage, route, and frequency of assault is a key factor for the success of immunization therapy. This a significant factor considered by drug companies when attempting to design the ideal vaccine. The dose should produce an optimum response. When the body is 'flooded' or 'overwhelmed' by too high a dose, the lymphocytes simply tolerate the vaccine rather than respond actively. An insufficient dose, by contrast, may also result in no response. Adjuvants are substances that can promote the specific immune response – they act as 'immune response boosters' when mixed with an antigen. They are useful as additives to a vaccine preparation that either does not generate a good immune response on its own (i.e. is not very immunogenic), or that, for one reason or another, can only be given in small amounts (e.g. because it is very expensive to manufacture, or toxic).

THE ROLE OF THE THYMUS

Cells destined to be T lymphocytes arise from the bone marrow and migrate to the thymus to be made functional. Within this relatively small organ, the optimum environment for T lymphocyte maturation is provided by a number of different cell types, some of which are called nurse cells. The thymic cells secrete hormones and display HLA-bound antigens to the 'virgin' T lymphocytes, which have just acquired their T cell receptors. Not all cells entering the thymus end up as functional cells, for those that actively recognize and respond to the dendritic cells and thymic epithelial cells are eliminated; hence many T lymphocytes do not leave the thymus alive. This is a safety mechanism to help guard against autoimmune disorders, in which the immune system attacks the body's own tissues (see Chapter 27).

In addition to the antigen receptors, T lymphocytes acquire either CD4 or CD8 markers in the thymus. These markers are necessary for the immune cell to adhere to its target (see Figure 24.6), and they have been used as a way of defining the different functional cell types – CD4 molecules are found on T helper cells, and CD8 molecules are found predominantly on cytotoxic T lymphocytes and T suppressor cells. However, as the subtypes are microscopically indistinguishable by conventional staining, commercially prepared antibodies raised against CD4 and CD8 are employed to visualize them. Clinicians have used the ratio of CD4+ and CD8+ cells as a way of judging the success of antiviral drugs, such as zidovudine, given to patients known to be HIV positive (see Chapters 18 and 28).

THE ROLE OF THE T-CELL RECEPTOR

T lymphocytes recognize antigens by way of the T-cell receptor. Antigen receptors on any individual T lymphocyte are all identical and specific for one antigen. However, unlike the immunoglobulins, T-cell receptors are not secreted but remain attached to the outer membrane. To be effectively displayed on the cell surface, the T-cell receptor needs a series of proteins, the CD3 complex. A T lymphocyte cannot display its T-cell receptors without CD3, and a CD3 complex needs a T-cell receptor in order to be displayed. This is particularly significant when considering the plight of patients with inherited T-lymphocyte immunodeficiency syndromes (see Chapter 28), whose cell surfaces are bare of antigen receptors.

The basic structure of T-cell receptors is similar to the immunoglobulins – it has four proteins bound together with constant regions and variable regions; in this instance, two alpha-chains and two beta-chains are used. Contained within their constant region is the anchor for attachment to the T-lymphocyte membrane, whereas the variable region at the opposite end of the T-cell receptor bears the site for binding to a HLA-bound antigen. This is the 'hot spot' – the T lymphocytes recognize not just the small peptide antigen, but the overall configuration (i.e. the HLA and the antigenic peptide slotted in its groove).

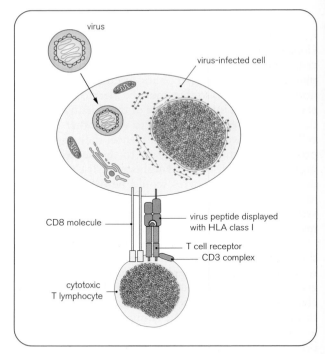

Figure 24.6 Binding of cytotoxic T lymphocyte to HLA-bound antigen. The binding is assisted by the adhesion properties of the CD8 marker.

MANUFACTURE OF AN ALMOST INFINITE NUMBER OF DIFFERENT T-CELL RECEPTOR MOLECULES

The T-cell receptors are encoded by a number of genes within the human genome. As with the immunoglobulins, a special genetic mechanism has evolved to provide variation in T-cell receptors so that one of them ought to recognize a specific antigen. However, there are only a finite number of T-cell receptor genes in the human genome, with the constant regions encoded by very few genes. Diversity in the variable regions is created by a series of V (variable), D (diversity), and J (joining) genes, which are cut by specific DNA enzymes and randomly shuffled. One of each type of gene is used to synthesize the variable regions of the T-cell receptor (i.e. one V gene, one D gene, and one J gene). Huge diversity is contrived by the addition or deletion of small sections of base sequence at the joining of the three genes or at the attachment with the constant region genes, or at both sites. The reading frames of the genes therefore may be altered by these additions and deletions (see Chapter 7), so there is the potential for an almost infinite number of different gene sequences for decoding and synthesis of T-cell receptors. The rearrangement of the variable region genes within any single T lymphocyte is, effectively, unique.

Once the genes have been shuffled and sorted, they do not mutate, for there is no somatic hypermutation allowed in the T lymphocytes. In fact, it is imperative that there is not, for if somatic hypermutation occurred, the thymus-educated T lymphocyte could turn into a 'mutant' that attacked the body rather than dangerous antigens.

THE TISSUE TYPE ANTIGENS – HLA CLASS I AND HLA CLASS II

The T-lymphocyte system for detecting and responding to foreign antigens is not unique to humans – it is used by many higher animals. The major histocompatibility complex (MHC) is the generic name for all species; the human MHC is referred to as HLA (human leukocyte antigen). The genes that code for HLA class I and class II are found close to one another on chromosome 6. HLA class I is encoded by three genes, HLA-A, HLA-B, and HLA-C; HLA class II genes are known as HLA-D. These genes are co-dominant, received from both parents; therefore the paternal and maternal inherited HLA are displayed concurrently on the surface of cells (see Chapter 7).

Both HLA class I molecules and HLA class II molecules are made up of four protein chains arranged into a distinct conformation, allowing them to signal to the T lymphocytes while at the same time remaining attached to the cell. At one end of the molecule is the anchorage site in the cell membrane, and at the opposite end is the distinct groove to slot antigenic peptides (i.e. the epitopes derived from antigen processing in the cell). The epitopes on HLA class I and class II are generally obtained from different sources – the epitopes on HLA class I are mainly synthesized by the cell's own intracellular machinery, whereas the epitopes on HLA class II are mainly derived from phagocytosed antigens.

The extensive analysis of HLA has revealed there is considerable diversity in gene sequence. Consequently, when decoded, the HLA proteins also exhibit distinct variation in the overall shape and electrical charge. Although only few genes are involved, sufficient minor 'wobbles' in the base sequence have arisen over many generations of humans to give rise to this diversity.

Diversity in the HLA genes means that the chances of finding two individuals with the identical HLA tissue type is remote, but this has a protective function in evolutionary terms. If we all had the same HLA, infectious microbes might mutate so that their antigens could not be displayed on the HLA, then the microbes would survive. Consider how hazardous this would be to public health if infectious agents could 'hide' from the immune system and multiply unchecked? The whole reason for the existence of HLA is to be a signalling mechanism and alert the immune system to the presence of a dangerous or foreign antigen.

HUMAN LEUKOCYTE ANTIGENS AND DISEASE

Many factors are considered when evaluating patients at risk of a disease, not least the family history and the environmental factors, which interact with each other. Some disorders caused by genetic mutations were discussed in Chapter 7. HLA proteins are highly polymorphic (derived from diverse genetic sequences), but each has the same function, namely to be the immunological sign boards to the T-lymphocyte arm of the immune system.

However, it is quite feasible that some HLA may display certain antigens more effectively than others because the antigenic peptides fit better in their groove. It is now well documented that distinct HLA types are linked with the predisposition to certain diseases. For example, in 1973 it was found that about 90 per cent of patients with ankylosing spondylitis are of the HLA-B27 type. That is not to say all individuals with HLA-B27 had the disease (in fact only around 4 per cent are sufferers), but this HLA-type is thought to contribute to the onset of the disease.

Following this discovery, more HLA links with disease were uncovered and, as might be supposed, many of them are associated with disorders of immune function. These disorders are generally chronic rather than life-threatening conditions (e.g. rheumatoid arthritis, diabetes mellitus). Nonetheless, not all patients with a particular disease have the HLA-type that has been linked with it – it is a predisposition rather than outright destiny. For instance, the erosive form of rheumatoid arthritis is strongly associated with the HLA-DR4 in Caucasians; however, not all patients with HLA-DR4 have rheumatoid arthritis, and not all people with rheumatoid arthritis have this tissue type. Similarly, insulin-dependent diabetes mellitus has an HLA association, but in this case two specific genes give rise to the highest risk (i.e. the presence of both HLA-DR3 and HLA-DR4).

It would seem that ethnic origins go some way to deciding HLA types, for population studies have revealed differences in tissue type between ethnic groups. One reason proposed for this is that, although the HLA genes are highly diverse, they do not mutate as fast as other genes. This has significant implications when evaluating prevalence of HLA-linked diseases in different populations.

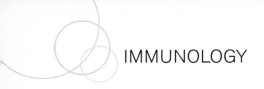

IMMUNOLOGY

FURTHER READING

Black CA (1997) A brief history of the discovery of the immunoglobulins and the origin of the modern immunoglobulin nomenclature. Immunol Cell Biol 75:65–8.

Frey AM (1991) The immune system and intravenous administration of immune globulin. Part I. The immune system. J Intraven Nurs 14:315–30.

Karius D, Marriott MA (1997) Immunologic advances in monoclonal antibody therapy: implications for oncology nursing. Oncol Nurs Forum 24:483–94.

Kuby J (1997) Immunology, 3rd edition. WH Freemen, New York.

Meyer MP, Malan AF (1993) Total IgM levels at birth and in early infancy. Ann Trop Paediatr 13:87–9.

Moodley D, Coovadia HM, Bobat RA, Gouws E, Munsamy Y (1997) Age-related pattern of immunoglobulins G, A and M in children born to HIV-seropositive women. Ann Trop Paediatr 17:83–7.

Reilly RM, Domingo R, Sandhu J (1997) Oral delivery of antibodies. Future pharmacokinetic trends. Clin Pharmacokinet 32:313–23.

Roitt I, Brostoff J, Male D (1997) Immunology, 5th edition. Mosby, London.

Stoll BJ, Lee FK, Hale E, et al. (1993) Immunoglobulin secretion by the normal and the infected newborn infant. J Pediatr 122:780–6.

COMMUNICATION BETWEEN IMMUNE CELLS AND TISSUES

LEARNING OBJECTIVES

After studying this chapter you will have a clearer understanding of:
- the mechanisms by which cytokines modify, control, and maintain the immune system
- the use of cytokines in clinical practice to manipulate the immune system
- the adverse symptoms provoked by cytokines and complement
- the role of the complement proteins in the clearance of microbes and immune complexes
- the clinical evaluation of the complement system and the adverse consequence of complement deficiency

INTRODUCTION

The organs, tissues, and cells of the immune system rely on a communication network to facilitate their efficient removal of unwanted antigens. The cells of natural immunity (e.g. phagocytes and mast cells) and specific immunity (lymphocytes) do not work effectively in isolation. Therefore, they must attract one another by means of chemotaxis for the appropriate cell types to appear in the area of infection or damage. Once the cells have arrived, the cellular activities must be co-ordinated and controlled to minimize the assault on surrounding healthy tissues and cells, because these activities are generally highly aggressive. To a certain extent, regulation of the immune response is achieved by the degree of antigen stimulation, (e.g. the number of microbes causing the infection). However, control of immune cell activation could not rely completely on the gradual decline in levels of the antigen (i.e. no stimulus, no action). Therefore, many different chemical messengers are secreted by immune cells and other tissues as the means of communication.

These messengers include a collection of hormone-like molecules called cytokines, whose functions are many and varied. Some cytokines recruit cells into a site of infection, others boost defence activities, and others have a more constraining influence. Numerous leukocytes are killed during the immune response, and they must be replaced. For example, neutrophils are easily used up during a bacterial infection. Accordingly, the stem cells in the bone marrow (the site of haematopoiesis) are stimulated by cytokines to differentiate and replenish the relevant cells for the maintenance of immune protection. Normal ranges have been estimated for all the different blood cell types, taking into account both age and sex (see Appendix 2). The mere existence of these values confirms that homeostatic mechanisms and signals must operate to ensure that the number of the various different blood cell types are kept within these physiological ranges.

The immune response does not happen instantaneously – it takes time for the lymphocytes to initiate a response and secrete immunoglobulins to a level that is effective. Therefore another series of soluble proteins, called complement, co-operate with the humoral arm of immunity for the removal of infectious microbes. When the immune complexes have been formed, complement proteins assist other cell types to clear them from body tissues and fluids. Cytokines and complement proteins are both secreted products that are dispersed throughout body fluids, where they serve as molecular signals to cells near to and distant from the cell that manufactured them. However, for cellular activities to be modified, a 'receiver' is needed (i.e.

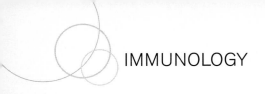
a specific receptor for the binding to complement or a cytokine) (Figure 25.1). Where there is no receptor on a cell or a cell's receptor mechanism is malfunctioning, that cell is insensitive to the stimulation.

The sequential influence of cytokines and complement proteins on the body has been analysed. Many cytokines and complement proteins form part of the natural response to injury and are responsible for eliciting the undesirable manifestations of a disease. In fact, often the symptoms caused by infection or other unwanted antigens, such as pollen, are the consequence of the cellular reactions to the cytokines and complement. For instance, fever and inflammation are common features of infection. Fever is provoked by the cytokines released by the immune cells; the raised body temperature has an antimicrobial effect. Similarly, an inflammatory response generated in response to the complement proteins has the therapeutic effect of immobilizing the wounded area. At the same time the swelling has a 'cushioning effect' against further injury, with cells recruited in to promote healing and repair, and to kill the microbes.

CYTOKINES

THE NAMING OF THE CYTOKINES

The cytokines are secreted proteins. When they were first discovered, they were classified according to the cell type synthesizing them. Thus, historically, cytokines made by the lymphocytes were collectively referred to as lymphokines, and monocyte-derived cytokines were called monokines. However, this terminology produced a certain degree of confusion when it was realized that a particular cytokine could be made by more than one cell type (e.g. a monokine could be produced by lymphocytes as well as monocytes). Many scientific groups became interested in investigating the structure, functions, and sources of these novel 'immunological hormones'. Each group that discovered a cytokine assigned it a name; therefore, if two or more groups discovered the same cytokine independently of one another, that cytokine was given more than one label. Imagine the confusion when it was later realized in scientific discussions that workers were in fact arguing about the same molecule!

The majority of the cytokines are now referred to by the generic term, interleukin (IL), and each is given a number to distinguish it (e.g. IL-1, IL-2). Other cytokines have kept their original label (e.g. the interferons) or a name that relates to one of their chief functions – for example, tumour necrosis factor-alpha (TNF-alpha) has anti-tumour activity.

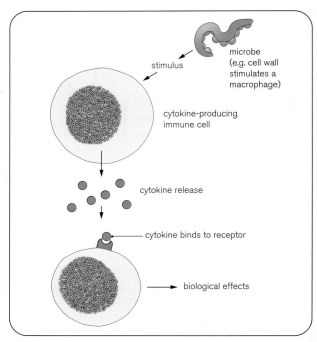

Figure 25.1. Release of cytokines by an immune cell in response to a stimulus. Cytokines disperse through the body fluids and bind to a specific receptor to elicit an effect.

GENERAL FUNCTIONS OF CYTOKINES

Cytokines have many properties similar to some of those of the endocrine hormones, in that they regulate the functions of cells that bear the correct receptor. Cytokine binding succeeds in eliciting an effect, which is generally short-lived. Individual cytokines do not work in isolation any more than the cells that secrete them, but operate 'in concert' by adjusting the intensity of the reactions and modifying the production of other cytokines (Box 25.1, Figure 25.2). If you think about how we communicate, it is not in the form of 'one-word answers' to 'one-word questions'; rather, a selection of words is used to convey a message. Much the same principles apply for directing immune activities.

Several cytokines from a number of different cell types co-ordinate the immune response, which is:
- initiated by stimulatory action;
- followed through and assisted; and then
- terminated by either an inhibitory or an antagonistic effect.

As a general rule, cells of natural immunity produce cytokines in response to the antigen's outer surface. For example, a macrophage secretes cytokines when it comes into contact with the endotoxin (lipopolysaccharide) of

BOX 25.1 CYTOKINES DO NOT WORK IN ISOLATION, INSTEAD TWO OR MORE CYTOKINES CAN ASSIST ONE ANOTHER IN A COMMON AIM

Consider the elements of the immune system employed to eliminate a parasitic infection. The cell types required include:

- IgE-secreting B lymphocytes (specific for the parasite),
- mast cells,
- eosinophils

- Select populations of B lymphocytes produce immunoglobulin E (IgE), and IL-4 stimulates the switch from the synthesis of IgM to IgE (see Chapter 24). IgE is released and binds the parasite.
- Mast cells are also needed in the area of infection, so another cytokine, IL-3 works synergistically with IL-4 to increase the number of mast cells available.

- Once the parasite–IgE complex has attached to the mast cell, the cell degranulates and releases chemotactic factors and chemical mediators of inflammation.
- The eosinophils are then recruited and, under the influence of IL-5, help to eliminate the parasite by the release of major basic protein.

Thus at least three different cytokines, IL-4, IL-3, and IL-5, operate together in advancing the overall antiparasitic effects provided by the immune cells (Figure 25.2).

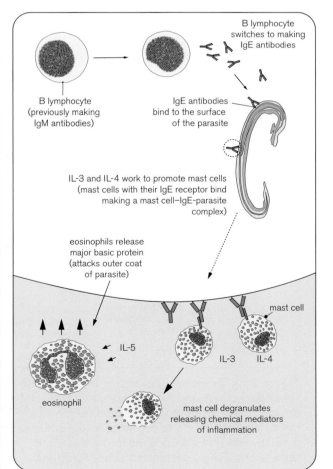

Figure 25.2 Events in the immune response to eliminate a parasite. A B lymphocyte that made IgM antibodies (primary immune response) switches to becoming a B lymphocyte that makes IgE antibodies (secondary immune response) – the cytokine stimulus for this switch is interleukin-4 (IL-4). The IgE molecules are released and bind to the parasite. IL-3 and IL-4 then work together to attract mast cells into the area. IgE receptors on the mast cell bind to the IgE molecules that are coating the parasite. This causes the mast cell to degranulate and release chemical mediators of inflammation. Eosinophils are attracted by IL-5 and release major basic protein that attacks the outer coat of the parasite.

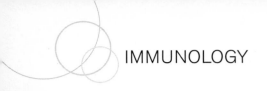
a microbial cell wall; a lymphocyte responds because it has made contact with the specific antigenic epitope that 'fits' its cell surface receptors, and one of their cellular activities also includes the secretion of cytokines.

Haematopoiesis and Specific Cytokines

Cytokines and colony stimulating factors, stimulate the differentiation of the immature stem cells. The different blood cell types are all derived from stem cells, which reside in the unique microenvironment of the bone marrow. Cytokines within this milieu promote their differentiation into mature cells. Some interleukins are involved, together with other more specific cytokines, the colony stimulating factors. For instance, monocyte colony stimulating factor (M-CSF) is one of this family of cytokines. It directs the development of monocytes from stem cells. The sort of blood cell that a particular stem cell becomes is dependent on the cocktail of cytokines stimulating the change. IL-7, for example, is instrumental in the production of B lymphocytes, and erythropoietin stimulates and regulates the formation of red blood cells (see Chapter 31).

Cytokines as Growth Factors

Some cytokines initiate cell division and others inhibit or even promote cell death. Many cell types, not just immune cells, may be influenced (e.g. TNF-alpha, as its name implies, induces necrosis of malignant cells and thus tumour regression). Likewise, interferons promote an internal environment that is not conducive to the survival of viruses, which includes the demise of the host cell harbouring the infection.

THE INFLUENCE OF SPECIFIC CYTOKINES

Originally, it was thought that each cytokine had its own singular function, but this idea has been rejected. It is now fully acknowledged that most cytokines fulfil many different functions and that the type of response elicited depends on the characteristics of the cell being modified.

Stimulation of More Than One Cell Type by a Single Cytokine

Consider IL-1, which is released by active macrophages during an infection. Several different cell types may be influenced by this one cytokine, whether they are close by or far distant from the original macrophage. For example, IL-1 promotes the antimicrobial activities of the macrophage by a positive feedback mechanism to stimulate the release of more IL-1. This is known as an autocrine response – a situation in which the cell produces a cytokine that acts on the same cell to stimulate more of the same activity. Alternatively IL-

1 released by a macrophage could modify the activities of a lymphocyte which was nearby – this is known as a paracrine response.

The neuroendocrine cells of the hypothalamus that control body temperature are sensitive to cytokine stimulation. Fever is a familiar symptom of infection; it is indirectly induced by IL-1. IL-1 stimulates prostaglandin synthesis, and prostaglandins act on the hypothalamus to produce the fever response. Aspirin is an effective treatment in reducing body temperature because it inhibits the synthesis of prostaglandins, (see Chapter 10). In these circumstances, IL-1 has exhibited endocrine hormone-like activities – a situation in which IL-1 secreted by a macrophage into the body fluids exerts a long-distance effect on the hypothalamus.

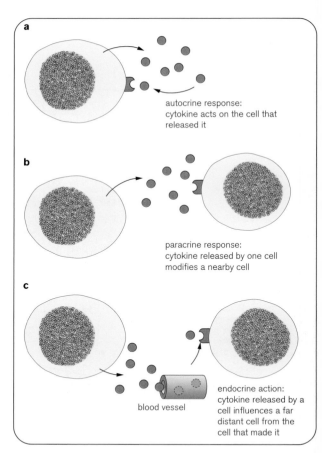

Figure 25.3 Autocrine, paracrine, and endocrine responses. (a) Autocrine response: a cytokine acts on the cell that releases it. (b) Paracrine response: a cytokine released by one cell modifies the activities of a nearby cell. (c) Endocrine response: a cytokine released by a cell disperses into body fluids and influences a cell far distant from the cell that made it.

Major Sources and Functions of Cytokines

Cytokine	Major sources	Functions
interleukin-1 (IL-1)	antigen-presenting cells (e.g. macrophages, dendritic cells)	induces fever; promotes activities of T and B lymphocytes, macrophages, and natural killer cells; induces acute-phase protein synthesis as opsonins for phagocytosis
interleukin-2 (IL-2)	T helper cells	promotes activities of T lymphocytes and natural killer cells (e.g. anticancer functions)
interleukin-6 (IL-6)	monocytes, macrophages, bone marrow stromal cells	stimulates production of immunoglobulin; replenishes supply of blood cells by the bone marrow stem cells; induces acute-phase protein synthesis as opsonins for phagocytosis
interleukin-7 (IL-7)	bone marrow stromal cells; thymic stromal cells	B lymphocyte production; T lymphocyte maturation
interleukin-10 (IL-10)	T helper cells	suppresses production of cytokine
interleukin-13 (IL-13)	T helper cells	controls the inflammatory response
tumour necrosis factor-alpha (TNF-α)	macrophages, mast cells	cytotoxicity, inflammation, cytokine-induced cachexia
transforming growth factor-beta (TGF-β)	macrophages, lymphocytes, mast cells, platelets	inhibit inflammatory response and promote wound healing
interferons (IFN-α, IFN-β, IFN-γ)	leukocytes (IFN-α); fibroblasts (IFN-β); T helper cells and natural killer cells (IFN-γ)	inhibit viral infections by promoting an antiviral state

Table 25.1 Major sources and functions of cytokines.

Two distinct cell types (the macrophages and hypothalamus) have responded differently as a result of stimulation by the same cytokine (i.e. IL-1) (Figure 25.3).

Similarly, IL-2 is known to be a potent stimulator of T lymphocytes (cells primarily involved in defence against the abnormal cell growth that occurs in tumours, and against intracellular infections) as well as being a modifier of the activities of natural killer cells and B lymphocytes. Moreover, the notion that a cytokine such as IL-2 is the product of only one cell type has been completely discredited. It is now fully appreciated that an individual cytokine is not unique to a specific immune cell type but may be synthesized by a variety of different cells (Table 25.1).

The Controlling Influence on the Immune System Exerted by Cytokines and Cytokine Inhibitor Molecules

Cells bathe in the internal environment, which is a composite of many different cytokines. Nonetheless, the stimulation provided by one cytokine does not persist indefinitely; it may be diminished by another cytokine with opposing or antagonistic properties. In addition, the immune cells have their own strategies to avoid being overexposed to a cytokine. A cytokine influences a cell only if that cell has functional receptors on the outer surface. Therefore, by reducing the number of receptors produced and displayed, the cell can curtail the modifying powers of the cytokine. The net effect of decreasing the receptor density may be achieved by the cell either (i) not synthesizing so many cytokine receptor molecules, or (ii) shedding them into the body fluids.

Another way of diminishing the effects of a cytokine is a competition between the cytokine and an inactive molecule that has the appropriate shape to bind to the cytokine receptor (i.e. a cytokine inhibitor). When the receptor site is blocked by the inhibitor, the active cytokine can not bind, thereby rendering the cell unresponsive (see Chapters 1 and 10). Similarly, a cytokine is unavailable for binding to a cell surface receptor if it is caught by an antibody in an immune complex. Novel treatments have exploited this strategy by using monoclonal antibodies to capture a cytokine, thereby reducing its pathological effects. An example of this is the use of monoclonal antibody against TNF-alpha in the treatment of rheumatoid arthritis.

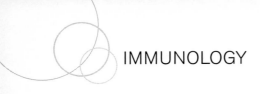

IMMUNOLOGY

TUMOUR NECROSIS FACTOR–ALPHA

TNF-alpha was discovered in the early part of the 20th century by a clinician called William Coley. Coley observed that tumours sometimes became necrotic when his patients suffered a Gram-negative bacterial infection. Therefore, in an effort to reduce the tumour size, he prepared bacterial supernatants (known as Coley's toxins) and injected them into his patients. Unfortunately, the name 'Coley's toxin' turned out to be rather apposite because it produced a number of undesirable side-effects. Later, it was realized that the active ingredients of Coley's toxin was endotoxin (lipopolysaccharide), which stimulated the release of the cytokine TNF-alpha.

TNF-alpha is a secreted product of activated immune cells (e.g. macrophages, lymphocytes). It is secreted in response to certain microbes. Once released into body fluids, it has a systemic effect and stimulates the liver to produce acute phase proteins for use as opsonins. Moreover, TNF-alpha is instrumental in eliciting some of the acute inflammatory symptoms

associated with diseases such rheumatoid arthritis and septic shock (see Box 25.2). Undoubtedly, though, these conditions are also caused by other cytokines that are sequentially released after TNF-alpha.

THE INTERFERONS

The interferons – interferon-alpha, interferon-beta, and interferon-gamma – are cytokines that are released in response to viral infections. Accordingly, one of the major functions of interferons is to induce an environment that is not conducive to the survival of viruses. They create an antiviral state at a number of levels. Interferons inhibit the replication of the virus itself and the replication of the viral host cell boost the synthesis of HLA class I molecules by the host cell, thus providing a greater number of 'immunological sign boards' on the cell surface. As a result, the viral peptides are more readily displayed to the cytotoxic T lymphocytes responsible for their demise. The natural immune system is also stimulated in that

---

BOX 25.2 SEPTIC SHOCK AND TUMOUR NECROSIS FACTOR-ALPHA

- Septic shock is a response to an acute bacterial infection caused by microbes that have gained access into the vascular compartment (e.g. via an intravenous catheter).
- Patients most at risk include:
  older adults,
  those who have suffered extensive trauma,
  the immunocompromised patient, or
  those who have an underlying pathology e.g. diabetes mellitus, malignant disease.
- Septic shock is also referred to as systemic inflammatory response syndrome. An apposite term for the infection stimulates the release of TNF-alpha in high concentrations, which provokes the symptoms of:
  hypotension,
  hypoglycaemia,
  bone marrow suppression,
  fever.

How does TNF-alpha produce these adverse effects?

- TNF-alpha induces smooth muscle relaxation. Thus, the resultant fall in blood pressure decreases the perfusion of blood to peripheral tissues and vital organs.

- Significant metabolic changes are also presented, like reduced blood glucose levels, which may be compounded if there is TNF-alpha-induced appetite suppression, and a wasting syndrome (cachexia).
- With bone marrow function suppressed:
  - fewer new white blood cells are produced to replenish an immune system already overwhelmed by infection.
  - platelet numbers are reduced, and this is exacerbated when TNF-alpha stimulates platelet aggregation and thrombosis. Consequently, disseminated intravascular coagulation (DIC), may be a complication of the infection, which is an acute and life-threatening bleeding disorder because platelets consumed in the clotting mechanism and not replaced by the bone marrow (see also Chapter 31).
- The cascade of cytokine is stimulated by TNF-alpha, so ultimately IL-1 and IL-6:
  - help restore bone marrow function,
  - induces a fever, which is not conducive to survival of the microbes that caused the sepsis.

PERSON-CENTRED STUDY: INTERFERON – ALPHA THERAPY FOR MULTIPLE MYELOMA

Eleanor, a 62-year-old patient, was being given recombinant interferon-alpha therapy as part of her treatment for multiple myeloma. However, she had suffered some adverse side-effects. An influenza-like disorder presented within days of starting her course of treatment. Eleanor was reassured that headaches, fever, myalgia, and the neurological manifestations of depression were quite common in the initial stages of treatment. It was also explained that interferon-alpha was released as part of the normal immune response to a viral infection – hence the symptoms. Blood specimens were taken to evaluate liver and gastrointestinal function (see Chapter 6) because previous studies had highlighted that high doses could have a detrimental effect on these systems. Similarly, full blood counts were also scrutinized regularly for evidence of anaemia and reduced numbers of leukocytes and platelets, in case the interferon-alpha therapy was suppressing her bone marrow function.

natural killer cell activity is increased for the elimination of the virus. But interferons are effective inhibitors of tumour growth and promote the antitumour activities of macrophages and other antigen-presenting cells (see Chapter 30).

THE USE OF CYTOKINES IN CLINICAL PRACTICE

Diseases persist either when the immune system has been overwhelmed or when the antigenic agents have eluded it. In these situations, an abnormal cell develops into a tumour or a microbe replicates unchecked. One treatment strategy has been to administer the specific cytokines that activate the particular part of the immune system most needed to eliminate the disease. Many of the immune modifications induced by the individual cytokines are known. Likewise, the types of infection and antigen that stimulate a particular part of the immune system have been broadly defined. Therefore, by knowing the 'cause and effect', ways of manipulating the immune system into being more efficient can be explored. Cytokine therapy is now a recognized part of clinical practice in the treatment of transplant rejection, autoimmune disorders, and cancers (see Person-Centred Study: Interferon – alpha Therapy for Multiple Myeloma).

Isolation and Preparation of Cytokines

The advent of deoxyribonucleic acid (DNA) technology has meant that cytokines can be produced by genetically manipulated cells (e.g. bacteria, yeasts). These cytokines are known as recombinant cytokines. Once synthesized by the microbe under controlled laboratory conditions, the recombinant cytokines are isolated and purified for pharmacological use. An obvious advantage of this technology is that there is no risk of contamination with blood-borne viruses such as hepatitis B virus and human immunodeficiency virus (HIV), because the cytokines have not been isolated from body fluids.

It must be emphasized that though DNA technology is relatively straightforward in theory, in practice it may take considerable time for the construction of a suitable compound with only the properties of the naturally occurring cytokine. Like other drugs, rigorous clinical trials must be carried out before recombinant cytokines are released for clinical use (see Chapter 8). Some preparations are still at the developmental stages because their immune modifying roles are merely a laboratory observation. For instance, the inhibition by IL-13 on the production of HIV in the macrophage and the potential anti-inflammatory effects of IL-10 for use as therapy are being investigated. Conversely, some cytokines are known to be a part of the pathological mechanism of a particular disease (e.g. IL-5 is known to elicit undesirable symptoms in asthma and transplanted graft rejection).

Recombinant Interleukins in Clinical Practice

The biological activities of some interleukins are exploited in clinical practice. Recombinant IL-1 has several known functions for manipulating immunity, not least in promoting haematopoiesis. One clear observation has been its ability to help preserve bone marrow function from the adverse effects of antitumour therapies. IL-2 is also used in the treatment of cancer; it exerts stimulatory effects on T and B lymphocytes and natural killer cells. However, some adverse symptoms have been documented – IL-2 treatment can be highly toxic and may induce cardiovascular and respiratory distress. Although the fever response caused by cytokine therapy may be effec-

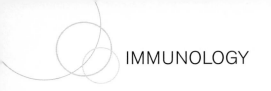
tively controlled with non-steroidal anti-inflammatory drugs, it may be advisable to discontinue treatment if there are neurological disturbances. Carpal tunnel syndrome is one of the neurological complications of IL-2 therapy. One case has been cited where the patient suffered paralysis of the right upper extremity and cognitive changes.

Recombinant Interferons in Clinical Practice

The antiviral and anti-tumour properties of the interferons are used with variable success as therapy for malignant disease, particularly those tumours in which a virus has been implicated in the aetiology. For example, the topical application of interferons in the treatment of cervical dysplasia resulting from infection with human papilloma virus has produced favourable results. Some success has also been achieved from giving interferon-alpha in conjunction with other cytotoxic and immunosuppressive drugs for multiple myeloma and leukaemias such as hairy cell leukaemia and chronic lymphocytic leukaemia. Interferon-alpha therapy has also been shown to inhibit the neoplastic cells in Kaposi's sarcoma, a tumour commonly seen in HIV-infected patients. A state of remission has been achieved in some patients with multiple sclerosis by the subcutaneous injection of interferon-beta. A latent virus in the central nervous system has been implicated in the aetiology and relapse of multiple sclerosis, and cytokine therapy that inhibits viral replication is therefore one possible reason why exacerbations of the disease are prevented in some patients (see Chapter 27). Another theory is that interferon-beta may help restore T suppressor cell activity in multiple sclerosis and so induce a state of remission by making the immune system more regulated.

COMPLEMENT

The role of complement in the immune response has often been met with a certain amount of apprehension by students of immunology. Almost certainly the fact that they feel honour-bound to remember how the 20 or so complement proteins interact has something to do with this. However, rather than learning the three pathways, it is perhaps more expedient to understand the fundamental roles of the activated complement proteins and their ability to assist the immune system (Figure 25.4).

FUNCTIONS OF COMPLEMENT

Many immune cell activities are either roused or supported by the activated complement proteins. The release of complement may promote the secretion of cytokines,

including IL-1, IL-6, and TNF-alpha. Furthermore, certain cytokines stimulate the release of complement proteins, and thus both types of communication molecules assist one another in the immune response.

Complement Proteins Act as Opsonins

Some complement proteins are opsonins and so promote the eradication of microbes by phagocytosis. This is particularly useful when immunoglobulin synthesis has not been fully established in the early stages of a primary infection. Consider the levels of immunoglobulin released during the primary and secondary immune response to an antigen (see Chapter 23, Figure 23.5). In the lag period following the first encounter with an

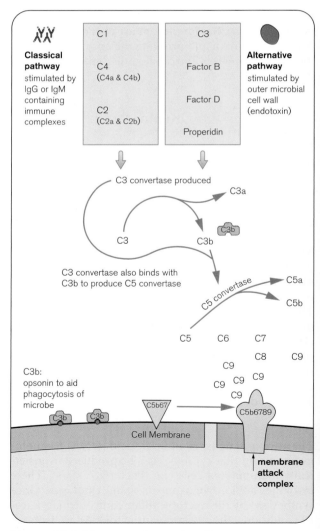

Figure 25.4 The complement pathways.

infection, it may take up to 2 weeks for the immune cells to produce antibodies up to a reasonable titre. If the immune system simply relied on antibodies as a source of opsonins, the microbe could continue to multiply unheeded and cause a rampaging infection. This is prevented to some extent because complement proteins are activated in response to the outer surface of the bacteria and provide opsonins to assist phagocytic clearance of the microbes. Furthermore, if any immune complexes a`re formed (i.e. microbe-immunoglobulin), their clearance is also assisted by complement.

Complement Encourages the Migration of Immune Cells

Immune cells are effective if they are in the vicinity of damage or infection, thus the complement proteins which are chemotactic agents encourage their migration. This favours the clearance of dead cells, which could otherwise provoke further tissue damage. Other complement fragments promote vasodilatation and vascular permeability, which further promote cellular transport into an area of infection. *But how does this happen?* Basophils and mast cells are some of the prime sources of chemical mediators of inflammation, and these cells degranulate and release substances such as histamine in response to complement binding to their cell surface. In fact, acute complement activation is in part responsible for the anaphylactic shock suffered by some patients with bacterial infections.

Complement Promotes Cell Death

Complement proteins are also directly involved in the elimination of antigens. A number of complement proteins may attack the surface of the 'foreign' cell by puncturing holes in the outer membrane and thereby causing death by lysis. Many of the functions of complement are aggressive, which, in common with other components of the immune system, has the drawback of contributing to some of the pathological symptoms of disease. Ischaemia activates the complement system, and periodically healthy cells are also injured by lysis if they are in close proximity to the 'action'.

WHAT ARE COMPLEMENT PROTEINS AND HOW DO THEY INTERACT?

Complement is a series of enzymes. These enzymes act on one another in the set order of a cascade pathway. They are synthesized by the liver and macrophages; therefore, the phagocytic cells, in effect, assist themselves by producing opsonins for phagocytosis and the removal of immune complexes.

Many of the complement proteins are identified by the letter 'C' (for complement) and a number (e.g. C3,

C4). However, they do not proceed along the cascade of pathways in an obvious numerical sequence; rather the numbers correspond to the order in which the proteins were discovered. Complement proteins are released into body fluids in an inactive form, and they become functional only when they split up into active fragments. This is a protective mechanism to prevent the spontaneous activation of complement and the subsequent adverse symptoms that would arise (see below). For instance, the protein C3 is inactive, but when worked on by proteins that precede it in the complement pathway, C3 is split into two fragments, C3a and C3b. These are active components of the immune response. Activated fragments diffuse through body fluids and attach to complement receptors on the surface of cells, or cover their target to promote damage by lysis or phagocytosis. The functions assigned to the complement proteins are listed in Table 25.2.

There are two major routes for activating the complement system – the classical and alternative pathways. These are initiated by different stimuli, either the presence of an immune complex or the presence of a microbe (see Figure 25.4). Thus, complement aids the removal of the foreign or dangerous antigen, whether it is the native encounter or as part of an immune complex.

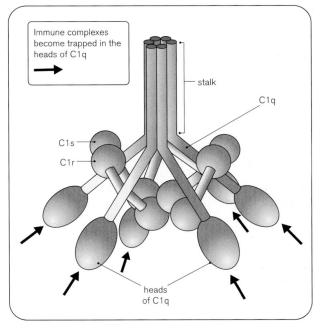

Figure 25.5 Structure of the C1 molecule. Part of the molecule resembles a bunch of six tulips in which the immune complexes become trapped. This sets off the classical complement pathway.

Functions of the Complement Proteins

Complement protein fragments	Functions of complement
C1	clearance of IgM- and IgG-containing immune complexes by initiating the classical pathway
C5a, C3a, C4a	inflammation and anaphylaxis
C3b, C4b	adherence of complement-coated immune complexes to red blood cells
C3b	opsonin to promote phagocytosis
C5b, C6, C7, C8, C9	membrane attack complex

Table 25.2 Functions assigned to the complement proteins.

The Classical Pathway

The classical pathway facilitates the removal of the immune complexes, which could themselves provoke pathological damage, and uses complement proteins C1, C4, C2, and C3 (in that order). It is triggered by immune complexes made up of IgM or IgG antibodies (Figure 25.5). As the immunoglobulin binds to the antigen:

- it encourages immune complex formation by the clumping together of other antigen–antibody structures, and
- it changes shape slightly to expose the binding-site for complement.

All this is a safety mechanism that guards against spontaneous complement activation in body fluids by single immunoglobulin molecules, which could be dangerous.

The Alternative Pathway

The alternative pathway is triggered by the outer cell wall of certain types of bacteria that contain lipopolysaccharide (endotoxin) and by yeasts, fungi, and some virus-infected cells. This part of the complement system provides many C3b molecules to cover microbial targets for efficient phagocytosis. The proteins that take part in the alternative pathway include C3, factor B, factor D, and a stabilizer molecule, properdin.

The Membrane Attack Pathway

The classical and alternative pathways share a common feature – they each assemble an enzyme, C3 convertase enzyme, to convert C3 into its active fragments (C3a and C3b). From the point where the C3 is activated, the classical and alternate pathways converge into the membrane attack pathway, which utilizes complement proteins C5, C6, C7, C8, and C9. These fragments aggregate together on the outer cell membrane to puncture holes in it and evoke the demise of the cell by osmotic lysis. Microbes such as yeasts with an outer coat that resists phagocytosis may be eliminated by this membrane attack strategy.

CONTROL OF THE AGGRESSIVE COMPLEMENT CASCADE

A fundamental property of the complement cascade is its tremendous capacity to produce many active complement fragments quickly. Once a single complement protein is split into its working fragments, it can activate not one but many molecules of the next protein in the sequence. Thus, when complement proteins make contact either with immune complexes (as in the classical pathway) or with microbial cell walls (as in the alternative pathway), it ensures that an abundant supply of active components are rapidly available to fulfil the various functions (e.g. clearance of immune complexes, inflammation, opsonization).

The immense expansion in the number of active complement fragments emerging from even a relatively small area of danger demands that the cascades must be controlled. Hence there are inhibitors at just about every stage of the cascade to prevent the spontaneous activation of complement. A breakdown in this regulation may provoke symptoms that could prove fatal without clinical intervention. For instance, patients with C1 inhibitor deficiency experience gastrointestinal disturbances, pharyngeal oedema, and respiratory distress when they suffer an acute attack (see below).

In healthy people, the inhibitors protect normal, healthy cells from complement lysis caused by 'friendly fire' in the immune response. But some pathogens have evolved mechanisms to block the lethal effects of complement by displaying molecules on the outer coat that mimic the complement inhibitors and regulators. This is a survival tactic that has also been demonstrated by some tumours, which attempt to evade the adverse attack by complement.

COMPLEMENT RECEPTORS IN HEALTH AND DISEASE

Cells with the appropriate receptors are able to work 'in concert' with the complement in the immunological defence. For example, red blood cells are invaluable for clearing immune complexes from body fluids and tissues by virtue of their cell surface complement receptors. The coating of immune complexes with complement proteins of the classical pathway provides a point of contact for attachment to red blood cells (i.e. immune complex–complement–red blood cell). However, this has a negative effect, for in 'shepherding' immune complexes to the spleen, red blood cells are rendered useless and so removed from the circulation. Some other immune cells (e.g. natural killer cells, mast cells) have their activities enhanced by complement.

Genetic disorders of the complement receptors bear witness to their valuable contribution to immunity. One complication that presents in patients with leukocyte adhesion deficiency is a reduced number of functional complement receptors; consequently, these patients suffer recurrent bouts of infections. However, certain complement receptors are not always beneficial to immunity, particularly when they are used by microbes. One example of this is seen in infectious mononucleosis, which results from the Epstein–Barr virus (EBV) infection. The EBV binds to cell surface complement receptors and infects the B lymphocytes.

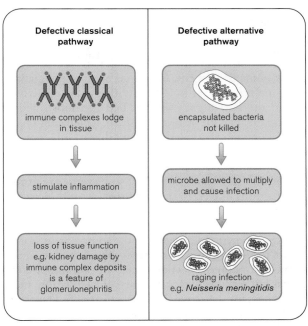

Figure 25.6 Defects in the complement pathways. Deficiency in proteins of the classical pathway results in excess immune complexes which deposit in tissue, leading to inflammation and loss of function. Deficiency in proteins of the alternative pathway result in decreased ability to combat encapsulated microbial infections.

DISORDERS OF COMPLEMENT

Genetic disorders of complement are comparatively rare, for they leave the patients open to infections and often lead to disorders which are potentially fatal. Diseases may arise when a complement deficiency is provoked because the proteins are used up more rapidly than they are synthesized. Generally, patients with disorders of the classical pathways do not seem to suffer recurrent infections. Instead, systemic lupus erythematosus-like disorders arise in patients with deficiency of one or more of the complement proteins in the classical pathway (e.g. C2, C4). One explanation for this is the decreased ability of these patients to clear immune complexes from body tissues. However, cause and effect is rather difficult to disentangle here, for more that half of the patients diagnosed with C2 and C4 deficiency also have systemic lupus erythematosus or some other autoimmune disease in which excess immune complex formation is part of the aetiology of their disorder (Figure 25.6, see also Box 25.3). In other words, is there really a complement deficiency, or has this mechanism for removing immune complexes been overwhelmed?

BOX 25.3 GLOMERULONEPHRITIS

Glomerulonephritis, a major renal disease, may be caused by immune complexes being formed more quickly than they can be cleared. Some patients suffer this disorder because they have developed nephritic factor, which is an antibody against complement fragments.

- The antigenic target of the nephritic factor is the C3 convertase enzyme of the alternative pathway.
- Binding of the antibody (nephritic factor) to its antigen (C3 convertase) results in the enzyme being stabilized and encourages the split of the C3 protein into its active fragments
- The complement pathways are perpetuated, leading to the formation of many active fragments, e.g. C3a and C3b
- Damage to the nephrons follows because the excess immune complexes are deposited in the kidney, and the many active C3a fragments released are potent inflammatory mediators.

Genetic deficiencies of one or more of the proteins in the alternative pathway lead to an increased susceptibility to the kind of infections that this part of the immune system controls. Therefore, patients suffer frequent bouts of pyogenic infections because phagocytosis is inefficient. It is noteworthy that reduced activity of the alternative pathway has been demonstrated in some patients with sickle cell disease, which could partly explain their increased susceptibility to infections.

In patients in whom the membrane attack pathway is compromised, the ability to deal with encapsulated bacterial infections is impaired, so patients are at risk of infections like *Neisseria meningitidis* and *Neisseria gonorrhoeae*, (see Chapters 15 and 16).

The regulatory mechanisms are essential to keep the pathways functional; otherwise the complement system could 'race along' and then the proteins would be rapidly used up. Moreover, when a microbe or immune complex is not responsible for complement activation, there is nowhere for the active fragments to attach. Therefore, the active fragments are inactivated within the body fluids, though this can leave the patient deficient of complement proteins and at risk of infections.

Hereditary Angioneurotic Oedema

In this scenario, a surplus of active complement fragments elicits adverse symptoms when they settle on healthy tissues. Hereditary angioneurotic oedema is an inherited deficiency of the C1 inhibitor that leads to uncontrolled activation of the classical pathway. Excess active complement fragments are released causing vasodilation and vascular permeability that results in inflammation and oedema. The symptoms of an attack, which include gastrointestinal disturbances, may persist for up to 72 hours. Any resultant oedema to the pharynx can cause obstruction to the airways, respiratory distress, and even death. Danazol (a drug often used to treat women with endometriosis) and methyltestosterone have been used in treatment, because they seem to stimulate the synthesis of C1 inhibitor and so reduce the incidence of relapse of the adverse symptoms. Attacks may be provoked at any time; but they are often induced by stress. These patients need to find ways of preventing an exacerbation of the symptoms.

Paroxysmal Nocturnal Haemoglobinuria

Complement regulators are attached to the outer membrane via an 'anchor'. Sometimes an inadequate supply of complement regulators arises, not because of a deficiency of the complement regulators as such, but because of the cell's inability to produce the anchor for its attachment on the cell. Patients with paroxysmal nocturnal haemoglobinuria have a genetic disorder – they lack the ability to make the membrane anchor that red blood cells use to display complement regulators. Most cells have a choice of anchor, but red blood cells produce only one type. Therefore, they are particularly vulnerable to complement-induced lysis, which leads to a haemolytic anaemia. Fortunately this is a comparatively rare disorder.

KEY POINTS

- Cytokines modify the immune system in a variety of ways, such as recruiting other cell types, stimulating haematopoiesis, and controlling immune cell activities.
- The functions of cytokines vary and the reactions provoked by cytokines depend on the cell type they are modifying.
- Tumour necrosis factor-alpha is a cytokine released in high concentration during an acute Gram-negative bacterial infection. It is responsible for many of the adverse symptoms of septic shock (e.g. hypotension, hypoglycaemia, thrombosis, disseminated intravascular coagulation, and bone marrow suppression).
- Recombinant cytokines are used to manipulate the immune system into being more efficient against diseases like cancer. However, in the initial stages of treatment, influenza-like symptoms may be elicited when administering interferon therapy.
- Complement is a series of proteins that proceed along a cascade of pathways. They have an integral role in the clearance of immune complexes and in the provision of many opsonins for the efficient phagocytic clearance of microbes.
- This system is highly aggressive and must be controlled; therefore, there are regulators at just about every stage of the complement pathways.
- The complement system may be assessed by screening tests for the pathways and estimations of individual complement proteins. Evaluation of the complement status is advised for patients who suffer recurrent bacterial infection or have a disorder that results in excess production of immune complexes (e.g. systemic lupus erythematosus).

Investigation of Complement Defects

Healthy people synthesize far more complement proteins than they actually need. Therefore, even if serum complement levels are below the normal range, it does not necessarily follow that the patient is at risk of infections; in fact they may well be asymptomatic. Clinical laboratory tests are available to evaluate the major pathways in the complement cascade. The CH50 test is used for investigating functional efficiency of the classical and membrane attack pathways. A screening test, the AP50 test, is also available for the alternative and membrane attack pathways. When an abnormality is exposed in either the CH50 or AP50 tests, then measurement of the individual complement proteins may be advised.

For instance, an abnormal CH50 test with low levels of C4 detected suggests that the classical pathway is 'racing along'. One possible explanation is an uncontrolled activation caused by reduced C1 inhibitor activity (as found in hereditary angioneurotic oedema; see above). It is worth regularly monitoring the plasma levels of complement proteins in the classical pathway in a patient with systemic lupus erythematosus, and others with disorders that generate large amounts of immune complexes, because the complement proteins are rapidly consumed in such conditions. Likewise, a complement deficiency should be investigated when a child or adolescent presents with recurrent bacterial infections such *Haemophilus influenzae* infections, sepsis, or infections with an encapsulated organism. This would indicate the need to investigate a possible defect in the alternative and membrane attack pathway of complement.

FURTHER READING

Adams DH, Lloyd, AR (1997) Chemokines: leucocyte recruitment and activation cytokines. Lancet 349:490–5.

Ahmed AE, Peter JB (1995) Clinical utility of complement assessment. Clin Diagn Lab Immunol 2:509–17.

Arend WP (1995) Inhibiting the effects of cytokines in human diseases. Adv Intern Med 40:365–94.

Aulitzky WE, Schuler M, Peschel C, Huber C (1994) Interleukins. Clinical pharmacology and therapeutic use. Drugs 48:667–77.

Boothman BR (1997) Interferon beta: the current position. Br J Hosp Med 57:277–9.

Caruso C, Candore G, Cigna D, et al. (1996) Cytokine production pathway in the elderly. Immunol Res 15:84–90.

Cornelis F, Montfort L, Osselaer JC, et al. (1996) Acute leukaemia in paroxysmal nocturnal haemoglobinuria. Case report and review of the literature. Hematol Cell Ther 38:285–8.

Fridman WH, Tartour E (1997) Cytokines and cell regulation. Mol Med 18:3–90.

Hecke F, Schmidt U, Kola A, Bautsch W, et al. (1997) Circulating complement proteins in multiple trauma patients – correlation with injury severity, development of sepsis, and outcome. Crit Care Med 25:2015–24.

Henderson B (1995)Therapeutic modulation of cytokines. Ann Rheum Dis 54:519–23.

Heyman B (1996) Complement and Fc-receptors in regulation of the antibody response. Immunol Lett 54:195–9.

Holden RJ, Pakula IS (1996) The role of tumor necrosis factor-alpha in the pathogenesis of anorexia and bulimia nervosa, cancer cachexia and obesity. Med Hypotheses 47:423–38.

Keating MM, Ostby PL (1996) Education and self-management of interferon beta-1b therapy for multiple sclerosis. J Neurosci Nurs 28:350–2.

Letizia M, Conway AM (1996) Interleukin-2 therapy for renal cell cancer: indications, effects, and nursing implications. Crit Care Nurs 16(5):20–6.

Lokki ML, Colten HR (1995) Genetic deficiencies of complement. Ann Med 27:451–9.

Mendell JR, Garcha TS, Kissel JT (1996) The immunopathogenic role of complement in human muscle disease. Curr Opin Neuro 9:226–34.

Michel M, Vincent F, Sigal R, et al. (1995) Cerebral vasculitis after interleukin-2 therapy for renal cell carcinoma. J Immunother Emphasis Tumor Immunol 18:124–6.

Morgan BP (1995) Physiology and pathophysiology of complement: progress and trends. Crit Rev Clin Lab Sci 32:265–98.

Neurath MF, Meyer zum Buschenfelde KH (1996) Protective and pathogenic roles of cytokines in inflammatory bowel diseases. J Invest Med 44:516–21.

Poignet JL, Degos F, Bouchardeau F, Chauveau P, Courouce AM (1995) Complete response to interferon-alpha for acute hepatitis C after needlestick injury in a hemodialysis nurse. J Hepatol 23:740–1.

Raymond BA, Haney PE, Gimesky J (1994) Interleukin-2 therapy: needs of the patient in a critical care setting. Crit Care Nurs 14(6):47–53.

Puduvalli VK, Sella A, Austin SG, Forman AD (1996) Carpal tunnel syndrome associated with interleukin-2 therapy. Cancer 77(6):1189–92.

Ratnoff WD (1996) Inherited deficiencies of complement in rheumatic diseases. Rheum Dis Clin North Am 22:75–94.

Sheeran P, Hall GM (1997) Cytokines in anaesthesia. Br J Anaesth 78:201–19.

Walport MJ, Davies KA, Morley BJ, Botto M (1997) Complement deficiency and autoimmunity. Ann N Y Acad Sci 815:267–81.

Ward PA (1996) Role of complement, chemokines, and regulatory cytokines in acute lung injury. Ann N Y Acad Sci 796:104–12.

Ward PA (1997). Recruitment of inflammatory cells into lung: roles of cytokines, adhesion molecules, and complement. J Lab Clin Med 129:400–4.

Williams CD, Linch DC (1997) Interferon alfa-2a. Br J Hos Med 57(9):436–9.

Zilow G, Zilow EP, Burger R, Linderkamp O (1993) Complement activation in newborn infants with early onset infection. Pediatr Res 34:199–203.

ALLERGY AND OTHER HYPERSENSITIVITY REACTIONS

LEARNING OBJECTIVES

After studying this chapter you will have a clearer understanding of:
- how and why an allergic reaction may present abruptly in an otherwise healthy person
- the investigative clinical tests, the possible treatments, and their limitations
- the differences in the immunological mechanisms that precipitate hypersensitivity types II, III, and IV and their significance in the clinical setting
- the characteristic features that may predispose a patient to a hypersensitivity reaction

INTRODUCTION

Hypersensitivity reactions represent the exaggerated or inappropriate activities mounted by immune system against an antigen. There are four types of hypersensitivity – type I, II, III, and IV. These were classified according to the type of immunological mechanism operating in the response – types I, II, and III reactions are caused by antibodies, whereas the type IV reaction is elicited by T lymphocytes. The pathological manifestations are generally experienced following the second or subsequent encounter with the offending antigen. Often, the tissue damage sustained seems incongruous when evaluating the antigen responsible – what is so dangerous about penicillin, pollen, or a simple insect bite? Yet each of these can stimulate an allergic reaction (also known as type I hypersensitivity), in which the symptoms range from an uncomfortable rash to the serious medical emergency of systemic anaphylaxis.

Other hypersensitivity reactions include the inappropriate immune response mounted to the patient's own otherwise healthy tissues in autoimmune disorders. Likewise, the haemolysis and other symptoms of a blood transfusion reaction seem ironic, considering the transfusion is given as replacement therapy for anaemia or blood loss. Yet the disease processes that cause the tissue injury in hypersensitivity are the same ones employed by the immune system to protect against pathogenic organisms. This chapter seeks to explain some of these mechanisms and the aetiological factors that precipitate them.

TYPE I HYPERSENSITIVITY (ALLERGIC) REACTIONS

Allergic reactions may arise when the immune system responds to an antigen by producing immunoglobulin E (IgE). The antigens that stimulate an allergic reaction are referred to as allergens. Pollen and nuts are well known examples of seemingly harmless antigens; some patients are allergic to antimicrobial drugs such as penicillin (see Chapter 13).

In the events preceding an allergic response, the immune cells are primed or sensitized because they have recognized and responded to the allergen in a previous encounter. Nevertheless, when the allergic response first presents, it invariably comes as a surprise since no such reaction was experienced in the past. An example of this is the patient who finds his or her skin covered in hives within hours of taking a second dose of penicillin because the drug had previously been perceived as dangerous by the immune system.

In some ways, allergy might be considered an aberration of nature and evolution, since IgE antibodies are also part of the antiparasitic response. Although people in developed countries are not generally infected by such pathogens, at least one-third of people living in developing countries are. As with many parasitic organisms, allergens often arise from the external environment and breach the physical barriers (the skin and mucosal surfaces). Many symptoms of allergy are therefore induced in organs such as the respiratory tract, gut, and skin; examples include rhinitis, shortness of breath, gastrointestinal disturbances, and hives. Once these surfaces have been penetrated, the allergen is transported to the spleen or the nearest lymph nodes, where the immune cells associated with the allergic reaction reside.

THE MECHANISM OF AN ALLERGIC REACTION

Consider the four major immune cell types involved in the allergic response: they include antigen-presenting cells, T helper cells, IgE-secreting B lymphocytes directed against the specific allergen, and mast cells. Now take the example of the college student who abruptly develops an allergy to peanuts. An alarming event, particularly if he or she has regularly consumed peanuts in the past without suffering any adverse symptoms. *So why did the allergy occur?*

On one of the occasions when peanuts were eaten before the allergic response, some undigested peanut protein breached the gut barrier and was engulfed by the antigen-presenting cells in the vicinity. After phagocytosis, the peanut allergen was processed and displayed on the HLA class II for recognition by T helper cells. The T helper cells then activated the B lymphocytes in an adjacent area of the lymph node to secrete the unique immunoglobulin that was able to bind the allergen. (This was essentially the primary response, and the IgM antibodies released do not elicit the allergic reaction.)

On the occasion when peanuts were eaten and the student suffered the allergic reaction, antigen-presenting cells and T helper cells were active again. However, this time the adverse outcome hinged on the isotype of immunoglobulins produced by the B lymphocytes. The onset of the allergy came about because, once stimulated, the B lymphocytes switched to synthesizing and secreting IgE (rather than IgG) against the peanut allergen, and the IgE bound to specific receptors on the surface of the mast cell. As the immune complex was formed on the surface of the mast cell (i.e. a mast cell–IgE–peanut allergen complex), it prompted the mast cell to degranulate. The consequent release of potent mediators of inflammation, such as histamine, leukotrienes, and prostaglandins, precipitated the pathological consequences of the allergy. For instance,

when histamine binds to the wall of blood vessels close to the surface of the skin, it may result in a rash. Respiration and blood pressure may also be adversely affected by histamine (Figure 26.1).

ATOPY AND PREDISPOSITION TO ALLERGY

People who suffer from allergies are said to be atopic. The word 'atopy' is derived from the Greek word meaning 'out of place'. Not everyone is affected by atopic diseases, but there are definitely familial links in the patients who are. If one or both of the parents suffered from an allergy (e.g. asthma, eczema) then the children are highly likely to be atopic. However, the organs affected may vary between parents and their children, for the children do not necessarily suffer the same allergic disorder as their parents. For instance, two people may have an allergic reaction to the same food, but the allergy may present as eczema in one person and as asthma in the other.

There is certainly an inherited component in the control of IgE antibodies, and plasma levels tend to be raised in patients who suffer allergic disorders. One reason given to explain this elevated IgE level is that atopic people tend to switch to making IgE in the secondary immune response, rather than IgG or IgA. This preference may be one reason for a person becoming allergic to two or more allergens. Raised plasma IgE levels are a diagnostic indicator of atopy, but it is by no means definitive, for a significant minority of patients who suffer from allergies have plasma IgE levels within the normal range (see also Person-Centred Study: A Wasp Sting in an Atopic Person).

The clinical presentation and intensity of an allergic reaction depends on the number of mast cells available and how sensitive the patient is to the inflammatory mediators that they release. Atopic patients generally have increased numbers of eosinophils, basophils, and mast cells residing in the vicinity of the skin, respiratory tract, and gut. Obviously, a persistent exposure to high levels of an allergen increases the risk of an allergic disorder erupting in susceptible people. But the allergens must penetrate the physical barriers to make contact with immune cells. Environmental pollutants such as sulphur dioxide and passive smoking encourage the infiltration of allergens because they promote membrane permeability to antigens.

INSECT BITES

According to the data collated by the Office of Population Censuses and Mortality Statistics 1988–1992, there were approximately four deaths per year

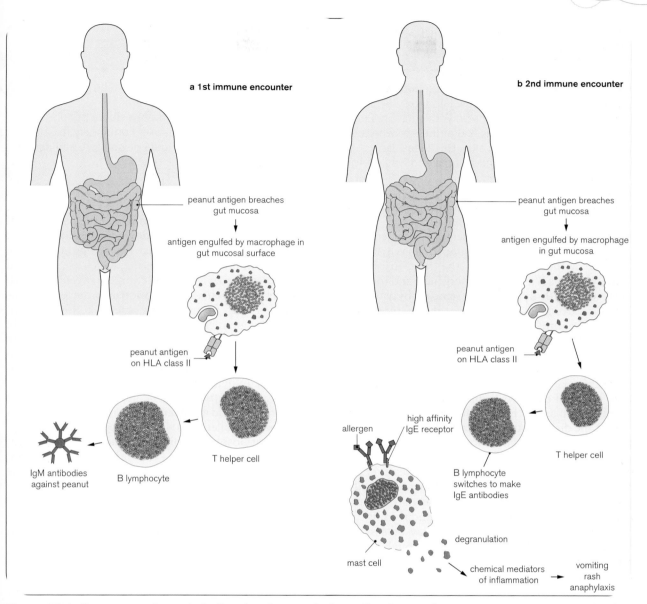

Figure 26.1 Sequence of events in the development of an allergic reaction to peanuts. (a)The first encounter of a peanut antigen with the immune system leads to the production of IgM antibodies. (b) The second encounter of a peanut antigen with the immune system leads to the production of IgE antibodies, mast cell degranulation, and the release chemical mediators of inflammation (e.g. histamine), which provoke the adverse symptoms.

caused by insect bites. The most serious allergic reactions are due to sensitivity to the venoms of wasps, hornets, or yellow jackets. These venoms are toxic. Bee stings are suffered mainly by bee keepers. Hornet stings carry the greatest risk of anaphylaxis to the general public in the UK. The venom may stimulate an IgE response, yet there does not appear to be an association between other atopic diseases and insect venom allergy.

The critical reason for the potentially lethal nature of insect venom is that:

• It can directly activate the alternative pathway of complement.

• In turn, the basophils and mast cells, which are instrumental in the acute inflammatory reaction, may be

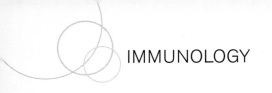

PERSON-CENTRED STUDY: A WASP STING IN AN ATOPIC PERSON

Alan was at a wedding. Just as the photographs were being taken, a wasp flew into the back of his shirt collar and stung his neck. Within minutes he experienced pain and swelling at the site where the insect had punctured his skin. Because Alan suffered from eczema and asthma and was allergic to cats, he was concerned in case the wasp sting stimulated an adverse reaction – he had heard reports about people dying following an insect bite. Fortunately for Alan, he suffered only a few hours discomfort, and he did not have an anaphylactic reaction.

degranulated when the activated complement proteins C3a and C5a bind to their outer surface.

- If the complement cascade releases sufficiently large quantities of these active fragments, anaphylaxis may occur within minutes of the first insect sting. Anaphylaxis is a medical emergency, and the patient presents with hypotension (caused by vasodilatation), cardiovascular distress, and respiratory distress. Treatment is with intravenous adrenaline (see Chapter 13).

ALLERGIC RHINITIS

This is one of the most common forms of allergy. It is often known as hay fever, although this is a misnomer in that the disorder is rarely caused by hay and, if anything, an allergic reaction produces a fall in body temperature rather than a fever. The nose is particularly susceptible to allergens not only because of its innate function but also its rich supply of surface blood vessels and secretory glands. The characteristic symptoms of itching eyes, sinusitis, wheezing, and rhinitis can be provoked by various stimuli that may be associated with a particular season of the year, though they may be perennial.

Patients demonstrating seasonal attacks of allergic rhinitis are generally sensitive to air-borne allergens like pollen. Perennial allergic rhinitis, however, is precipitated by allergens that are around throughout the whole year (e.g. house dust mites, smoke, domestic pets), and even emotional stress can precipitate the symptoms of allergy. Antihistamine therapy and decongestants are the most effective pharmaceutical treatments, but 'detective work' to find out and exclude the causative allergen from the patient's natural environment is the most effective way of dealing with an allergy. (It is worth noting that the drug terfenidine, an antihistamine, was recently found to be contraindicated if used with erythromycin and some other antimicrobial agents, because of the potential for serious cardiac effects.)

ASTHMA

Asthma is an atopic disease in which the pathological manifestations present lower down the respiratory tract than those of allergic rhinitis. The symptoms include shortness of breath and wheezing, which are provoked by reversible airways obstruction. Between 5 and 10 per cent of the general population are affected by asthma. Their lungs become hyper-reactive following stimulation by an allergen (see Chapter 33). The bronchi and bronchioles of people who suffer from asthma are more sensitive to the inflammatory mediators (e.g. histamine, leukotrienes) released by mast cells than non-asthmatic individuals.

An asthma attack may be induced by extremes of temperature (cold air, steam), exercise, stress, infectious microbes, and allergies to food (e.g. eggs). Some patients react to atmospheric pollutants, such as smoke, dust, and laboratory odours. As with other allergic diseases, the frequency of attacks may be seasonal, and some patients can even pinpoint their attacks to a particular month of the year. Occupational asthma has recently gained considerable publicity, and several hundred different agents have been implicated in its aetiology. Workers in industries that either use or generate particulate matter (e.g. wood dust, flour, plastics) are particularly susceptible. Such occupations may exacerbate the condition in people who are either predisposed to allergies or who already suffer from asthma, because of the continuous stimulation by allergens to the lungs.

The Sequence of Events in an Asthma Attack

There are two types of asthma attack, the early-phase attack and the late-phase attack. Both of these are elicited by immune cell activities. The early-phase attack happens soon after allergen stimulation, and the late-phase attack is delayed.

In the early-phase attack, the bronchi are constricted, rather than inflamed, following release of chemical mediators of inflammation. Shortness of breath and wheezing are experienced within about 15 minutes of allergen stimulation, and they are treatable with bronchodilators (see Chapter 10).

The late-phase asthma attack may occur as long as 5 hours after exposure to the allergen; it consists of an inflammatory reaction and bronchospasm. The symptoms are precipitated by mast cells, eosinophils, and neutrophils, which induce oedema and immunological injury to the epithelial cells. Consequently, the lungs are less efficient at clearing the mucus secretions, which exacerbate the respiratory distress (Figure 26.2).

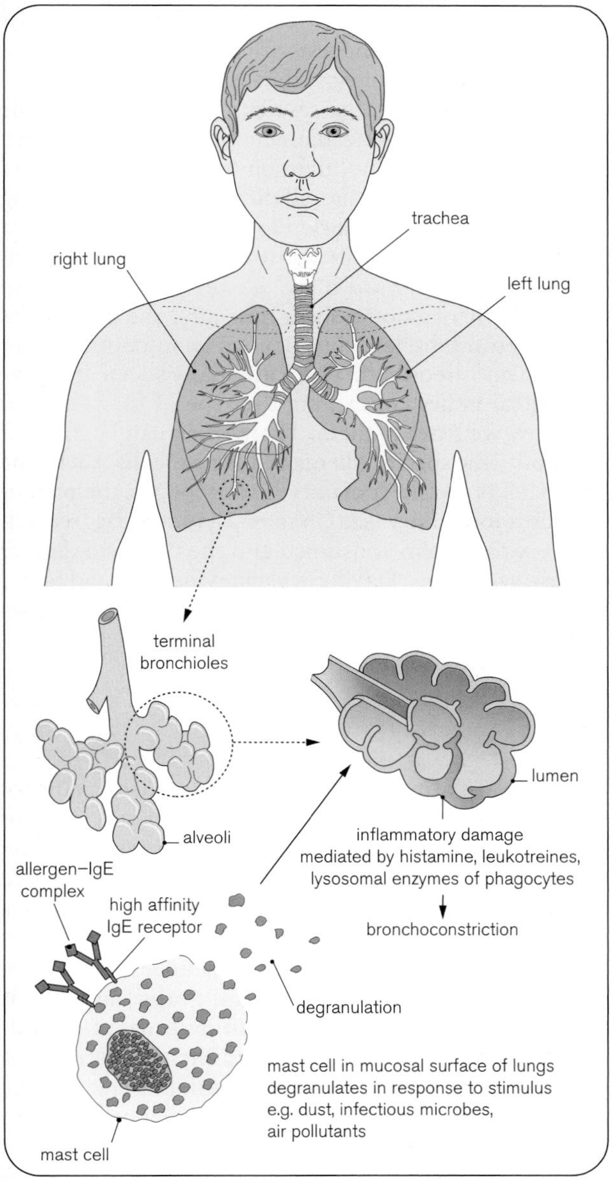

The real dilemma is that many asthmatics suffer both types of asthma attack, and the late-phase is particularly dangerous owing to the lag period between stimulation by the allergen and the bronchial reaction. The patient may then suffer an attack when it is least expected (e.g. during sleep). As a the result the attack may not be promptly treated and could lead to a fatal outcome.

Treatment of Asthma

Treatment is generally palliative – the bronchial hyper-reactivity itself is not treated, only the symptoms. Therefore, therapy is prescribed to relieve the bronchospasm and promote the dilation of the bronchi. The chemical mediator of the attack must be identified because this has implications for the choice of therapy. For instance, if antihistamines are given for an asthma attack provoked by leukotriene release, the lungs generate a thicker mucus, which exacerbates the symptoms. Bronchodilators, such as salbutamol, are given to relieve bronchospasm. Drugs like sodium cromolyn are effective because they stabilize the mast cells and inhibit the degranulation that prompts the attacks. Inhaled corticosteroids are also prescribed to block the production of inflammatory mediators and immune cell activation. Adequate delivery of the drugs is one of the practical problem, especially when treating young children and older adult patients. Getting the correct dosage is also an issue, for the ability to metabolize drugs is suboptimal in these patients.

Asthma can present at any age and it is sometimes difficult to make a firm diagnosis. In children under 5 years, it may be indistinguishable from other childhood respiratory disorders. In older adults, their symptoms can overlap with chronic obstructive pulmonary disease (see Chapters 33 and 40).

ECZEMA

Eczema is a form of skin allergy with characteristic erythematous skin lesions that cause local irritation. As a result, the chronic desire to scratch leads to tissue damage, which may in turn become infected, with scarring and dyspigmentation of the skin. Eczema is most prevalent in patients with family history of atopic disease. It mainly affects children, and around 90 per cent of patients are clear of symptoms by adulthood. The causative agents are largely an enigma, though cow's milk has been implicated – goat's milk may be used as an alternative in people allergic to cow's milk. Palliative care with topical corticosteroid creams and antihistamine drugs is the main line of treatment. In extreme cases, corticosteroid therapy may be prescribed as an oral drug or an ointment.

Figure 26.2 Hyper-reactive lungs of a person with asthma. The hyper-reactivity leads to the production of inflammatory mediators that provoke bronchospasm, inflammation, and mucosal damage.

trachea

right lung

left lung

terminal bronchioles

lumen

alveoli

inflammatory damage mediated by histamine, leukotreines, lysosomal enzymes of phagocytes

allergen–IgE complex

high affinity IgE receptor

bronchoconstriction

degranulation

mast cell in mucosal surface of lungs degranulates in response to stimulus e.g. dust, infectious microbes, air pollutants

mast cell

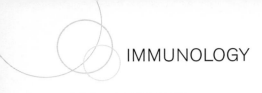

IMMUNOLOGY

FOOD ALLERGIES

An allergic reaction to food ought to be an unlikely event since our nutritional intake is central to survival, yet it may arise at any age. Children are more susceptible than adults because an immature gut does not provide the same effective barrier to allergens.

Food allergy should not to be confused with food intolerance, which is caused by other mechanisms. For instance, patients with a lactose intolerance have a deficiency of the gut enzyme, lactase and are therefore inefficient at digesting lactose, the sugar found in milk products. Consequently, the undigested lactose attracts water into the gut (i.e. is osmotically active) and this results in the adverse symptoms of abdominal pain, bloating and diarrhoea. Migraine has been linked to foods such as cheese and chocolate, but this is thought to be the result of a pharmacological reaction rather than an immunological one (see Chapter 38).

The mechanism that precipitates a food allergy is much the same as the mechanisms that precipitate other allergic disorders – a partially digested allergen breaches the physical barrier (in this case the gut) and stimulates an IgE response. Gastrointestinal disturbances are caused when the gut mucosa is sensitive to the histamine released by local mast cells. However, other areas can react – skin rashes, eczema, and asthma may be precipitated by allergies to food. Protein-containing foods are especially allergenic (e.g. cow's milk, peanuts, shellfish), as are some food flavourings and additives. Raw foods are more likely to cause a reaction, for cooking has been shown to inactivate some food allergens. Occasionally, even breast-fed infants present with a food allergy. The main explanation for this is that the passage of allergens from the mother in the breast milk may sensitize the infant's immune cells.

There seems to be an increased public awareness of the foods and additives that cause allergies, with self-help groups emerging to provide support and information. For instance, 'Gut Reaction' is an organization that was set up to help sufferers of irritable bowel syndrome. The causes of this disorder in many patients remain an enigma, but some patients have gained relief and control of the adverse symptoms with antihistamine drugs, which suggests that an immunological mechanism is involved. There is also some evidence to suggest that diseases with known immunological mechanisms (e.g. rheumatoid arthritis) are treatable with diet.

CLINICAL DIAGNOSIS OF ALLERGY

There are a number of clinical tests available for evaluating patients suspected of being atopic and for identifying the specific allergens. Raised levels of plasma IgE is one diagnostic indicator, and this can be used with some confidence in Westernized society. However, it is of limited use in developing countries because IgE antibodies are raised in response to parasitic organisms. The specific IgE antibodies may be evaluated for their reactivity to an allergen by means of the radioallergosorbent (RAST) test.

Intradermal testing may also be employed to confirm that IgE antibodies are indeed provoking the disorder. In this instance, allergens are administered intradermally to the forearm, and the area is observed for the development of a reaction such as a weal or erythema. Although the tests are performed under controlled clinical conditions, they are by no means conclusive; for example, the results may suggest multiple allergies when only one allergen is the causative agent.

Characterizing the allergen responsible requires 'detective work', but it is still difficult even after taking a stringent clinical history. How does one seek out a food allergen that causes an atopic disease? This is relatively straightforward if the person vomits or has an anaphylactic reaction a short time after the meal but if the symptoms are less conspicuous an in-depth dietary assessment is required. There are many social and psychological issues controlling the type of foods we eat and how we react to them. Therefore it can be difficult to identify the specific allergen causing the disorder. One approach is to take a dietary history or ask the patient to keep a food diary (see Chapter 2), in which is recorded every food item consumed and the time and date of adverse symptoms. Having evaluated this data and found the potential allergen, exclusion and provocative testing should verify or refute the suspected food.

TREATMENTS FOR ALLERGY
Palliative Therapy

Generally, treatment is a palliative measure to control the symptoms rather than cure the hyper-reactivity of the affected organ. Excluding the allergen from the patient's immediate environment is the most effective approach, but this is difficult if the atopic disease has a seasonal component (e.g. pollen that provokes allergic rhinitis or asthma). In these instances, the symptoms may be controlled with oral antihistamines. It should, in theory, be far easier to exclude an offending food from the diet, and certainly the nutritional information provided by food manufacturers is useful for patients who are sensitive to a particular food, but accidents still happen occasionally. This may occur, for example, when friend provides a meal or the patient eats at a restaurant or canteen. There is also the possibility of processed food becoming contaminated with allergens in the factory production line.

Desensitization Therapy

Desensitization is one of the treatment strategies used for reducing the risk of repeated attacks, particularly when they are acute and possibly life threatening. The basic mechanism of the therapy is to manipulate the immune system into producing IgG against the allergen, rather than IgE which provokes mast cell degranulation. The allergen is therefore administered by a different route from its usual route of entry to the body (e.g. subcutaneous injection of an allergen that is normally inhaled or eaten) in order to stimulate specific IgG-secreting B lymphocytes. The rationale is that, when the allergen is encountered, IgG antibodies should be rapidly synthesized and bind the allergen before IgE antibodies can do so.

Desensitization has been used with success in patients who suffer anaphylaxis following an insect bite. One schedule has recommended once-weekly subcutaneous injections for about 4 months, followed by one maintenance injections every 4–6 weeks for 3 years. There are some side-effects of desensitization, such as inflammation, swelling, and pain at the site of injection, and there is a risk of anaphylaxis during treatment. Therefore, desensitization must be conducted at a specialist allergy centre where the patient can be closely observed and there is a resuscitation facility at hand if needed.

TYPE II HYPERSENSITIVITY REACTIONS

Type II hypersensitivity reactions are precipitated by pre-existing antibodies in the patient's body fluids. However, the pathological mechanisms differ from atopic disorders in that IgE is not instrumental in the attack. Instead, IgG or IgM antibodies raised against cell surface antigens are involved; these bind to their target tissues or cells to form immune complexes. This results in activation of the complement cascade and recruitment of neutrophils, which contribute to the inflammation and cellular destruction. Such injury may be inflicted on the patient's own cells or on foreign tissues and cells (e.g. cells given in a blood transfusion). The mechanism that mediates the cellular damage is sometimes referred to as antibody-dependent cell mediated cytotoxicity. The ultimate consequences of a type II hypersensitivity reaction depend on the characteristics of the cells targeted by the antibodies.

BLOOD TRANSFUSION REACTIONS

Blood transfusion reactions caused by ABO incompatibility are extremely rare. Even in emergencies, patients are given blood that is compatible with their own ABO blood group, although samples of the donor blood are retained in the laboratory for testing retrospectively. Only in life-threatening situations (e.g. a ruptured aortic aneurysm or a severed femoral artery) is unmatched group O rhesus-negative blood used. Depending on the patient's blood group, naturally occurring anti-A or anti-B antibodies may be present in body fluids; these antibodies are generally of the IgM isotype, though it is worth remembering that there are numerous blood group systems other than the ABO system. (see Chapters 24 and 31)

Immune cells may actively respond to transfused blood cells if they display a blood group antigen that is not normally on the surface of their own cells. Therefore, before an elective blood transfusion, serum of the patient to be transfused is mixed with the donor's red blood cells in a serological test (a cross-match) to ensure that there are no antibodies in the patient's serum that could react with the donated cells (i.e. to ensure compatibility) (see Chapter 31).

Patients must be observed throughout a blood transfusion in case an adverse reaction is provoked, because such a reaction may be life threatening. The symptoms include fever, hypotension, nausea, vomiting, a sensation of chest compression, and lower back pain. In the sequence of events that accompany these physical manifestations, the donated cells are coated with pre-existing antibodies in the recipient's plasma. The cells agglutinate (clump together) as part of the immune complexes that are formed, complement is activated, and haemolysis results. Acute tubular necrosis of the kidney is a possible outcome of the red blood cell destruction because the kidney is inadvertently damaged by the immune system ('caught in the cross-fire') during elimination of the incompatible transfused cells.

HAEMOLYTIC DISEASE OF THE NEWBORN
Rhesus Incompatibility Between Mother and Fetus

Before the introduction of anti-D therapy, haemolytic disease of the newborn (HDN) was found in the second rhesus D positive (RhD-positive) infant born to rhesus D negative (RhD-negative) mothers. [For a RhD-negative mother to have a RhD-positive baby, the father must be RhD-positive]. HDN is caused by the agglutination and destruction of fetal red blood cells *in utero* by IgG antibodies that pass across the placenta from the mother (Figure 26.3). However, since the fetal and maternal circulations do not mix but are juxtaposed, *how can the mother make antibodies against the red blood cells of her fetus?*

Invariably a few fetal cells will migrate into the maternal circulation, but these are of little consequence in the first pregnancy. However, more fetal blood cells pass

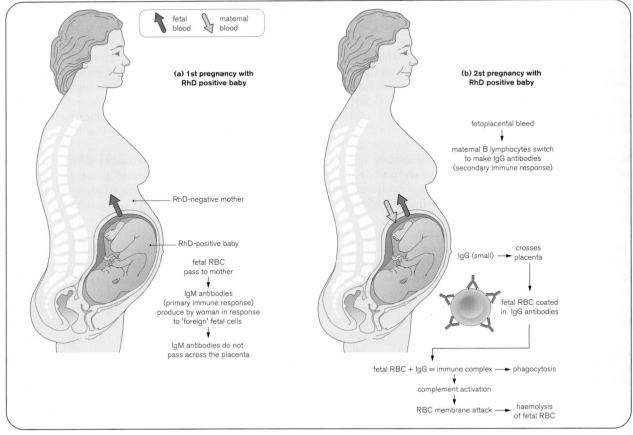

Figure 26.3. Haemolytic disease of the newborn. (a) When an RhD-negative woman is carrying her first RhD-positive fetus, fetomaternal bleeding in the third trimester and at birth sensitizes the mother to produce IgM antibodies in response to fetal red blood cells (RBC). IgM antibodies are too large to cross the placenta. (b) When the same RhD-negative woman is carrying her second RhD-positive fetus, fetomaternal bleeding in the third trimester and at birth sensitizes the mother to produce IgG antibodies in response to fetal RBC. Unlike IgM antibodies, IgG antibodies are small enough to cross the placenta and provoke complement-induced lysis of fetal RBC.

across with the transplacental bleed which happens during labour and delivery. The fetal cells that are RhD - positive are recognised as foreign by the immune cells of the RhD-negative mother. She then becomes sensitised and produces IgM antibodies in a primary immune response. The IgM antibodies do not translocate across an intact placenta whilst the child is *in utero*, and obviously do not affect the newborn infant. If she were to conceive a second child which happened to be RhD-negative, then this child would not suffer HDN. However, should the mother conceive another RhD-positive baby, then the child would be at risk of HDN.

As the pregnancy with the second RhD-positive child progresses, a few fetal red blood cells pass across the placenta. These are detected by the mother's immune cells which subsequently react and mount a rapid secondary immune response. The IgG antibodies cross the placenta and agglutinate the fetal cells, resulting in haemolysis. If the fetus is severely affected, it could even die of anaemia *in utero* (i.e. *hydrops fetalis*). Therefore when indicated, an intrauterine blood transfusion may be performed until it is considered safe to deliver the infant by elective induction of labour. Once the baby is delivered the raised plasma bilirubin levels and jaundice may be treated by an exchange transfusion. A physical examination often indicates that the infant has an enlarged liver and spleen, as these are the organs most involved in red blood cell production and destruction.

Today, HDN due to a rhesus incompatibility of mother and fetus is extremely rare since a RhD- negative mother delivering a RhD-positive infant is given an intramuscular injection of anti-D immunoglobulins (i.e passive immunity) (see Chapter 23). Similarly, RhD-negative females who have a pregnancy termination are also given anti-D immunoglobulin as prophylaxis to reduce the risk of HDN in subsequent conceptuses. The antibody targets the fetal RhD-positive cells that enter the maternal circulation. But the timing of the injection is critical for it must be given within 72 hours of delivery, to remove the fetal cells from the maternal circulation before her immune system can be sensitised into a response, (see Box 26.1).

ABO Incompatibility Between Mother and Fetus

Jaundice is often present in neonates, and one of the possible causes is blood group incompatibility between the mother and fetus. However, such cases of HDN rarely demand the medical intervention of an exchange transfusion. Mothers who are blood group O are more likely to deliver an infant with jaundice. If the maternal blood has high titres of naturally occurring anti-A and anti-B antibodies. These antibodies cross the placenta, they can cause haemolysis of the fetal red blood cells. Infants who are blood groups A or B are the most at risk. Unlike HDN caused by rhesus incompatibility, ABO incompatibility may arise in the first pregnancy because anti-A and anti-B are naturally occurring antibodies. If these antibodies are of the IgG isotype, they are small enough to cross the placenta into the fetus. Ultraviolet light therapy is prescribed for neonatal jaundice.

AUTOIMMUNE HAEMOLYTIC ANAEMIA

Autoimmune haemolytic anaemia is precipitated when the patient's own red blood cells are lysed because they have been caught up in an immune complex. The immunoglobulins responsible are called autoantibodies and may be detected following an infection. Molecular mimicry is one reason for the autoimmune disorder – the antigen-binding site of the immunoglobulin recognizing the microbe may also fit and bind to an epitope on the surface of the red blood cells (see Chapter 27). But there is an alternative immunological mechanism that results in haemolysis, in which the red blood cell is inadvertently damaged in complement 'cross-fire'. Some drugs, including penicillin and methyldopa, are known to trigger an autoimmune haemolytic anaemia. In this instance, the drug 'sticks' to the surface of the cell, and as a foreign molecule it is perceived as dangerous, so it elicits an immune response. Consequently, when the immunoglobulins bind the drug, the red blood cells are captured in the immune complex and either lysed or sequestered to the spleen.

TYPE III HYPERSENSITIVITY REACTIONS

Type III hypersensitivity is an inflammatory reaction provoked by excess immune complexes which lodge in tissues. Normal healthy people are generally able to solubilize immune complexes and remove them rapidly from the circulation. However, the mechanisms for clearance may be either inefficient or overwhelmed. For instance, if the synthesis of immunoglobulin is continually stimulated because the patient is persistently assaulted by an antigen within the work environment, many immune complexes are formed and these, if not efficiently cleared, may be deposited on tissues. The complement cascade is therefore activated and gives rise to inflammatory damage.

BOX 26.1 ANTI-D IMMUNOGLOBULIN THERAPY

Haemolytic disease of the newborn still occurs. Why?

- Some women develop IgG antibodies against the red blood cells of the developing fetus because occasionally the guidelines for postnatal anti-D therapy are not followed and there is leakage of fetal blood into the maternal circulation in the third trimester of pregnancy i.e. fetomaternal bleed.
- A Kleihauer test is performed on maternal blood which assesses the number of fetal cells present. This provides evidence for the extent of the transplacental bleed from baby into mother, for additional anti-D injections may be necessary.
- Following spontaneous/therapeutic abortion, a RhD-negative woman should also receive anti-D immunoglobulins, and a Kleihauer test requested, where gestation was 20 weeks or more.

At a conference of the Royal College of Obstetricians & Gynaecologist and Royal College of Physicians of Edinburgh in 1997, it was agreed that anti-D immunoglobulin therapy given to the mother in the third trimester could reduce the incidence of rhesus D haemolytic disease of the newborn caused by fetomaternal bleeding.

There are a number of factors that predispose to immune complex deposition. It is particularly encouraged by vascular permeability and changes in blood flow (e.g. as found in hypertensive patients). The size of the immune complexes is another consideration, for larger complexes are more readily detected and removed by the liver, whereas smaller immune complexes tend to lodge in tissues like the kidney and blood vessels. Furthermore, most molecules and tissues bear some sort of electrical charge, and this can be another factor, because 'opposites attract'. Thus, positively charged immune complexes are more likely to 'home in' on negatively charged tissues like the glomerular basement membrane in the nephron.

A number of tissue-damaging mediators are released in response to immune complex deposits by the activation of the classical pathway of complement. For instance, the C5a fragment is a potent stimulator of vasodilatation and vascular permeability, and these changes allow immune cells to gain access to areas where they perpetuate the inflammation and incite injury. As capillaries become leaky and dilated, they expose collagen, an integral part of the vessel wall, which encourages the aggregation of platelets and thrombus formation. Further damage may be instigated by phagocytes as they engulf the immune complexes if lysosomal enzymes overflow on to adjacent tissues and cause damage. The release of cytokines (e.g. TNF-alpha, IL-1) also contributes to the inflammatory process.

ARTHUS REACTION

The Arthus reaction is a local inflammatory reaction that most frequently presents as a raised and inflamed skin lesion that wanes within about 2 days. It can be experimentally induced if an antigen is injected into the skin of a patient with a high titre of specific immunoglobulin in the body fluids. The characteristic lesion appears at the injection site within 10 hours and eventually becomes ulcerated. Bruising may be seen if the blood vessels burst; tissue necrosis and ischaemia may be precipitated if the local circulation is interrupted. An example of the Arthus reaction is the delayed skin reaction that occurs 4–10 hours after an insect bite. The lesion is likely to be diffuse and at least 50 mm in diameter (Figure 26.4).

SERUM SICKNESS

Before the advent of antibiotics, patients with potentially fatal diseases were given antibody therapy. It was the final strategy for treating patients who would otherwise have died. Antisera were prepared for therapeutic use by injecting larger domestic animals such as horses with the bacteria or toxins. Accordingly, the animals made a substantial antibody response, which could be harvested. Diphtheria was treated with massive doses of antidiphtheria antibodies raised in horses. However, this treatment was not without its side-effects, for many patients developed a local Arthus reaction at the injection site, and a few patients developed a systemic type III hypersensitivity reaction called serum sickness. They presented with lymphadenopathy, joint pain, and fever. In most cases, however, symptoms persisted only for a few days, after which the healing and repair mechanisms took control.

The systemic deposition of immune complexes in joints, blood vessels, or other tissues precipitated an inflammatory reaction. Consequently, an arthritis-like disorder erupted if the deposition was in joints, arteritis occurred if the blood vessels were involved, and glomerulonephritis occurred if the deposition was in the basement membrane of the glomerulus. It is noteworthy that these pathological features are often found in patients with systemic lupus erythematosus (see

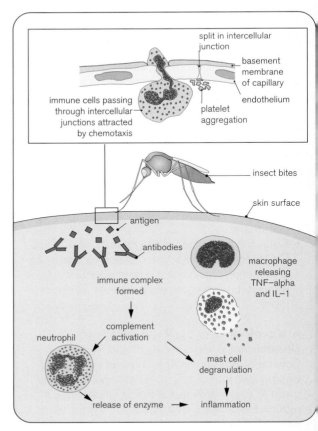

Figure 26.4 Type III hypersensitivity reaction to an insect bite. (Arthus reaction.)

Chapter 27), for this autoimmune disorder is mediated by a massive load of immune complex and very much parallels chronic serum sickness.

GLOMERULONEPHRITIS

Glomerulonephritis may be precipitated by a vast range of antigens (e.g. *Toxoplasma*, *Candida*, and viruses such as hepatitis B virus, measles virus and Epstein–Barr virus). It is also a renal complication found in susceptible patients about 1–3 weeks after a streptococcal infection – in this instance, the immunoglobulin response mounted against the infection results in excess immune complex formation. Because these particular microbes tend to adhere to the glomerular basement membrane, the kidney is damaged as the immunoglobulins bind their streptococcal targets.

FARMER'S LUNG

Mucosal surfaces may be injured by type III hypersensitivity reactions if they are persistently bombarded with antigens that stimulate an immunoglobulin response. Industrial workers who are exposed to vast quantities of air-borne particulate matter or microbes are especially vulnerable. A classic example is farmer's lung, a chronic respiratory disorder suffered by farm workers who persistently inhale air-borne spores of fungal moulds on hay (see Chapter 33). If these spores stimulate an unremitting immunoglobulin response, it can result in the formation of immune complexes at a rate that outstrips their clearance. The complexes are deposited in the lungs, causing immunologically induced tissue damage that leads to impaired gaseous exchange.

TYPE IV HYPERSENSITIVITY REACTIONS

This type of hypersensitivity differs from the other types by being mediated by T lymphocytes rather than by immunoglobulins. It is also referred to as a delayed hypersensitivity reaction because it proceeds at a much slower pace. The causative antigens can be as innocuous as a brand of cosmetics that produces contact dermatitis. However, when microbes are the stimulus it is rather more serious, since they are generally intracellular organisms such as *Mycobacterium tuberculosis*, which is a difficult infection to control. One of the notable problems of such infections is that, although T-lymphocyte-derived cytokines enhance phagocytic activities, the outer surfaces of these microbes are not easily degraded by phagocytes. Consequently, when

they are engulfed during phagocytosis, they passively acquire their new host (i.e, the phagocyte) when it surrounds them in the phagosome.

CONTACT DERMATITIS

Contact dermatitis is an inflammatory skin disorder that may be elicited by metals (e.g. nickel), topical drugs, or cosmetics; some people may have a reaction to contact with plants on a country walk. The affected area becomes swollen and, if an exudate is released, it may become a focus for microbial growth. The site of the skin lesion can provide clues to the causative agent.

Langerhans' cells (the major antigen-presenting cell in the skin) engulf the antigen for display to the T lymphocytes. As a result, the specific immune cells are sensitized to recognize and respond to any subsequent encounter with the antigen. As the sensitized T lymphocytes migrate through the lymphatic circulation and peripheral blood, they trigger a skin lesion at any location where the antigen makes contact again. However, the intensity of the reaction is highly variable between patients. Once reactivated, the cells release cytokines that recruit other immune cell types to the area. Neutrophils arrive within about 4 hours of antigen contact, and T lymphocytes and macrophages migrate within about 12 hours. An inflammatory reaction ensues, with the cytokines encouraging the adherence of immune cells to the capillary surfaces.

Being a delayed hypersensitivity reaction, the lesion does not normally present until about 12–24 hours after contact with the antigen. If it is an antigen that is difficult to phagocytose (e.g. talc or silica), the macrophages become activated and release cytokines to recruit more cells into the area to assist and to encourage the neighbouring macrophages to coalesce (combine together) and form giant cells, which are huge, multinucleated cells. Although these giant cells are highly efficient phagocytes, they form a hard 'lump' called a granuloma. The main course of treatment is topical preparations (e.g. corticosteroid creams) to reduce the symptoms and prevent the open wound becoming infected (Figure 26.5).

INTRACELLULAR INFECTIONS THAT PROVOKE TYPE IV HYPERSENSITIVITY

Intracellular microbial infections can stimulate delayed hypersensitivity reactions, and *Mycobacterium tuberculosis* and *Mycobacterium leprae* are two examples which result in the development of granulomas. Mycobacterial infections are major stimulators of giant

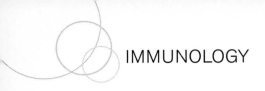
cell formation, and together with the tissue fibrosis occurring, the physiological functions of organs involved are severely affected. There is evidence that *Mycobacterium paratuberculosis* is implicated in the aetiology of Crohn's disease, a chronic inflammatory bowel disorder. The fistulae that occur in Crohn's disease are caused by granulomas. Similarly with leprosy there is a wide spectrum of pathological features, ranging from hypopigmented skin lesions to inflamed lesions containing the *Mycobacterium leprae* organisms. Not all cases of leprosy result in gross anatomical malformations such as the loss of digits, but when the Schwann cells of myelinated nerve fibres are infected with *Mycobacterium leprae*, these nerves are less effective at propagating action potentials, owing to granuloma formation. Consequently, there is numbness in peripheral tissues and insensitivity to damage.

The Mantoux Test

A positive result of the screening test for tuberculosis immunity hinges on the development of a delayed hypersensitivity reaction. In the Mantoux test, a protein preparation, referred to as purified protein derivative (PPD), is made from a culture of *Mycobacterium tuberculosis*. This is given intradermally using a multiple puncture injector that discharges small amounts of the PPD in a characteristic pattern. A positive result is detected as a raised and inflamed skin lesion within about 18 hours of the injection. This reaction indicates that the patient's T lymphocytes have remembered a previous encounter with *Mycobacterium tuberculosis* and have responded to the PPD. The red swollen vesicles are generally gone within about 7 days (see Figure 26.5). Individuals do not need to have suffered tuberculosis to become immune, for those who have previously been immunized or who have lived on a farm and drunk untreated milk may have a positive Mantoux test. Patients with a negative result are offered an intradermal injection of Bacille Calmette–Guérin (BCG), which is an avirulent strain of *Mycobacterium*. The BCG vaccine is recommended for people who have been in contact with tuberculosis and for those are likely to come into contact with the disease.

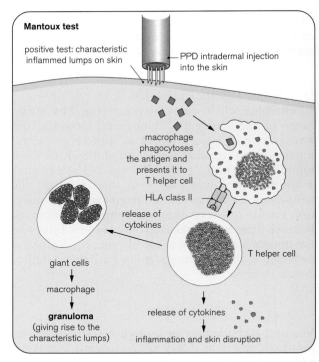

Figure 26.5 Sequence of events in the production of a positive Mantoux test (type IV hypersensitivity).

KEY POINTS

- Type I hypersensitivity reactions (allergy) may arise after the immune system responds to allergens and produces an IgE antibody response.
- Most allergens are from the patient's external environment and breach the physical barriers (the skin and mucosal surfaces); hence the symptoms of allergy are often induced in organs such as the respiratory tract, the gut, and the skin.
- Atopic people share some common characteristics – in comparison to non-atopic people, they have raised plasma levels of IgE; increased numbers of eosinophils, basophils, and mast cells; and hyper-reactivity to the chemical mediators of inflammation.
- The clinical tests available for evaluating patients suspected of being atopic include estimating total and specific plasma IgE levels, intradermal testing with suspected allergens, and exclusion and provocative testing to verify or refute the causative agent.

- Treatments for allergy are generally palliative and aim at controlling the symptoms rather than curing the hyper-reactivity of the organ affected.
- Type II hypersensitivity reactions are precipitated by pre-existing antibodies in the patient's body fluids, which provoke antibody-dependent cytotoxicity (e.g. blood transfusion reactions).
- Type III hypersensitivity reactions are inflammatory reactions that are provoked by excess immune complexes, which lodge in tissues. The reaction may affect one organ, as in glomerulonephritis, or it may be systemic, as in serum sickness.
- Type IV hypersensitivity is also referred to as delayed hypersensitivity since the progress of the reaction is slower than in the other types of hypersensitivity because it is elicited by T lymphocytes. Type IV hypersensitivity may be stimulated by chemicals (e.g. talc) or intracellular microbial agents e.g. *Mycobacterium tuberculosis*.

FURTHER READING

Ashworth L (1997) Is my antihistamine safe? Home Care Prov 2:117–20.

Duguid JKM (1997) Antenatal serological testing and prevention of haemolytic disease of the newborn. J Clin Pathol 50:193–6.

Ferguson A, Gillett H, O'Mahony S (1996) Active immunity or tolerance to foods in patients with celiac disease or inflammatory bowel disease. Ann N Y Acad Sci 778:202–16.

Fireman P (1996) Cytokines and allergic rhinitis. Allergy Asthma Proc 17:175–8.

Gelder C, Harris J, Williams D (1996) Allergy to bee and wasp venom. Br J Hospi Med 55:349–52.

Myers JD, Ind PW (1996) Bronchial hyperresponsiveness and bronchial provocation tests. Br J Hosp Med 55:107–10.

Nelson RJ, Demas GE (1996) Seasonal changes in immune function. Q Rev Biol 71:511–48.

Norman PS (1996) Current status of immunotherapy for allergies and anaphylactic reactions. Adv Intern Med 41:681–713.

Parikh A, Scadding GK (1997) Seasonal allergic rhinitis. BMJ 314:1392–5.

Peters S (1997) Food allergies. Identification and prevention techniques. Adv Nurs Pract 5:45–9.

Rietschel RL (1997) Occupational contact dermatitis. Lancet 349:1093–5.

Robinson DS, Durham SR, Kay AB (1993) Cytokines. 3. Cytokines in asthma. Thorax 48:845–53.

Rumsaeng V, Metcalfe DD (1996) Food allergy. Semin Gastrointest Dis 7:134–43.

Ruffilli A, Bonini S (1997) Susceptibility genes for allergy and asthma. Allergy 52:256–73.

Tsuyuguchi I (1996) Regulation of the human immune response in tuberculosis. Infect Agents Dis 5:82–97.

Thomas WR (1996) Recombinant allergens for immunotherapy. Adv Exp Med Biol 409:85–93.

van Dijk B (1997) Preventing RHD haemolytic disease of the new born. BMJ 315:1480–1.

Vercelli D (1993) Regulation of IgE synthesis. Allergy Proc 14:413–16.

Waters J (1997) Latex gloves: still a serious occupational hazard. Nurs Times 93:56–8.

Waters MF, Jacobs JM (1996) Leprous neuropathies. Baillieres Clin Neurol 5:171–97.

AUTOIMMUNITY

For a broader understanding of this chapter you should read the first four chapters of the Immunology section (Chapters 22, 23, 24, 25).

INTRODUCTION

The immune system evolved to protect the body at just about every site where a foreign antigen could gain entry. However, occasionally a fault arises in the system and lymphocytes attack the body to cause an autoimmune disorder. Rheumatoid arthritis and pernicious anaemia are two examples of this type of disorder. Most people remain free of autoimmune diseases, thanks to the molecular signals and selection procedures aimed at controlling the lymphocyte activities. This control prevents a constant attack from occurring on the body's anatomical structures and molecules. The antigens on body tissues and in body fluids are collectively referred to as autoantigens, or 'self'. The enigma to be unravelled is how the lymphocytes distinguish between an autoantigen and a foreign or dangerous antigen. Recently, immunologists have closely re-examined this contentious issue after Professor Polly Matzinger put forward her theories on the subject. This chapter seeks to provide information on how lymphocytes are controlled, the risk factors that pre-

dispose to autoimmune diseases, and the causes and manifestations of some of these disorders.

IMMUNOLOGICAL TOLERANCE

The specific immune system seems to be selective in healthy people, knowing when to react and when to be tolerant. However, the lymphocytes are not oblivious of the presence of autoantigens – they recognize them but do not mount a tenacious response. In a way, this is analogous to being accidentally assaulted by a policeman – one is more inclined to be tolerant, owing to prior knowledge that retaliation could have possible legal implications! Now, returning to the case of the lymphocytes – they persistently attack antigens only when they are given clear signals to direct and provoke activation. When an autoantigen is encountered, not all the signals are emitted, and so lymphocytes that could recognize them do not persistently respond; instead these lymphocytes are inactivated and ultimately die.

This is known as immunological tolerance and is an essential part of our protection strategy, for when it breaks down an attack is mounted on otherwise healthy cells. For example, Hashimoto's thyroiditis is caused by the release of antibodies whose specific targets are parts of the thyroid gland (see below). In patients with Hashimoto's thyroiditis, the thyroid-specific lymphocytes have escaped the tolerance process and, when activated, they secrete harmful antibodies against autoantigens. The anti-thyroid antibodies are examples of autoantibodies.

WHEN MUST OUR IMMUNE SYSTEM BE TOLERANT?

A considerable part of the immune response is involved in tolerating rather than attacking. Lymphocytes must tolerate many changes in the human body throughout its life cycle because a different array of antigens are expressed throughout human growth and development (i.e. from life as a neonate, through childhood to puberty, the fertile years, and then the decline with ageing). Many of the antigens that occur in a new phase of the life cycle may not have been previously detected. For instance, consider the lactating breast that produces milk under the influence of pituitary hormones. It is well known that immune cells and immunoglobulins are present in breast milk, for they are part of the passive immunity conveyed by the mother to the neonate. In spite of the fact the mother's lymphocytes have not encountered milk in the breast tissue before lactation, antibodies against the milk are not produced because it is not considered dangerous.

It is not only 'self' tissues that are tolerated; foreign antigens may also be spared if they are not perceived as hazardous. The gut is a major site for immunological tolerance; in its physiological function it is exposed to a vast number of different foreign antigens in the diet. Although a significant minority of patients suffer food allergies, most people do not make an immune response to dietary constituents. Likewise, commensal microbes reside and multiply in the gut (they are not eradicated); this is advantageous because they crowd out pathogenic organisms which could precipitate an infection. However, these commensals do not fulfil the same role if they migrate into the genitourinary tract; instead, they are perceived as dangerous and precipitate an inflammatory response as immune cells are attracted to the area of infection to eliminate them. Hence, cystitis caused by a bacterial infection is treated with antimicrobial drugs, such as trimethoprim, and the recommendation to drink plenty of fluids (see Chapters 19 and 36).

HOW IS IMMUNOLOGICAL TOLERANCE ACHIEVED?

Immunological tolerance is a concerted effort by the immune system to inactivate or kill cells that would respond to autoantigens. To a certain extent the T suppressor cells have a restraining influence on the immune response. However, it would not be enough to rely on one cell type being at the right anatomical location to curb this type of aggression. Tolerance is therefore also achieved by a number of other mechanisms.

Central tolerance

Central tolerance occurs in the primary organs of the immune system as the lymphocytes develop and mature. For instance, B lymphocytes differentiate from stem cells in the bone marrow to become functionally active immune cells. The maturation process generates many cells that are specific for dangerous antigens and vital in the immune defence. However, some B lymphocytes arise whose specific targets are autoantigens (e.g. hormones, cell surface receptors). Most of these autoreactive (self-attacking) cells never leave the bone marrow because they are deleted by a programmed cell death called apoptosis. This type of cell death is not unique to the lymphocytes – it is employed throughout the body by different tissue types during healing, repair, and replenishment of cells (see Chapter 4). In healthy people, the few autoreacting B lymphocytes that 'slip through the net' are thought to be rendered inactive by tolerance induced in the periphery.

Cells destined to be T lymphocytes arise from the bone marrow and migrate to the thymus. What happens once they reach the thymus is very much open to debate. The general view is that a selection process occurs as the immature T lymphocytes (also known as thymocytes) are made functional. The thymocytes encounter dendritic cells, which are highly professional antigen-presenting cells that display the patient's unique tissue type in the form of the human leukocyte antigen (HLA). Within the groove of the HLA is one of a vast array of self-antigen peptides (autoantigens) that might be encountered by mature T lymphocytes outside the thymus. Cells that would actively respond to the HLA are deleted, and a large proportion of thymocytes never reach the peripheral circulation as mature T lymphocytes because they are considered unsafe and likely to precipitate damage or autoimmunity.

Peripheral tolerance

The induction of immunological tolerance in the bone marrow and thymus is by no means the whole story, for some lymphocytes escape central tolerance in the bone marrow. In any case, it would be almost impossible for the thymus (which is little more than 30 g in weight) to cope with a flood of every possible 'self' peptide. Therefore, a certain amount of tolerance must take place in the periphery, by way of the cytokine network and distress signals alerting the immune system to possible danger.

Therefore, unless the lymphocytes in the periphery receive two signals as they encounter an antigen, they are inactivated and die – this is peripheral tolerance (see Box 27.1). The two signals required are HLA-displaying peptide (signal one) and a distress signal (signal two), for example a cytokine released from a neighbouring antigen-presenting cell, or a distress signal emitted by a cell in the periphery (Figure 27.1).

BOX 27.1 THE IMMUNE RESPONSE TO A VIRUS INFECTION ON THE LIP

- Virus-infected cells on the lip need to be eliminated, but there are also many other healthy cells which are not infected. Therefore, immunological tolerance is required for selectivity in the immune response i.e. persistent assault of virus-infected cells rather than uninfected lip cells.
- Most of the lymphocytes reside in the lymphatic organs i.e. lymph nodes and spleen, so they need to be alerted to the presence of the virus.
- The antigen-presenting cells circulating in the lip engulf the virus-infected targets. A specific immune response is mounted by T helper cells when they migrate to the nearest lymph node and display their engulfed virus which they have processed and displayed on HLA class II.
- In the engulfing process, the antigen-presenting cells become activated and secrete the cytokines.
- T helper cells prompt the B lymphocytes to secrete anti-virus antibodies, and cytotoxic T lymphocytes to migrate out of the lymph node to eliminate the infection in the lip.
- After a round of killing has been completed, they return to the lymph node and revert to the resting state and probably become memory cells.
- While the infection rages, the viral-infected and dying cells emit distress signals, and there is a continuous trafficking of immune cells between the lymph node and lip, until the virus is finally eliminated (i.e. antigen-presenting cells display to the resting T lymphocytes, which are reactivated and return to the lip for a further round of action before retreating back to rest in the lymphatic organs).
- During the immune attack on the viral infection, cellular debris of healthy lip antigens may also be engulfed by the antigen-presenting cells.

- It is possible that autoreactive T lymphocytes against lip antigens could have evaded the central tolerance mechanisms and be residing in the lymph node. However, there is little danger of an autoimmune disorder erupting because of a limited supply of second signals to activate them, since normal lip cells are not perceived as dangerous.

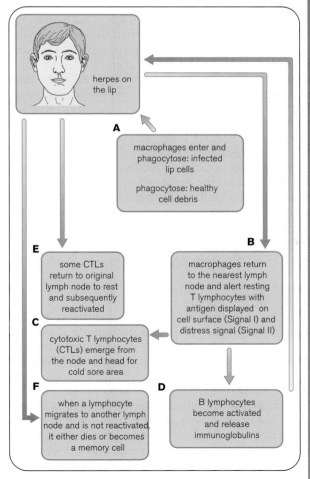

Figure 27.1 Peripheral tolerance.

The cell lysis induced by the cytotoxic T lymphocytes is not considered dangerous for it is already part of the immune defence. However, cell death induced by a source of stress (e.g. infection, fever) may result in the release of a danger signal, as may heat shock proteins, which are secreted in response to stressors other than raised body temperature. Distress signals may include the exposure of an intracellular component such as deoxyribonucleic acid (DNA), which is normally hidden inside cells but released by a damaged or infected cell as it dies.

AUTOIMMUNITY

Autoimmunity occurs when there is breakdown in the stringent mechanisms that generate immunological tolerance. As a result, autoreactive lymphocytes (lymphocytes that should have either been deleted or inactivated) are available to become reactive against body cells and molecules. Cellular injury and loss of physiological function follows in otherwise healthy tissues, owing to the damage elicited by autoreactive T lymphocytes and autoantibodies secreted by autoreactive B lymphocytes. Immune complexes are formed from autoantibodies bound to tissues, and these complexes stimulate inflammation and complement-mediated cell lysis. Other immune cells bearing Fc receptors (antibody receptors) are also prompted into action (e.g. phagocytes, natural killer cells) by the presence of autoantibody-coated tissues.

Consequently, the injured cells are efficiently phagocytosed because the autoantibodies act as opsonins. Where natural killer cells are involved in forming immune complexes (injured cell–autoantibody–natural killer cell), they eliminate the distressed cell by releasing cytotoxic granules. This type of killing is an example of antibody-dependent cell mediated cytotoxicity.

MECHANISMS OF AUTOIMMUNITY

There are a number of different mechanisms to explain why some people develop autoimmune disorders. Certainly, the chances of making autoantibodies increase with age as the thymus involutes and its activity is diminished. The increased incidence of autoimmune disorders found in older patients is evidence to support this (see Chapter 40). Similarly, when the regulatory pathways that control the immune system are impaired by a disease or by drugs, it provides an opportunity for autoreactive lymphocytes to emerge. Patients who have an immunodeficiency syndrome or are given immunosuppressive drugs are therefore at risk of acquiring an autoimmune disorder (see Chapters 28 and 29).

'Friendly Fire'

Lymphocytes caught in 'friendly fire' have been considered significant in the progress of autoimmune disease, according to Professor David Isenberg and Dr John Morrow. This amounts to autoreactive lymphocytes being in the 'wrong place at the wrong time'. Just suppose that a restrained autoreactive B lymphocyte is in the same vicinity as another B lymphocyte that was specific for a dangerous antigen, when along comes an immune cell that secretes the appropriate cytokine to activate *both* cells. The cytokine stimulus was intended to activate the lymphocyte involved in the defence, but the autoreactive cell was also, inadvertently, stimulated. Consequently, when immunoglobulins are released, the autoantibodies may cause tissue damage. This is not a rare event, for most of us have a low level of autoantibodies circulating in the body fluids. These autoantibodies are relatively harmless; if anything, they are beneficial because they assist as opsonins for the phagocytes to scavenge cellular debris, which could otherwise cause inflammation. Destruction on a larger scale is inflicted when there is a high titre of autoantibodies with the potential to precipitate an autoimmune disease.

Microbial Infection

Microbial infections can stimulate the production of autoantibodies by a number of mechanisms. For instance, when a B lymphocyte is infected by an Epstein–Barr virus (EBV), it becomes activated and secretes immunoglobulins. If it is a cell that manufactures autoantibodies and is normally inactive, the EBV infection can stimulate the release of these autoantibodies, and ultimately result in an autoimmune response. In fact, a reactive arthritis is quite common in patients with infectious mononucleosis (glandular fever in young adults caused by EBV).

Molecular Mimicry

Molecular mimicry is a classic cause of autoimmunity, in which an external source of antigen (e.g. a microbe or vaccine) mimics an autoantigen. This can occur because the number of different shapes that the B lymphocytes might encounter as epitopes must be finite. Therefore, an epitope on the surface of a microbe may quite easily be the same shape as a cell surface component. Consequently, when the B lymphocyte is activated by the infection and secretes immunoglobulin whose antigen-binding sites happen to fit the 'self-mimicking' epitope on the microbe, it has, in effect, made an autoantibody. The cardiac complications of rheumatic fever are the consequence of molecular mimicry (see below).

Foreign Antigen Adhering to Cell Surfaces

Some drugs and viruses have been known to elicit an autoimmune response because of their tendency to adhere to cell surfaces. Autoimmune haemolytic anaemia is one of the complications of methyldopa, an anti-hypertensive drug that is inclined to stick to red blood cells. If this happens, the cell surface appears foreign to the immune system, and so it precipitates a response. Unfortunately, the red blood cell is lysed (haemolysis) when it becomes caught up in the immunological assault meant for the drug molecule (see Chapter 26).

Cellular Damage

Cellular damage in itself can stimulate the release of autoantibodies when the intracellular contents are exposed. Cellular organelles (e.g. the mitochondria and the nucleus) in the cytoplasm are not normally encountered by the immune system so could be perceived as 'foreign'. For instance, one of the diagnostic features of systemic lupus erythematosus is the presence of antinuclear antibodies. Similarly, pericarditis suffered by patients after a myocardial infarct may be caused by autoantibodies raised in response to the ischaemic injury (see also Chapter 32).

FACTORS PREDISPOSING TO AUTOIMMUNE DISEASES

Patients with autoimmune diseases and their families have been extensively studied in an effort to evaluate any common characteristics that may be causative factors. A hormonal influence is presumed, since autoimmune diseases are generally more common in females than males, particularly during the child-bearing years. Another significant feature is the association between specific HLA types and distinct autoimmune diseases (e.g. HLA-DR4 with rheumatoid arthritis, HLA-DR3 and HLA-DR4 with insulin-dependent diabetes mellitus) (see Chapter 24). HLA are the 'immunological sign boards' and are inherited from the parents. One of the ideas put forward to explain these links is that certain HLA types display autoantigens more readily that others (Figure 27.2).

This is a plausible explanation because some autoimmune diseases have been experimentally induced in animals with a specific genetic makeup. For instance, autoimmune thyroiditis may be caused by injecting thyroid antigens into genetically susceptible mice. Furthermore, genetic and environmental influences are difficult to disentangle because the production of autoantibodies is considered to be antigen-driven. Hence, the patient's environment is viewed as a key factor, for close relatives often have an autoimmune disease affecting the same organ. Unfortunately, in patients with a tendency to make autoantibodies, one autoimmune disorder seems to predispose to another. For instance, autoantibodies against the thyroid gland may be detected in patients with pernicious anaemia (see Person-Centred Study: Pernicious Anaemia).

SPECIFIC AUTOIMMUNE DISORDERS

Autoimmune disorders are a consequence of immunological damage to the body's own cells and physiological molecules. The presentation and symptoms of an auto-

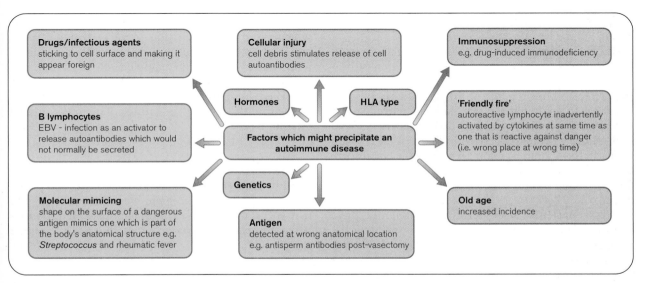

Figure 27.2 Factors that might precipitate an autoimmune disease.

Ruth was a 55-year-old who had been finding life rather tough going, having little energy and feeling emotional at the slightest provocation. The persistent 'pins and needles' in her hands and feet became so uncomfortable that she finally went to her general practitioner, who listened and took some blood for a full blood count and estimations of serum levels of vitamin B12 and folate.

The results showed that her serum and red blood cell folate levels were normal, but that her serum vitamin B12 level was very much reduced (84 ng/l). The full blood count revealed a raised mean cell volume of 103 fl and a reduced haemoglobin concentration of 9.3 g/dl.

Therefore, an appointment was made for Ruth to have a Schilling test at the local hospital to assess absorption of vitamin B12. She was requested to fast overnight before the appointment. At the clinic she was given an oral dose of radioactive vitamin B12 (1 mg of ^{58}Co-vitamin B12), and an intramuscular injection of the non-radioactive form (1000 mg of vitamin B12). She was asked to collect all the urine she passed for the next 24 hours.

No radioactive vitamin B12 was detected in the urine, which suggested that she had a malabsorption syndrome. Therefore the test was repeated with oral intrinsic factor given as capsules, but still no radioactive vitamin B12 was detected in the subsequent 24-hour urine specimen. A blood test confirmed that Ruth had serum intrinsic factor antibodies and a diagnosis of pernicious anaemia was made.

She was advised that treatment was straight-forward – she simply needed regular 3-monthly intramuscular injections of vitamin B12 because she was unable to absorb the vitamin from her diet. (A normal range of serum vitamin B12 is 150–1000 ng/l with a mean cell volume of 78–97 fl and a haemoglobin concentration of 12–16 g/dl.)

immune disorder depends on the nature of the immunological attack and its target. Therefore some diseases affect a specific organ (e.g. autoimmune thyroiditis); other disorders may be systemic if immune complexes are deposited on several different tissue types and cellular injury results (e.g. systemic lupus erythematosus).

PERNICIOUS ANAEMIA

Pernicious anaemia is a vitamin B12 malabsorption syndrome caused by autoantibodies which subsequently affect vitamin transport in the gut. Generally it is detected after the age of 40 years, with a higher incidence found in females (see Person-Centred Study: Pernicious Anaemia). In healthy people, gastric parietal cells release a protein called intrinsic factor (IF), which forms an IF–vitamin B12 complex. The efficient absorption of the vitamin depends on this complex docking into a specific receptor on the surface of the terminal ileum.

Most patients with pernicious anaemia have detectable autoantibodies whose targets are either the intrinsic factor itself or the gastric parietal cells. As a result, intrinsic factor that is bound to the autoantibodies is no longer usable for vitamin B12 transport, so the vitamin is not absorbed (Figure 27.3).

Patients with vitamin B12 deficiency present with symptoms such as fatigue, sore tongue, changes in hair colour and texture, and paraesthesia. The gastric changes caused by the autoimmune reaction leads to achlorhydria and functional loss owing to cellular destruction. The resultant nutritional deficiency leads to defective production of erythrocytes (see Chapter 31). Sometimes neurological symptoms are found even when erythrocyte production appears to be unaffected, and irreversible damage may result without treatment with vitamin B12. Dietary supplements of vitamin B12 would be useless because they could not be adequately absorbed, but pernicious anaemia can be successfully treated with regular intramuscular injections of vitamin B12.

RHEUMATIC FEVER

Rheumatic fever is a childhood disorder that was prevalent in the pre-antibiotic era in Westernized society and it is still found in developing countries. It follows a beta-streptococcal throat infection, but not all patients with such an infection develop rheumatic fever. However, those who do, have detectable serum levels of anti-streptococcal antibodies. These antibodies bind to an epitope on the heart valves as well as to one of

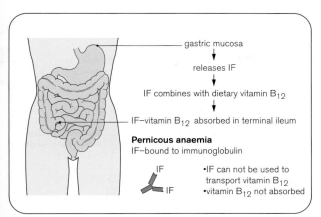

gastric mucosa
↓
releases IF
↓
IF combines with dietary vitamin B$_{12}$
↓
IF–vitamin B$_{12}$ absorbed in terminal ileum

Pernicious anaemia
IF–bound to immunoglobulin

IF
IF
• IF can not be used to transport vitamin B$_{12}$
• vitamin B$_{12}$ not absorbed

Figure 27.3 Intrinsic factor antibodies and malabsorption of vitamin B12. Mechanism by which the antibodies cause the malabsorption of vitamin B12.

the bacterial cells – this is an example of an autoimmune disease caused by molecular mimicry. The clinical features are, to a large extent, brought on by these antibodies; they include endocarditis and heart valve defects. Neurological symptoms and polyarthritis may also erupt. The joints most often affected are the knees, ankles, wrists, and elbows (see also Chapter 32).

RHEUMATOID ARTHRITIS

The characteristic symmetrical joint deformities and nodules of rheumatoid arthritis would suggest that this is a disease of skeletal tissue. Destruction of cartilage and bone erosion is a feature of this debilitating disease. It is caused by immune complex formation and damage within the joints. However other systems may be affected – wherever immune complexes are deposited, the resultant inflammation causes loss of tissue function. Neurological diseases such as polyneuropathy or carpal tunnel syndrome may be present, and renal and pulmonary manifestations are not uncommon. Lung involvement produces inflammation of the alveoli and bronchioles and fibrosis, resulting in a reduced oxygen supply, so more tissues are compromised. Occasionally, large rheumatoid nodules emerge in the lungs; these resemble tumours on X-ray.

The activities of the different immune cell types precipitate the hyperplasia and hypertrophy of the synovial linings of the joints. Macrophages, T lymphocytes, and B lymphocytes migrate into the area and start releasing cytokines, including IL-1 and TNF-alpha. The cellular actions and cytokines have been implicated as some of the mediators of joint damage. In addition, B lymphocytes in the joint produce autoantibodies, called

'rheumatoid factor'. The antigenic target of rheumatoid factor is the Fc region of IgG molecules. Therefore, there is no shortage of antigen to form immune complexes, for any IgG molecule may be captured. Immune complexes stimulate the complement pathways, so an inflammatory reaction ensues. Macrophages and other phagocytes are attracted into the joint by chemotaxis to assist in the removal of the immune complexes. However, in this endeavour they release free radicals and spill lysosomal enzymes that cause further damage to the joint.

Rheumatoid arthritis is about three times more prevalent in females than males, particularly in the child-bearing years. An intriguing observation is that a significant number of patients experience remission of symptoms during pregnancy, only to relapse in the postnatal period. Some patients may develop rheumatoid arthritis following pregnancy. This evidence suggests that there is a hormonal influence in the progression of the disease. As with other immunological diseases, an HLA-association has been identified. Patients who are of the HLA-DR4 and HLA-DR1 tissue type are more likely to suffer the erosive form of the disease.

The effects of the pain, morning stiffness, and immobility are particularly stressful, and dependence on carers has a profound effect on the patient's self esteem. Analgesia and anti-inflammatory drugs control some of the symptoms (see Chapter 39). If the reason why the immune cells were attracted into the joint were known, this could provide some ideas for treatment. Physical injury following an accident has been proposed, as have infectious organisms such as *Mycobacterium tuberculosis* and the rubella virus. Novel therapies have recently emerged to help reduce the immune cell activation. Since cytokines are some of the significant mediators of joint damage, capturing them by antibody therapy is a possible treatment and this is presently being pioneered. Monoclonal antibodies against TNF-alpha have been used in clinical trials and given promising results because they significantly reduce the cytokine levels and immune cell activities causing the joint damage. Nutritional intervention using marine fish oils has also been shown to produce a modest beneficial effect for patients with rheumatoid arthritis. This is thought to be due to the effects of the oils on the cytokine profile.

Other Forms of Arthritis Disease

There are several other forms of arthritic disease. Still's disease is an HLA-linked childhood disorder. It is sometimes referred to as juvenile chronic arthritis. In addition a number of conditions are known to be caused by infections.

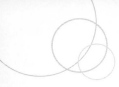

Ankylosing spondylitis is a connective tissue disease that affects young adults; males are three times more likely to be affected than females. Up to 90 per cent of patients with ankylosing spondylitis are of the HLA-B27 tissue type. Certain infections (e.g. enteric infections with *Klebsiella* species) have been associated with onset of the disorder in susceptible people.

Similarly, Lyme disease is a form of arthritis caused by a spirochaete, *Borrelia burgdorferi*, which is treatable with antimicrobial therapy. The resultant inflammation affects many organs besides the joints, with T lymphocytes and macrophages responsible for some of the immunological mechanisms (see Chapter 39).

SYSTEMIC LUPUS ERYTHEMATOSUS

Systemic lupus erythematosus (SLE) is an immune-complex-mediated disease. It has a higher incidence in Asian and black African people than in Caucasians, and nine times more common in females than males. Many women are diagnosed during the child-bearing years, which suggests a hormonal trigger as an aetiological factor of the disorder. A distinguishing clinical feature of SLE is a light-sensitive 'butterfly rash', a skin lesion on the cheeks, eyelids, and bridge of the nose. One of the diagnostic indicators is the presence of anti-DNA antibodies and rheumatoid factor in body fluids. These autoantibodies encourage the deposition of immune complexes at various sites, including the skin, blood vessels, joints, and kidneys (Figure 27.4). Certain anomalies in the immune system of some SLE patients contribute to the immune complex load in the body:

- deficiencies of complement proteins of the classical pathway (a system needed for the clearance of immune complexes) (see Chapter 25); and
- a limited control of the immune response, owing to reduced T suppressor cell activity (promoting the formation of immune complexes).

Many of the clinical manifestations of SLE are caused by the immunological assault mounted against the immune complexes. Symptoms vary between patients depending on where the immune complexes are deposited. Vasculitis may erupt when they lodge in small blood vessels; this leads to thickening and occlusion of the capillaries. There may also be haematological problems if the clotting mechanism is affected, there is an increased risk of thrombosis. Ischaemic damage may result in tissues served by the blocked vessels, owing to an inadequate blood supply. The inflammation and erosion in the joints resembles rheumatoid arthritis. Renal failure is one of the major causes of mortality. Patients with SLE have periods of relapse and remission, exacerbations being precipitated by

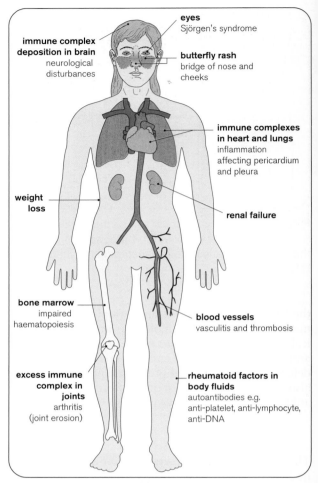

Figure 27.4 **Clinical features of systemic lupus erythematosus.**

diverse types of environmental stressors (e.g. infection, exposure to sunlight, emotional stress). It is noteworthy that certain drugs (e.g. procainamide, hydralazine) induce an SLE-like disease, which is reversible when the drug treatment is withdrawn.

Further investigation into the aetiology of the disease is compelling – one study has provided the intriguing observation that the pet dogs of some SLE sufferers have higher serum levels of anti-DNA antibodies than the dogs of healthy people! A transmissible factor within the environment (perhaps a virus) is one possible explanation for these findings.

Anti-inflammatory and immunosuppressive drugs are prescribed, and complications are treated as they arise (see also Box 27.2). For instance, the anaemia

BOX 27.2 SJÖGREN'S SYNDROME

Sjögren's syndrome is a disorder which may occur alone or as a complication associated with SLE and rheumatoid arthritis.

- Rheumatoid factor and anti-nuclear antibodies are detectable in the body fluids of patients with Sjögren's syndrome.
- One of the prominent features is lymphocyte infiltration into the lacrimal and parotid glands which results in a lack of saliva and tears; consequently patients suffer from dry mouth and eyes.
- Digestion is affected and patients must be meticulous in their dental hygiene to reduce the frequency of caries. The lack of tears produces itching and burning eyes and can lead to corneal ulceration, conjunctivitis, keratinization of the cornea, and even blindness.
- The Schirmer test is used to assess the amount of tear flow. Artificial tears may be prescribed, however, some patients develop allergies to the preservatives in these preparations.

and abnormality in clotting mechanisms must be monitored by regular haematological investigations (see Chapters 6 and 31).

AUTOIMMUNE DISORDERS OF THE NERVOUS SYSTEM

Multiple Sclerosis

The media have heightened public awareness of multiple sclerosis (MS), a major neurological disorder that often affects young adults, particularly females. It is a debilitating disease owing to the demyelination within the central nervous system, which severely affects the transmission of nerve impulses. An autoimmune mechanism is thought to be responsible for the demyelination. Genetic factors cannot be excluded – an association has been identified between susceptibility to MS and HLA-DR2, and first-degree relatives of a person with MS have an increased risk of the disease. Again, though, the influences of genes and environment on disease onset are difficult to evaluate. In addition, a rather bizarre association has been found – the incidence of MS within a population seems to be related to the latitude where they live – more cases are found in countries lying nearer the North and South poles. An infectious agent such as a retrovirus has been proposed as a causative factor, although no conclusive evidence has been found. Ethnicity is also thought to have a role in patient susceptibility, since more Caucasians have MS than black and Asian people – this might partly explain reduced incidence of MS near the equator.

An assessment of the immune status of MS patients has connected the phagocytic cells with the demyelination process. However, lymphocytes are also implicated, for they have been detected within the white matter of the central nervous system. One of the diagnostic criteria for MS is the presence of oligoclonal bands in the cerebrospinal fluid (CSF), which are found in up to 90 per cent of patients. These bands are immunoglobulins derived from a few B lymphocytes. Unlike the polyclonal antibodies found in blood (which are raised against a wide variety of antigens), the oligoclonal bands in CSF are made up of a few different immunoglobulin molecules. It was speculated that the nature of the antigenic targets of the oligoclonal bands might provide clues to the cause of MS. Unfortunately, however, no conclusive evidence has been drawn, although anti-measles antibodies have been detected, and T lymphocytes that are specific for myelin basic protein, a protein in the myelin sheath, have also been found.

The disease mechanisms may be the outcome of an inadequately controlled immune system, for reduced T suppressor cell activity (the cell involved in immunological tolerance) has been identified in some patients with MS. Recent clinical evidence has supported this idea by demonstrating that T suppressor activity could be boosted by interferon-beta therapy, with subsequent control of the cycles of relapse and remission.

There appears to be no specific regimens for the treatment of MS. Vitamin and mineral supplements in the diet have been used with some success, but it is not known whether the remission of symptoms is due to a nutrition-induced manipulation of the immune system or to a placebo effect (see Chapter 8). Recent experimental evidence has indicated that changing the type of dietary fats consumed can dampen the immune activities in rodents that have an experimental disease resembling MS. Clinical trials are now underway to ascertain whether this dietary modification could be effective therapy for humans with MS.

Guillain–Barré Syndrome

Named after two French military clinicians, Guillain–Barré syndrome is a disease that can attack any neurone outside the brain and spinal cord. Demyelination of the peripheral nervous system is found, but in contrast to the situation with MS, up to 70 per cent of patients with Guillain–Barré syndrome make a complete recovery.

The characteristic features are oedema and inflammation in the myelin sheath and Schwann cells. The disease commonly follows an infection (e.g. with Epstein–Barr virus or *Campylobacter jejuni*), although occasionally it is a complication of surgery, pregnancy, or immunization.

Molecular mimicry between an infectious agent and a component of the myelin sheath on peripheral neurones has been proposed as one of the mechanisms of the disease with the subsequent release of autoantibody. Inflammation and destruction by activated macrophages spilling enzymes and free radicals is another possible damage mediator.

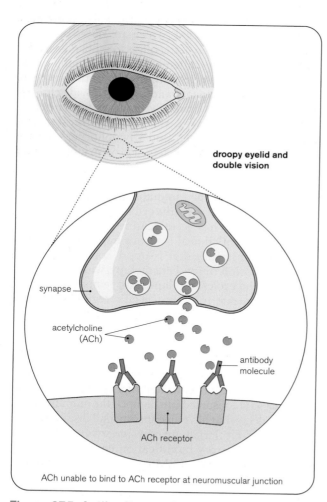

droopy eyelid and double vision

synapse

acetylcholine (ACh)

antibody molecule

ACh receptor

ACh unable to bind to ACh receptor at neuromuscular junction

Figure 27.5 Antibodies against acetylcholine receptors at neuromuscular junctions in myasthenia gravis. The antibodies mean that acetylcholine is unable to bind to the receptors, resulting in the symptoms of myasthenia gravis such as droopy eyelids and double vision.

Myasthenia Gravis

Myasthenia gravis results in defective nerve impulse transmission at the synapse of neuromuscular junctions. It can erupt at any age, and like most other autoimmune disorders, it is more prevalent in females, especially between adolescence and 30 years. When it occurs in males, it tends to occur at a later age. In healthy people, a muscle responds to a nerve impulse because acetylcholine diffuses across the synaptic cleft and binds the acetylcholine receptors on the postsynaptic membrane at the neuromuscular junction – this forms the interaction between the nerve impulse and the muscle fibre. In people with myasthenia gravis, the acetylcholine receptors are blocked by autoantibodies, and so neurotransmission to the muscle is impeded (Figure 27.5).

The symptoms of the disease depend on which of the neuromuscular junctions are affected. If the eye muscles are involved, the patient may have drooping eyelids and experience double vision. When the muscles affected by the autoantibodies lead to respiratory distress or dysphagia (swallowing difficulties), the condition becomes more serious.

The reason why these autoantibodies are raised is not known, but a T lymphocyte trigger has been considered, since around 40 per cent of patients have an enlarged thymus. Several therapies have been used with some success to weaken the effects of the autoimmune disease. These include:

- thymectomy;
- plasmapheresis to remove the autoantibodies from body fluids; and
- anticholinesterase drugs (e.g. neostigmine) (see Chapter 10) to increase the activity of acetylcholine at the neuromuscular junction.

Myasthenia gravis is diagnosed by the edrophonium (Tensilon) test, in which a short-acting acetylcholinesterase inhibitor, that conserves the acetylcholine levels at the neuromuscular junction, is given intravenously. A positive result is found when muscle function is restored or improved.

FERTILITY AND THE PRESENCE OF AUTOANTIBODIES

One of the causes of human subfertility is the presence of antisperm antibodies in the genital tract (either male or female). When men synthesize and secrete these antibodies into seminal fluid, their sperm are agglutinated (clump) and unable to swim up the Fallopian tube and fertilize an ovum. A significant number of vasectomized men make these autoantibodies because the sperm are delivered into an alternative intercellular space, where they are considered 'foreign'. This is one of the reasons for limited success restoring fertility when the surgical procedure is reversed. Likewise females with anti-sperm antibodies in cervical mucus have problems conceiving because the antibodies halt the sperm soon after sexual intercourse (see Chapter 37). It is notable that autoantibodies raised against other areas of reproductive tract can affect fertility. Menopause before the age of 40 years has been attributed to premature ovarian failure caused by autoimmune responses against the ovary (see also Box 27.3).

AUTOIMMUNE THYROID DISEASES

A spectrum of autoimmune disorders affect thyroid function, but it depends on the nature of the immunological attack as to whether the result is an underactive thyroid (hypothyroidism) or an overactive thyroid (hyperthyroidism).

Hashimoto's Thyroiditis

Hashimoto's thyroiditis is a chronic disease arising in middle age and is four times more common in females than males. It produces hypothyroidism and is caused by autoantibodies generated against the components of the gland required to synthesize thyroxine and tri-iodothyronine. These active hormones are manufactured from thyroglobulin and iodine, and the enzyme thyroid peroxidase catalyses the reaction. Thyroglobulin and thyroid peroxidase are the two main antigenic tar-

gets of the autoantibodies commonly found in Hashimoto's thyroiditis, and thus hormone synthesis is severely affected. The gland itself is often enlarged (producing a goitre), and it may be infiltrated with plasma cells secreting the autoantibodies. An antibody-dependent cell mediated cytotoxicity is one of the mechanisms thought to cause the tissue damage. Classic symptoms of hypothyroidism are present, including weight gain owing to a reduced metabolic rate, mental slowness, and intolerance to changes in ambient temperature.

Graves' Disease

Graves' disease is an autoimmune hyperthyroid state, which seems to be more prevalent in populations with a high dietary intake of iodine. It is a disease of middle age and it may be induced by stress. Raised thyroxine levels lead to symptoms of weight loss owing to an increased basal metabolic rate, tachycardia, diarrhoea, and nervous irritability. The immunological mechanism involves autoantibodies whose antigenic targets are receptors on the thyroid gland that stimulate the release of excess hormone. In healthy people, the pituitary-derived thyroid-stimulating hormone (TSH) controls the synthesis and release of thyroxine via TSH receptors on the surface of the thyroid gland (see Chapter

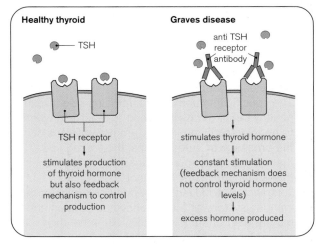

Figure 27.6 Anti-TSH-receptor antibodies in Graves' disease. In the normal situation, TSH stimulates production of thyroid hormone but there is also a feedback mechanism to control production of thyroid hormone. In Graves' disease, the anti-TSH-receptor antibodies bind and stimulate the thyroid gland, which then releases excess amounts of thyroid hormone. Feedback mechanisms are ineffectual along the hypothalamus–pituitary–thyroid axis owing to the blocking of the TSH receptor by the autoantibodies. (TSH: thyroid-stimulating hormone.)

BOX 27.3 MATERNAL AUTOIMMUNE DISORDERS AND THE FETUS

It is natural to assume that maternal-derived antibodies passing across the placenta to the fetus will offer immune protection during the vulnerable period of neonatal life. However, if the mother has an autoimmune disorder, then her autoantibodies may cross the placenta to the fetus (if they are of the IgG isotype) and precipitate a transient form of the disease. Nevertheless, since these antibodies are passively acquired rather than the product of the neonate's own immune cells, symptoms are generally short-lived and do not persist after 6 months of age. Neonates need to be observed if born to mothers with Graves' disease, Hashimoto's thyroiditis, myasthenia gravis, autoimmune haemolytic anaemia, or systemic lupus erythematosus.

35). In Graves' disease, autoantibodies bind the TSH receptor, so perpetually priming the gland to release hormone (Figure 27.6). Immune destruction of the thyroid is not a general feature of the disease, although there is some lymphocyte infiltration into the thyroid gland.

INSULIN-DEPENDENT DIABETES MELLITUS

Insulin-dependent diabetes mellitus (IDDM) is one of the most common diseases of carbohydrate metabolism. It occurs after the progressive immunological destruction of beta-cells in the islets of Langerhans in the pancreas. As long as a few cells remain, they take on the role of synthesizing enough insulin to maintain glucose homeostasis. The onset of IDDM occurs abruptly when all the beta-cells have been destroyed. An exogenous source of insulin is required for the rest of the patient's life, which is unfortunate considering that the disease so often presents in children between the ages of 10 and 13 years. There is a seasonal association with IDDM – more cases are diagnosed in the autumn and spring than in other seasons of the year.

It has been suggested that infectious agents may act as a mimic to precipitate the disease. Certain vaccines (e.g. mumps, rubella) have also been implicated – some studies have pointed to an association between immunization schedules and the subsequent appearance of the disease. However, this is debatable. Similarly, a Swedish study suggested that children born to mothers who suffer an enteroviral infection during pregnancy were at risk of this type of diabetes mellitus. One possible cause is an autoimmune response raised against a heat shock protein released as a stress signal by cells. Part of this molecule is a molecular mimic of a protein localized in the beta-cells. Other immunological mechanisms thought to be deployed in beta-cell destruction include enzymes released by macrophages, cytokine-mediated damage by IL-1 and TNF-alpha, and infiltration of the pancreas by T lymphocytes.

KEY POINTS

- Occasionally a fault arises in the immune system and lymphocytes attack the body and cause an autoimmune disorder (e.g. rheumatoid arthritis, pernicious anaemia).
- The specific immune system remains selective in healthy people, knowing when to react and when to be tolerant. Lymphocytes are not oblivious of the presence of autoantigens; they recognize them but do not mount a tenacious response – this is immunological tolerance.
- Tolerance is achieved in the primary organs of the immune system as the lymphocytes develop and mature (i.e. central tolerance). Tolerance also takes place in the periphery via the cytokine network controlling the immune response, and distress signals alerting the immune system to possible danger (i.e. peripheral tolerance).
- Autoimmunity is caused by a breakdown in the stringent mechanisms that generate immunological tolerance. As a result, lymphocytes that should have either been killed or inactivated are available to become reactive against body cells and molecules – these are autoreactive lymphocytes.
- There are a number of factors that predispose to the development of autoimmune disorders (e.g. age, immunodeficiency syndromes, the use of immunosuppressive therapy).
- Microbial infections can stimulate an autoimmune response by mimicking a body component (e.g. streptococcal infection preceding the onset of rheumatic fever).
- Patients with autoimmune diseases and their families have been extensively studied. Some of the causative factors identified include an association between specific HLA types and a hormonal influence, since autoimmune diseases are generally more common in females than males, particularly during the child-bearing years.
- The symptoms of an autoimmune disorder depend on the nature of the immunological attack and its target. Some diseases are organ-specific (e.g. autoimmune thyroiditis). Other disorders are systemic when immune complexes are deposited on several different tissue types and cellular injury results (e.g. systemic lupus erythematosus).

FURTHER READING

Akama H, Tanaka H (1992) Autoantibodies in pet dogs of patients with systemic lupus erythematosus. Lancet 340:303–4.

Ament LA (1994) Anticardiolipin antibodies. A review of the literature. J Nurse Midwifery 39:19–24.

Baker JR Jr (1997) Autoimmune endocrine disease. JAMA 278:1931–7.

Butler RB (1996) Immune tolerance: a nursing perspective. Vox Sang 70 (Suppl 1):70–1.

Calder PC (1998) Dietary fatty acids and the immune system. Nutr Rev 56:(1 Pt. 2) 570–83.

Dahlquist GG, Ivarsson S, Lindberg B, Forsgren M (1995) Maternal enteroviral infections during pregnancy as a risk factor for childhood IDDM. A population-based case-control study. Diabetes 44:408–13.

Davis D, Charles PJ, Potter A, Feldmann M, Maini RN, Elliott MJ (1997) Anaemia of chronic disease in rheumatoid arthritis: *in vivo* effects of tumour necrosis factor alpha blockade. Br J Rheumatol 36:950–6.

Davies KA (1996) Michael Mason Prize Essay 1995. Complement, immune complexes and systemic lupus erythematosus. Br J Rheumatol 35:5–23.

Eigler A, Sinha B, Hartmann G, Endres S (1997) Taming TNF: strategies to restrain this proinflammatory cytokine. Immunol Today 18:487–92.

Hahn AF (1998) Guillan–Barré syndrome. Lancet 352:635–41.

Hardy EM, Rittenberry K (1994) Mysthenia gravis: an overview. Orthop Nurs 13:37–42.

Hawa M, Rowe R, Lan MS, *et al.* (1997) Value of antibodies to islet protein tyrosine phosphatase-like molecule in predicting type I diabetes. Diabetes. 46: 1270–5.

Isenberg DA, Morrow WJW (1995) Friendly fire: explaining autoimmune disease. Oxford University Press, Oxford.

Kernich CA, Kaminski HJ (1995) Myasthenia gravis: pathophysiology, diagnosis and collaborative care. J Neurosci Nurs 27:207–15.

Kuby J (1997) Immunolgy 3rd edition WH Freeman Co, New York.

Leslie RDG, Elliott RB (1994) Early enviromental events as a cause of IDDM: evidence and implications. Diabetes 43:843–50.

Lindsbaum J, Healton EB, Savage DG, *et al.* (1988) Neuropsychiatric disorders caused by cobalamin deficiency in the absence of anaemia or macrocytosis. N Engl J Med 318:1720–8.

Matzinger P (1994) Tolerance, danger and the extended family. Annu Rev Immunol 12:991–1045.

Nadelman RB, Wormser GP (1998) Lyme borreliosis Lancet 352:557–65.

Ogilvy-Stuart AL (1995) Endocrinology of the neonate. Br J Hosp Med 54:207–11.

Prummel MF, Van Pareren Y, Bakker O, Wiersinga WM (1997) Anti-heat shock protein (hsp) 72 antibodies are present in patients with Graves' disease (GD) and in smoking control subjects. Clin Exp Immunol 110:292–5.

Rasmussen HB, Clausen J (1997) Possible involvement of endogenous retroviruses in the development of autoimmune disorders, especially multiple sclerosis. Acta Neurol Scand Suppl 169:32–7.

Rees J (1995) Guillain–Barré syndrome. Clinical manifestations and directions for treatment. Drugs 49:912–20.

Sawcer S, Goodfellow PN, Compston A (1997) The genetic analysis of multiple sclerosis. Trends Genet 13:234–9.

Sigal LH (1997) Lyme disease: a review of aspects of its immunology and immunopathogenesis. Annu Rev Immunol 15:63–92.

Sleasman JW (1996) The association between immunodeficiency and the development of autoimmune disease. Adv Dental Res 10:57–61.

Timbers KA, Feinberg RF (1997) Recurrent pregnancy loss: a review. Nurse Pract Forum 8:77–88.

Weyand CM, Goronzy JJ (1997) Pathogenesis of rheumatoid arthritis. Med Clin North Am 81:29–55.

HEREDITARY AND ACQUIRED IMMUNODEFICIENCY

LEARNING OBJECTIVES

After studying this chapter you will have a clearer understanding of:
- the clinical consequences of an immunodeficiency and its relationship to a defective part of the immune system
- the way that immunodeficiency in one part of the immune system can affect the functional activities of the other components
- the fact that most inherited immunodeficiencies are rare but some are potentially life-threatening without medical intervention
- the fact that acquired immunodeficiencies may be caused by infections, metabolic disorders, surgical or medical interventions, or malnutrition – acquired immunodeficiency syndrome is only one example of an acquired immunodeficiency
- the mechanism by which human immunodeficiency virus causes immunodeficiency, the progress to AIDS, and its treatment

For a broader understanding of this chapter you should read the first four chapters of the Immunology section (Chapters 22, 23, 24, 25).

INTRODUCTION

With the potential threat that acquired immunodeficiency syndrome (AIDS) will reach epidemic proportions, the general public as well as health care professionals have an increased awareness of the part our immunological defences play in the maintenance of health, and the devastating effects of immunodeficiency. But AIDS is only one type of immunodeficiency and is caused by infection with human immunodeficiency virus (HIV). Immunodeficiency exists in many forms and is the outcome of an irregularity in one or more of the components of the immune system. Immunodeficiency may be inherited or acquired.

An inherited immunodeficiency arises where there is an irregularity or absence of a gene that encodes part of the immune system. This results in an immune factor being malfunctioning, absent, or in short supply. An acquired defect may be the consequence of a clinical situation – certain infections, malignancy, malnutrition, and medical interventions may suppress normal immune function. Whatever the basis for the immunodeficiency, the result is the same – an increased susceptibility to the infections and cancer one would be protected from if the immune system were functionally intact.

No two patients necessarily present with the same clinical symptoms and diseases – the outcome of an immunodeficiency is related to the part of the immune system affected and the extent of the defect. Because both the natural and specific immune systems work together, one component being suboptimal means that other parts of the immune system are highly likely to be affected as well. The severe deficiencies attract the most attention, but far more common are the partial defects that result in certain people being more susceptible than others to repeated mild infections, such as upper respiratory tract infections or troublesome conditions such as recurrent candidiasis (thrush) (see Chapter 23).

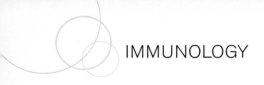

IMMUNOLOGY

HEREDITARY IMMUNODEFICIENCIES

Immunodeficiency syndromes caused by a fault which is inherited are called primary deficiencies. They may be classified according to the part of the immune system affected – phagocytic system (neutrophils and macrophages), complement system (see Chapter 25); antibody-mediated (B lymphocyte) immunity, or cell-mediated (T lymphocyte) immunity.

Defective phagocytosis may be due to low numbers of phagocytes, malfunctioning cells, or possibly reduced levels of opsonins available to promote phagocytosis (see Chapters 22 and 23). Since immunoglobulins act as opsonins, a defect in the B lymphocytes or plasma cells that produce them may reduce the competence of the phagocytes and ultimately lead to an increased risk of bacterial infections (e.g. infections due to *Haemophilus influenzae*, *Staphylococcus aureus*, and *Streptococcus pneumoniae*).

In contrast, patients with impaired T lymphocyte activities are susceptible to developing cancers and infections that grow inside cells (e.g. infections with viruses and intracellular bacteria such as *Mycobacterium* species) as well as opportunistic infections, which are not easy to treat.

There is a congenital disease called reticular dysgenesis, in which haematopoietic stem cells fail to produce granulocytes, monocytes, and lymphocytes; affected infants die within hours of birth. Mercifully, it is a rare condition.

DEFECTIVE PHAGOCYTES AS A CAUSE OF IMMUNODEFICENCY

For phagocytes to fulfil their role in natural immunity they must be attracted to the area of infection by chemotaxis. Therefore, having adhered to the endothelial cells that line the capillaries, they must squeeze through the junctions between these cells to where phagocytosis is required. The phagocyte must be functionally active to engulf the microbes and effectively produce the enzymes and free radicals necessary to kill those organisms in the phagosome. If there is an insufficiency of an essential component at any one of these individual stages, the result is defective phagocytic function and an increased tendency to contract the infections that this immunological mechanism controls.

Leukocyte Adhesion Deficiencies

Immune cells must stick to their target, whether it is the endothelial cell wall at a site of an infection or an infected cell to be killed. There are some inherited disorders, collectively named leukocyte adhesion deficiencies, in which this does not happen effectively. This may be due to an abnormal synthesis of the adherent molecules or to impaired action of the immune cells. In some severe cases, a bone marrow transplant is the only successful treatment to replace the defective cells (see Figure 28.1).

Lazy Leukocyte Syndrome

The inherited diseases that cause these various defects are rare but nevertheless they are extremely dangerous. One such condition, lazy leukocyte syndrome, is when there is a fault in neutrophilic chemotactic response either because the cells are insensitive to the attractant or the attractant itself is at a reduced level or inactive. Prophylactic antibiotic therapy is necessary to avert recurrent bacterial infections, thus emphasizing the importance of these cells in removing bacteria to prevent an infection.

Chronic Granulomatous Disease

In chronic granulomatous disease (CGD), the killing ability of phagocytes is hindered by inadequate production of hydrogen peroxide, caused by a deficiency of an enzyme such as NADPH oxidase. As a result, low levels of hydrogen peroxide promote the survival of bacteria within the phagosome. CGD is not just one disorder, but a group of inherited disorders, which may be X-linked or autosomal recessive (see also Chapter 7). Affected children tend to suffer recurrent and prolonged infections such as pneumonia, abscesses in the skin and liver, and osteomyelitis. The clinical management is to treat the infections when they arise and give leukocyte infusions to supply functional cells, but this is just a temporary measure – the only real cure is a bone marrow transplant (see Chapter 29). To confirm a diagnosis of CGD or to test for carrier status in the family of an affected patient, the functional competence of the phagocytes is examined. This is a simple procedure in which the cells are given a dye (nitroblue tetrazolium) to 'eat'; if the cells are active then a colour change will be seen when they are viewed down a microscope.

HUMORAL DEFICIENCIES

Immunoglobulins pass from mother to fetus before birth, but it is some time before the baby's own production gets going effectively. Children under the age of 2 years often have transient low levels of immunoglobulins before normal levels are attained while their immune system matures as it is assaulted by a wide variety of antigens. However there are a number of known inherited defects of B lymphocytes that affect the various stages of development:

- defective cell production by the bone marrow;
- impaired ability of B lymphocytes to mature into plasma cells;
- an insensitivity to the assistance provided by the T helper cells; and
- a block in the intracellular pathway affecting the production and/or secretion of one or more classes or subclasses of immunoglobulin (Figure 28.2).

An infant born at full term is protected, at least in part, by the passive immunity of immunoglobulins acquired *in utero*, but these have a short half-life. Thus, from around the age of 6 months, children are 'on their own' as far as immunoglobulins are concerned, relying solely on the capabilities of their own immune cells. Any humoral deficiency is therefore likely to be exposed at this age, when the child might attend a clinic with a failure to thrive and recurrent infections. Inevitably, the nature and severity of the inadequate immunoglobulin production will influence when and how the adverse clinical symptoms are presented.

Selective Immunoglobulin A Deficiency
The most common inherited defect of humoral immunity is selective immunoglobulin A (IgA) deficiency. It

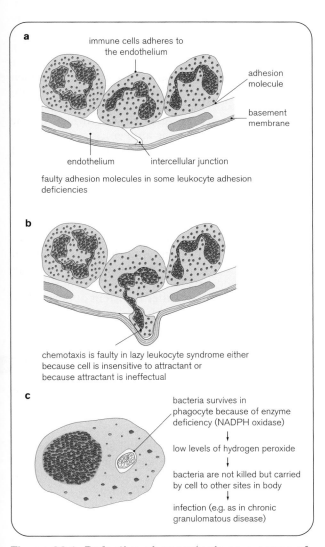

Figure 28.1 Defective phagocytosis as a cause of immunodeficiency. Defective phagocytosis can be due to (a) defective leukocyte adhesion; (b) defective chemotaxis; or (c) defective killing ability.

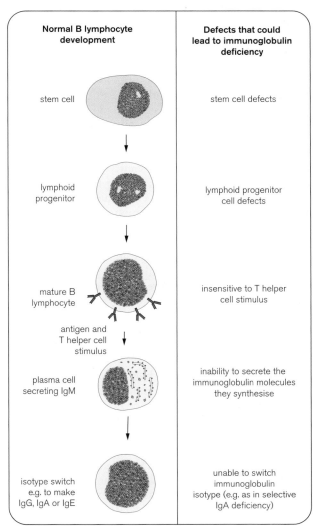

Figure 28.2 Defects of B-lymphocyte development that lead to immunoglobulin deficiency.

affects around one in 700 people. It results in low levels of IgA in body fluids and it is a disorder of B lymphocytes bearing the membrane-bound IgA; these cells do not develop into plasma cells and therefore do not secrete IgA upon antigen stimulation. This may well be one of the diseases in which the B lymphocytes are insensitive to the action of T helper cells.

A consequence of IgA deficiency is inadequate immune protection at the mucosal surfaces. Thus, environmental substances and microbial infections gain entry more easily. Patients tend to suffer recurrent episodes of pneumonia and other bacterial infections. Allergic diseases are also a problem because mucosal surfaces are inadequately protected. Therefore potential allergen can breach these barriers and elicit an IgE response. When this occurs in the gut it may result in malabsorption and reduced body weight (see Person-Centred Study: Selective IgA Deficiency). After all, the food we eat is immunologically foreign. Immunoglobulins made against these antigens may cross-react and also bind to tissues within the body, resulting in immunoglobulin-related diseases such as autoimmune disorders and type III hypersensitivity reactions.

Bruton's Hypogammaglobulinaemia

Patients with selective IgA deficiency produce the other classes of immunoglobulin, unlike the patient with hypogammaglobulinaemia examined by Bruton in 1952. This patient had few B lymphocytes in the blood, although there were normal populations of cells detectable in the bone marrow. Moreover, when other areas within the lymphatic system were investigated (areas where immunoglobulins are produced), they were also found to be depleted of B lymphocytes. This was one of the first immunodeficiency diseases to be rationalized and was named Bruton's hypogammaglobulinaemia. Like several other inherited disorders of immunity, the genetic defect was later identified on the X chromosome and therefore the disease affects males. The inability to produce mature B lymphocytes means patients require gammaglobulin replacement therapy to reduce the risk of infections.

INHERITED T LYMPHOCYTE DEFICIENCIES

The effects of defective T lymphocytes vary in their clinical severity for quantitative and qualitative deficiencies of these cells have different outcomes. There are three main types of T lymphocyte (i.e. cytotoxic T lymphocytes, T helper cells, and T suppressor cells). These cells have diverse actions, so the immune response is affected differently when there is a deficit of any one of them. Functionally, defective T lymphocytes may develop because of a reduction in:

- T-cell receptor expression on the cell surface (i.e. the cells cannot recognize the antigen);
- the signalling within the cell that follows antigen binding (i.e. the cells cannot respond effectively to the antigen); or
- the levels of the cytokine action (i.e. regulation of the immune response is affected).

Furthermore, even if cytokines are adequately produced, if the cell surface receptor levels are low or if they fail to induce the appropriate response on receptor binding, they are of little use.

As a result, patients suffer recurrent opportunistic

PERSON-CENTRED STUDY: SELECTIVE IgA DEFICIENCY

Throughout her life, Donna had had recurrent ear, nose, and throat infections and gastrointestinal disturbances; about once a month she would suffer a cold, and she regularly had bouts of diarrhoea. At the age of 32 years, she became ill with symptoms like those of glandular fever – fatigue, malaise, fever, and lymphadenopathy. Her general practitioner prescribed a course of amoxycillin to reduce the risk of a secondary bacterial infection in addition to what seemed to be a viral infection. When, after 1 month, her symptoms had not improved, blood was taken for microbiological investigation, and cytomegalovirus was detected.

Donna was severely affected by the cytomegalovirus infection and was unable go to work for about 9 months. During this time it was decided that further tests were needed. More blood was taken to evaluate her immunoglobulin status, for the general practitioner suspected a possible immunodeficiency. The results indicated that she had selective IgA deficiency. Donna was relieved that (at last) there was an explanation for her persistent problems, and was advised that the preferred treatment strategy was simply to deal with any infections when they occurred.

infections, and when T lymphocytes are functionally inadequate, a combined immunodeficiency may develop. Immunoglobulin production is affected as well, if it is dependent on T helper cell activity, which happens to be ineffectual.

Severe Combined Immunodeficiency Syndrome

Of particular concern are the heterogeneous group of inherited diseases collectively known as severe combined immunodeficiency syndrome (SCID). As the name implies, these are deficiencies in both cellular and humoral components of immunity, which may be caused by either a X-linked gene or an autosomal-recessive gene. Normal immune cells are extremely active, requiring high levels of nucleic acid production for growth and mitosis. But some SCID patients have either mutant (malfunctioning) enzymes or frank deficiencies of enzymes involved in nucleic acid synthesis. Two of the enzyme anomalies that have been identified in SCID patients are:

- a deficiency in adenosine deaminase, which leads to an increase in deoxyadenosine triphosphate levels in lymphocytes, resulting in a block in the synthesis of DNA;
- a deficiency in purine nucleoside phosphorylase, which affects the production of the nucleotide base, guanine, needed for the synthesis of DNA and RNA.

The net effect on immune cells is that their mitotic ability and response to antigen stimulation are significantly reduced. Consequently, T and B lymphocytes are reduced in number, and low plasma levels of immunoglobulins can be found (Figure 28.3). It is therefore dangerous to give these patients live-attenuated vaccine (e.g. polio vaccine), because their immunity is compromised. Infants with this syndrome present with a failure to thrive and an increased susceptibility to a wide spectrum of infections, some being potentially life-threatening.

Di George Syndrome

Di George syndrome (thymic hypoplasia) is a rare condition, which has been identified as a gene deletion on chromosome 22; it therefore affects males and females equally. Other irregularities include characteristic facial and ear deformities, and an abnormal aortic arch, parathyroid gland, and thyroid gland. These anatomical structures develop at around 6–10 weeks' gestation and share the same embryonic origins as the thymus.

These patients have a thymus that is either small or absent, and the degree of immunodeficiency is linked to the level of thymic activity. The resultant inadequate thymic education means T lymphocytes numbers are diminished in Di George syndrome compared with normal people. Hence, patients have an increased susceptibility to infection with viruses, fungi, and, in particular, *Pneumocystis carinii* and other opportunistic infections. The thyroid and parathyroid glands are often absent, and so metabolic activities and calcium homeostasis may be disturbed as well. Indeed, hypocalcaemia and tetany are often the first clinical symptoms of this condition. Because of the impaired immunity of these patients, caution is again required when considering the normal childhood immunization schedules, because giving live-attenuated vaccines could be life-threatening.

ACQUIRED IMMUNODEFICIENCIES

The acquired immunodeficiencies, also called secondary immunodeficiencies, may be considered to be the result of an extrinsic factor compromising an otherwise normal immune system. The immune cells and tissues are highly metabolically active and are therefore sensitive to changes in the internal environment caused by reduced nutritional status as well as by the infections or tumours it is trying to eliminate. Certain medical therapies (surgical and pharmaceutical) may also affect the normal immune function (Figure 28.4). It is now realized that stress, whether psychological (as encountered by students taking final examinations, for example) or physical (e.g. excessively strenuous athletic training) may lead to immunodeficiency sufficient to allow the development of infectious diseases (see Chapter 23).

IMMUNOSUPPRESSION CAUSED BY METABOLIC AND GENETIC DISORDERS

Diseases in which the homeostatic controls of the internal environment are disturbed may lead to dysfunction of the normal defence mechanisms. Such changes may occur in metabolic disorders, whether they are inherited or acquired as a consequence of a pathological process. For instance, phagocytosis is often impaired in alcoholic cirrhosis because the liver is a major source of opsonins (i.e. complement and acute phase proteins). A protein-losing syndrome in the gastrointestinal tract or kidney may result in a chronic loss of immunoglobulins (e.g. as occurs in patients with ulcerative colitis, Crohn's disease, and chronic renal failure). An acute loss of immunoglobulins may ensue in patients who have sustained severe burns.

Insulin-dependent diabetes mellitus is a common disorder of carbohydrate metabolism which has an abrupt onset once all the beta-cells in the islet of Langerhans are destroyed. Although lymphocyte

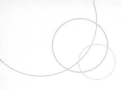

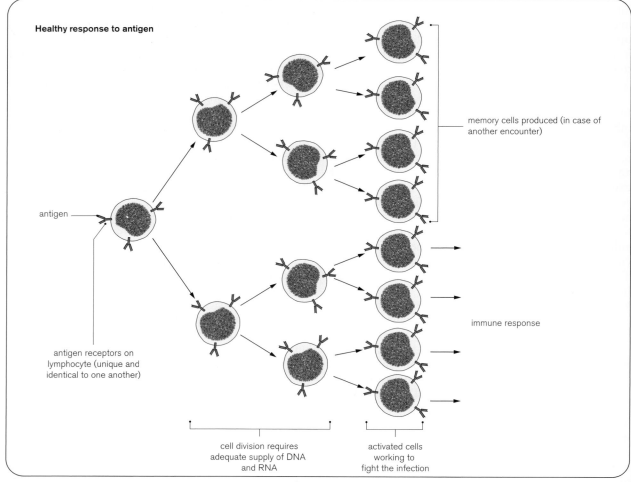

Figure 28.3 Enzymes deficiencies in severe combined immunodeficiency syndrome. (a) The healthy response to antigen. (b) The deficiencies in severe combined immunodeficiency syndrome reduce the numbers of both T and B lymphocytes, owing to the build-up of toxic metabolites that inhibit DNA and RNA synthesis and thus cell division.

function in diabetes remains normal, people with poorly controlled diabetes have an increased incidence of bacterial and fungal infection, which may be partly attributable to an impaired chemotactic response by their phagocytes. Unfortunately, a problem for these and other patients with an autoimmune disease is that one autoimmune condition often co-exists with another (e.g. a person with autoimmune thyroiditis may also develop pernicious anaemia) (see Chapter 27).

Certain inherited diseases may result in immunodeficiencies even though the defective gene does not encode for part of the immune system (see Box 28.1).

A defective alternative pathway of the complement

system has been described in sickle cell disease (see also Chapter 25). This makes patients liable to recurrent bacterial infections because of the lower levels of opsonins available for phagocytosis. Unfortunately, certain pathogens may gain entry to the body from microinfarction in mucosal surfaces (see Chapter 31). Appropriate management of wounds is therefore vital in the postoperative period for these and every other patient.

Some groups are more at risk of prolonged healing than others. The newborn, older adults, and malnourished patients are obvious candidates, as well as cachectic patients with an underlying critical pathology.

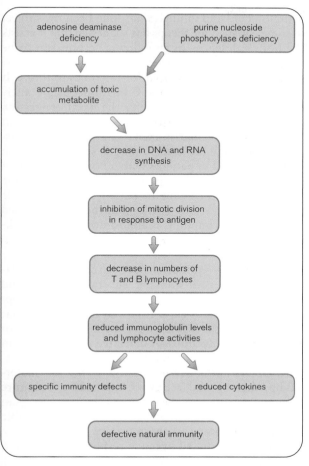

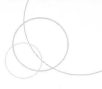

In some genetic abnormalities, compromised bodily defences have been exhibited even when the defective gene does not encode part of the immune system. Down's syndrome is an example of this:

- In Down's syndrome there is an increased frequency of gastrointestinal and respiratory tract infections.
- The reasons for the down-regulated immunity are not fully known, a reduced ability to kill bacteria due to impaired chemotaxis and phagocytic activity have been given as possible explanations.
- Natural killer cell and T lymphocyte activities are also defective (particularly T helper cells), where thymic abnormalities are presented. Certainly the association between Down's syndrome and childhood leukaemia (e.g. ALL), together with the increased incidence of autoimmune thyroid disease could be partially explained by these anomalies.
- It is also noteworthy that an increased incidence of hepatitis B has been reported in Down's patients, but this is more likely to be due to the effects of institutionalized living conditions rather than the trisomy 21 *per se*.

Figure 28.3b Severe combined immunodeficiency syndrome. (See previous caption for explanation.)

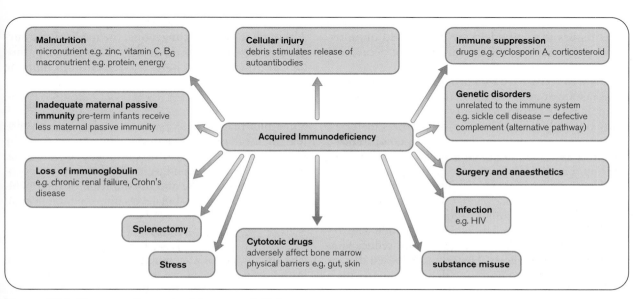

Figure 28.4 Causes of acquired immunodeficiency.

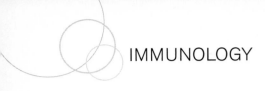

MALNUTRITION AND IMMUNODEFICIENCY

Tragic scenes of children and adults with malnutrition are depicted in the media, but this is not confined to the developing countries – it may also be seen in Westernised societies. Many examples are encountered in clinical practice – inactive and bored hospitalized patients given the typical hospital diet rarely have voracious appetites, so the nutritional value of the meals they consume may well be suboptimal. Patients prescribed nasogastric or parenteral feeding may be inadequately nourished if their feed is not regularly and effectively administered. Children encouraged to eat bulking agents, such as dietary fibre, which promote appetite satiety may consume insufficient calories, protein, vitamins, minerals, and trace elements for growth, development, and the maintenance of an active immune response. The tissues and cells of the immune system, like other rapidly dividing and metabolically active tissues, require these nutrients as cofactors for enzymes and the synthesis of secretory products, including immunoglobulins and cytokines (see Chapter 23). The down-regulation of the immune response in these patients may be worsened if a gastrointestinal infection erupts and provokes malabsorption.

In advanced stages of malnutrition, the vital organs (the heart, liver and brain) are maintained at the expense of other systems. Humoral immunity appears to be relatively preserved, with normal B lymphocyte numbers and circulating levels of immunoglobulins in body fluids. However, T lymphocyte function is affected, and reduced cytokine stimulation and thymic changes are probably responsible for this. In addition, the steroid hormones released in times of stress can precipitate thymic atrophy. Unfortunately, although other tissues (e.g. muscle) may be restored on nutritional rehabilitation, the thymus may not necessarily be fully regenerated.

It is well recognized that drugs used to treat chronic diseases can alter nutritional status – an obvious example is the cytotoxic agents that provoke nausea, anorexia, and changes in taste perceptions of foods. These symptoms compound the already compromised immunity as a result of the suppression of normal bone marrow function.

Certain therapies have an adverse effect on specific nutrients; for instance phenytoin, an anticonvulsant drug, increases the patient's requirement for vitamin D. Both aspirin and corticosteroids, which are frequently used as anti-inflammatory drugs, reduce vitamin C levels in the body. Hence an increased dietary intake is necessary to prevent a deficiency, particularly if these drugs are used long term. The effects of high doses of vitamin C for treating and preventing the common cold and influenza has long been the subject of some debate. One theory has suggested that it assists the body's defences by mobilizing serum iron to be stored in organs like the liver, so it is not so freely accessible as an essential nutrient for microbes to thrive. It is also thought that vitamin C might act as an 'alternative antihistamine' to reduce the nasal congestion of a cold. However, aspirin (freely available without prescription) is regularly taken to alleviate the unpleasant symptoms of these infections, so supplementation may be required in patients with a borderline vitamin C status. Smoking is well known as an irritant to the respiratory tract, leaving the patient more vulnerable to infections. It is noteworthy that the recommended daily intake of vitamin C is almost doubled for smokers, who metabolize the vitamin much faster than non-smokers do.

Fetal growth retardation has been examined in relation to the effects of smoking, substance misuse, and maternal malnutrition. These have become highly topical issues in health care. It is well documented that low birth weight infants have an increased risk of opportunistic infections. A defective placenta (e.g. in pre-eclampsia), which causes impairment of IgG transport, results in the newborn baby having less maternal IgG than normal (see also Chapter 23). Premature babies will have received less passive immunity than full-term infants. Even after reaching a respectable body weight, some of these infants demonstrate a reduced cell-mediated immune response and delayed hypersensitivity reactions.

IMMUNOSUPPRESSIVE EFFECTS OF MEDICAL INTERVENTION

Although it seems incongruous, the medical and surgical interventions used in the treatment of pathological processes can induce a depletion in immune activities.

Drugs

Some pharmacological agents modulate one physiological mechanism but at the same time alter the immune system. Phenytoin, an anticonvulsant drug, has an adverse effect on IgA levels; the effect is dependent on both the dose and the duration of treatment. By reducing the dose, IgA levels approaching normal may be achieved.

Postoperative Immunodeficiency

The advantages of a secondary immunodeficient state in the catabolic response of the postoperative period have been mentioned (see Chapter 23). Generally, the effects of the trauma of elective or emergency surgery on the immune system are considered to be less than the effects of accidental stress, because surgery is under some degree of medical control. Even so, the effects are dependent on the nature of the pathology and the organ or body system involved.

Splenectomy

A splenectomy is often advised to prolong red blood cell survival in haematological disorders such as sickle cell disease and beta-thalassaemia major (see Chapters 7 and 31). Yet the spleen is a vital organ for filtering blood-borne antigens; hence some splenectomized patients are prescribed prophylactic antibiotic therapy to avoid conditions such as septicaemia.

Malignancy

Patients with a malignancy have an incredible obstacle from an immunological point of view – they are being treated for a condition that, by definition, has eluded the immune system (see also Chapters 5 and 30). The therapies used to eliminate a tumour together with the stress of a potentially life-threatening disease can dampen the immune response. A reduced sensitivity to cytokines is one of the mechanisms proposed for the secondary immunodeficiency seen in these patients. Antiproliferative drugs, like cyclophosphamide and azathioprine, which inhibit DNA and RNA synthesis in malignant cells may also diminish B lymphocyte activities. The immunoglobulin response appears to be blunted in some oncology patients, as demonstrated when serum antibody titres have been measured after immunization. Selective immunoglobulin defects have also been described with certain tumours (e.g. secondary IgA deficiency in oesophageal carcinoma).

Radiotherapy and chemotherapy, used to reduce the size of tumours, have a deleterious effect on other rapidly dividing tissues, such as the skin and the gastrointestinal tract, which leaves them open to microbial attack. This is compounded by their suppressive effects on bone marrow function, which lead to reduced leukocyte numbers. Sadly, chemotherapeutic agents used in the treatment of one tumour have been found to be instrumental in causing other malignancies (e.g. leukaemia) at a later date.

Immunosuppressive Therapy to Prevent Transplant Rejection

Total body radiation therapy is sometimes advised to prevent rejection episodes in transplant patients. The immunosuppressive therapies used to prevent graft rejection and to treat inflammatory and immunological disorders leave patients at risk of opportunistic infections. Generally, the drugs selectively target a specific arm of the immune system. However, their actions have adverse consequences on cellular activities other than the T lymphocytes and macrophages, some of the main cell types responsible for transplant rejection. Corticosteroids, for example, affect the ability of neutrophils to adhere to the endothelial cell wall and inhibit the release of cytokines (notably IL-2, IL-3, IL-4, IL–5), and therefore sequentially affect other immune cells, with the result that systemic Gram-negative infections may occur. Cyclosporin A is another well known immunosuppressant with inhibitory activity on T and B lymphocytes, but it is also potentially nephrotoxic (Box 28.2) (see Chapter 29).

IMMUNODEFICIENCIES AS A CONSEQUENCE OF INFECTIONS

Many of the pathological symptoms resulting from infections are caused by the body's own reaction to an intruder rather than to the direct effects of the organism. In order to survive, microbes have evolved a number of survival strategies, some of which can stimulate an immunosuppressive mechanism. For example, some bacteria inhibit the body's bactericidal response by impeding phagocytosis (see also Chapters 16 and 18). Some infections (e.g. malaria) modify the immune response of the host as a means of protection from attack. These inhibitory effects leave the patient vulnerable to other infections because of the microbe-induced immunodeficiency. This is probably one reason why mass immunization schedules (e.g. for tetanus and *Salmonella* infections) appear to be of limited use in areas where infections such as malaria are endemic, since infected patients do not respond as effectively to certain vaccines.

Infections alter the immune system in different ways, depending on the nature of the infectious agent; this is certainly true for different viruses. For instance, patients with infectious mononucleosis often present with a reduced natural killer cell activity and reduced lymphocyte numbers (the cell types that are generally involved in the disposal of viruses). The disease is caused by Epstein–Barr virus (EBV), which enters and infects B lymphocytes. In turn these cells are subsequently killed by cytotoxic T lymphocytes. Although cytokines (especially interferons) may be generated to promote an antiviral state, EBV can also counteract this by stimulating the secretion of an interleukin-10-like substance, which has an inhibitory effects on immunity.

Other viruses, such as the influenza virus, may alter the immune system in another way. Influenza virus elevates natural killer cell activity but causes a transient reduction in the number of lymphocytes (lymphopenia). One reason for this may be that there are relatively more

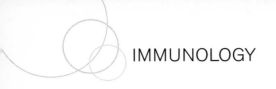

> ### BOX 28.2 IMMUNODEFICIENCY AS A CONSEQUENCE OF CHRONIC RENAL FAILURE AND ITS TREATMENTS
>
> Chronic renal failure may be the result of a congenital abnormality (e.g. congenital nephrotic syndrome), or following a streptococcal infection, or it may be caused by an autoimmune disease affecting the kidney, such as Goodpasture's syndrome or glomerulonephritis.
>
> Chronic renal failure patients:
> - lose plasma proteins in urine, such as albumin and immunoglobulins which pass through the glomerular filtrate. In particular IgG and IgA antibodies (IgM antibodies are generally too large to be filtered through), thus their humoral immunity is depleted.
> - The extent and duration of uraemia that follows impaired renal function has adverse consequences on immunity. Uraemia affects the physical barriers including the skin and mucosal surfaces, which become friable and open to microbial growth, so patients are more prone to infections and pruritus.
> - With dialysis therapy (haemodialysis or continuous ambulatory peritoneal dialysis) there is an increased risk of infections. This may be partly exacerbated because impaired neutrophil function has been reported in patients with chronic renal failure. Additionally, the loss of blood and nutrients like zinc and iron required for the maintenance of an active immune response, further compromise the defence mechanisms (see also Chapter 36).

T suppressor cells around to dampen the response because the virus induces a change in the ratio of different subpopulations of T lymphocytes. (T suppressor cells then inhibit cytokine production, and so T lymphocyte proliferation is impaired.) Patients are therefore vulnerable to other infections when they suffer influenza; hence antibiotics may need to be prescribed even though they have no therapeutic value for the viral infection itself.

Chronic fatigue syndrome, otherwise known as 'yuppy flu', has gained considerable media attention as a rather enigmatic disease whose causative agents are not really known. A virus has been suggested because of the prevailing influenza-like symptoms, and EBV has been implicated. Allergic reactions and a variety of esoteric noxious substances have also been proposed as the aetiological factors. A number of immunological anomalies have been demonstrated, including reduced lymphocyte activities and impaired phagocytic function by monocytes. However, the many therapies prescribed and advocated make it difficult to judge whether the depressed immune response is induced by an infectious agent, the long-term medical interventions, or the psychological stress of the syndrome.

ACQUIRED IMMUNODEFICENCY SYNDROME (AIDS)

AIDS really came to light when, in the summer of 1981 a cluster of homosexual men in Los Angeles were diagnosed as being infected with *Pneumocystis carinii* with palpable, generalized lymphadenopathy. Cytomegalovirus and herpesvirus were initially considered as possible causative agents, but it has since been conclusively identified that AIDS is the result of infection with HIV. The population groups most at risk of infection with HIV include people who come into contact with blood products infected with the virus, the sexual partners of HIV-positive patients, and intravenous drug users who share needles. Vertical transmission of HIV from the infected mother to her fetus also occurs. Because HIV infection nearly always leads to a fatal outcome, there have been world-wide efforts at national and international levels to prevent the spread of the virus and decrease the impact of the disease.

WHAT HAPPENS TO THE HUMAN IMMUNODEFICIENCY VIRUS AFTER ENTERING THE BODY?

Like all viruses, HIV must enter a cell to survive, and the major cell types to become infected are those possessing the CD4 marker. The T helper cells and other immune cells that bear this marker – macrophages, monocytes, Langerhans' cells, dendritic cells, and even stem cells in the bone marrow – are therefore targets of the virus (see Chapters 18 and 24). The reason for this is that the CD4 marker acts as a receptor for the virus to gain entry into the cell. On the surface (or outer envelope) of HIV are two proteins, which aid access of the virus into cells. One of these proteins is gp120, which binds to the CD4 marker; the other protein is gp41, which assists the process by acting as a 'sucker' to ensure the virus adheres to the outer plasma membrane of its target cell.

As the virus invades the cell the outer envelope is lost, and viral enzymes and RNA are released into the host cell. The RNA is then converted to single-stranded DNA using the enzyme reverse transcriptase. (A number of anti-HIV drugs, including zidovudine, act by inhibiting this enzyme to limit the replication of the virus.) A second complementary strand of DNA is synthesized using the first strand as a template, and this strand is then incorporated into the host genome to form a provirus. The provirus may remain dormant or, by using the host intracellular machinery, it may reproduce RNA and viral proteins to propagate the infection. The virus spreads by 'budding' particles from its host; these particles then circulate and infect other cells. Low levels of budding are conducive to host cell survival; if intense budding takes place, the host cell will almost certainly die. In the period when budding HIV particles are detectable by the immune system, a humoral response can be made to produce anti-HIV antibodies.

CAUSES OF IMMUNODEFICIENCY IN HIV INFECTION

The main cell types to be infected with HIV are CD4+ cells. The immunological functions of infected cells are impeded. For example, once HIV has penetrated a T helper cell, ability of the cell to work with the antigen-presenting cells is impaired. Similarly, HIV-infected macrophages are inefficient at being antigen-presenting cells. Unfortunately, although HIV can be controlled by the immune system for a time, it is not completely destroyed, and so a balancing act exists between host and virus. The extent of immuno-deficiency becomes progressively worse as the number of active cells are reduced. In particular, a reduction in the number of T helper cells causes deterioration in immune function, since these cells assist other immune cells.

A number of mechanisms have been proposed for the reduction in CD4+ cells, including:

- killing of infected cells by cytotoxic T lymphocytes;
- binding of anti-HIV antibodies to the infected cells, which promote antibody-dependent cytotoxicity; and
- stimulation of apoptosis (programmed cell death) by HIV of the cell it has infected (Figure 28.5).

The greatest risk of contracting AIDS is by contact with the body fluids of an infected person, yet the levels of the free virus are remarkably low (as HIV needs to be inside cells to survive). Macrophages are a major vehicle for HIV transmission because they harbour the virus and they are found in body fluids other than

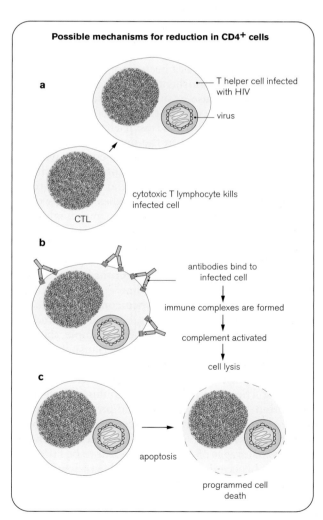

Figure 28.5 Possible mechanism of reduction in CD4+ cell count in HIV infection. (a) Infected cells can be eliminated by cytotoxic T lymphocytes. (b) Infected cells can undergo antibody-dependent lysis. (c) Infected cells can undergo programmed cell death.

blood. Although the CD4 marker provides one way for the virus to enter cells, it is not the only one – phagocytosis of HIV-infected cells and immunoglobulin-coated HIV particles are thought to be the main route into macrophages. Since macrophages express CD4 at a much lower level than T helper cells, they probably do not become as heavily infected, so acting as a reservoir for HIV because they are not killed.

TESTING FOR THE HUMAN IMMUNODEFICIENCY VIRUS

There are two viruses that cause AIDS, HIV-1 and HIV-2, and it seems that people who are infected with HIV-2 remain stable and healthier for longer than those infected with HIV-1. Conventional screening detects both viruses, so there should be no concern about a wrong diagnosis of the patient's HIV status because the strain of virus has not been recognized by the test. An enzyme immunosorbent assay is used for the test, but it can give a false-positive result so Western blot analysis is used to confirm the presence of HIV antibodies (see Chapter 24). The test itself detects IgG antibodies against proteins on the outer envelop of HIV, and so there is a time lapse between contact with the virus and the immune system mounting the antibody response that is detected. The initial infection stimulates the production of IgM antibodies (like any other primary immune response); once the immunoglobulin class switches to IgG, the HIV status of the patient can be confirmed. There could be a lag period of up to 3 months between a patient's contact with HIV and a positive test result. Detection of IgG antibodies against HIV is known as seroconversion.

Particular care is needed when considering the test results for a patient's HIV status, because an evaluation of the whole patient is required. For example, the anti-HIV IgG antibodies can be vertically transmitted from mother to fetus. Therefore, a neonate may be identified as positive when tested even though not infected with the virus. The maternal-derived immunoglobulins are lost within 18 months of birth, and provided the virus was not transmitted across the placenta or during labour, the infant has not been infected. Conversely, patients in the terminal stages of AIDS may appear to be HIV-negative simply because they are incapable of synthesizing detectable amounts of immunoglobulins.

Selection of People for Screening

Mandatory testing is required before the donation of blood, of organs for transplant, and of gametes for assisted reproduction programmes. For hospital patients, the policies for HIV testing is generally hosital unit-dependent, although there is a certain balance between a person's right to privacy and public welfare. There is compulsory testing for certain institutionalized people, particularly if there is the possibility of intravenous drug misuse or homosexual practices (e.g. in prisons). The confidentiality of the patient should be preserved if the decision to be screened is voluntary and ideally a full counselling service is advised where the implications of a positive result can be discussed. In some states of the USA, there are tracing agencies to ensure that partners of HIV-positive patients are informed of their status.

HIV infection is frightening because of the almost certain fatal outcome, but it is comforting to note that seroconversion may not necessarily occur after the first contact with body fluids containing the virus. This has been amply demonstrated in studies of the partners of HIV-infected haemophiliacs, many of whom had not seroconverted after 4 years, and in the risk analysis of occupational hazards such as needle-stick injuries (see also Chapter 20).

CLINICAL PICTURE OF HIV INFECTION IN RELATION TO THE IMMUNOLOGICAL MANIFESTATIONS

No clear time scale has been defined between the first infection with HIV and the clinical manifestations and signs of immunodeficiency. Some studies have indicated a period of around 10 years between the start of HIV carrier status and the development of AIDS. The clinical presentation of AIDS is governed by the level of immune competence, and thus the progression of the HIV infection may be classified by the diseases presented (see Chapter 18). The majority of patients are asymptomatic after the initial encounter with HIV and seroconversion, although by around 4–8 weeks after exposure to the virus some individuals suffer with influenza-like symptoms of malaise, muscle weakness and neurological symptoms such as headaches and photophobia. The acute phase proteins are generally elevated in the initial response to HIV, and this causes an elevated erythrocyte sedimentation rate (ESR).

The progress of the HIV infection is paralleled by a decrease in the functional activities of T helper cells and other immune cells. Clinicians use the number of $CD4^+$ cells in blood as an indicator of immunocompetence, but this has been recently considered rather an imprecise parameter. The number of T helper cells in peripheral blood amounts to only about 2 per cent of the total number of T helper cells – the rest are found within the lymphoid organs. Therefore, the $CD4^+$ cell count may not represent what is going on in the body as a whole. An alternative test is an assessment of virus load by molecular biological techniques using the polymerase chain reaction (see Chapter 7).

As the disease progresses, the lymphoid organs, including the spleen and lymph nodes, are the major sites where HIV-infected cells reside and replicate. Therefore, symptoms of splenomegaly and persistent lymphadenopathy are presented because of the virus overload. However, in full-blown AIDS, as the immune system gradually becomes exhausted and unable to respond to antigen stimulation, the lymph nodes are frequently no longer palpable. Furthermore, as the virus enters the thymus, it affects the maturing T helper cells, and the immune surveillance for abnormal cells is also gradually diminished. Therefore, there is an increased risk of malignancy [e.g. Kaposi's sarcoma (Figure 28.6) and lymphomas] and this is exacerbated by the impaired activity of the natural killer cells.

Many AIDS patients suffer from some degree of dementia. This is not merely a psychological manifestation of a terminal disease, but a significant clinical condition that can be visualized by imaging techniques such as magnetic resonance imaging. HIV infection of the brain is referred to as AIDS encephalopathy or AIDS dementia complex. The microglial cells (macrophages in the brain) are considered the main route by which the virus transverses the blood–brain barrier. Patients then become vulnerable to the infections that cause encephalitis and meningitis.

Similarly, the alveolar macrophages are a major source of HIV to the lungs. Tuberculosis, which had been controlled, at least in part, by the mass immunization of schoolchildren, has re-emerged as a major disease. There has been a profound rise in the incidence of the disease in the UK, particularly in the homeless and AIDS populations. In a significant number of cases, tuberculosis may be diagnosed before patients are aware of their HIV status.

As in other immunodeficiency states, AIDS carries the risk of multiple infections persisting simultaneously. An added difficulty in AIDS is that the typical signs that indicate the presence of the infections (e.g. fever) are not always apparent because the immune cells are not functionally competent. The gastrointestinal symptoms of nausea and vomiting further complicate the clinical management. The weight loss with or without diarrhoea found in HIV infection is sometimes referred to as Slim's disease. The metabolic effects of cachexia that are seen in AIDS have been partially attributed to tumour necrosis factor-alpha (see Chapter 25), which compounds the problems of reduced body weight and may partly account for the emaciated appearance of AIDS patients. Colitis caused by microorganisms such as cytomegalovirus may arise. Cytomegalovirus may also be responsible for the impaired vision found in some patients with AIDS.

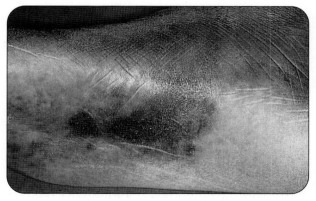

Figure 28.6 Kaposi's sarcoma. This is a common lesion in patients with AIDS. (By kind permission of Professor A Dalgleish, St George's Hospital Medical School, London, UK.)

MANAGEMENT OF AIDS

The main strategies for treating HIV-infected patients are inhibiting the infectious agent (i.e. HIV) as well as the other micro-organisms and their associated symptoms as they arise. The aim is to prevent other microbial infections from taking hold and multiplying, because AIDS patients do not die from HIV infection as such but from the diseases that they are unable to fight as a result of the HIV infection-induced immunodeficiency. This is done by extensive antimicrobial therapy. The holistic approach in preserving the psychosocial well-being, together with dietary advice, also helps to sustain these patients.

Clinical Management of Patients with AIDS

Research groups and drug companies are racing to find an effective anti-HIV drug, and many drug designs are based on inhibiting some of the essential HIV enzymes. One of these drugs is saquinavir, which restrains the activities of HIV proteases used in the budding mechanism of the virus (see Chapter 19). The enzyme in HIV, reverse transcriptase, catalyses the conversion of the viral RNA into DNA for replication using the host cellular machinery, and zidovudine works by inhibiting this enzyme. A major problem associated with the long-term use of zidovudine and other anti-HIV therapies is that their efficacy diminishes with time. As with other chemotherapeutic agents, viral resistance may develop, and hence not one drug but a combination of drugs is given to reduce the risk of untreatable HIV mutants emerging. The anti-HIV drugs also produce side-effects. For example, patients prescribed zidovudine experience nausea, vomiting, headaches, and myalgia. Regular blood transfusions are also needed to treat the resultant anaemia. Neutropenia may arise, and thrombocytopenia which may lead to clotting disorders, are other additional clinical complications, but they are reversible when the therapy is changed.

As their immune system becomes progressively less efficient, HIV-infected patients are prone to infections (as are other immunocompromised patients). Thus antimicrobial agents come to be required for longer durations since they are probably the only means of completely eradicating infections. More than one type of antibiotic may be needed. As the normal indicators of a disease are often somewhat blunted, the response to treatment is less obvious, which leads to further uncertainties. Infection control is therefore of paramount importance in the nursing care of AIDS patients in order to obliterate sources of infection and prevent transmission of infections from other patients. Patient compliance to therapies is essential to themselves and the community at large. This is particularly important when treating diseases such as tuberculosis, in order to prevent its spread and ensure that a drug-resistant strain does not evolve (see Chapters 16 and 18).

Another major issue in caring for AIDS patients is pain management – the causes of pain are multifactorial and may be due to a diagnostic procedure or surgery; to the localized pain of an infection or tumour; or to an inflammatory process (e.g. myopathy, persistent headaches). The appropriate analgesic drug and dose are necessary, taking into consideration the patient's perception of the nature and intensity of the pain (see Chapter 14). Some patients also complain of insomnia, which may be partly explained by the stress of the disease or by AIDS-related dementia. However, the environment is a contributory factor, particularly for in-patients, since a hospital ward is a notoriously difficult place to try to sleep.

Dietary Management of Patients With AIDS

Maintenance of body weight in conjunction with the other clinical interventions can improve quality of life and serve to retard the progression of the disease. Accordingly, the weight loss seen in AIDS is often used in the diagnostic criteria for it closely follows the advance to the later stages of the disease. End-stage AIDS patients may have a 30–40 per cent reduction in their previous body weight. They are often in negative energy balance, (their energy intake is less than their energy expenditure), which seems almost impossible considering the symptoms of lethargy and fatigue. Anorexia has significant effects on dietary intake and is partly related to drugs such as zidovudine, which evokes changes in taste perception. Moreover, HIV infection is known to affect gastrointestinal absorption, which has been accounted for by changes in structure and function of the villi. Gut infections that cause malabsorption reduce the nutritional intake still further (e.g. *Entamoeba histolytica*).

The public view of a healthy diet is low-fat with the correct caloric intake to protect from diseases like cardiovascular disease. However, this is contrary to the requirements for AIDS patients, whose dietary regimens should be high in energy-giving nutrients to sustain body weight and therefore could be perceived as 'unhealthy'. Appetite stimulants may be offered, but if there is evidence of malabsorption, formulated feeds may be advised to boost the calorific intake and promote absorption. In the earlier stages of HIV infection, body weight can be maintained by giving high-protein and high-energy nutritional supplements, especially where there is no underlying secondary infections. However, the decision to feed enterally may be considered when the inadequate dietary intake causes dramatic weight losses (e.g. in patients with nausea and persistent anorexia). Only in cases where the gut is non-functional should total parenteral nutrition be advised, but this form of artificial feeding carries the risk of infections.

OCCUPATIONAL RISK AND HIV INFECTION

When HIV-positive and AIDS patients were first seen in the early 1980s, there was grave concern expressed by health care professionals regarding the personal danger of infection. In the assessment of the occupational exposure, it is now realized that the risk of becoming infected with HIV is less than for other infections such as hepatitis B, because HIV itself is not a robust micro-organism. Yet the same care is needed for all patients, and health care professionals should be ever aware of the asymptomatic carrier of HIV. Therefore, there are universal precautions to be practised when handling body tissue and fluids:

- it is essential that gloves are worn when handling all body fluids;
- good practice must be implemented in the disposal of sharps such as hypodermic needles – it is advised that syringe and needle are immediately disposed of in a designated bin for incineration, because replacing the needle guard increases the danger of a needlestick injury;
- where the centrifugation of body fluids is required, the use of a face mask is necessary to prevent the spread of HIV via aerosols.

Although pre-operative testing for HIV has been advocated in the USA, there has been no conclusive policy agreed by the UK Government. However, when a surgical patient is known to be HIV-positive, the case is usually put to the end of the theatre list as an extra precaution to prevent cross-infection to other patients (see Chapter 20).

Many carers (not only the clinical workers but also ancillary staff in clinics, wards, and other public institutions) are still fearful of becoming infected with HIV. It is reasonable to question the risk of handling blood-soiled linen or cleaning a wash basin or work surface contaminated with blood. The responsibility lies with health care workers to educate themselves and the general public, in order to allay fear about the transmission of HIV. There is also the need to counsel carers as well as AIDS sufferers – it is stressful to treat patients who are ill with a disease for which there is no real cure or vaccine.

KEY POINTS

- An inherited immunodeficiency arises when an irregularity or absence of a gene that encodes part of the immune system leads to that part malfunctioning, being in short supply, or missing.
- Defective phagocytosis may be the result of inadequate levels of the opsonins that promote the function of phagocytes, reduced cell numbers, or malfunctioning cells.
- An inherited humoral deficiency may be the outcome of defective haematopoiesis or the inability of B lymphocytes to develop into plasma cells, which can be due to their insensitivity to T helper cell activity.
- Humoral deficiencies persist if one or more of the different classes (e.g. IgA, IgG) of immunoglobulin are not effectively produced.
- Production of immunoglobulins by B lymphocytes may be impaired due to inadequate synthesis or to a fault in the intracellular pathway that blocks the cell surface expression or secretion of immunoglobulins.
- Inherited deficiencies of T lymphocytes result in patients being more susceptible to opportunistic infections because their cell-mediated immunity is functionally inadequate.
- An acquired immunodeficiency may result when clinical intervention (e.g. surgery, drugs) for some other pathology affects the functional capacity of the immune system.

- HIV produces symptoms of immunodeficiency because it infects the immune cells, which are then impeded in their defence activities, leaving the patient at risk of infections and malignancies.
- HIV enters and infects immune cells that possess CD4, a cell surface marker, and cells capable of phagocytosing HIV-infected cells and antibody-coated HIV particles.
- Macrophages are thought to be a major vehicle of HIV transmission since they are found in body fluids other than blood, and they act as a reservoir to harbour the virus.
- The HIV test detects IgG raised against the outer coat of HIV; a positive test is known as seroconversion.
- The treatments for AIDS patients are much the same as for other immunocompromised patients (i.e. antimicrobial drugs and dietary supplements). In addition, counselling and appropriate therapies are given for symptoms of depression and pain.
- Good practice must be observed when treating all patients, being ever aware of the asymptomatic carrier of HIV (i.e. gloves must be worn when handling body fluids, sharps must be disposed of appropriately and safely, and face masks must be used during centrifugation to prevent inhalation of aerosols).

FURTHER READING

Barre-Sinoussi F (1996) HIV as the cause of AIDS. Lancet 348:31–5.

Beiser C (1997) Recent advances. HIV infection-II. BMJ 314:579–83.

Bogstedt AK, Nava S, Wadstrom T, Hammarstrom L (1996) *Helicobacter pylori* infections in IgA deficiency: lack of role for the secretory immune system. Clin Exp Immunol 105:202–4.

Cochran J (1995) Primary immunodeficiency disease in children: recognizing problems in primary care practice. J Am Acad Nurse Pract 7:33–8.

Coyle TE (1997) Hematologic complications of human immunodeficiency virus infection and the acquired immunodeficiency syndrome. Med Clin North Am 81:449–70.

Dalakas MC, Cupler EJ (1996) Neuropathies in HIV infection. Baillieres Clin Neurol 5:199–218.

Gleeson M, Cripps AW, Clancy RL, Hensley MJ, Henry RJ, Wlodarczyk JH (1995) The significance of transient mucosal IgA deficiency on the development of asthma and atopy in children. Adv Exp Med Biol 371B:861–4.

Fleisher TA (1996) Evaluation of the potentially immunodeficient patient. Adv Intern Med 41:1–30.

Hegde HR (1995) Anergy, AIDS and tuberculosis [Review]. Med Hypotheses 45:433–40.

Hirasawa A, Sato T, Nishikawa T, *et al.* (1995) An adult diagnosed as hyper-IgM immunodeficiency syndrome. Intern Med 34:640–2.

Ickovics JR, Meisler AW (1997). Adherence in AIDS clinical trials: a framework for clinical research and clinical care. J Clin Epidemiol 50:385–91.

Kappes DJ, Alarcon B, Regueiro JR (1995) T lymphocyte receptor deficiencies. Curr Opin Immunol 7:441–7.

Kosko DA (1997) Dermatologic manifestations of human immunodeficiency virus disease. Lippincotts Prim Care Pract. 1(1): 50–61.

Krown SE (1997) Acquired immunodeficiency syndrome-associated Kaposi's sarcoma. Biology and management. Med Clin North Am 81:471–94.

Kuby J (1997) Immunology WH Freeman and Co. New York.

Lee ML, Gale RP, Yap PL (1997) Use of intravenous immunoglobulin to prevent or treat infections in persons with immune deficiency. Annu Rev Med 48:93–102.

Lewis P, Smith R (1996). The management of HIV-positive pregnant women. Mod Midwife 6:26–8.

Mawle AC, Nisenbaum R, Dobbins JG, *et al.* (1997) Immune responses associated with chronic fatigue syndrome: a case-control study. J Infect Dis 175:136–41.

Ming JE, Stiehm ER, Graham JM Jr (1996) Immunodeficiency as a component of recognizable syndromes. Am J Med Genet 66:378–98.

Moscardini C, Touger-Decker R, Ostrowski MB (1997) Nutritional needs in the AIDS patient. Recognizing and treating wasting syndrome. Adv Nurse Pract 5:34–7.

Nokes KM, Kendrew J, Rappaport A, Jordan D, Rivera L (1997) Development of an HIV educational needs assessment tool. J Assoc Nurses AIDS Care 8:46–51.

O'Brien SJ, Dean M (1997) In search of AIDS-resistant genes. Sci Am 277(3):28–35.

Odeleye OE, Watson RR (1991) The potential role of vitamin E in the treatment of immunologic abnormalities during acquired immune deficiency syndrome. Prog Food Nutr Sci 15:1–19.

Ramesh S, Schwartz SA (1995) Therapeutic uses of intravenous immunoglobulin (IVIG) in children. Pediatr Rev 16:403–10.

Roitt I, Brestoff J, Male D (1997) Immunology 5th edition. Mosby, London.

Schietinger H, Daniels EM (1996) HIV infection. What nurses need to know. The consumer perspective. Nurs Clin North Am 31:137–52.

Shyur SD, Hill HR (1996) Recent advances in the genetics of primary immunodeficiency syndromes. J Pediatr 129:8–24.

Soucy MD (1997) Fatigue and depression: assessment in human immunodeficiency virus disease. Nurse Pract Forum 8:121–5.

Stein CM (1996) Immunodeficient states and associated rheumatic manifestations. Curr Opin Rheumatol 81:52–6.

Tossing G (1996) Immunodeficiency and its relation to lymphoid and other malignancies. Ann Hematol 73:163–7.

Wahn U (1995) Evaluation of the child with suspected primary immunodeficiency. Pediatr Allergy Immunol 6:71–9.

Warren RP, Odell JD, Warren WL, *et al.* (1997) Brief report: immunoglobulin A deficiency in a subset of autistic subjects. J Autism Dev Disord 27:187–92.

Weyer D (1997) Skin: a window to the immune system. Recognizing and treating HIV-related lesions. Adv Nurse Pract 5:22–6.

Winter H. Chang TI (1996) Gastrointestinal and nutritional problems in children with immunodeficiency and AIDS. Pediatr Clin North Am 43:573–90.

Zenone T, Souquet PJ, Cunningham-Rundles C, Bernard JP (1996) Hodgkin's disease associated with IgA and IgG subclass deficiency. J Intern Med 240:99–102.

TRANSPLANTATION AND IMMUNOSUPPRESSIVE THERAPY

INTRODUCTION

Transplantation is the term used to describe the surgical transfer of cells, tissues, or organs from one location to another. This repositioning may be an autologous transplant, in which tissue is transplanted within the body of the same patient (e.g. skin grafted from the thigh to the face) (Figure 29.1), more often an allogeneic transplant is performed, involving the transfer of an organ donated by another person (e.g. a kidney taken from a donor who is not related to the recipient). Transplantation is used in the clinical management of patients with end-stage organ failure and certain haematological malignancies (e.g. acute myeloid leukaemia), and for treating some inherited disorders.

Nevertheless, though the donated tissue (often referred to as the graft) is meant to provide a better quality of life for the recipient, the recipient's immune system does not always perceive it as harmless. Peter Medawar was one of the first immunologists to cite observations on transplant patients; these were the fighter pilots who suffered extensive burns in the Second World War. It became clear that the incidence of mortality was related to the severity of burn injuries, and skin grafting improved patient survival. However, what Medawar particularly noted was that skin grafted from one anatomical site to another on the same patient's body was not rejected. However, if the skin was donated by an unrelated donor, the graft did not 'take'. Furthermore, if a subsequent operation was performed with more 'foreign skin', the second graft was rejected even faster than the first. Medawar began to realize that the reason behind the rejection was connected with how the immune system operated.

SOURCES OF DONATED ORGANS FOR TRANSPLANTATION

The physiological function of the tissue or organ required for transplantation effectively dictates whether the donor is alive or is a cadaver. Sometimes donations are anonymous – blood transfusion must be the best-established transplant procedure in health care but the identity of the donor is not generally known to either the hospital staff or the patient. However, stringent records are kept by the National Blood Service, and each unit of blood assigned a number so the donor may be traced in the unlikely event of a complication.

AUTOLOGOUS DONATION

Patients of some faiths (e.g. Jehovah's Witnesses) profess beliefs that prohibit the transfusion of blood

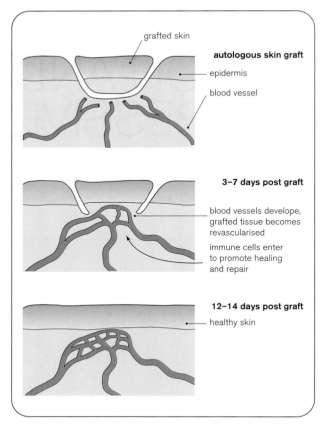

autologous skin graft

grafted skin

epidermis

blood vessel

3–7 days post graft

blood vessels develope, grafted tissue becomes revascularised

immune cells enter to promote healing and repair

12–14 days post graft

healthy skin

Figure 29.1 Sequence of events in an autologous skin graft. By 3–7 days, the grafted tissue is being revasularized. By 12–14 days, healing and repair have taken place and the tissue should be resolved and functional.

products or the transplant of organs from another person. In a situation where such people require elective surgery that demands cross-matched blood, they may donate their own blood for storage in case a transfusion is needed. (This is an example of an autologous transplant, in which tissue or cells are removed then put back into the same individual at a later date.) However, a dilemma arises in an emergency when a blood transfusion is refused. Intravenous saline and intravenous iron supplement may be given instead of blood for minor transfusion needs, but inevitably the time taken for rehabilitation is prolonged. Ultimately the decision of an adult patient must be respected, but in a life-threatening situation in which the patient is under 18 years, the clinician may apply for a court order to enable treatment to go ahead against the wishes of the parents.

ALLOGENEIC DONATION FROM CADAVERS

A graft acquired from a donor who is genetically unrelated to the recipient is known as an allogeneic donation. For example, vital organs such as the heart may be obtained from an otherwise healthy person who died following a fatal accident or was in a coma and confirmed to be brain dead (see also Box 29.1).

Although cadaver donors are an obvious and convenient source of organs, their use is only feasible and ethical if there is a minimal risk of cross-infection from donor to recipient. Septicaemia and malignancy are serious postoperative complications for patients prescribed immunosuppressive therapy. Hence transplantation of organs is contraindicated when there has been evidence of:

- bowel perforation;
- gangrene in the intra-abdominal tissues;
- infectious contamination with other organs; (e.g. overspill of bowel contents)
- metastatic tumours.

Organ donation from a cadaver is a highly sensitive issue and therefore respect and an awareness of the feelings of the relatives of the donor are essential. In fact, sometimes the donor may still be alive and on a life-support system when the family is approached and asked to consider organ donation. Likewise, the recipient is likely to be acutely aware that their improved quality of life is at the cost of another person's life.

BOX 29.1 CORNEAL GRAFTING

Corneal grafting is one of the most common transplant procedures. It is used to treat patients with obstructed vision due to misshapen or opacified corneas (e.g. patients with keratoconus). Patients are generally given topical drugs: antibiotics to prevent infection, and corticosteroids to reduce any postoperative inflammation and possible immune rejection. Prevention of scar tissue formation is essential, as it would limit the transparency of the newly transplanted cornea. As with other transplant procedures there is the possible risk of cross-infection between donor and recipient. There have been case reports of Creutzfeldt–Jakob disease being transmitted to the transplant patient from the cadaveric donation of cornea grafts.

LIVE DONORS

There are distinct advantages in obtaining a graft from a live donor. With both donor and recipient prepared and the donation and transplantation procedures co-ordinated, the physical conditions of both parties can be optimized before elective surgery. In addition, the short time between operations means the physiological function of the newly grafted organ is quickly re-established. Conversely when the organ is obtained from a cadaver, surgery is generally performed as an emergency, often following a protracted wait for the suitable donor. Likewise, deterioration in tissue function is inevitable where there has been a delay owing to transportation and storage of the graft, or the need to contact and prepare the transplant patient for theatre.

Who might be a suitable live donor? A patient with a monozygotic twin is fortunate in having a genetically identical sibling who could provide a syngeneic graft. Alternatively, another first-degree relative may also be approached, but this is not generally a routine practice for solid organ donation in the UK. Graft donation by a relative is a highly sensitive issue. Genuine feelings of goodwill are likely to prevail where the tissue is one which can be replenished (e.g. bone marrow). However, conflicting emotions may emanate in the case of an organ donation (e.g. kidney). The donor may feel pressurized to co-operate, knowing that the organ donation would greatly improve their relative's quality of life, but he or she may also be concerned about living with one kidney instead of two in case renal complications should develop at a later date.

One of the real problems in transplant medicine is that there are more patients in need of transplant surgery than there are organs available. Financial rewards have been offered in exchange for organ and tissue donation, but this is an extremely dubious practice. One particular case, involving Turkish nationals and kidneys donated for money, ended in a High Court battle. Parliament in the UK was therefore compelled to intervene and legislate, so the Human Organ Transplant Act (the 'HOT' Act) was passed. Consequently it has been advised that donation of a solid organ for transplant by a live donor may only be provided by a person who is either genetically related to the recipient or the recipient's partner.

XENOGENEIC GRAFTS

An alternative strategy that has been suggested for reducing the waiting lists is to use the organs from non-primate donors. These are referred to as xenogeneic grafts, but this is merely at the clinical trial stage and by no means routine practice. Obviously, the issue of breeding animals to provide organs for donation is highly controversial. Pigs have been considered as a suitable source since their organs are of similar dimensions to human organs, so there is no real size problem for grafting into the body cavity. An added advantage of using pigs is that they breed rapidly and produce large litters, so there would be a plentiful supply of organs.

However cross-species donations carries the significant risk of infection, which in itself is life-threatening to the immunocompromised transplant patient. In addition, there is the possibility of transplant rejection. In order to challenge this problem, genetic engineering techniques (transgenics) are being used to modify the genetic material of embryos and produce transgenic animals. For example, animals have been created that possess human complement inhibitor proteins on the cell surface, to block organ rejection mediated by the complement system.

TRANSPLANT REJECTION

Surgical techniques and immunosuppressive therapies are continually being developed and improved. This, together with the appropriate protocols for the preservation of donated organs, has led to a better prognosis for transplant patients. Nonetheless, unlike most types of surgery, the success of a transplant is not just dictated by the dexterity of the surgeon, but also by how well the donor and recipient have been matched from an immunological perspective. It must be appreciated that the immune system recognizes and responds to potentially dangerous antigens. A transplant operation involving a donated organ is more likely to be rejected if it is grafted into a genetically non-identical patient. Immune cells do not distinguish between a foreign molecule or organ of clinical benefit and one that could be harmful (see Chapter 24).

TESTING DONORS AND RECIPIENTS
Human Leukocyte Antigen Status

Like the blood group antigens on the surface of red blood cells, the HLA molecules present on the surface of nucleated cells do not change but remain the same throughout life, for they are genetically determined. Matching the HLA type of donor and recipient in conjunction with prescribing the appropriate immunosuppressive drugs regimen are clear objectives of the transplant medical team, particularly for bone marrow transplants. A good match helps prevent a hyperacute graft rejection and sustains the functional life of the graft. However, the HLA type varies greatly between individual members of a population and also between populations (see Chapter 24). Therefore,

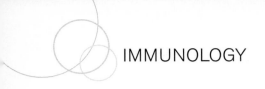

unless the patient has an identical twin, the probability of a near-perfect HLA match between two unrelated individuals is remote.

Two types of histocompatibility screening test are routinely performed before a transplant operation is considered. Cells are collected to determine the HLA class I and class II of both donor and recipient, and serum is collected for use in the cross-match technique. A 20 ml blood sample is required for HLA typing the surface of white blood cells. (White blood cells are used because they are simple to isolate from a blood sample and they display the HLA molecules found on other cell types.) The conventional immunological assays have used commercially prepared antibodies that distinguish between the different HLA molecules. However, tissue-typing laboratories have recently chosen more rapid and sensitive molecular biological techniques because they seem to give a more definitive result. Matching the HLA type of donor and recipient is particularly crucial for the successful outcome of a bone marrow transplantation. In solid organ transplantation a good HLA match is not so critical, but all patients must be screened via a serological test called a cross-match.

The principles of the cross-match for tissue or organ transplantation are the same as for blood transfusion (i.e. to assess whether there are antibodies in the transplant recipient's serum that could recognize and respond to the donor cells). The technique used is a cytotoxicity test, in which white blood cells from the donor are mixed with serum from the recipient. A positive result indicates the presence of serum HLA antibodies that could react with the foreign HLA antigens present on a new graft. Therefore, the cross-match provides sufficient evidence to suggest that a particular donor–recipient combination is contraindicated. In order to investigate the nature of the antibodies and their precise targets, further immunological tests are performed.

Blood Grouping

ABO blood group compatibility between donor and recipient is advised in solid organ transplantation, since the kidney, liver, and heart are all blood reservoirs. Any blood remaining in the graft could evoke the equivalent of a transfusion reaction if it was serologically incompatible.

Cytomegalovirus status

It is essential that the cytomegalovirus (CMV) status of the donor and recipient are known, since a CMV-negative transplant patient acquiring an organ from a CMV-positive donor may produce a life-threatening cross-infection. CMV infection is a serious complication

for patients prescribed immunosuppressive therapy (Figure 29.2).

The hepatitis B virus and human immunodeficiency virus (HIV) status of both donor and recipient are evaluated; HIV-positive patients are not generally offered transplantation.

CLINICAL INDICATORS OF TRANSPLANT REJECTION

One of the clinical indicators of a transplant rejection is a massive infiltration of immune cells into the grafted tissue. Clearly, the surgical procedure prompts a certain amount of tissue damage. Likewise, cellular death results from a long delay between removing the tissue from the donor and grafting it into the patient. Therefore, as immune cells are attracted into the graft to deal with the tissue damage, they also orchestrate the immunological rejection. Some of these mechanisms resemble the hypersensitivity type II and type IV reactions (see Chapter 26). As with other specific immune responses, there are two main stages: recognition of the transplanted tissue and reaction to it. Antigen-presenting cells (e.g. macrophages) migrate into the graft and engulf any cell debris. Once engulfed, the antigens are processed and presented to T helper cells. Subsequently, the macrophages and T helper cells become activated and release the cytokines, which have a significant role in the rejection episode. Other parts of the immune system are then stimulated, graft-specific B lymphocytes and cytotoxic T lymphocytes are

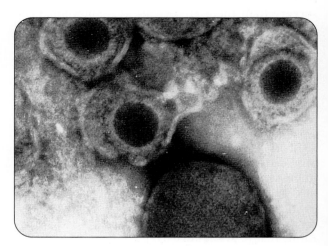

Figure 29.2 Electron micrograph of a cytomegalovirus (CMV) particle. CMV infection a common problem in the first year post-transplantation, probably because CMV is a latent infection found in about one-third of the population.

triggered, and some non-specific immune damage is elicited by natural killer cells.

Most transplanted tissues contain a certain amount of blood. Some of the major problems in rejections are on account of the donor dendritic cells and other antigen-presenting cells in the graft. Following surgery, these 'non-self leukocytes' migrate between the lymphatic system, body tissues, and fluids of their new host. As a result, the transplant patient's immune system is alerted to danger because the donor's dendritic cells have entered areas where they are able to be detected. Depleting grafts of dendritic cells before surgery reduces the incidence of rejection because the transplant patient does not mount a dramatic immune response.

DETECTION AND TREATMENT OF REJECTION

Graft rejection may develop almost immediately after the operation (hyperacute rejection), or it may take weeks (acute rejection) or even years (chronic rejection). The immunological mechanisms differ according to when after surgery rejection presents. Immunoglobulin and complement-mediated lysis are mainly responsible for hyperacute and chronic rejections. Cytokines that encourage the production and display of HLA molecules [e.g. interferons and interleukin-2 (IL-2)], also have an integral role. For example, graft-specific T lymphocytes are activated by both IL-2 and recognition of the HLA-bound antigens of the graft. The T lymphocytes detect both the antigen in the groove and the HLA. Consequently, if the antigen or the HLA (or both) are perceived as foreign, the immune cells respond and launch an attack. With the rapid cell division that ensues, many specific immune cells are provided in combination with the release of cytokines that recruit other parts of the immune system (Figure 29.3).

Hyperacute Graft Rejections

Hyperacute graft rejections are rare but, when they develop, the transplanted tissue becomes inflamed and malfunctioning within hours of surgery. These rapid rejection episodes are generated because of pre-existing antibodies in the body fluids of the transplant patient that bind the newly donated graft. Immune complexes (graft and immunoglobulins) are formed as a result, and these initiate the complement cascade. The inflammatory cells are attracted into the graft and the clotting mechanism is stimulated. Consequently, the tissue is inadequately perfused with blood because of the thrombus formation and cellular haemolysis that follows (Figure 29.4). Patients at risk of a hyper-

acute rejection episode, who therefore need to be closely observed postoperatively, are ones who have:
• previously undergone a transplant;
• previously received a blood transfusion; or
• been pregnant and developed antibodies against the partner's HLA.

In all these cases, the patients have been exposed to the HLA molecules of another person – the previous donor or the partner. Consequently, their immune cells are primed to respond to cell surface antigens on the graft (see Chapter 26).

Acute Graft Rejections

Acute graft rejections erupt within weeks of the transplant surgery. Even so, the functional integrity of the graft may be conserved provided that the onset of a rejection is rapidly detected and controlled with

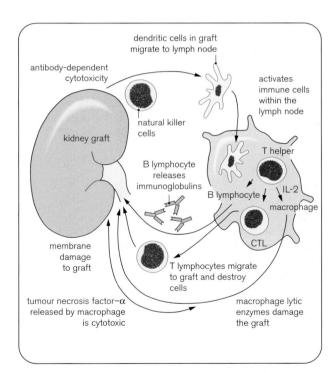

Figure 29.3 The immune response in graft rejection. Dendritic cells arise from the graft and migrate to a nearby lymph node. T helper cells are activated and in turn release interleukin-2. Cytotoxic T lymphocytes are activated, which then cause membrane damage to the graft. B lymphocytes release immunoglobulins that bind the graft (i.e. immune complexes form). Thus, complement is activated and natural killer cells provoke cytolytic damage.

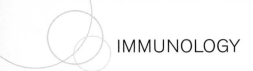

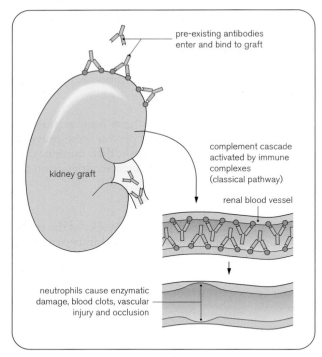

Figure 29.4 Hyperacute graft rejection. This occurs when there are pre-existing antibodies in the donor's body fluids that bind the graft. Complement is activated by the immune complexes formed, and vascular injury results from enzymatic damage and thrombi. Thus the graft never becomes adequately perfused with blood.

immunosuppressive therapy. Hence needle biopsy aspirates are taken for histological examination in the postoperative period, and one predictive indicator of rejection is the presence of large numbers of lymphocytes and macrophages. These cells incite inflammation and immunological damage on recognition of surface antigens and cellular debris of the graft.

Chronic Graft Rejection

Chronic graft rejection develops months or even years after successful transplantation despite immunosuppressive therapy. Therefore, since grafts do not necessarily have an indefinite life-span, younger patients are liable to require a second transplant. Regrettably, patients who previously suffered an acute rejection episode in which the blood vessels of the graft were damaged are a high risk for chronic rejection episodes at a later date. Unlike acute rejections, the clinical management is not as straightforward. Chronic rejections

are caused by damage mediated by immune cells and immunoglobulins. When graft-specific immunoglobulins are raised after transplantation, the resulting immune complexes are deposited and stimulate complement-mediated damage. In the sequence of events, blood vessels eventually become blocked because thrombi are formed, and this leads to tissue ischaemia and fibrosis (Figure 29.5).

IMMUNOSUPPRESSIVE THERAPY

Although donors and recipients are tested for compatibility, immunosuppressive therapy is still essential for the survival of an allogeneic graft (i.e. tissue or cells derived from another person). However, it is a fine balance – if transplant patients were completely immunosuppressed they would be at risk of life-threatening infections (see Chapter 18). Thus, the ideal treatment strategy is to restrain the parts of the immune system that would attack the graft while maintaining the rest of the immune surveillance network intact. A cocktail

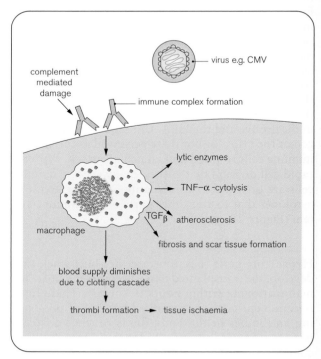

Figure 29.5 Chronic graft rejection. This results in a steady decline in the functional capacity of the graft. This type of rejection is mediated by infection and immunoglobulins. Blood supply is diminished owing to thrombus formation and atherosclerosis. Tissue ischaemia and fibrosis lead to loss of tissue function.

of drugs is therefore prescribed that operates at a number of levels to reduce the immune cell activities. Some immunosuppressive drugs inhibit DNA synthesis and mitosis, thereby inhibiting the rapid cell division mounted by graft-specific lymphocytes (i.e. one of the significant parts of the immune response). Other drugs modify the expression of cell surface antigen receptors, therefore when the receptors are either not displayed or non-functional, the immune cells are unable to recognize and respond effectively to the graft. Certain immunosuppressive drugs modify the release of cytokines to inhibit the immune response (Figure 29.6). Note: Anti-inflammatory and immunosuppressive drugs are also used to treat other immunological disorders e.g. asthma, rheumatoid arthritis.

TOTAL BODY IRRADIATION

Total body irradiation is used mainly as part of the regimen to ablate the patient's own bone marrow prior to bone marrow transplantation. Treatment involves the irradiation of the spleen, lymph nodes, and thymus with multiple exposure to X-rays. This damages DNA so the cells die during mitotic division. T-lymphocyte activities are particularly affected, and as this type of immunosuppression is non-selective, lymphocytes other than the graft-specific cells are restrained. Therefore, caution is essential in prescribing the appropriate dose, because excessive irradiation may leave the patient severely immunocompromised and vulnerable to virus infections and malignancy. It is also preferable that the radiation be given as two smaller doses a day rather than as one large dose, in order to reduce the incidence of adverse gastrointestinal disturbances (see Person-Centred Study: Bone Marrow Transplant for Acute Myeloid Leukaemia).

IMMUNOSUPPRESSIVE DRUGS

Azathioprine, methotrexate, and cyclophosphamide inhibit cell division and reduce lymphocyte numbers where mitosis has been blocked. There follows a restraint in T and B lymphocyte activities and potent inhibition of antibody production. Some unwanted side-effects of these drugs include bone marrow suppression, skin rashes, gastrointestinal disturbances, and hepatotoxicity.

Corticosteroid Therapy

With corticosteroid therapy, much of their control of immune function is focused on modification of cytokine levels – this class of drug has proved particularly useful in the management of acute rejection episodes. Prednisolone, which inhibits the production and release of cytokines, is often used. Corticosteroids reduce the activities of T and B lymphocytes and the functional efficiency of the phagocytic cells.

Caution is essential when changing the dose regimen or cessation of therapy because this may cause adverse withdrawal symptoms. For example, patients may experience a fall in blood pressure (hypertension is a known side-effect of corticosteroid therapy). In addition, the influence of corticosteroids have on electrolyte and water balance needs to be considered, particularly in patients where these metabolic indices are being monitored (e.g. patients who have had a kidney, liver, or heart transplant). The glycaemic control of diabetic patients is generally improved when the dose is reduced or therapy withdrawn, since corticosteroids tend to be diabetogenic (see also Box 29.2 and Chapter 35).

Cyclosporin A

Perhaps the best-known immunosuppressive drug is cyclosporin A, which is a natural metabolite derived from a fungus. It was discovered to have an inhibitory influence on immune cell activities. One of its main functions hinges on its effect on the cytokine, IL-2. Cyclosporin A provokes a decrease in the production of IL-2 itself and also in the number of available cell

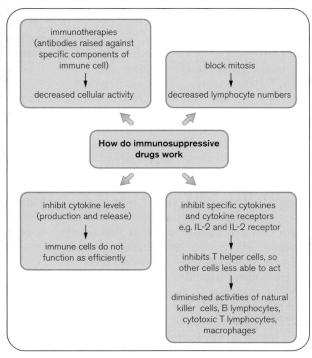

Figure 29.6 Mechanisms by which immunosuppressive drugs inhibit immune activities and help prevent graft rejection.

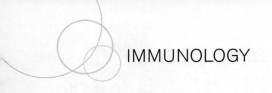

PERSON-CENTRED STUDY: BONE MARROW TRANSPLANT FOR ACUTE MYELOID LEUKAEMIA

Grace was a 52-year-old woman with acute myeloid leukaemia (AML) who was recommended to have a bone marrow transplant. A 20 ml specimen of blood was taken to evaluate her HLA-type and cytomegalovirus status. Her relatives were tested but were found not to be HLA-compatible, so a genetically unrelated donation was required. The Anthony Nolan Bone Marrow Trust was contacted and a suitable donor was found.

About 6 days before the transplantation, she was given therapy to ablate her own bone marrow. This consisted of cyclophosphamide (a cytotoxic drug) and total body irradiation, which was given twice daily in two small doses rather than as one large dose, in order to reduce the incidence of

adverse symptoms like nausea and vomiting. Then, 3 days before the infusion of the donated bone marrow, Grace commenced immunosuppressive therapy with cyclosporin A, methotrexate, and Campath (a monoclonal antibody) to prevent graft-versus-host disease (see below).

The bone marrow transplant procedure was straightforward, for it was given as an intravenous infusion. In the first weeks after her transplant, Grace suffered gastroenteritis and mucositis, which gradually subsided. She was discharged from hospital when her liver function, renal function, and white blood cell count were confirmed to be satisfactory.

BOX 29.2   TRANSPLANTATION OF ENDOCRINE GLANDS

Transplantation of endocrine glands has been proposed as a useful treatment for patients who require an exogenous supply of hormones. A number of donor sources of endocrine tissues have been pursued, including organs from first-degree relatives and fetal tissue from pregnancies terminated in the first trimester, though there is a huge ethical debate over the use of fetal tissues as a source of organs. Pancreatic transplantation has been considered for insulin-dependent diabetes mellitus to improve the metabolic control of glucose and reduce the incidence of microvascular complications such as retinopathy, and nephropathy. In the surgical procedure, the donated pancreas is inserted into the kidney capsule (i.e. a heterotopic site), but this has not proved to be a permanently effective form of treatment. The transplantation of fetal-derived adrenal glands as a source of dopamine has had limited success for treating the tremor of Parkinson's disease.

surface IL-2 receptors. Therefore, with the 'signal' and 'receiver' levels reduced, the influence of IL-2 on the immune system is diminished. Since this cytokine is a stimulator of T helper cells, other areas of the immune response are also modified as a result (e.g. natural killer cells, B lymphocytes, cytotoxic T lymphocytes, and macrophages are inhibited). In addition to IL-2 inhibition, cyclosporin A stimulates the release of cytokines that deplete immune function (e.g. transforming growth factor-beta).

Unlike other immunosuppressive drugs, cyclosporin A does not suppress bone marrow function; however it is nephrotoxic, and prolonged treatment may ultimately lead to renal failure. Unfortunately, in kidney transplant patients it is sometimes difficult to distinguish between a graft rejection and an adverse drug reaction. Therefore renal function tests are an essential part of the regular monitoring protocol.

Two other fungal-derived immunosuppressive drugs have been prepared, tacrolimus (also called FK506) and rapamycin, which have a more potent therapeutic effect and so can be given at a lower dose than cyclosporin A. However, although these newer drugs have a reduced risk of known side-effects, their value will only be confirmed when the results of clinical trials have been fully evaluated.

ANTIBODY THERAPY

Immunotherapies in the form of antibodies for infusion have emerged for the control of transplant rejection. For example, anti-lymphocyte immunoglobulins raised and harvested from rabbits and horses that have been previously immunized with human lymphoid cells are sometimes used to control acute rejection episodes. Thus T-lymphocyte function and, to a lesser extent, B-lymphocyte and antibody responses are diminished. But anti-lymphocyte immunoglobulins are not very specific – they will bind to one of the many different epitopes on the lymphocyte surface.

A monoclonal antibody called Campath has been raised against human lymphocytes and monocytes. It is being used with some success to prevent graft-versus-host disease (Box 29.3).

Precise functional areas of the lymphocytes can be targeted and inhibited by raising immunoglobulins against a distinct cell surface protein. One of the most significant markers is the CD3 complex, whose function is linked with the presentation of T-cell receptors on the cell surface (see Chapter 24). Therefore a monoclonal anti-CD3 antibody called OKT3, has been prepared for intravenous infusion. When CD3 complex is bound up in an immune complex with OKT3, the cellular activities are inhibited. However, the therapy has a major disadvantage in that, because a mouse produced the monoclonal antibody, it is deemed foreign by the human immune system. Therefore, about 75 per cent of patients respond by developing antibodies against the OKT3, which renders the treatment less effective. There are also a number side-effects, such as fever and myalgia, produced as the antibody therapy stimulates the release of cytokines that precipitate the adverse symptoms (see Serum Sickness, Chapter 26).

SIDE-EFFECTS OF PROLONGED IMMUNOSUPPRESSIVE THERAPY

By definition, immunosuppressive therapy reduces the immune surveillance mechanisms, and consequently it causes an increased risk of malignancy. Skin cancer, cervical cancer, and Kaposi's sarcoma are recorded examples, and non-Hodgkin's lymphoma is more prevalent in transplant recipients than in the general population. The increased risk of infection is another obvious complication (see Chapter 18). CMV infection is a common problem in the first year after a transplant, probably because CMV is a latent infection found in about one-third of the population. Therefore, to reduce the risk of cross-infection, blood for transfusion into transplant patients is selected which is CMV-negative (this testing is performed by the National Blood Service), then this blood is cross-matched to confirm blood group and rhesus compatibility.

Some immunosuppressive drugs do not only target the immune cells – other rapidly dividing cells can be adversely affected (e.g. the gut, the skin, the hair, and bone marrow). From another perspective, serum lipid abnormalities arise with long-term administration of immunosuppressive drugs (e.g. the combination of prednisolone, azathioprine, and cyclosporin A). Raised serum cholesterol and triglyceride levels tend to increase the risk of atherosclerosis and could affect the viability of the graft. Lipid-lowering agents are prescribed to reduce the risk of ischaemia, but rhabdomyolysis may be produced when these are given with cyclosporin A.

CLINICAL APPLICATIONS OF TRANSPLANTATION

HEART TRANSPLANTATION

Heart transplantation may be offered to patients with end-stage cardiac failure (e.g. as caused by idiopathic or ischaemic cardiomyopathy), provided that there is no evidence of malignancy or infection (see Chapter 32). The age limit for surgery is both controversial and

---

BOX 29.3 GRAFT-VERSUS-HOST DISEASE (GvHD)

Acute GvHD develops about 7 days after the bone marrow transfusion.

Chronic GvHD is the term used when this disease occurs 100 or more days after the transplant. Patients could suffer GvHD which develops into chronic GvHD.

Clinical evaluation or staging of the GvHD (stages I–IV) is based on the number of organ systems affected and the severity of the symptoms.

Symptoms include:
- Progressive and painful erythematous rash with marked exfoliation
- Nausea, vomiting, and abdominal cramps
- Severe watery diarrhoea; blood is detected with the progression of the GvHD
- Protein-losing enteropathy
- Abnormal liver function tests
- Hepatosplenomegaly

dependent on the particular hospital unit. Some surgeons prefer not to operate on patients aged 60 years or older, since these patients may be less able to tolerate such radical surgery. Cardiac transplantation is also contraindicated where there is a co-existing pathology that could affect the graft (e.g. impaired hepatic or renal function). When a donor becomes available, donor and recipient organ size may also be matched – this is because of the limited capacity of the thorax. An orthotopic transplantation is preferable, in which the diseased heart is removed and replaced. However, if the size of the donated organ is inadequate for the size of the thorax or if the recipient's pulmonary arterial pressure is high, the graft may be anastomosed in parallel to the diseased heart.

HEART AND LUNG TRANSPLANTATION

Heart and lung transplantation is rather more complex and not so frequently performed, since the transplantation of lungs alone is increasingly successful for the treatment of chronic obstructive pulmonary disease and cystic fibrosis (see Chapter 33). The lung may be transplanted singly or as a double-organ transplant. However, because the donated lungs are likely to be from cadavers that have sustained trauma, the lungs must be confirmed as functional, intact, and without infectious contamination (e.g. fungal infections).

Postoperatively, lung function, cardiac output, and arterial gases are used to assess the physiological integrity of the grafted organs. Since lungs have an extensive mucosal surface, it is critical that their function should be rapidly restored in order to re-establish an immunological barrier, for infections are a major cause of mortality in lung transplant patients. Haemorrhage and acute respiratory failure are other frequent complications in the postoperative period.

RENAL TRANSPLANTATION

Renal transplantation is a well-established treatment for patients in chronic renal failure who have a functioning lower urinary tract (e.g. patients with diabetic nephropathy, polycystic renal disease, systemic lupus erythematosus, or glomerulonephritis) (see Chapter 36). Regrettably, the pathological mechanisms that were responsible for the organ failure invariably affect the donated graft. For example, patients with systemic lupus erythematosus who have suffered immune complex-mediated damage to their own kidneys are likely to suffer damage to the donated kidney at a later date.

A number of factors exclude a patient from renal transplantation, including persistent substance misuse, HIV infection, and terminal malignant disease. Patients with active hepatitis B or hepatitis C are also closely evaluated before surgery is advocated because of the risk of hepatic failure.

While on the waiting list for surgery, renal patients may be managed and stabilized with haemodialysis or continuous ambulatory peritoneal dialysis and diet (electrolyte, protein, and fluid restrictions). When the kidney is grafted, it is not placed in the normal anatomical location but in the iliac fossa (or retroperitoneally if it is a small child) – this is an example of a heterotopic transplant.

Renal function and urinary output are assessed in the postoperative period. Needle biopsy specimens are taken so the onset of a rejection episode may be identified and treated. Urinary tract infections are a common problem owing to the presence of an indwelling catheter. Hepatitis B and hepatitis C virus infections are a significant cause of mortality. Hence there is rigorous monitoring of the hepatitis status of patients, visitors, and staff working on a renal unit to prevent cross-infection. Post-transplant patients are prescribed a diet in which protein and electrolytes (sodium and potassium) are moderately restricted. Energy and saturated fat intake are also modified to stabilize body weight, since certain drugs (e.g. steroids) stimulate a voracious appetite. Moreover, cardiovascular disease is a frequent complication; this is exacerbated by some immunosuppressive drugs because they alter serum lipid profiles (see Chapters 6 and 36).

LIVER TRANSPLANTATION

Liver transplantation may be used in the clinical management of end-stage hepatic disease in patients who have remained unresponsive to other forms of therapy. Patients with an inborn error of metabolism that affects the liver (e.g. glycogen storage disease type I or type IV) may also be referred for liver transplantation. Patients with metastases, renal, or cardiac dysfunction, however, are not generally offered this type of treatment; and, although this is rather controversial, people who persistently misuse alcohol may also be excluded. Liver grafts are often given to patients with hepatic failure caused by paracetamol overdose.

One of the innate advantages of the liver is its capacity to regenerate itself. Recent progress in surgery has permitted the use of individual lobes from a single liver to provide grafts for more than one patient. In some cases a lobe donated by a live donor has proved effective for treating small children with a restricted capacity in the abdominal cavity for the newly donated organ.

Impaired immune function in hepatic failure and post-transplantation is a notable complication, for the healthy liver has significant role as part of the mononuclear phagocytic system and in the production of complement proteins. Therefore, in impaired liver function the supply of opsonins is depleted and so phagocytic function may be suboptimal. In addition, patients with cirrhosis are likely to be malnourished, and this further compromises immunity. Thus, liver transplant patients are especially vulnerable in the immediate postoperative period while the physiological functions of the liver are being re-established. A pre-operative evaluation is therefore advised to assess for any infections at the mucosal surfaces, since infections are a significant cause of mortality in the first year after surgery. Some hospital units routinely immunize patients against hepatitis B and *Pneumococcus* before surgery.

Liver function tests, clotting screens, and fine-needle biopsies are performed routinely after surgery to give a clearer indication of graft viability and to detect any possible signs of rejection. Postoperative complications include leakage of bile, obstructive jaundice, and intraperitoneal bleeding, which may result in hypovolaemic shock. About 3 per cent of liver transplant patients suffer from graft-versus-host disease (GvHD), a disorder caused by the immune cells within the donated liver (i.e. the donor's white blood cells), which emerge and attack the tissues of their new host. The gut and skin are particularly affected. When GvHD arises, it carries a significant risk of mortality (see Box 29.3).

SMALL BOWEL TRANSPLANTATION

Most of the organs used in small bowel transplantation come from cadaveric donations, although occasionally organs from live donors may be resected. Postoperatively the graft is assessed by radiological and endoscopic examinations, together with estimations of metabolic indices (e.g. serum urea, electrolytes, glucose levels). Normal physiological function is restored gradually, for there is usually a delay in electrolyte and water absorptive powers while neurological control of the small bowel is re-established and while the lymphatic system adapts to the presence of the new graft. Since the gut is both a physical and immunological barrier, a rapid recovery of physiological function reduces the risk of infection. If normal function is not restored, the patient is maintained on total parenteral nutrition. However, this form of nutritional support carries the significant risk of sepsis to the already immunocompromised patient.

BONE MARROW TRANSPLANTATION

Bone marrow transplantation is a standard therapy for the treatment of inherited disorders of haematopoiesis,

including some immunodeficiency syndromes (e.g. chronic granulomatous disease). However, the majority of transplants are offered as treatment for haematological malignancies (see Person-Centred Study). In many cases an autologous transplant is preferred, in which bone marrow is aspirated, purged of malignant cells then given back to the patient. Although there is no risk of HLA incompatibility, there is the potential for contamination with malignant cells and a relapse of the disease at a later date. Grafts may also be acquired from a first-degree relative or an unrelated donor, but a reasonable HLA match between the donor and recipient is essential.

There are two registers of bone marrow donors who have been screened for infections (e.g. hepatitis, HIV, CMV) as well as for HLA type. The British Bone Marrow Registry is co-ordinated by the National Blood Service, and their bone marrow donors are also usually regular blood donors in the UK. The other register is a charity called the Anthony Nolan Bone Marrow Trust. In addition there is access to about 4 000 000 donors through a world-wide cross-referencing register to trace a suitable donor for a patient with a rare HLA type. If the donor and recipient reside in different countries, arrangements are made for the bone marrow to be aspirated and sent by courier to its destination for transplantation.

The donor is given a general anaesthetic, and bone marrow obtained from the iliac crest by multiple needle aspirations (10–20 ml/kg body weight is taken). The bone marrow is then put into heparinized tissue culture medium and strained through a fine mesh to remove particulate matter such as tissue and bone.

The transplant procedure is far simpler than in other transplantations, for the cells are given as an intravenous infusion, which subsequently 'homes in' to the bone marrow micro-environment (e.g. within the sternum and iliac crest). Generally the recipient's own bone marrow is ablated (destroyed) with chemotherapy (e.g. cyclophosphamide) to provide a location into which the new bone marrow can migrate. In cases such as the one described in the Person-Centred Study, it is hoped that the patient's diseased bone marrow has been completely removed so that a relapse does not recur.

Bone marrow is different from other types of transplant in that the donor has given haematopoietic stem cells, which will ultimately differentiate into immune cells (i.e. the immune system of another person is being donated). Consequently, a significant post-transplant complication is the situation in which the acquired bone marrow rejects the body into which it has been donated – graft-versus-host disease (GvHD). This type of rejection is extremely difficult to treat. The donated T lymphocytes play a significant role in the immunological attack on the healthy tissues of the host. One preventative strategy, which has been undertaken in some hospitals, is to deplete the bone marrow of post-thymic T lymphocytes.

In order to distinguish between postoperative infections and GvHD it is therefore essential to take body tissue and fluid samples for microbiological examination. For example, is the patient's diarrhoea being caused by an infection? Is the skin rash the symptom of an adverse drug reaction? Nonetheless, when allogeneic bone marrow is donated for the treatment of leukaemia, a low grade GvHD is an asset in the immediate post-transplant period. Here the cytotoxic activities of the donated cells that cause GvHD can be put to good use – namely, to kill any residual malignant cells in the bone marrow which were not removed when the bone marrow was ablated.

KEY POINTS

- Transplantation is the term used to describe the surgical transfer of cells, tissues, or organs from one location to another within the same patient (an autologous graft), or the implantation of cells, tissues, or organs donated by another person.
- Donated tissues and organs may be acquired from a number of different sources – a first-degree relative, a living, unrelated donor, or a cadaveric donor.
- Prior to solid organ transplantation, patients and donors are screened for HLA type, HLA antibody status, CMV status, ABO blood grouping, and a number of infectious diseases including HIV-1, HIV-2, hepatitis B, and hepatitis C.
- A cross-match is a screening test that detects the presence of serum antibodies (e.g. HLA antibodies) that could attack the graft.
- Routine postoperative examination of the graft is essential for the detection and treatment of a possible rejection episode (e.g. by needle biopsy aspirate to detect the infiltration of immune cells, and by organ function tests).
- Immunosuppressive drugs are prescribed in order to restrain parts of the immune system that would attack the graft, but at the same time endeavouring to maintain the immune surveillance network intact.
- Modes of drug action that inhibit immune function include inhibiting DNA synthesis or cell division, blocking the activities of functional cell surface proteins, and modifying the release of cytokines and their influence on immune cells.
- Prolonged immunosuppressive therapy generates some undesirable side-effects (e.g. increased risk of infection, malignancy, serum lipid disorders, and organ toxicity – for example, cyclosporin A is nephrotoxic).

FURTHER READING

Baldwin WM 3rd, Pruitt SK, Brauer RB, *et al.* (1995) Complement in organ transplantation. Contributions to inflammation, injury, and rejection. Transplantation 59:797–808.

Barone GW, Sailors DM, Hudec WA, Ketel BL (1997) Trauma management in solid organ transplant recipients. J Emerg Med 15:169–76.

Cho YW, Terasaki PI, Cecka JM, Gjertson DW (1998) Transplantation of kidneys from donors whose hearts have stopped beating. N Engl J Med 338:221–5.

Cohen B, D'Amaro J, De Meester J, Persijn GG (1997) Changing patterns in organ donation in Eurotransplant, 1990–1994. Transpl Int 10:1–6.

Cossio FG, Alamir A, Yim S *et al.* (1998) Patient survival often renal transplantation I. The impact of dialysis pre-transplant. Kidney Int 53:(3) 767–72.

De Mario MD, Liebowitz DN (1998) Lymphomas in the immunocompromised patient. Sem Oncol 25:(4) 492–502.

Epstein S, Shane E, Bilezikian JP (1995) Organ transplantation and osteoporosis. Curr Opin Rheumatol 7:255–61.

Fung JJ, Starzl TE (1995) FK506 in solid organ transplantation. Ther Drug Monit 17:592–5.

Giacomini M (1997) A change of heart and a change of mind? Technology and the redefinition of death in 1968. Soc Sci Med 44:1465–82.

Halloran PF (1997) Immunosuppressive agents in clinical trials in transplantation. Am J Med Sci 313:283–8.

Heckmann JG, Lang CJ, Petruch F, *et al.* (1997) Transmission of Creutzfeldt-Jakob disease via a corneal transplant. J Neurol Neurosurg Psychiatry 63:388–90.

Hurley C (1997) Ambulatory care after bone marrow or peripheral blood stem cell transplantation. Clin J Oncol Nurs 1:19–21.

Jindal RM, Sidner RA, Milgrom ML (1997) Post-transplant diabetes mellitus. The role of immunosuppression. Drug Saf 16:242–57.

Kobashigawa JA, Kasiske BL (1997) Hyperlipidemia in solid organ transplantation. Transplantation 63:331–8.

Lanza RP, Cooper DKC, Chick WL (1997) Xenotransplantation. Sci Am 277:54–9.

Lucas KG, Pollok KE, Emanuel DJ (1997) Post-transplant EBV induced lymphoproliferative disorders. Leuk Lymphoma 25:1–8.

Murray BM (1997) Management of cytomegalovirus infection in solid-organ transplant recipients. Immunol Invest 26:243–55.

Riether AM, Mahler E (1995) Organ donation. Psychiatric, social, and ethical considerations. Psychosomatics 36:336–43.

Shapiro R Tacrolimus (FK-506) in kidney transplantation. Transplant Proc 29:(1–2) 45–7.

Shaw LM, Kaplan B, Kaufman D (1996) Toxic effects of immunosuppressive drugs: mechanisms and strategies for controlling them. Clin Chem 42:1316–21.

Winkler M, Christians U (1995) A risk–benefit assessment of tacrolimus in transplantation. Drug Saf 12:348–57.

Woodward JM, Mayer D (1996) The unique challenge of small intestinal transplantation. Br J Hosp Med 56:285–90.

Woo SB, Lee SJ, Schubert MM (1997) Graft-vs-host disease. Crit Rev Oral Biol Med 8:201–16.

Zaia JA (1996) Prophylaxis and treatment of CMV infections in transplantation. Adv Exp Med Biol 394:117–34.

THE IMMUNE SYSTEM AND CANCER

30

LEARNING OBJECTIVES

After studying this chapter students should have a clearer understanding of:
- the anti-tumour mechanisms of the immune system
- how cancer cells hide from the immune surveillance network
- the people who are most at risk of developing cancer
- newer therapeutic strategies being designed to boost the immune response to cancers

INTRODUCTION

The advancement in antimicrobial therapies and the widespread administration of immunizations during this century has meant that mortality from infectious disease has declined dramatically in Western countries. Therefore, people in these countries tend to live longer and cancer has replaced infection as a major cause of death. Cancers generally arise because one or two abnormal cell clones have proliferated out of control and then evaded immune recognition. Healthy cells contain tumour-suppressor genes, which are stretches of genetic sequence that are believed to control cellular proliferation. Although the precise mechanisms by which they operate are as yet not fully understood, when these genes are inactivated or defective, cell division becomes more erratic. (The properties of abnormal growth and aetiological factors that predispose to malignancy are discussed at length in Chapters 3 and 5.)

An intriguing revelation from post-mortem examinations has highlighted that many more tumours arise than are actually detected. Some tumours emerge and then regress because the patient's own defences have detected and eradicated them. This chapter explains the mechanisms used by the immune system to recognize and respond to abnormal cells, and the ways in which the tumour attempts to escape the immune surveillance network. Because a healthy immune system is already equipped to be tumouricidal, treatments are being

designed to up-regulate its activities. The immunotherapies being explored for use in clinical oncology practice will be explained in this chapter along with some of the pitfalls of these treatment regimens.

ANTI-TUMOUR STRATEGIES OF THE IMMUNE SYSTEM

The natural and specific immune systems operate 'in concert' to provide an immune surveillance network for the recognition and elimination of abnormal cells. In particular, this involves the activities of the natural killer cells, macrophages, and lymphocytes and their secretory products (the immunoglobulins and cytokines) (Figure 30.1).

NATURAL KILLER CELLS

Natural killer cells are involved in the non-specific defence against malignant (and virus-infected) cells. Unlike the lymphocytes, they are not limited to simply killing cells which display human leukocyte antigen (HLA)-bound antigens. Therefore, since they are not HLA-restricted, natural killer cells appear to be less discriminatory. However, it needs to be acknowledged that an element of selectivity does exist, for many types of virus-infected and tumour cells are not killed by natural killer cells.

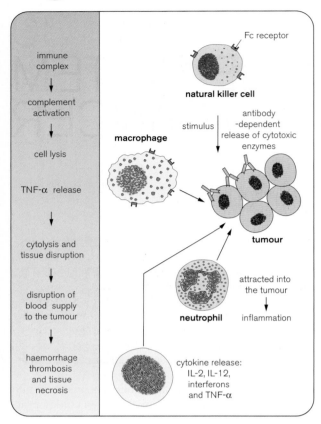

immune
complex
↓
complement
activation
↓
cell lysis
↓
TNF-α release
↓
cytolysis and
tissue disruption
↓
disruption of
blood supply
to the tumour
↓
haemorrhage
thrombosis
and tissue
necrosis

Fc receptor

natural killer cell

stimulus

antibody
-dependent
release of cytotoxic
enzymes

macrophage

tumour

attracted into
the tumour

neutrophil   inflammation

cytokine release:
IL-2, IL-12,
interferons
and TNF-α

Figure 30.1 Anti-tumour strategies of the immune system. Immunoglobulins released in response to a tumour stimulate complement and antibody-dependent cytotoxic activities by cells bearing Fc receptors (e.g. natural killer cells and macrophages). Neutrophils attracted into the tumour cell cause inflammatory damage. Cytokines potentiate the immune cell functions and cause cytolytic damage. Blood supply to the tumour is disrupted, leading to haemorrhage, thrombosis, and tissue necrosis.

Some malignant cells attempt to escape immune surveillance by depleting the number of HLA molecules present on the cell surface. This may be achieved by either not synthesizing so many HLA molecules, or by impeding part of the intracellular pathway through which they move (see Chapter 24). Even if this strategy means the cytotoxic T lymphocytes are not able to recognize abnormal cells easily, natural killer cells can distinguish cells with a sparse distribution of surface HLA. In fact, if very few or no HLA molecules are displayed, it is a significant activating signal for natural killer cells. Once a cell has been recognized as abnormal, the tumouricidal activity of the natural killer

cells is prompted by cell–cell contact. In many ways the killing is similar to the action of the cytotoxic T lymphocytes, for when the contents of cytoplasmic granules are released, the enzymes and the substance perforin puncture holes in the membrane and the cell bursts (cell lysis). Apoptosis (programmed cell death) is also mediated by the natural killer cells and is thought to contribute to their cytotoxic influence.

Natural killer cell function in immune surveillance should not be underestimated – patients with Chediak–Higashi syndrome (in which the activities of the natural killer cells and the phagocytic cells are impaired) have an increased incidence of cancer. Extrinsic factors also influence their function; for instance, nutritional intervention studies have found a positive correlation between reduced micronutrient status and diminished natural killer cell function. Supplementation with selenium and vitamin E has been shown to increase their activity. Another interesting and possibly disturbing observation has been the suppressed immune function of patients with silicone breast implants. This reduction seems to be attributable to the presence of the silicone gel, for natural killer cell activity is restored when the implant is removed.

MACROPHAGES AND LYMPHOCYTES

Macrophages and lymphocytes are frequently detected as clusters around tumours, and they are known to be instrumental in tumour regression. Indeed, their presence in the abnormal tumour cell mass of a tissue biopsy is a good indicator that the immune system has responded to the cancer. These infiltrating cells are a significant source of cytokines. Some of these cytokines, such as tumour necrosis factor-alpha (TNF-alpha) have a direct cytotoxic effect, others, such as interleukin-2 (IL-2) and interferons, recruit and activate immune cells in the vicinity of the tumour. The damage to the tumour cells following the release of lytic enzymes and free radicals by the macrophages results in the formation of cell debris. Healthy cells readily inactivate free radicals using the enzyme superoxide dismutase. Conversely, tumour cells do not generally synthesize enough of this enzyme, so they are more likely to be affected by the highly energetic and damaging activities of free radicals.

Lymphocytes residing in the lymph nodes need to be alerted to the presence of cancer cells in other parts of the body. For this reason, one of the key functions of macrophages is to roam through the body tissues and fluids to pick up and display antigens for the activation of other immune cells. The macrophages engulf and process tumour cell debris (i.e. the tumour antigens), which they would have been instrumental in generating. Then they migrate to the nearest lymph node, having processed the antigens for presentation to the T helper cells on HLA class II. Although T helper cells are not directly involved in the killing of the tumour, they do secrete cytokines like interferon-gamma and TNF-alpha, which up-regulate the activities of other immune cells. Thus, in due course the natural immune system has contributed to the stimulation of lymphocytes for a round of killing by tumour-specific T lymphocytes and B lymphocytes secreting anti-tumour antibodies.

Cancer cells that display the appropriate antigen on HLA class I are eliminated by specific cytotoxic T lymphocytes. Once the tumour antigens have been synthesized, they are presented on the outer surface of mutant cells in much the same way as a virus infection (see Chapter 24). It is especially important that cytotoxic T lymphocytes respond to viruses because these infections are a known aetiological factor in the development of certain types of tumours (e.g. hepatitis B virus and hepatocellular carcinoma) (see Chapters 5 and 34).

IMMUNOGLOBULINS

Immunoglobulins released in response to a cancer facilitate the cells of natural immunity to perform antibody-dependent cytotoxic damage, thereby reducing the size of the tumour. Once bound to their specific surface antigens, the immunoglobulin molecules become a point of attachment for immune cells possessing Fc receptors (antibody receptors) (i.e. macrophages and natural killer cells). In effect, they form a 'bridge' (tumour–immunoglobulin–immune cell) to facilitate the delivery of enzymes that perforate the target cell membrane. Furthermore, when the cancer is caught up as immune complexes, the complement cascade is stimulated, and so the cells are lysed with the sequential development of the membrane attack complex (see Chapter 25).

CYTOKINES

Cytokines have a fundamental role in the co-ordination of the anti-tumour immune response, for a precise cascade of different cytokines is required to orchestrate the immune surveillance network. Natural killer cells release a number of cytokines (e.g. interferon-gamma). In turn, the activities of the natural killer cells are stimulated by the presence of IL-2, IL-12, and the interferons, particularly interferon-alpha and interferon-beta – these cytokines are produced by other immune cell types (like T lymphocytes and macrophages) that were activated in response to the tumour.

The effects of tumour necrosis factor-alpha (TNF-alpha) were some of the first anticancer mechanisms of the immune system to be identified. It followed the observation that tumours became necrotic when patients suffered Gram-negative infections. The main sources of TNF-alpha include the macrophages, T lymphocytes, and activated natural killer cells. In addition to the systemic influences, the elevated levels of TNF-alpha have a toxic effect on the tumour itself and the associated blood vessels (see Chapter 25). It is assumed that, on binding to the tumour, TNF-alpha becomes internalized within the cells, where it destroys the architecture of the cells and tissues. The shape and integrity of a tissue is maintained by the junctions (e.g. the gap junctions between cells) (see Chapter 1), and TNF-alpha interferes with these structures. Both the tumour cells and its blood vessels are disrupted, and this leads to haemorrhagic necrosis due to inadequate blood perfusion. Activation of the clotting cascade results in thrombus formation; an inflammatory reaction also ensues when neutrophils are recruited into the tumour. Metabolic disturbances arise, and hypoglycaemia and the physical manifestation of cachexia are symptoms that are seen in cancer patients in response to high levels of TNF-alpha (see Chapter 25).

ANTIGENS DETECTED BY THE IMMUNE SYSTEM
Tumour Antigens

Tumour antigens are synthesized by cancer cells, and these antigens may be processed and displayed on the outer membrane or released into the body fluids. Some tumour antigens are proteins made from the decoding and translation of a specific oncogene (see Chapter 5). The protein called Neu is one such example; it is detectable in patients with breast cancer but it is only found in minute quantities in healthy breast tissue. Likewise, it is well established that certain antigens are tumour-specific (e.g. the ovarian tumour antigen, CA-125) (see also Chapter 37).

Other tumours synthesize large quantities of an antigen that it would have been produced in fetal life but not detected in adult tissues. For example, alpha-fetoprotein (AFP) is synthesized by the fetal liver, and elevated AFP levels are a recognized prenatal indictor that there is a high risk that the developing fetus may have neural tube defects (see Chapter 7). But raised serum AFP levels may be also found in patients with liver cancer. Similarly, the carcinoembryonic antigen (CEA), which is a protein synthesized by the fetal gut, is a marker of colorectal cancers in adults. As far as its pathophysiological role in the tumour is concerned, it is thought that CEA promotes their binding in the abnormal cell mass. However, it is not a tumour-specific antigen since raised serum levels are found in patients with other types of cancer (e.g. cancer of the breast, lung, pancreas) and in patients with inflammatory diseases (e.g. pancreatitis and colitis). Despite the lack of tissue specificity of many tumour antigens, clinicians have realized the value of estimating levels of these antigens in the serum of patients with cancer in order to assess the effectiveness of treatment – a fall in the serum level is a useful diagnostic marker of tumour regression.

HOW DO CANCERS HIDE FROM THE IMMUNE SYSTEM?

The presence of a cancer suggests that the internal environment of the body had been conducive to tumour cell proliferation. This may occur if the cancer either:
• has not been perceived as dangerous; or
• has eluded the immune system.

It is possible that the tumour would not be perceived as dangerous since the disease has arisen from a few cells that were originally part of a normal healthy tissue. If the malignant cells do not emit distress signals, they may be overlooked and so continue dividing. It is acknowledged that T lymphocytes require two signals for activation, the first signal being the HLA-bound peptide (e.g. HLA displaying a tumour-derived antigen) and signal two being the danger or distress signal required for co-stimulation (this may be a cytokine released by another immune cell; an intracellular component released during cell lysis has also been suggested) (see Chapter 27). If the two signals are not forthcoming, then the abnormal cells will not be aggressively eliminated. If the T and B lymphocytes do not respond to malignant cells, it may mean the cancer is not very immunogenic or that the immune surveillance by these cells is suboptimal. Tumours that are immunogenic are more readily recognized and attacked by an active immune system. Moreover, if antigen-presenting cells are not attracted into the tumour, then resting lymphocytes in the lymph node will not be alerted to eliminate the abnormality (Figure 30.2).

When an anticancer response has been raised, some tumours try to counterbalance the attack by various mechanisms. One mechanism is the synthesis and secretion of cytokines that inhibit the immune cell activities or at least counteract the effects of the cytokines. For example, release of transforming growth factor-beta inhibits the activities of lymphocytes and macrophages. It is also evident that tumours have evolved various strategies to avoid being recognized by the immune

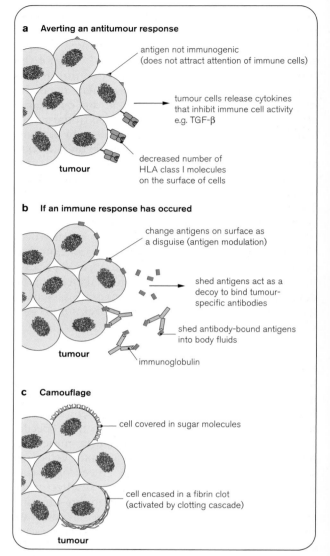

Figure 30.2 Mechanisms used by tumours to evade immune attack.

system. Some cancer cells have a much lower density of HLA molecules on their cell surface than their normal healthy counterparts. With the diminished number of immunological sign boards available, it is possible for them to proliferate undetected by the lymphocytes.

When an antigen has been the target of an attack, the tumour may vary the types of antigen it synthesizes – this is known as antigenic modulation. It is envisaged that without the specific antigen being detectable there should be a decline in the anti-tumour antibody levels and T lymphocyte activity, owing to diminished antigenic stimulation.

Damage limitation approaches can also be adopted when an antigen has elicited an antibody response. Cancer cells may:

- shed the immune complexes from the outer surface of the tumour (i.e. the tumour antigen–antibody complexes are cast off like a snake sheds its skin!);
- release the target antigens alone from the tumour surface – then the free antigens act as a decoy by binding to the antibodies in the body fluids, thereby averting a direct antibody-mediated attack on the tumour mass;
- use antibody-binding to disguise their outer surface so as to deflect the immune activities of the T lymphocytes;
- camouflage their outer surfaces by synthesizing sugar molecules to cover the outer surface – a phenomena known as antigen masking; or
- shield themselves by stimulating the coagulation pathway and become encased in a fibrin clot to avoid being recognized as abnormal.

WHO IS AT RISK OF CANCER?

People most vulnerable to developing a tumour include patients who have an inadequate immune surveillance network. Thus, very young children whose immune system is naïve, and older patients whose immune cells have become less active, are at higher risk of developing cancer than young adults.

Regrettably, the cytotoxic agents given to treat some malignancies have been implicated in the aetiology of haematological malignancies at a later date. Some people carry genes that predispose to certain types of malignancy (e.g. BRCA1 gene may be responsible for up to 5 per cent of breast cancer) (see Chapter 7). A patient's genetic make-up may lead to compromised immune function, for individuals with inherited immunodeficiency syndromes have an increased incidence of cancers (see Person-Centred Study: The Anti-Tumour Properties of the Immune System Make Headline News!). Acquired immunosuppression also carries a significant risk, and many patients with AIDS develop Kaposi's sarcoma (see Chapter 28). Likewise, the fact that transplant patients who are prescribed long-term immunosuppressive therapy develop lymphoma at a rate 400–700 times that of the normal population is confirmation of this fundamental role of immunity (Figure 30.3).

There is evidence that psychosocial factors (e.g. anxiety, depression, and stress) affect the immune surveillance of the defence system. The effects of stress and the levels of endocrine hormones on immune function are developing fields of interest, but they are highly controversial and open to much speculation. Nonetheless, although experimental data on immune cell function and stress is limited, there seems to be a plausible link between physical health and psychological well-being (see Box 30.1). For instance, one study, which evaluated the immunocompetence of healthy, independently living Italian centenarians, demonstrated high activities of natural killer cells and T lymphocytes.

The possible role of personality types and stressors have also been reviewed in relation to possible association with cancer development. In the quest to understand these influences, it has been postulated that stress may facilitate carcinogenesis by a number of mechanisms, including diminishing the ability to repair deoxyribonucleic acid and increasing the tendency to express proto-oncogenes (see Chapter 5). Together these factors could precipitate genetic mutations in a cell, and thus create an abnormality which is compounded by an inadequate ability of immune detection.

HOW DO TREATMENTS FOR CANCER WORK?

Chemotherapeutic drugs and radiotherapy are well-recognized treatments of malignancy that inhibit tumour cell growth, but the treatments are not always completely effective. Therefore, if a few malignant cells remain, they may develop into another tumour at a later date. Moreover, healthy cells are often adversely affected by these highly toxic regimens, not least the bone marrow, which is responsible for immune cell replenishment.

Therefore, therapeutic approaches that have been designed to manipulate the immune response and preserve bone marrow function are being investigated.

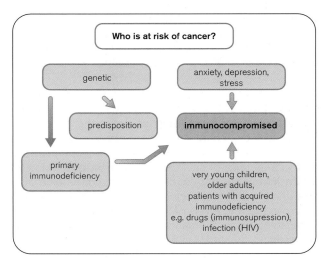

Figure 30.3 Who is at risk of cancer?

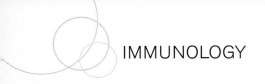

PERSON CENTRED STUDY: THE ANTI-TUMOUR PROPERTIES OF THE IMMUNE SYSTEM MAKE HEADLINE NEWS!

A young boy with severe combined immunodeficiency syndrome (SCID) was given weeks to live – he had suffered numerous infections, and now tumours had been detected in his liver, skin, bone, and spleen. The paediatricians rejected the idea of using conventional anticancer therapy (cytotoxic drugs and radiotherapy) since they were considered too aggressive for this vulnerable child. However, it was realized the reason why he had succumbed to multiple infections and cancer was because he had an inadequate immune system. Furthermore, the condition was not likely to improve on its own since SCID is a genetically acquired condition. Therefore, the last hope was to perform a bone marrow transplantation (i.e. give him a new immune system). Although bone marrow transplantation carries certain risks, the parents gave their consent, a suitable donor was found, and the bone marrow infusion was carried out (see Chapters 28 and 29).

Within weeks, the tumours had disappeared! The added benefit was that because the boy's new immune system had eradicated the tumour, a specific immunological memory had been generated. Therefore if the tumours were to re-emerge, then a rapid immune attack would be mounted to kill them.

Everyone who had cared for this remarkable child – family, clinicians, and all the other health care professionals – was delighted with the success of the bone marrow transplantation. However, think of the cascade of different emotions that the parents and family had gone through in the preceding weeks, from utter despair at the thought of losing the boy, to the elation of knowing that he was now cured and healthy.

However, it must be emphasized that many of these techniques are merely at the stage of clinical trials and are not routinely used in clinical practice. Treatments that stimulate the patient's own immune system are aimed at making the defences more acutely aware of a tumour that has either: (i) not been recognized, or (ii) considered harmless and so not eliminated. The added advantage of this type of therapy is that, if the malignancy is eradicated by an attack, a specific immunological memory is created. Accordingly, if the cancer cells were to emerge again at the same site or a different location, a rapid secondary immune attack would be mounted. The transfer and infusion of immune cells or their secretory products from another external source are also being evaluated (e.g. recombinant cytokines with known specific anticancer activity); some have given promising results.

BOX 30.1 PSYCHO-SOCIAL FACTORS, THE IMMUNE SYSTEM AND CANCER

In 1979 there had been media reports of a nuclear accident at Three Mile Island in the USA. Obviously the inhabitants of the surrounding areas were extremely anxious about the possible threat to their health, particularly for those living closest to the nuclear plant. The worst fears were confirmed when the number of newly diagnosed cases of cancer escalated. In particular, the incidence of patients diagnosed with non-Hodgkin's lymphoma increased in the population living nearest to the disaster. Yet no change was found in the frequency of new cases arising in those living further away but still within a 10-mile radius of the plant. Environmental data of the area around the time of reported nuclear accident was analysed. This was to see if the weather conditions might have exacerbated the alleged disaster. However, investigators went on to prove that the levels of radiation released were very small, and unlikely to have been responsible for the ensuing rise in the cancer incidence. It was therefore advised that the high level of distress and anxiety resulting from information suggesting that a nuclear disaster had occurred so close to their home was the more important aetiological factor in these patients.

ADOPTIVE CELLULAR IMMUNOTHERAPY

Adoptive cellular immunotherapy has been attempted, in which immune cells are given as an infusion. The cells may be derived from the patient suffering the tumour or donated from another source. Natural killer cells with tumouricidal activity may be generated in the laboratory by stimulating the isolated cells in culture with IL-2 before administration – the cells so-produced are called lymphokine-activated killer cells (LAK cells). When the patient's own immune cells are isolated and activated for therapy, it is termed an autologous transfer of cells. However, this treatment has only really been attempted in patients with metastases. As with drug therapies, there needs to be strict evaluation of the cells retrieved and the patient's reactions; thus the following details require in-depth consideration:

- the sources and optimal dose of cells used in the treatment;
- delivery to the patient (e.g. should the cells be given as a local or systemic infusion?);
- selection criteria for patients who would most benefit from the therapy; and
- methods for assessing the effectiveness and adverse effects of treatment.

There are some inherent problems with adoptive cellular immunotherapy; many of these are due to an incomplete understanding of the physiology of the LAK cells. One of the significant complications is the fact that the cells do not automatically identify and migrate into the tumour mass. Furthermore, although their ability to kill tumours may have been amply demonstrated in the laboratory, the microenvironment within the patient may affect the functions of the LAK cells. Equally important are the patients themselves, for the success of treatment also seems to depend on their own baseline immune status.

CYTOKINE THERAPY

The use of specific recombinant cytokines to up-regulate the anti-tumour defence mechanisms in a patient with cancer is seen as one way of promoting tumour regression. Commercially prepared recombinant cytokines may be prescribed for administration as subcutaneous or intramuscular injections. In particular, interferon-alpha therapy has given effective results in the treatment of a number of haematological malignancies (e.g. chronic myeloid leukaemia, lymphoma), although influenza-like symptoms have been documented (see Chapter 25). Extensive investigations of such therapies are essential in order to ascertain both the type of pathology that the cytokine is best used for and the route of administration and dose regimen.

Safety testing to evaluate the benefits in comparison to the toxicity is also required.

Naturally, the dosage, route, and length of administration vary depending on the condition being treated. However, a significant problem is that a naturally occurring cytokine released *in vivo* does not work in isolation but as part of a cascade of cytokines emerging and increasing then diminishing their levels with the progress of the immune response. However, when a single recombinant cytokine is injected, it may well be perceived by the host immune system as having arrived 'out of the blue' and therefore not produce the desirable anti-tumour effects. A further consideration is the effect of the internal environment on immune function, for a cytokine may be immunosuppressive in some conditions and stimulatory in others. For instance, although TNF-alpha has a well-known role in tumour regression (see Box 30.2), recent evidence has suggested that it can also promote the metastatic spread by impairing natural killer cell activities.

Prostaglandins released by macrophages have an inhibitory influence on the anti-tumour activities of the macrophages, and elevated levels of prostaglandins are now being suggested as a possible marker of the increased metastatic potential of a tumour. This seems logical, because if these soluble factors suppress the immune defences, this could favour the proliferation of malignant cells. A study of patients with breast cancer has added credence to these observations because its showed that the anti-tumour activity of macrophages was *diminished* when their secretion of prostaglandins was increased, yet *enhanced* by indomethacin, an antiprostaglandin drug. Even so, the outcome of indomethacin treatment seems to be variable, depending on the type of immune cell it modifies and the stage of the tumour spread. An intriguing observation has highlighted that indomethacin may decrease LAK cell activity in patients where tumours have metastasized. However, the cells may be stimulated if the tumour has not undergone metastatic spread. Unlike the situation with macrophages, the effects of indomethacin on LAK cells are considered to be due to a mechanism that is unrelated to its ability to inhibit prostaglandin metabolism. However the effect of indomethacin on tumour progression is disturbing since it is also prescribed as an analgesic – therefore such information demands further investigation, for it might well have significant implications for treating pain in oncology patients in the future (see Chapters 10 and 14).

CANCER VACCINES

Cancer vaccines are being considered as a way of initiating an active response to a tumour by the patient's

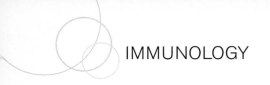

BOX 30.2 RECOMBINANT TNF-ALPHA THERAPY

Recombinant TNF-alpha has been used in a number of clinical trials to investigate its potential as an anticancer therapy. In one trial, involving patients with renal carcinoma, there were reports of rather toxic and severe side-effects of TNF-alpha. Several reasons have been suggested for the limited success of TNF-alpha treatment, including:

- its short half-life, which necessitates treatment being administered as frequent intravenous injections;
- its adverse side-effects, which mean that it can be given only in small amounts – it is possible that the optimal dose for the anti-tumour effect is extremely toxic;
- the potential for some tumours to develop resistance to the therapy; and
- the fact that the activities of TNF-alpha in the patients relies on the cascade of cytokines operating in concert to produce the anti-tumour activities (e.g. synergistic effects of TNF-alpha and IL-1 – indeed, *in-vitro* studies have demonstrated this).

Other trials with TNF-alpha have included the use of combination therapy of drugs and other cytokines (e.g. IL-2, TNF-alpha, and indomethacin – where IL-2 is an activator of lymphocytes and natural killer cells, and indomethacin can indirectly potentiate the tumouricidal effects of macrophages by its antiprostaglandin effects).

---

immune system. Unlike most immunization schedules, which are generally given to prevent disease occurring, cancer vaccines are often given to initiate or potentiate a response against a disease that already exists. Nonetheless, there is an element of prophylaxis – because the immunological memory is generated, the vaccine may be offered as a preventative measure against a recurrence of the tumour. It is also realized that people who have been identified as being at high risk of a particular type of cancer ought to benefit from cancer vaccine therapy by way of helping avert the evolution of a tumour.

The vast amount of information available on conventional vaccine design has proved valuable for devising suitable antigens to be used in anticancer therapy. Specific antigens may be obtained from the patient's tumour. However, the cells retrieved for use in vaccine preparation must be modified so that they are unable to divide – it would be inconceivable to inject active cancer cells into a patient if those cells could subsequently form a tumour elsewhere in the body. Therefore, the isolated cells are irradiated to prevent mitosis, then mixed with an adjuvant such as the Bacille Calmette-Guérin, an immune response booster (see Chapter 24) to increase the likelihood of a good immune reaction by the patient. This procedure is an example of an autologous tumour vaccine, and has been used with some success for the remission of malignant melanoma. As with all vaccine therapies, the key issue is to identify the precise antigenic target that will mimic the disease. Using an autologous source assures that the antigen is specific for the patient suffering the tumour.

Synthetic derived antigens have been prepared as an alternative antigen. Investigations have characterized a number of distinct epitopes that are specific for certain tumours, including melanoma. This in turn has led to the production of novel peptide vaccines that are capable of stimulating a tumour-specific response by the lymphocytes. The advantages of peptide vaccines include:

- the precise chemical composition of the vaccine is known, because it has been synthesized in a laboratory;
- an unlimited supply can be produced, making it relatively inexpensive to prepare;
- the ability to undertake quality control in the batch processing of vaccine;
- it is possible to devise peptides that are able to stimulate the appropriate immune cells to respond (i.e. cell-mediated and antibody-mediated attack on the tumour); and
- it is possible to carry out safety testing to ensure that the peptide selected will not stimulate unwanted side-effects (e.g. autoimmune diseases) and that it is not contaminated with infection.

However, one of the chief problems of synthetic vaccines is choosing the precise peptide for the therapy. As mentioned above, cancers can modify their outer surface by changing the expression of epitopes (i.e. antigenic modulation), so some antigens may be lost and others emerge as the disease progresses. Therefore, if the treatment is to have a favourable therapeutic outcome, it is necessary to confirm that the peptide to be used as a vaccine is detectable on the tumour. Analysis of a tissue biopsy is one way of acquiring such information.

MONOCLONAL ANTIBODIES

Monoclonal antibody technology has allowed the development of antibodies with specific target epitopes. These can be applied in the treatment of haematological cancers, in which the malignant cells display distinctive cell surface markers. Again, the dosage and length of administration vary depending on the condition being treated. Monoclonal antibody preparations may be given as an infusion to target and 'coat' the tumour surface. They effectively stimulate a response by immune cells bearing the appropriate Fc receptors and the complement cascade, because immune complexes are formed from the monoclonal antibodies binding to the tumour. Some other immunotherapies operate by cutting off the blood supply to the tumour mass by means of antibody-mediated toxicity acting on the blood vessels (Figure 30.4).

As more information becomes available regarding the nature of the signals required for cell growth and

cell death, monoclonal antibodies have another possible role – for example, to bind a precise surface component and signal the cancer cell to die or simply to stop proliferating. In a recent trial, a monoclonal antibody raised against CD20 marker, a surface protein of B lymphocytes, was given to transplant patients who developed lymphoma as a side-effect of their immunosuppressive drugs. It was soon realized that the anti-CD20 therapy would destroy the normal B lymphocytes as well as the malignant cells. However, by about 6 months after treatment, healthy B lymphocytes were detectable, because all the monoclonal antibody had been cleared from the body. Patients did not seem to suffer any significant ill effects of being temporarily without a B lymphocyte immune system.

Magic bullet therapy

Magic bullet therapy is an adjunct of immunotherapy, in which monoclonal antibodies are coupled with toxic molecules to target and kill the tumour. Ricin is one such molecule – it enters the tumour cell and provokes its demise by disrupting the ribosomes. Radioactive isotopes and drugs have also been coupled to antibodies to promote cell death by inhibiting protein synthesis or cellular replication. A significant consideration in the design of such treatments is to ensure that the 'magic bullet' binds only to the cancer cells and not to healthy cells. Therefore, a thorough knowledge of the mechanism of cytotoxicity and the tumour-penetrating power of the magic bullet is required. Even so, there have been reports of side-effects caused by the toxic reagents adversely affecting organs like the liver. As with other forms of antibody therapy, there is the possible complication of the treatment itself stimulating an immune rejection episode. For example, if the monoclonal antibody has been synthesized in an animal cell, it is deemed foreign by the human immune system and so eliminated (Figure 30.5)

GENE THERAPY

Gene therapy involves the introduction of a known gene into a cell to change its genetic composition, either on a temporary basis or permanently. It has been used to try to alleviate one of the problems with conventional cytotoxic regimens, the toxic effects on bone marrow function. Thus, a gene-directed multiple-drug resistance has been devised to protect the bone marrow from chemotherapeutic damage. This then allows the clinician to prescribe higher doses of cytotoxic drugs than would normally be tolerated by the haematopoietic cells, and at the same time it helps to preserve immune function. Using a similar technique,

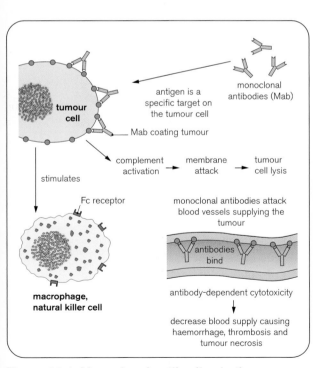

Figure 30.4 Monoclonal antibodies in the treatment of cancer. Monoclonal antibodies may be raised to stimulate complement and antibody-dependent cytotoxic activities on tumour cells or blood vessels.

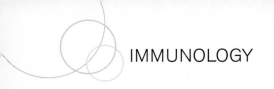

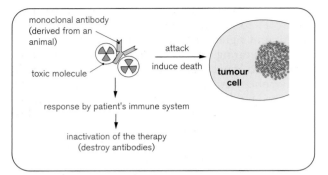

Figure 30.5 Magic bullet therapy. A monoclonal antibody with toxic molecules attached targets the tumour cells and induces death. The disadvantage of this form of therapy is that the monoclonal antibody is derived from an animal, and is therefore deemed foreign; consequently the patient's immune system responds and destroys it.

genes inserted into cancer cells are being seen as a possible way of inducing a programmed cell death. Additionally, genetic manipulations are being explored to find ways of making tumours more sensitive to anti-cancer drugs.

From another perspective, gene insertion into cells is being examined as a means of encouraging the patient's own defences to eradicate the disease. Genes have therefore been inserted:

- into the tumour cells, to improve their immunogenicity and make them more recognizable to the immune system, and
- into the immune cells, to enhance their anti-tumour capabilities. However, the latter strategy relies on the modified cells actually 'homing into' the tumour. In addition, tumour cells have been transfected with genes to secrete TNF-alpha, IL-2, and other cytokines that have been shown to elicit an immune response and encourages an augmented local attack. Again, this is only at the experimental stage.

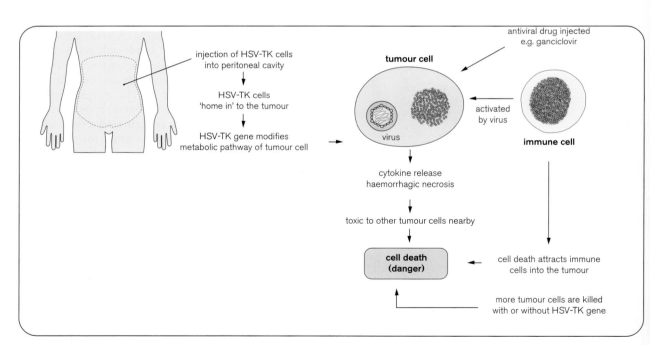

Figure 30.6 The bystander effect. Cells containing the herpes simplex thymidine kinase gene (HSV-TK gene) are injected into the peritoneal cavity. These cells home in on the tumour, modify the metabolic pathways of the tumour cells and make the tumour cells appear as virus-infected cells to the patient's immune system. Antiviral drugs (e.g. ganciclovir) will act on these 'virus-infected' cells and kill them. This death of tumour cells is toxic to other cells. Immune cells are now attracted into the tumour because of the cell death, and these immune cells identify and kill tumour cells both with and without the herpes simplex thymidine kinase gene.

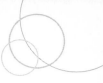

Suicide Gene Therapy

Suicide gene therapy involves modifying cancerous cells so that they express a gene that will lead to their demise. This has been given alone and in conjunction with recombinant cytokine therapy (e.g. interferon-alpha, IL-2). One of the genes used in experimental trials has been the herpes simplex thymidine kinase gene (HSV-TK gene). This gene operates by modifying a metabolic pathway within the tumour cells to make them sensitive to antiviral drugs. Thus, following treatment with ganciclovir, an antiviral agent, the transfected cells die.

Interestingly, a significant level of tumour regression was achieved by this method, even though only about 10 per cent of the cells contained the virus-derived gene. It was therefore presumed that the dying cells provoke a toxic effect on other cells nearby. This phenomenon is now referred to as the 'bystander effect', which may be enhanced by the cytokines such as interferon-alpha that improve tumouricidal activities (Figure 30.6). These observations add credence to the concepts of 'danger' and 'distress', which were discussed in Chapter 27. Inevitably, cells containing the suicide gene and treated with ganciclovir are likely to release their intracellular contents once they die. This type of lysis may be perceived as a danger signal by the immune system. As a result, the migration of immune cells into the area would be encouraged, so tumour cells other than the ones carrying the herpes gene may be perceived as abnormal and therefore eliminated.

IMMUNOLOGY

KEY POINTS

- The activities of the natural killer cells, macrophages, and lymphocytes and their secretory products (immunoglobulins and cytokines) provide an immune surveillance network for the recognition and elimination of abnormal cells.
- The anticancer activities of natural killer cells prompt lysis and apoptosis of the tumour cells.
- Macrophages and lymphocytes are frequently detected as clusters around the tumour. They release lytic enzymes and free radicals, which result in tissue damage and cell debris formation.
- Immunoglobulins produced in response to a cancer are able to stimulate the complement cascade and facilitate the anticancer role of immune cells that possess Fc receptors. In effect, a 'bridge' is formed (tumour–immunoglobulin–immune cell) to aid the delivery of enzymes to perforate the target cell membrane.
- Tumour antigens synthesized by the mutant cells may be present on the cell surface in much the same way as a virus infection, using HLA.
- Tumour antigens may be released into body fluids; serum levels may be estimated for evaluating the effectiveness of treatment.
- Some tumours try to counteract the anticancer immune response by a number of mechanisms, e.g. secreting inhibitory cytokines reducing the cell surface density of HLA molecules.
- If an anti-tumour response has been raised, some cancers disguise their outer cell surface (e.g. with sugar molecules, fibrin clot), or shedding the immune complexes from the outer surface, or releasing the tumour antigens into body fluid to act as a decoy and so avert a direct antibody-mediated attack on the tumour mass.

- People most vulnerable to developing a tumour include patients who have a suboptimal immune surveillance network – very young children, older adults, those with an inherited immunodeficiency syndrome or an acquired immunodeficiency (e.g. infection with HIV, immunosuppressive drugs).
- There is evidence to suggest that psychosocial factors (e.g. anxiety, depression, stress) affect the immune surveillance ability of the defence system.
- Therapeutic approaches that manipulate the immune response and preserve bone marrow function are being investigated. The transfer and infusion of immune cells, or the recombinant cytokines with known specific anticancer activity are also being evaluated.
- Monoclonal antibody preparations may be given as an infusion to target the surface of a tumour. This stimulates a response by immune cells bearing the Fc receptors, and the complement cascade.
- Magic bullet therapy is an adjunct of immunotherapy, in which monoclonal antibodies are coupled with toxic molecules (e.g. ricin, radioactive isotopes) to target and kill the tumour.
- Gene therapy involves the introduction of a known gene into a cell to change its genetic composition, either on a temporary basis or permanently. It has been used to try to alleviate the toxic effects of anticancer therapy on bone marrow function.
- Genetic manipulations are being explored to find ways of making tumours more sensitive to anticancer drugs or to encourage the patient's immune defences to eradicate the disease.

FURTHER READING

Ballen K, Stewart FM (1997) Adoptive immunotherapy. Curr Opin Oncol 9:579–83.

Ben-Efraim S (1997) Cancer immunotherapy: potential involvement of mediators. Mediators Inflammation 6:163–73.

Blaese RM (1997) Gene Therapy for Cancer. Sci Am 276:(6) 111–5.

Buckingham JC, Gillies GE, Cowell AM (1997) Stress, Stress Hormones and the Immune System. John Wiley and Sons, Chichester.

Dermime S, Barrett J, Gambacorti-Passerini C (1995) The role of the immune system in anti-tumour responses. Potential for drug therapy [Review]. Drugs Aging 7:266–77.

Freeman SM, Ramesh R, Marrogi AJ (1997) Immune system in suicide-gene therapy. Lancet 349:2–3.

Freeman SM, Abboud CN, Whartenby, KA, et al. (1993) The 'bystander effect': tumour regression when a fraction of the tumour mass is genetically modified. Cancer Res 53:5274–83.

Glotz D, Antoine C, Garnier JL, et al. (1997) Preliminary observations on the treatment of post-transplant lymphoma by multi-Fc chimeric antibodies. Tumor Targeting, in press.

Hafner M, Orosz P, Krüger A, et al. (1996) TNF promotes metastasis by impairing natural killer cell activity. Int J Cancer 66:388–92.

Hatch MC, Wallerstein S, Beyea J, et al. (1991) Cancer rates after Three Mile Island nuclear accident and proximity to residence to the plant. Am J Pub Health 81:719–24.

Holden RJ, Pakula IS (1996) The role of tumour necrosis factor-alpha in the pathogenesis of anorexia and bulimia nervosa, cancer cachexia and obesity. Med Hypotheses 47:423–38.

Kammerer R, von Kleist S (1996) The carcinoembryonic antigen (CEA) modulates effector–target cell interaction by binding to activated lymphocytes. Int J Cancer 68:457–63.

Mackensen A, Lindemann A, Mertelsmann R (1997) Immunostimulatory cytokines in somatic cells and gene therapy of cancer. Cytokine Growth Factor Rev 8:119–28.

Okuno SH, Tefferi A, Hanson CA, et al. (1996) Spectrum of diseases associated with increased proportions or absolute numbers of peripheral blood natural killer cells. Br J Haematol 93:810–12.

Raso V (1990) Antibodies in diagnosis and therapy. The magic bullet–nearing the century mark. Semin Cancer Biol 1:227–42.

Salgaller ML (1997) Monitoring of cancer patients undergoing active or passive immunotherapy. J Immunother 20:1–14.

Shephard RJ, Shek PN (1995) Cancer, immune function, and physical activity. Can J Appl Physiol 1995 20:1–25.

Stiller CA, Parkin DM (1996) Geographic and ethnic variations in the incidence of childhood cancer. Br Med Bull 52:682–703.

Susser M (1997) Consequences of the 1979 Three Mile Island accident continued: further comment. Environ Health Perspect 105:566–70.

Vojdani A, Campbell A, Brautbar N (1992) Immune functional impairment in patients with clinical abnormalities and silicone breast implants. Toxicol Ind Health 8:415–29.

Zeller JM, McCain NL, Swanson B (1996) Psychoneuroimmunology: an emerging framework for nursing research. J Adv Nurs 23:657–64.

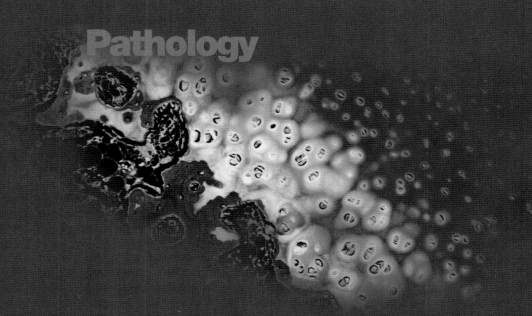

Pathology

BLOOD AND ITS DISORDERS

ANATOMY AND PHYSIOLOGY OF THE BLOOD

Blood functions as a transport system, carrying molecules and cells around the body. It is composed of a liquid medium, plasma, and cellular components, namely:
- the red blood cells (erythrocytes);
- the white blood cells (leukocytes); and
- the platelets.

Plasma

Plasma accounts for approximately 55 per cent of the blood volume and the blood cells making up the remaining 45 per cent, of which 99 per cent are red blood cells. The volume of blood taken up by the red blood cells is known as the haematocrit or packed cell volume.

Plasma consists of approximately 93 per cent water, and it contains a number of different molecules. The most important of these are the electrolytes and the plasma proteins. The electrolytes are inorganic ions, such as sodium, potassium, and chloride, which are important in keeping water in the bloodstream and also act as buffers to help keep the pH of blood within a healthy physiological range (see Chapter 2). Plasma proteins are grouped into three types – fibrinogen, albumin, and globulins. Fibrinogen and some of the globulins are important in blood clotting. Serum is plasma that has been allowed to clot, and it therefore lacks fibrinogen and some of the other clotting proteins.

Another important type of globulin is the immunoglobulins or antibodies (see Chapter 24). Albumin is important in maintaining the fluid compartments in the blood and, by binding a variety of compounds in the blood, it aids in their transport of molecules. The plasma also transports nutrients and waste products, hormones, and small amounts of blood gases.

Red Blood Cells

Oxygen is not particularly soluble in plasma and almost all of it is transported in the erythrocytes. These are small, disc-shaped cells with a characteristic biconcave shape, and they lack a nucleus. Such features allow the erythrocyte to squeeze through narrow capillaries in the tissues. These cells contain high concentrations of haemoglobin, the oxygen-binding protein, which gives the cells their characteristic red colour. Each haemoglobin molecule consists of four subunits. A subunit consists of a haem group, which contains iron and binds oxygen, and a polypeptide or globin molecule. The haemoglobin molecule binds oxygen efficiently in the lung and delivers it to the tissues.

White Blood Cells

The leukocytes consist of five types of cells – neutrophils, eosinophils, basophils, monocytes, and lymphocytes – all of which are important in defence against disease (see Chapter 22) Three of these cell types, the neutrophils, eosinophils, and basophils, are often

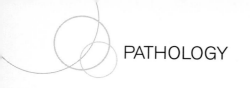

referred to as polymorphonuclear granulocytes, since the nucleus of these cells is divided into lobes and the cytoplasm contains numerous antimicrobial granules.

Platelets

Platelets are small cell fragments which are produced by budding from a large precursor cell in the bone marrow, called a megakaryocyte. Platelets are important in blood clotting and their function is discussed later in this chapter.

HAEMATOPOIESIS

Haematopoiesis refers to the production of blood cells, which takes place in the bone marrow (see Chapter 22). In children, almost all of the bone marrow produces blood cells, but in adults haematopoiesis is restricted to particular sites, such as the ends of the long bones, the iliac crest, and the sternum. All of the cell types in the blood arise from the pluripotential stem cells. These

stem cells divide and replicate and, according to the type of soluble factor influencing their development, become committed to differentiate into a particular cell type. Stem cells (and the more committed progenitor cells) are morphologically indistinguishable in that they look like small primitive cells. On the other hand, the more differentiated precursor cells are recognizable as belonging to a particular lineage (Figure 31.1).

The production of cells in the bone marrow proceeds at a rapid rate. For example, a red blood cell only survives for about 120 days in the circulation, and more than 2 000 000 of these cells need to be replaced every second. Nevertheless, the number of each type of blood cell in the circulation remains remarkably constant over a period of time. Blood cell production is controlled by soluble haematopoietic growth factors, which are released by other cell types in the bone marrow (i.e. the stromal cells). The stromal cells are distinct from the stem cells, and they include macrophages, fat cells, endothelial cells and

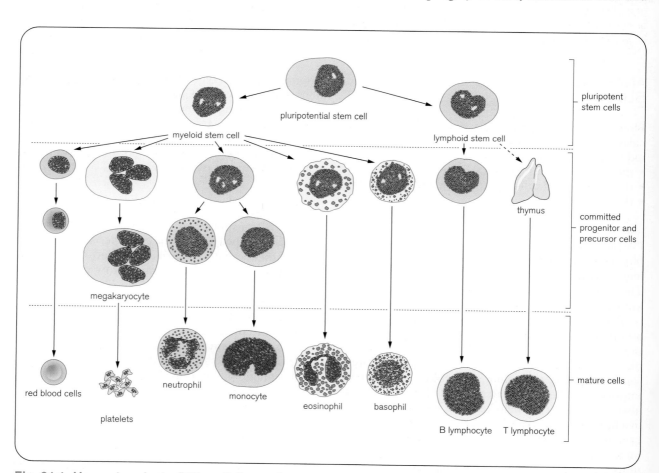

Fig. 31.1 Haematopoiesis. Differentiation and maturation of stem cells in the bone marrow for the formation of blood cells.

fibroblasts. Erythropoietin, which is produced by the kidney, is a growth factor that regulates red blood cell production, the colony stimulating factors regulate the production of granulocytes and monocytes, and the interleukins play a role in the development of lymphocytes (see Chapter 25).

LABORATORY INVESTIGATIONS

The haematology laboratory performs a large number of diagnostic tests. Some of these are specialized tests for the investigation of particular haematological diseases, while others form part of a general medical evaluation. A few of the commonly requested tests are listed below; many of these are now performed by automated blood analysers (see alsoChapter 6).

Blood Counts and Blood Smears

The full blood count provides information about the blood cells in the circulation. The more important parameters measured are:

- the white blood cell count, which measures the total number of leukocytes;
- the haemoglobin concentration; and
- the platelet count.

In addition, the full blood count also gives information about the size, shape, and number of the red blood cells. Not only is the total number of white blood cells important, but it is also necessary to evaluate the relative numbers of the different types of leukocyte. This is called the differential white cell count.

The blood film is usually examined in cases where the cell counter yields abnormal results – for example, a low haemoglobin concentration (anaemia) or a high white cell count (leukocytosis). To examine the nature of the abnormality, a drop of blood may be smeared on a glass slide then fixed and stained with dyes that are taken up and colour the different features of the blood cells (e.g. the nucleus, the cytoplasmic granules). This is called the blood film, which is scrutinized under a microscope for the appearance (morphology), size, and shape of red blood cells, white blood cells, and platelets. In a similar way, a sample of bone marrow can be obtained by needle aspirate from the iliac crest and examined for the morphology of the haematopoietic cells.

Erythrocyte Sedimentation Rate

If a blood sample is allowed to stand on the bench in a tube, cells that are normally maintained in suspension by the movement of the blood through the blood vessels will begin to sediment to the bottom of the tube. The rate at which they do this is dependent on the relative concentration of proteins in the plasma. The concentration of these proteins changes in the course of the majority of disease processes; therefore this phenomenon is useful in providing a non-specific evaluation of the progression of disease. Blood is drawn up into a long thin tube and allowed to stand for one hour. Normal blood sediments at a very slow rate – the normal erythrocyte sedimentation rate (ESR) is less than 10 mm/hour, and an increase in the ESR is an indication of an underlying pathology.

ANAEMIA

Anaemia is defined as a haemoglobin concentration in the blood of less than 13.5 g/dl in adult males, and less than 11.5 g/dl in adult females. The reduction in haemoglobin concentration results in a reduction in the oxygen-carrying capacity of the blood. Anaemia may arise as a consequence of a change in erythrocyte numbers owing to a decline in their manufacture, increased destruction or loss of cells, decreased production of haemoglobin, or a combination of these factors (Box 31.1). The effective production of erythrocytes requires an adequate supply of minerals (the most important of which is iron), vitamin B12, folic acid, and hormones (in addition to erythropoietin, thyroid hormone, and adrenocortical hormones are also important). Furthermore, defects in the genes encoding alpha-globin or beta-globin may lead to impaired haemoglobin synthesis and anaemia (see Chapter 7).

Anaemia is often accompanied by a change in the size and shape of the erythrocytes; hence a useful classification of anaemias is based on the red blood cell indices that are calculated as part of the full blood count. These indices include:

BOX 31.1 CAUSES OF ANAEMIA

Decreased production of red blood cells
- vitamin (folate, B12) deficiency
- iron deficiency
- decreased levels of erythropoietin or thyroxine
- genetic disorders of haemoglobin production
- bone marrow failure

Loss of red blood cells
- bleeding, either acute or chronic
- accelerated breakdown of red blood cells (haemolysis)

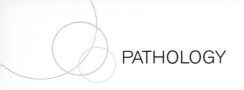

- the mean cell volume (MCV), which refers to the size of the red blood cells; and
- the mean cell haemoglobin (MCH) and the mean cell haemoglobin concentration (MCHC), which refer to the haemoglobin content in the cell.

Hence a microcytic hypochromic anaemia is one in which the red blood cells are small (microcytic) and have a low haemoglobin content (hypochromic), a picture typical of iron deficiency anaemia.

IRON DEFICIENCY ANAEMIA

Iron is essential for the synthesis of the oxygen-carrying pigment, haemoglobin; iron-deficiency anaemia is the most common cause of anaemia world-wide and a major public health problem. Factors that may be contributory to iron-deficiency anaemia include poor diet, malabsorption from the gut, increased demands of growth, and pregnancy. Moreover, iron deficiency anaemia is often associated with chronic blood loss, particularly from the gastrointestinal tract and the uterus. Identification of the underlying cause is important.

Clinical features may include general features of anaemia (e.g. tiredness, lethargy, breathlessness) and the particular features of iron deficiency, such as spoon-shaped nails (koilonychia), sores at the corners of the mouth (angular stomatitis), and unusual dietary habits (pica).

Laboratory investigation reveals that the erythrocytes are smaller than normal (microcytic) and have less haemoglobin than normal (hypochromic). By the time anaemia develops, iron stores are depleted and serum iron levels are low. Treatment involves identification of the underlying cause, as well as the replenishment of the iron stores, usually by prescribing oral iron supplements (see also Box 31.2). However, they may cause indigestion or constipation, so it may be necessary to try several of the compounds available on the market before finding one that the patient will tolerate. In rare cases, it may be necessary to give iron as intramuscular injections or even as an intravenous infusion (which carries the risk of an anaphylactic reaction).

MEGALOBLASTIC ANAEMIA

Megaloblasts are the cells that are characteristically seen in the bone marrow in vitamin B12 or folate deficiency. Folic acid is needed for the synthesis of deoxyribose nucleic acid (DNA), as is vitamin B12, which is required for the conversion of dietary folate to folate polyglutamate, the form used by the cell in the synthesis of nucleic acids. Any reduction in the capacity of the body to support cell division first affects tissues with a rapid rate

---

BOX 31.2 DIETARY IRON

- There are two forms of iron: ferrous (Fe^{2+}) and ferric (Fe^{3+}), ferrous iron is more readily absorbed than the ferric form.
- Dietary iron consists of two main forms – haem iron, found in meat products containing haemoglobin and myoglobin and is more readily absorbed than the non-haem iron found in vegetables and cereals.
- Vitamin C can enhance the absorption of iron.
- Iron absorption is inhibited by:
  phytates (e.g. in foods rich in dietary fibre), phosphates (e.g. in dairy foods), and tannic acid in beverages, (e.g. tea and coffee).

---

of cell proliferation, such as the bone marrow; hence the development of anaemia in vitamin B12 or folate deficiency. The anaemia is characterized by the presence of abnormal erythrocyte precursors (megaloblasts) in the bone marrow; in the blood, the red blood cells are large (macrocytic) and the neutrophils may show an increase in the number of lobes in the nucleus (hypersegmented neutrophils). Vitamin B12 is produced by bacteria and is acquired in the human diet by eating foodstuffs of animal origin. Folic acid is present in many foods, particularly liver, green leafy vegetables, and fortified cereals, but it is easily destroyed by cooking. Megaloblastic anaemia may arise from deficiency of either or both of these factors in the diet, and it may occur in vegans whose diet lacks foodstuffs of animal origin.

Pernicious Anaemia

The most common cause of vitamin B12 deficiency in Western countries is pernicious anaemia. This is an autoimmune disease in which the parietal cells in the stomach are destroyed, resulting in the failure to produce intrinsic factor. Intrinsic factor is a protein secreted by the stomach; it is essential for absorption of vitamin B12 – in the absence of intrinsic factor, vitamin B12 cannot be absorbed even if dietary sources are adequate.

The anaemia may be extreme in these patients (with a haemoglobin concentration as low as 3–4 g/dl), but because of the insidious onset over 2–3 years, they may have relatively mild symptoms. The leukocyte count and platelet count may also be depressed, giving a blood picture known as pancytopenia. The diagnosis of pernicious anaemia is confirmed by performing a Schilling test, in which the absorption of radioactive-labelled vitamin B12 is measured in the presence and absence of intrinsic factor (see the Person-Centred Study in Chapter 27).

Folate Deficiency

Folate deficiency is usually due, at least in part, to inadequate diet. In Western societies, coeliac disease (gluten-sensitivity enteropathy) is a major cause of folate deficiency (see Chapter 34), while in tropical countries, sprue can cause a general malabsorption syndrome in which folate deficiency is a prominent feature. It is also important to remember that folate stores may also be depleted as the physiological demand increases (e.g. as a result of pregnancy and lactation, and in patients with haemolytic anaemia such as sickle cell disease and hereditary spherocytosis).

Treatment

Treatment of the megaloblastic anaemias involves replacing the deficient factor. Folic acid supplements are given orally, but because the underlying cause of vitamin B12 deficiency is often an inability to absorb the vitamin, supplements are normally given by intramuscular injection. Fortnightly injections of vitamin B12 are required for up to 6 weeks in order to replenish stores, after which 3-monthly injections are usual.

INHERITED DISORDERS OF HAEMOGLOBIN SYNTHESIS

The predominant haemoglobin in the adult is haemoglobin A, in which the globin protein consists of two types of peptide chain, alpha-globin and beta-globin. Each haemoglobin molecule contains two alpha-globin and two beta-globin chains, encoded by four alpha-globin genes and two beta-globin genes (see Chapter 7).

Each globin chain is attached to a haem group, which contains iron. The rate of synthesis of the alpha- and beta-globin chains is regulated, so that equal amounts are produced.

In the inherited disorders of haemoglobin, synthesis may occur, but the actual haemoglobin produced may be abnormal or malfunctioning (e.g. sickle cell disease), or there may be a deficiency in haemoglobin synthesis that leads to an imbalance between alpha-globin and beta-globin chain synthesis (e.g. beta-thalassaemia; see Person-Centred Study: Beta-Thalassaemia Major). Another inherited anaemia due to a problem with haemoglobin production is sideroblastic anaemia, in which there are defects in the enzyme pathway of haem synthesis.

Sickle Cell Disease

In sickle cell disease, an abnormal beta-globin chain is produced; this differs from the normal beta-globin by just one amino acid – glutamine is replaced by valine at the sixth position on the peptide chain. This amino acid substitution is caused by a single base change in the DNA coding for beta-globin. It results in the formation of an abnormal haemoglobin molecule, haemoglobin S (HbS), which becomes insoluble when the haemoglobin molecule gives up oxygen in the tissues. The insoluble haemoglobin molecule precipitates in the erythrocytes to form long crystals, which results in the characteristic 'sickle' shape of the cells. These sickle cells are more rigid and do not pass through the capillaries very easily, so they become lodged in blood vessels. This leads to tissue anoxia followed by ischaemic cell death.

This pathological process is reflected in the clinical presentation of sickle cell crisis, which occurs in patients who are homozygous for the disease and may cause

---

PERSON-CENTRED STUDY: BETA-THALASSAEMIA MAJOR

A physical examination of Costas, a boy aged 8 years, revealed he had splenomegaly. He was of Greek origin and had been diagnosed as having beta-thalassaemia major within months of birth. Throughout his relatively short life, his spleen had needed to be highly active to cope with erythrocytes (red blood cells) with a reduced life span; therefore it had become enlarged. Regular blood transfusions were given to suppress the ineffective erythropoiesis caused by the lack of functional genes, and this helped to maintain his haemoglobin levels above 10 g/dl.

However, his need for transfused blood had become more frequent and with it had come iron overload. It was now advised that he should have a splenectomy. Although the increased risk of infections (such as pneumonia) for splenectomized patients was appreciated, this treatment would prolong erythrocyte survival. He was over the age of 6 years, so his immune system was considered sufficiently mature to cope without a spleen. However, he was given anti-pneumococcal vaccine about 3 weeks before the surgery and prescribed long-term prophylactic penicillin therapy to reduce the risk of blood-borne infections.

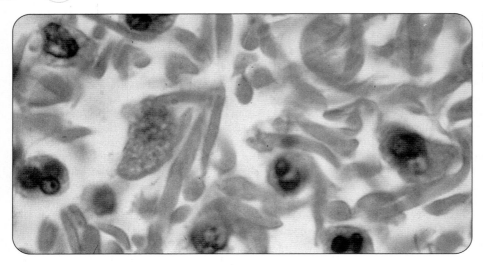

Figure 31.2 Sickling red blood cells in lung tissue. ©Medical Illustration, Addenbrooke's NHS Trust, Cambridge, UK.

acute pain. The haemolysis or premature destruction of the red blood cells leads to anaemia, and this is exacerbated during sickling crises (Figure 31.2). Complications result from tissue ischaemia following repeated episodes of vascular occlusion. Thus patients may have bony infarcts (which may lead to osteomyelitis), renal impairment, and retinal damage.

The gene for sickle cell haemoglobin is particularly prevalent in people from parts of central and west Africa. Patients who are heterozygous for HbS (sickle cell trait) do not normally demonstrate symptoms of the disease, but may develop problems at low oxygen levels (e.g. under general anaesthesia). Hence a sickle cell screening test is advocated preoperatively for patients from ethnic origins where the gene is prevalent. It is noteworthy that sickle cell trait is thought to confer some protection against *Plasmodium falciparum* malaria, which may partly

explain why the gene is comparatively common in these populations.

Laboratory investigation reveals a low haemoglobin (6–8 g/dl) and the characteristic sickle-shaped cells on the blood film. Haemoglobin electrophoresis on cellulose acetate allows the identification of the different types of haemoglobin (Figure 31.3). A sickle test to demonstrate the insoluble haemoglobin detects the presence of the sickle gene, but it does not distinguish between sickle cell anaemia (homozygous) and sickle trait (heterozygous). The symptoms of anaemia are comparatively mild considering the haemoglobin level, partly because HbS has a lower affinity for oxygen than normal haemoglobin does and so is able to release oxygen more readily to the tissues.

Successful management of this condition requires patient education as to how to avoid crises (by keeping warm and well hydrated) as well as how to manage mild

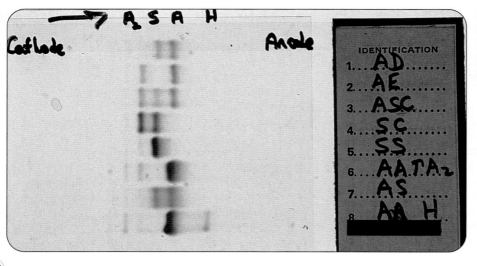

Figure 31.3 Electrophoresis of haemoglobin used in the investigation of haemoglobinopathies.

attacks at home. Severe crises are often precipitated by infection. The treatment may demands hospitalization for intravenous hydration, opiate analgesia, antibiotics, and even blood transfusion. Penicillin and pneumococcal vaccine are often prescribed as prophylaxis against pneumococcal infection. Patients who experience frequent crises and need pain relief such as pethidine are sometimes labelled as addicts. Some do become addicted, and this adds to the morbidity of this chronic illness; however, many simply request the analgesia for control of their symptoms. Exchange transfusions may be necessary to replace the HbS with normal haemoglobin and to decrease the overall level of HbS to help reduce the incidence of crises. The spleen becomes shrunken and non-functional, owing to repeated splenic infarcts; folate supplements are also important because of the chronic haemolysis. Retinal infarcts lead to the growth of new vessels; however, these may cause retinal detachment and loss of sight. The hip joint is particularly vulnerable to infarcts, and chronic loss of blood supply can cause avascular necrosis of the femoral head, a painful and crippling bone deformity. Most patients with sickle cell disease do not require regular transfusions, an exception being patients who have suffered a stroke or another complication of the disease such as renal failure, and pregnant patients.

Some patients with sickle cell disease have a comparatively mild clinical course owing to the presence of another gene that leads to the persistence of fetal haemoglobin (HbF). HbF is able to ameliorate some of the deleterious pathological effects of homozygous sickle cell disease. A new therapy for this disease is hydroxyurea, which increases the levels of HbF. Recent trials have shown that hydroxyurea is able to decrease the frequency and severity of crises in patients with sickle cell disease.

Other sickling disorders arise when a patient inherits one sickle (S) gene together with a gene for another abnormal haemoglobin, usually haemoglobin C (HbC) or haemoglobin D (HbD). This results in HbSC or HbSD. HbC is common in West Africa, and results from a genetic mutation that is similar to sickle cell disease. Again it is an amino acid substitution at the sixth position of the beta-globin chain. HbSC disease occurs in patients who have inherited one C together with one S gene, and it is generally a milder disease than homozygous HbSS (sickle cell disease). Patients have a mild anaemia and infrequent crises, but they may suffer complications such as necrosis of the femoral head or retinal detachment. Patients with HbC disease (homozygous) have a mild anaemia that requires no treatment. HbD includes several haemoglobin variants that migrate in the same position as HbS on electrophoresis. HbE is the most common haemoglobin variant in south-east Asia, and it results in a mild anaemia.

The Thalassaemia Syndromes

Beta-thalassaemia

The thalassaemia syndromes arise from reduced or absent synthesis of either alpha-globin or beta-globin chains. The beta-thalassaemias are the more important clinically. They occur in a geographical belt from the Mediterranean area through the Middle East and Indian subcontinent to south-east Asia. In beta-thalassaemia major, the patient is either homozygous for a molecular defect that leads to absent beta-globin chain synthesis or heterozygous for two different molecular defects with the same result; in either case, no beta-globin chains are produced. These gene defects are termed beta^0 thalassaemia. Production of alpha-globin chains proceeds at a normal rate, giving rise to excess alpha-globin chains. These are unstable and precipitate out, damaging the developing erythrocyte precursors in the bone marrow. The result is severe haemolysis and a failure to make enough erythrocytes (ineffective erythropoiesis).

The severity of the disease reflects the level of beta-globin production. Severe anaemia begins about 3 months after birth. The liver and spleen become enlarged, owing to increased erythrocyte destruction, and the amount of bone marrow devoted to haematopoiesis is enlarged, leading to characteristic skeletal abnormalities, particularly in the skull.

Treatment involves regular blood transfusions to maintain an adequate level of haemoglobin as well as to suppress the abnormal erythropoiesis. Iron overload is the major cause of morbidity and mortality in this disease, and it is the consequence of both the ineffective erythropoiesis and repeated transfusions. Iron is toxic, particularly to the liver, endocrine organs, and heart, and iron overload leads to premature death from cardiac failure unless the iron can be removed. Therefore, iron-chelating agents, such as desferrioxamine, are used to prevent or delay the problems associated with iron overload.

The heterozygous state, beta-thalassaemia trait or beta-thalassaemia minor, does not normally present with symptoms. Laboratory investigation reveals hypochromic, microcytic red blood cells and mild anaemia, if any.

Alpha-thalassaemia

Alpha-thalassaemia results from deletion of one or more of the genes encoding alpha-globin. There are four of these genes, two on each chromosome; deletion of all four is incompatible with life and results in intrauterine death. If three genes are deleted and there is only one producing alpha-globin, four beta-globin chains form a new haemoglobin molecule, HbH. The patient survives but the haemoglobin is unstable, which leads to haemolysis and a moderate anaemia. If only one or two alpha-globin genes are deleted, anaemia is not normally present because there are enough remaining alpha-globin genes to be decoded for haemoglobin synthesis.

ANAEMIA DUE TO BONE MARROW FAILURE

Anaemia of Chronic Disease

This commonly occurs in the context of a systemic illness, such as chronic infection (e.g. tuberculosis, endocarditis, osteomyelitis), a chronic inflammatory disease (e.g. rheumatoid arthritis, polymyalgia rheumatica) (see Chapter 39), or advanced malignancy. In chronic renal failure, there is failure of erythropoietin production by the diseased kidneys, leading to a failure of erythropoiesis. These anaemias are collectively termed anaemias of chronic disease.

Laboratory investigation reveals a mild anaemia with erythrocytes of normal appearance (normocytic, normochromic), but a low serum iron level is detected. These patients are not iron deficient, but there is a defect in the ability to use the iron in the bone marrow.

Other Causes of Bone Marrow Failure

Other causes of bone marrow failure include treatment with drugs (idiosyncratic reactions to antibiotics; chemotherapy used for malignant disease), radiotherapy, and viral infections, which can cause a transient suppression of erythropoiesis in the bone marrow (e.g. parvovirus).

Primary Bone Marrow Failure

Primary bone marrow failure (aplastic anaemia) may occur at any age, and is considered to be due in part to immune dysfunction. Infiltration of the bone marrow, either with leukaemia (see below) or with cancer cells from other organs, such as the lung, breast, or prostate, may also give rise to failure of erythrocyte production, with resultant anaemia.

HAEMOLYTIC ANAEMIA

Ageing erythrocytes are destroyed by mononuclear phagocytic cells, mainly in the spleen; this is a natural process, and the life span of erythrocytes is about 120 days. This destruction process can be accelerated (producing haemolytic anaemia) if:

* there is an intrinsic abnormality of erythrocyte structure – this is often a hereditary trait, such as in sickle cell disease, hereditary spherocytosis, or glucose-6-phosphate dehydrogenase deficiency;
* there are extraneous factors in the blood that alter the life span of the erythrocytes.

One example of the latter case is the presence of antibodies directed against the erythrocytes, which lead to their premature destruction. These antibodies may either be directed against the patient's own cells (autoimmune haemolytic anaemia), or against transfused blood that is incompatible (a transfusion reaction, with haemolysis of the red blood cells) (see also Chapters 26 and 27). Finally, in the condition known as disseminated intravascular coagulation, inappropriate activation of coagulation results in the deposition of fibrin strands in the small vessels and capillaries. These cause damage to the red blood cells flowing through these blood vessels, producing cellular fragmentation and an intravascular haemolytic anaemia.

LEUKAEMIA

ACUTE LEUKAEMIA

Leukaemia results from the uncontrolled proliferation of an abnormal clone of haematopoietic cells in the bone marrow, which arises because of the malignant transformation of a primitive cell. When this transformed cell undergoes proliferation without differentiation, normal haematopoietic tissue becomes replaced with these malignant immature blast cells within the space of weeks. This is acute leukaemia, which may be either lymphoblastic or myeloblastic depending on whether the malignant blasts express more lymphoid or myeloid features.

The patient typically has a short history of being unwell, with symptoms of anaemia, abnormal bleeding and bruising (owing to decreased platelet production), and infections (owing to defective production of neutrophils).

The distinction between acute lymphoblastic leukaemia (ALL) and acute myeloblastic leukaemia (AML) is important because the chemotherapy regimens employed are different in the two conditions, as is the eventual prognosis.

AML is rare in children and the incidence increases with age. Sometimes there is a preceding period of myelodysplasia (which used to be called 'preleukaemia') or a history of previous cytotoxic chemotherapy; such cases are called 'secondary AML'.

Broadly speaking there are two forms of ALL – childhood ALL, which responds well to treatment and has a cure rate of around 80 per cent, and adult ALL, which has a much lower cure rate of around 30 per cent.

Acute leukaemia is fatal without treatment, and much work has gone into determining the combination and treatment schedules of cytotoxic drugs that are most effective in the different forms of the disease. The prognosis for a patient with acute leukaemia depends not only on the subtype, but also the presence or absence of certain chromosomal abnormalities. Bone marrow transplantation is used to treat patients whose disease does not respond easily to cytotoxic drugs alone. The ideal donor is a sibling who has the same histocompatibility antigens (see Chapter 29).

CHRONIC LEUKAEMIA

Chronic leukaemia is also a disease of the bone marrow, but the clone produces predominantly mature or partly differentiated cells, which often circulate in high numbers in the blood stream.

Chronic lymphocytic leukaemia is a disease of older adults. It runs an indolent course in some two-thirds of patients. Chronic myeloid leukaemia occurs in younger patients (aged 30–50 years) and invariably transforms into an acute leukaemia, at which point the outlook is extremely poor. The malignant cells in chronic myeloid leukaemia possess the Philadelphia chromosome, a characteristic chromosome translocation in which the ends of chromosomes 9 and 22 are switched over (see Chapter 7).

Both forms of chronic leukaemia may be treated with oral chemotherapy, but most centres aim to cure younger patients with chronic myeloid leukaemia by bone marrow transplantation. In all forms of leukaemia, management consists not only of chemotherapy aimed at eliminating the malignant clone, but also of supportive therapy, including erythrocyte and platelet transfusions and the prophylactic use of antibiotics.

LYMPHOMA

Lymphomas include Hodgkin's disease and the different forms of non Hodgkin's lymphoma (NHL). These diseases result from the abnormal proliferation of lymphocytes (usually B lymphocytes) in lymphoid organs (lymph nodes, spleen, liver), and sometimes in non-lymphoid tissues as well. The lymphomas may be classified according to the histological appearance, cell type, and pattern of organ involvement. Today it is customary to refer to NHL as being either low grade or high grade, and Hodgkin's disease is subdivided into different histological types.

NON-HODGKIN'S LYMPHOMA

NHL is the most common haematological malignancy and it can occur at any age. Essentially it is a disease of lymph nodes, but up to one-third of patients present with extranodal disease (i.e. disease outside the lymphoid tissue). In most cases, the aetiology is unknown, but some forms of NHL arise in immunodeficient patients (e.g. patients with acquired immunodeficiency syndrome or after an organ transplantation). Infection with the Epstein–Barr virus (EBV) is also known to predispose to NHL in some people.

Typical presentation is with enlarged nodes in the neck and axillae and an enlarged liver or spleen. There is a form of NHL in which the disease arises in the lymphoid tissue of the gastrointestinal tract (MALT lymphomas); these have a relatively good prognosis. The EBV virus has also been implicated in another type of malignancy, Burkitt's lymphoma, particularly in those suffering from the disorder in parts of Africa.

Low-grade lymphomas generally have an indolent course, and although the initial response to single agent chemotherapy is good, the disease repeatedly relapses and median survival is seldom more than 8 years. High-grade lymphomas require combination chemotherapy to induce a response, and about one-third of patients will be cured after completing six or so cycles of treatment. In both forms of NHL, patients whose disease is confined to one group of lymph nodes and who have no systemic symptoms (such as weight loss, sweats, or fevers) can be treated with radiotherapy to the affected area. Relapsed or resistant disease has a poor outlook, and often cure is only attained by bone marrow transplantation.

HODGKIN'S DISEASE

Hodgkin's disease occurs in adults in their third decade and in people over the age of 60 years. It is more common in men. A typical presentation is with enlarged nodes in the neck or in the chest. Extranodal involvement is less common than in NHL. Patients may have systemic symptoms, including weight loss, fever, and sweats.

Treatment depends upon the stage of disease; and this is determined by the extent of disease, whether it involves the bone marrow, and whether there are systemic symptoms. Early disease has a relatively good prognosis, with up to 75 per cent cure rates, and it may be treated with local radiotherapy, whereas advanced stage disease requires combination chemotherapy.

MYELOMA

Multiple myeloma is a malignancy of plasma cells and arises in the bone marrow, where the malignant cells secrete an abnormal protein (called a paraprotein) and produce cytokines that cause bone destruction (see Chapter 24). Myeloma is predominantly a disease of older adults, and it can cause considerable bone pain.

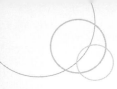

Infiltration of the bone marrow by malignant plasma cells results in anaemia and thrombocytopenia, and infections are common because the malignant clone suppresses the production of normal immunoglobulins (immunoparesis). Other complications include hypercalcaemia, renal failure, and amyloid deposits.

Myeloma is diagnosed on the basis of there being more than 10 per cent plasma cells present in the bone marrow, a monoclonal protein in the serum or urine, and characteristic osteolytic lesions on X-ray. Although myeloma may be diagnosed by chance on laboratory screening, many patients have clinical evidence of bone disease, including bone pain and pathological fractures.

Treatment is directed at the complications, and includes local radiotherapy for bone lesions, biphosphonates for hypercalcaemia, prompt treatment with antibiotics for intercurrent infections, and appropriate therapy for renal failure. Chemotherapy is given in an attempt to halt the progression of the disease, but cure is only possible with high dose therapy and bone marrow transplantation.

HAEMOSTASIS AND THROMBOSIS

Coagulation is the process by which soluble proteins in plasma take part in a series of reactions in which the end-point is the conversion of fibrinogen, a soluble plasma protein, into fibrin, an insoluble polymer. The sequence of reactions involves several clotting factors, each of which functions as an enzyme to activate the next factor along the pathway, thus forming a 'cascade'.

The coagulation pathway has traditionally been divided into the intrinsic and the extrinsic pathways (Figure 31.4). The intrinsic pathway is activated when the blood vessel wall is damaged, exposing collagen. Activation of factor XII leads to the sequential activation of factors XI, IX, X, and II; factors VIII and V are cofactors in this process. In the extrinsic pathway, tissue factor, a protein that is present on tissues of the vessel walls, binds factor VII, and this activates factors X and II. Factor II is prothrombin, which is converted to thrombin, which in turn converts fibrinogen to form an insoluble colt of fibrin.

When the lining of a blood vessel is breached, the steps in the formation of a haemostatic plug are as follows:

- the circulating platelets adhere to the exposed subendothelial tissues; these platelets become activated in response to collagen in the tissues and undergo aggregation;

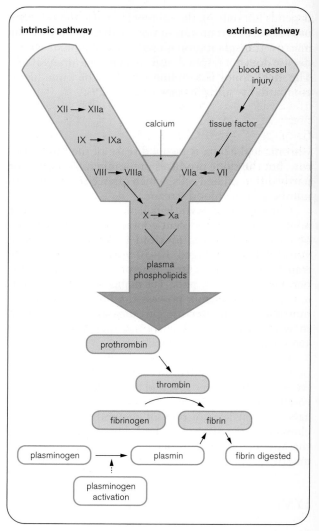

Figure 31.4 The clotting cascade. Flow diagram of the clotting and fibrinolytic pathways.

- the membrane surface of these activated platelets facilitates the rapid development of the coagulation cascade, with the resultant formation of fibrin, which acts to consolidate the initial platelet plug.

Thus, platelet deficiency (thrombocytopenia), as well as deficiencies of the various clotting factors or their reduced synthesis in liver failure, may lead to a bleeding tendency (Box 31.3).

Fibrin is dissolved (fibrinolysis) by an enzyme called plasmin. Fibrinolysis occurs after healing has taken place and in order to prevent the occlusion of small blood vessels. An inactive plasma protein, plasminogen, is activated by the presence of fibrin, and converted to plasmin by a plasminogen activator. The main sources of plasminogen activator are the endothelial cell lining of the vessel walls and the kidney, where it helps avert microthrombus formation in the small vessels serving the nephrons. Thrombolytic agents (e.g. streptokinase) are available as treatment to dissolve clots (e.g. in deep vein thrombosis and after myocardial infarction) (see Chapter 32). However, one of the problems with this type of therapy is that it carries the risk of haemorrhage.

LABORATORY TESTS

A coagulation screen consists of the tests that are performed to determine the ability of the plasma to clot in the presence of specific activators of the clotting pathway – the prothrombin time, the activated partial thromboplastin time, and the thrombin time.

The prothrombin time estimates the time for a clot to form in a test tube when thromboplastin is added to plasma in the presence of calcium; this tests the activity of the patient's extrinsic pathway in the coagulation cascade.

The activated partial thromboplastin time measures the time taken for clot formation in response to phospholipid and calcium. It is an indicator of the intrinsic pathway activity.

When information about the plasma fibrinogen content is needed, the thrombin time is used, in which the formation of clot in the presence of excess thrombin is evaluated.

A general estimation of the overall clotting mechanism may be determined by an assessment of the bleeding time. In this test, several small punctures on the forearm are made with a lancet, and the time taken for the bleeding to stop is recorded with a stop watch.

BLEEDING DISORDERS

Bleeding disorders can arise because of an anomaly affecting the coagulation pathway, which may be due to a defective gene or an acquired abnormality induced by disease (e.g. the decreased production of coagulation factors in liver disease).

Haemophilia

Haemophilia A is a sex-linked disorder, in which there is a mutation in the gene for factor VIII (located on the X-chromosome). It results in low levels or even an absence of this factor in the plasma. The activated form of factor VIII serves to amplify the coagulation pathways and eventually leads to the production of fibrin, and thus it is important in the stabilization of a clot.

> **BOX 31.3 CAUSES OF BLEEDING DISORDERS**
>
> Inherited bleeding disorders
> - haemophilia A (factor VIII deficiency)
> - haemophilia B (factor IX deficiency)
> - von Willebrand disease
> - platelet disorders (e.g. Bernard–Soulier syndrome)
>
> Acquired bleeding disorders
> - liver disease
> - disseminated intravascular coagulation
> - vitamin K deficiency
> - iatrogenic disorders (e.g. warfarin overdose)
> - thrombocytopenia (e.g. caused by cytotoxic therapy; vitamin B12 deficiency, folate deficiency)

Severe factor VIII deficiency results in spontaneous bleeds, often into joints and muscles.

The diagnosis is confirmed by the prolonged activated partial thromboplastin time and specific factor VIII assays. Severe cases are those where circulating factor VIII levels are less than 1 IU/l (normal range 70–150 IU/l). Patients with severe haemophilia suffer from spontaneous bleeds, usually into joints or muscle, while patients with mild disease have problems only after trauma or surgery.

Haemophilia is treated with specific factor concentrates made from plasma pooled from many blood donations. Unfortunately, some batches of factor VIII used to treat patients before 1985 were contaminated with viruses such as human immunodeficiency virus and hepatitis C. Today, stringent screening of all donors and the availability of recombinant factor VIII has minimized the risk of virus transmission.

Haemophilia B, or Christmas disease, is a disorder similar to haemophilia A. It results in a failure to produce adequate amounts of factor IX. Like haemophilia A, it is an inherited disorder caused by a defective gene, and is diagnosed by the presence of an abnormal clotting screen and low levels of plasma factor IX. The only effective treatment is a regular exogenous supply of factor IX.

Von Willebrand's Disease

Von Willebrand's disease is the most common inherited bleeding disorder. It is an autosomal dominant disorder and is caused by abnormalities in the gene encoding von Willebrand factor (vWF). The vWF is important for platelet adhesion and aggregation, and it also binds and stabilizes factor VIII in the circulation. Thus a deficiency of vWF manifests as a platelet defect (with prolonged bleeding time) together with a prolonged activated partial thromboplastin time (owing to the lack of stability of factor VIII). Von Willebrand's disease is characterized by gum bleeding, nose bleeds, and, in women, heavy menstrual periods. The main treatment is with a vasopressin analogue, 1-desamino-8-*d*-arginine-vasopressin (DDAVP), which stimulates release of vWF from endothelium.

Acquired Abnormalities of Bleeding

Frequently the causes of an abnormal bleeding tendency are acquired abnormalities, such as occur in liver disease. The liver is the site for the production of many coagulation factors, including fibrinogen, the precursor of fibrin. Patients with advanced liver disease, typically caused by alcohol misuse or hepatitis, have prolonged clotting times as measured in the laboratory and a bleeding tendency. Patients with renal failure also have a (mild) bleeding tendency, owing to defective platelet function.

The clotting cascade is under stringent control, but it occasionally becomes highly activated. Disseminated intravascular coagulation is a clinical condition in which uncontrolled activation of coagulation leads to fibrin being deposited in small vessels. This fibrin is broken down, and the rapid consumption of clotting factors and platelets leads to widespread bleeding (e.g. from cannulation sites). Thrombotic events can also occur. Predisposing factors include septicaemia (see Chapter 25, Septic Shock and TNF-alpha), obstetric emergencies, or an ABO-incompatible blood transfusion (Figure 31.5).

THROMBOTIC DISORDERS

An increased tendency to form clots may lead to inappropriate thrombosis, with its attendant clinical consequences. As a general rule, abnormalities in the plasma factors that regulate coagulation lead to clots in veins, unlike the diseases of the vessel wall, such as arteriosclerosis, which leads to thrombosis in arteries. Plasma contains several natural anticoagulants, which serve to prevent clots forming in blood vessels. These anticoagulants include antithrombin III, protein C, and protein S. Genetic deficiencies of each of these proteins have been described, and the inheritance of an abnormal gene for any one of these proteins leads to a slight increased risk of venous thrombosis, a state referred to as thrombophilia. A recently identified cause of thrombosis is the inheritance of an abnormal factor V gene, which renders factor V less susceptible to the anticoagulant action of protein C. This is called factor V Leiden, and is the commonest known cause of inherited thrombophilia, with a prevalence of about 5 per cent in western Europeans.

However, it is the interaction of two or more of these deficiencies, together with other risk factors (e.g. pregnancy, use of the oral contraceptive pill, abdominal surgery) that usually results in actual thrombosis. Homozygous inheritance of any one of these genetic defects may produce a severe clinical picture of perinatal thrombosis with high mortality (purpura fulminans).

The management of a patient who has suffered a thrombosis consists of identifying any inherited risk factors (such as those mentioned above) and then instituting appropriate anticoagulant therapy. It is advisable to investigate for inherited thrombophilia if the patient has developed thrombosis at an early age (less than 30 years old) or sustained several thromboses; women who have more than one stillbirth should also be investigated.

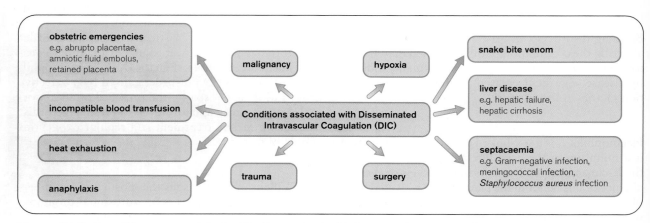

Figure 31.5 Conditions associated with disseminated intravascular coagulation.

The main anticoagulant drugs used in the prevention of a thrombosis formation or to extend the time taken for clot formation, are heparin and warfarin. Heparin may be given subcutaneously and operates by increasing the natural anticoagulant action of antithrombin III, which in turn inhibits the actions of thrombin and factor X. Low-molecular-weight heparin has recently been developed, and is considered to carry less risk of bleeding than standard heparin. It is used both as prophylaxis during major abdominal or orthopaedic surgery and to treat venous thrombosis.

Warfarin is an anticoagulant drug that works by preventing the synthesis of the Vitamin K-dependent clotting factors, namely factors II, VII, IX, and X. Warfarin is an oral drug used to treat thrombosis; however, it takes several days to work and hence heparin and warfarin are given together when therapy is started, and heparin is withdrawn once warfarin levels are satisfactory. The treatment is assessed by the international normalized ratio (INR), which compares the prothrombin time of the patient with that of normal healthy controls and expresses the result as a ratio. If a warfarinized patient travels abroad or attends another clinic because of a bleed while away from home, the international normalized ratio may be compared and the anticoagulant therapy re-evaluated (see also Chapter 10).

BLOOD TRANSFUSION

BLOOD GROUP ANTIGENS AND ANTIBODIES

The surface membrane of a red blood cell contains more than 400 antigens. Red blood cell antigens are divided into groups, so that antigens in one group are inherited in a linked fashion but independently of antigens in other groups. Antibodies against the red blood cell surface antigens are immunoglobulins, mainly of the IgG or IgM isotype (see Chapter 24). Antibodies combine with their corresponding antigens; this is a reaction that can be observed in the laboratory and that may also give rise to clinical problems in the patient. The blood group of the patient is assigned on the basis of the antigens present on their red blood cells. Conversely, the blood group antibodies present in a patient's serum are directed against antigens that are not expressed on his or her own red blood cells (obviously, or the patient would suffer long-term haemolysis).

The most important blood group system is the ABO system. People with blood group A have red blood cells expressing the A antigen but no anti-A antibodies in their serum; instead they have anti-B antibodies, which will react with any group B cells that are inadvertently transfused. Group O red blood cells do not express either blood group A or blood group B. However, naturally occurring anti-A and anti-B antibodies are detectable in the serum of people who are blood group O. Table 31.1 shows the relative frequency of the ABO groups in the UK.

There are also other, minor blood group antigens, including the rhesus, Kell, Duffy, and Kidd groups. Antibodies directed against these antigens are formed only when a patient is exposed to red blood cells expressing these antigens (e.g. as a result of an incompatible blood transfusion or pregnancy). These are termed 'immune antibodies' and are usually of the IgG subclass. The most important of these blood groups is the rhesus group, which is a major cause of haemolytic disease of the newborn, since IgG antibodies can cross the placenta and harm the unborn child (see Chapter 26).

Compatibility Testing

Compatibility testing is performed to determine the ABO and rhesus group of the patient. In the crossmatch, the serum of the patient to receive the transfusion is mixed and incubated with the red blood cells

The ABO Blood Groups

Blood group	Antibodies in serum (naturally-occurring)	Frequency in the Caucasian population of the UK (%)
A	anti-B	42
B	anti-A	8
O	anti-A and anti-B	47
AB	none	3

Table 31.1 Relative frequency of ABO blood groups in the Caucasian population of the UK.

of the donor and then observed for cell agglutination (clumping of red blood cells). This is a test to establish whether there are antibodies present in the serum of the recipient that may recognize and respond to antigens on the surface of the donor cells. In many cases, the patient's serum would have been tested for atypical antibodies prior to the selection and cross-matching of units of blood for transfusion. The use of the Coombs' reagent, which is anti-human globulin, allows the detection of immune antibodies directed against minor blood group antigens. If 'incompatible' red blood cells are transfused into a patient, the cells are caught up with the antibodies to form an immune complex, and so are destroyed. This is termed a haemolytic transfusion reaction, and in cases involving the ABO system it is potentially fatal.

BLOOD COMPONENTS FOR TRANSFUSION

Red blood cells for transfusion are depleted of plasma and resuspended in an isotonic medium containing sucrose and amino acids. This gives the cells a shelf-life of up to 40 days.

Other products obtained from a donation of blood include platelets, plasma, and plasma constituents. Platelets are transfused into a patient with a low platelet count (thrombocytopenia), whether due to bone marrow disorders like leukaemia, to cytotoxic drugs or radiotherapy, or to a massive blood loss in which platelets are also lost (e.g. post-operative bleeding, ruptured aortic aneurysm). Platelets for transfusion have a shelf-life of only 5 days.

Plasma contains albumin, fibrinogen, clotting factors, and immunoglobulins, all of which are of potential therapeutic use. Fresh frozen plasma contains all the clotting factors, including factors V and VIII, and is used to treat patients with bleeding problems caused by a deficiency of clotting factors, liver failure, or substantial blood loss. Concentrates of factor VIII and factor IX are used to treat the specific clotting factor deficiency states of haemophilia A and haemophilia B. Cryoprecipitate contains fibrinogen and is prepared from fresh frozen plasma by slow thawing. Human serum albumin may be prepared by fractionation of pooled plasma, and is available as either 4 per cent or 20 per cent human albumin. It is generally used to replace plasma protein loss in severe burns, renal failure, or liver failure. Specific immunoglobulins are used in passive prophylaxis against infections such as tetanus and varicella–zoster or to prevent haemolytic disease of the newborn (anti-rhesus D immunoglobulin). Non-specific immunoglobulins are used for passive prophylaxis against infections such as hepatitis A and in the treatment of inherited immunodeficiency disorders (see Chapters 23 and 28).

HAZARDS OF TRANSFUSION

Immediate Transfusion Reactions

The adverse effects of blood transfusion may be essentially grouped as immediate and delayed. Generally, immediate reactions to transfusion have an immunological basis. The most important of these are haemolytic transfusion reactions. For example, if red blood cells bearing the blood group A antigen are transfused into a patient who is blood group O, the anti-A antibodies in the patient's serum will activate complement. In turn the complement will destroy the transfused cells by puncturing holes in the membrane, so they are haemolysed (see also Chapters 25 and 26). In addition toxic substances and red blood cell membrane components will be released into the circulation. The result is hypotension, renal damage, and uncontrolled activation of the coagulation system. The patient becomes rapidly unwell with fever, tachycardia, hypotension, loin pain, restlessness, and confusion.

Hence, patients must be regularly observed throughout a blood transfusion, and especially in the first 30 minutes. If a haemolytic transfusion reaction is suspected, the transfusion should be stopped and replaced with a saline infusion. The clinician should be informed, and the unit of blood taken down and returned to the blood bank, together with a sample of the patient's blood for testing. Management of the patient requires specialist advice and often intensive care. The mortality in ABO-incompatible transfusions is anything up to 50 per cent. Unfortunately, the most common cause of incompatible blood transfusions is clerical error, in which a unit of blood cross-matched and assigned to one patient is given to another patient by mistake or in which the original recipient's blood sample was labelled with the wrong patient's name before being sent to the blood bank for cross-matching.

Delayed Transfusion Reactions

Delayed haemolytic transfusion reactions frequently involve a minor blood group antigen mismatch. They are rarely severe and occur about 1 week after the transfusion. In these cases, the patient has probably been previously transfused with donated blood and raised antibodies against a minor blood group antigen, but the level of antibody in the serum was probably too low for detection in the cross-match. However, with the subsequent infusion of cells bearing the antigen they had formerly encountered and recognized as foreign, antibody levels were boosted over the ensuing few days to cause the eventual destruction of transfused cells. These reactions commonly occur in the spleen, and result in fever, jaundice and anaemia. The patient should be tested for the presence of the antibodies in the blood, which should also be identified in order that any future transfusion can be with blood that does not bear the antigens.

Patients who require regular transfusions (e.g. patients with beta-thalassaemia major – see Person-Centred Study: Beta-Thalassaemia Major) are liable to raise antibodies against one or more of the minor blood groups. This is a dilemma for the blood transfusion laboratory, for many units of blood may need to be cross-matched in order to select compatible blood for transfusion.

Reactions to Contaminating Leukocytes

Immune reactions to contaminating leukocytes within red blood cells and platelet transfusions are generally directed at human leukocyte antigens (HLA), and they can precipitate fever and tachycardia. These are usually managed by slowing down or stopping the transfusion and administering antihistamine drugs and hydrocortisone. Then the transfusion can generally be re-commenced once the symptoms have subsided. Up to one-third of patients who receive repeated transfusions will become 'sensitized' to donor leukocytes and so will need blood products specially selected and prepared so that the number of contaminating leukocytes are minimal. Such blood products are termed 'leukodepleted' and are available from the transfusion centres.

Some patients suffer immunological reactions to plasma proteins, and the symptoms that result include itching, sometimes fever, and occasionally wheezing and anaphylaxis.

Infectious Complications

Infectious complications of blood transfusion include the transmission of bacteria, parasites, and viruses. Bacterial contamination can occur at the time of opening a unit of blood, and that is why blood for transfusion should be given within 4 hours of being connected to a giving set. All blood donations are screened for syphilis. Parasites which can be transmitted in blood products include malarial parasites and trypanosomes. Therefore, donors are not accepted if they have recently travelled to areas where these infections are endemic (see Chapter 29). Hepatitis B and C can be transmitted in blood products, as can HIV-1 and HIV-2. All donations are therefore screened by the National Blood Service and confirmed negative for hepatitis B, hepatitis C, and HIV. In the USA and some European countries, testing for human T cell leukaemia virus-1 is also carried out.

PATHOLOGY

FURTHER READING

Buswell C (1996) Beta thalassaemia. Prof Nurse 12:145–7.

Embury SH, Hebbel RP, Mohandas N, *et al*. (1994) Sickle Cell Disease: Basic Principles and Clinical Practice. Raven Press, New York.

Epstein FH (1998) Respiratory function of haemoglobin N Engl J Med 338:239–47.

Fielding AK, Ager S, Russell SJ (1997) The future of haematology, molecular biology and gene therapy. BMJ 314:1396–9.

Grijseels EW, Bouten MJ, Lenderink T, *et al*. (1995). Pre-hospital thrombolytic therapy with either alteplase or streptokinase. Practical applications, complications and long-term results in 529 patients. Eur Heart J 16:1833–8.

Hoffbrand V, Provan D (1997) ABC of clinical haematology. Macrocytic anaemias. BMJ 314:430–3.

Kroft SH, Finn WG, Peterson LC (1995) The pathology of the chronic lymphoid leukaemias [Review]. Blood Rev 9:234–50.

Majno G, Joris I (1996) Cells, Tissues and Disease: Principles of General Pathology. Blackwell Science, Oxford.

Mollison PL, Engelfriet CP (1997) Blood transfusion in clinical medicine 10th ed. Blackwell Science, Oxford.

Proven D, Henson A (1997) ABC of clinical haematology. BMJ Books, London.

Sergent G (1997) Sickle-cell disease. Lancet 350:725–30.

United Kingdom Haemophilia Centre Directors Organisation Executive Committee (1997) Guidelines on therapeutic products to treat haemophilia and other hereditary disorders. Haemophilia 3:63–77.

van Leeuwen FE (1996) Risk of acute myelogenous leukaemia and myelodysplasia following cancer treatment [Review]. Baillieres Clin Haematol 9:57–85.

DISEASES OF THE CARDIOVASCULAR SYSTEM

LEARNING OBJECTIVES

After studying this chapter students should have a clearer understanding of:
- the risk factors for developing atherosclerosis and the clinical features associated with atherosclerosis in different vessels
- the pathophysiology of essential hypertension and its clinical complications
- the pathophysiology of heart failure

It is expected that you should have a basic understanding of:
- the names and courses of the major blood vessels, the anatomy of the heart and circulation
- the control mechanisms of the cardiovascular system.

ATHEROSCLEROSIS

Arteriosclerosis is the general term for hardening of the arteries, of which atherosclerosis is the most frequent cause. It is the most common cause of death in the Western world, far exceeding deaths from cancer. The basic pathological feature of atherosclerosis is an abnormal plaque of fatty and fibrous tissue on the lining of the artery, known as atheroma. As this plaque thickens, it narrows the artery, interfering with the blood flow.

Depending on which artery is affected, the clinical features will vary, although the underlying problem is that of ischaemia, lack of blood flow. The plaque may become calcified and the surface may ulcerate. This weakens the vessel wall and is also the source of emboli, clots that break off and travel in the circulation to lodge in narrower arteries, causing further ischaemia (Figure 32.1).

RISK FACTORS FOR ATHEROSCLEROSIS

Extensive research has identified several risk factors for developing atherosclerosis. The most important factor is cigarette smoking, which has recently been shown to increase the risk to up to five times that of non-smokers. Uncontrolled hypertension and high levels of serum cholesterol are also associated with an increased risk. Patients who have diabetes mellitus or who are obese also have a higher incidence of atherosclerosis. The Health of the Nation campaign has directed resources and attention to each of these factors in an attempt to reduce the incidence of coronary heart disease in the UK, by encouraging people to stop smoking, to eat a low-cholesterol diet, and to have their blood pressure and cholesterol level checked (Boxes 32.1 and 32.2).

This tactic is known as primary prevention and is directed at stopping the atherosclerosis developing in the first place. Secondary prevention involves patients who have already developed atherosclerosis, and attempts to minimize their further risk from the disease [e.g. by strict control of diabetes and hypertension, diet, drug treatment of hypercholesterolaemia (raised serum cholesterol), and drugs and surgery for the atherosclerosis, when appropriate].

ATHEROSCLEROSIS OF THE CORONARY ARTERIES

The coronary arteries are commonly affected by atherosclerosis. Initially, the reduced blood flow through the narrowed vessels means that areas of heart

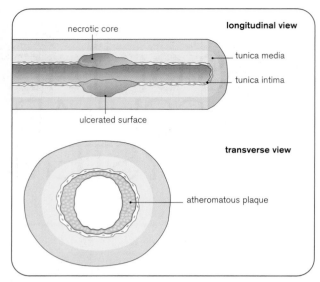

longitudinal view

necrotic core

tunica media

tunica intima

ulcerated surface

transverse view

atheromatous plaque

Figure 32.1 Atheromatous plaque narrowing the vessel lumen. Ulcerated surface can act as focus for thrombus and source of emboli.

BOX 32.1 RISK FACTORS FOR ATHEROSCLEROSIS

Smoking
Hypertension
Hypercholesterolaemia
Diabetes
Obesity

BOX 32.2 HEALTH OF THE NATION TARGETS

By the year 2000:
- in people aged under 65 years, to reduce death rates from coronary heart disease and stroke by at least 40 per cent
- in people aged 65–74 years, to reduce death rates from coronary heart disease by at least 30 per cent
- in people aged 65–74 years, to reduce stroke death rates by at least 40 per cent

---

muscle are poorly oxygenated and the patient will experience episodes of angina, a tight band-like pain around the chest, caused by ischaemia of the heart muscle. This is worse on exercise, when the heart muscle requires more oxygen, and will subside when the patient rests.

As the disease becomes more severe, the patient may experience angina at rest, which is a significant symptom requiring urgent treatment. A myocardial infarction occurs when the blood flow to the heart muscle is reduced by so much (or is interrupted altogether) that the heart muscle dies owing to oxygen starvation. This usually happens when an atheromatous embolus breaks off and completely blocks the artery further down. In this situation, the chest pain is usually more severe and is not relieved by resting or by taking anti-anginal medication. There is a critical time period between the artery being blocked and the muscle cells actually dying, and a thrombolytic drug (a drug that dissolves the thrombus or clot) should be administered as soon as possible. In some remote areas, the thrombolytic drug (e.g. streptokinase) is given at home by the general practitioner to avoid fatal delay.

The major cause of death within the first 2 hours of a myocardial infarction, however, is due to rhythm disturbances, and treatment of this may require a defibrillator or specialized drugs.

If the patient survives the heart attack (myocardial infarction), the muscle that has died heals as an area of fibrous tissue, which does not have the same contracting properties as heart muscle (see Chapter 4). This may lead eventually to heart failure, particularly if the patient suffers more than one myocardial infarction. At the site of the infarct, a ventricular aneurysm, which is a non-contracting dilatation of the heart wall, may form. Thrombus can develop within the aneurysm and subsequent emboli may be carried round the circulation and cause obstruction in other blood vessels of the body.

Coronary angioplasty and coronary artery bypass grafts are surgical techniques to open up constricted vessels or replace them altogether with vessel grafts if the damage is too severe for balloon angioplasty (see Person-Centred Study: The Complications of a Heart Attack).

CEREBROVASCULAR ATHEROSCLEROSIS

Atherosclerosis also commonly causes narrowing of the carotid arteries supplying the brain and sometimes affects arteries within the brain. An early symptom of this is a transient ischaemic attack (see Chapter 38). Reduction in the blood flow to one area of the brain causes symptoms such as sudden loss of speech or paralysis of a limb. The brain does not have pain sensation as such, so the symptom is experienced as a loss of function rather than as pain.

By definition, the symptoms have to completely resolve within 24 hours for the episode to be labelled as a transient ischaemic attack, which is the equivalent of angina in the coronary vessels (i.e. there is no significant cell death). After a critical period of time of being deprived of oxygen, however, the brain cells will die and the loss of function will then be permanent. The patient has then suffered a stroke, or cerebrovascular accident. Atherosclerosis is not the only cause of strokes, and sometimes they are caused by haemorrhage into brain tissue rather than by ischaemia, although the clinical end result is the same.

In the same way as surgery is used to prevent further damage in coronary heart disease, some patients benefit from carotid endarterectomy, in which the layer lining the carotid artery and containing the atheromatous plaques is stripped out to try to prevent further problems.

AORTIC ATHEROSCLEROSIS

The earliest appearances of atheroma, fatty streaks, can be seen in the aortas of teenagers who have died from other causes. The plaques may become more extensive and ulcerate, leading to weakness of the aortic wall. This dilatation is known as an aortic aneurysm; sudden leakage from and rupture of an aortic aneurysm is a common cause of sudden death, particularly in older men. Sometimes, the patient may get an early warning of leakage by developing sudden severe back pain, but even with urgent surgery at this stage, patients often die. Current research suggests that if the aneurysm can be detected before it leaks and is surgically replaced with an artificial fibre aortic graft, mortality will be reduced. However, the only way of detecting an aneurysm over 6.5 cm, which is the diameter suitable for operation, is to use abdominal ultrasound, which would make it a very costly screening programme.

PERIPHERAL VASCULAR DISEASE

When atherosclerosis affects the main arteries of the legs, a characteristic symptom known as intermittent claudication is produced. Like angina, this is pain originating in a muscle; in this case it is the lack of blood flow to the calf muscle that produces the intense cramp on walking, which eases off when the patient stops (Box 32.3).

Peripheral vascular disease is very strongly associated with cigarette smoking, and stopping smoking may, alone, significantly relieve symptoms. These patients are at serious risk of gangrene of the foot if the circulation reaches a critically low level. Warning of this is given by the patient developing rest pain in bed, when the minimal change in gravity of lifting the foot into bed critically reduces the flow. The patient has to dangle the foot out of bed to relieve the pain. Gangrene can suddenly occur if an embolus breaks off a plaque further up the artery and lodges in a smaller vessel supplying the foot (see also Chapter 4). This requires urgent surgery to prevent the need for an amputation, or at least to limit the damage.

HYPERLIPIDAEMIA

There are two main groups of circulating fats or lipids in the blood, triglycerides and cholesterol. Both have an important role to play in the normal metabolism of the body. Cholesterol levels can be subdivided further by measuring its transport molecules, high-density lipoproteins (HDL), low-density lipoproteins (LDL), and very low-density lipoproteins (VLDL) (see Chapter 6). There has been enormous publicity given to the effects of cholesterol since research began to show that abnormally high cholesterol levels were associated with an increased risk of heart disease.

The clinical signs of hypercholesterolaemia may include xanthelasmata (fatty yellow skin deposits under lower eyelids) and corneal arcus (white deposits around the rim of the iris).

A small proportion of the population has an inherited defect of an enzyme that metabolizes cholesterol, which means that they have very high levels of circulating cholesterol and are at high risk of atherosclerosis at an early age – familial hypercholesterolaemia. These patients and their families will usually require drug treatment to lower their cholesterol levels to try to prevent the onset of coronary heart disease. This is why great emphasis is placed on a history of a family member suffering heart disease at an early age, since identifying this group is very important.

A far greater number of people have mildly raised cholesterol levels, which can be lowered to some extent by reducing total dietary fat intake. Confusion has abounded over dietary recommendations and the relative benefits of treating mildly raised cholesterol levels, particularly if lifelong drugs are required.

When evaluating the plasma cholesterol level it is important to measure the HDL and LDL levels as well as the total level. The optimum total cholesterol level is 5.2 mmol/l, but whatever the level a high proportion of HDL is a relatively good sign because HDL is inversely related to coronary heart disease. Drug therapy is required if dietary manipulation does not succeed. Some doctors are aggressive in their management and introduce drugs at cholesterol levels of 6.8 mmol/l; others take a level above 7.5 mmol/l as an indication for drug therapy. However, a wide range of studies have shown that managing other risk factors, such as smoking, which still remains the single most significant risk factor for developing atherosclerosis, is equally important.

HYPERTENSION

In the general population, levels of blood pressure vary in a normal distribution, and the definition of high blood pressure (hypertension) has been based on observations of increasing risk of complications as the level rises. There is no definite cut-off point but, in the UK, levels above 160(systolic)/90(diastolic) mmHg are considered to put the individual at risk.

Hypertension may be secondary to other disorders, including:
- renal disease (e.g. polycystic kidneys);
- endocrine disease (e.g. phaeochromocytoma);
- drugs (e.g. corticosteroids).

However, the majority of patients (up to 2 per cent of the UK population) have essential hypertension – raised blood pressure for which no underlying cause can be found.

CLINICAL FEATURES OF HYPERTENSION

In itself, hypertension does not cause any symptoms and is often diagnosed on opportunistic health checks. The risks of hypertension lie in its complications. Sustained raised arterial pressure means that the heart is having to contract harder to force the blood through the vessels, leading to hypertrophy (thickening) of the

---

BOX 32.3 CLINICAL FEATURES OF AN EMBOLUS IN THE LEG

Pain with sudden onset
Pallor (whiteness)
Pulselessness
Paraesthesia (loss of sensation)
Paralysis
Perishing cold

heart muscle. Eventually, the heart muscle can no longer sustain the overload, and the patient goes into heart failure. The abnormal pressure on the cerebral vessels may cause rupture and bleeding into the brain – a stroke caused by cerebral haemorrhage rather than ischaemia. Hypertension accelerates the development of atheroma and in turn leads to coronary artery disease, increasing the risk of angina and myocardial infarction. In the kidney, the raised pressure causes thickening of the small blood vessel walls which can lead to kidney failure. Uncontrolled hypertension is one of the reasons why a patient may ultimately require renal dialysis. This small blood vessel damage may also be seen in the retinal blood vessels in the eye, where haemorrhages and loss of vision may result.

MANAGEMENT OF ESSENTIAL HYPERTENSION

Before resorting to drug treatment of hypertension, there are many changes in people's lifestyles that can lower their blood pressure. Stopping smoking, regular exercise, weight control, and reducing alcohol intake will all reduce blood pressure and may mean that drugs are not required at all.

Deciding at which level to add drug therapy can be difficult. When the diastolic pressure is above 115 mmHg, the benefits of treatment far outweigh the risks. When the diastolic level is over 100 mmHg or the systolic is above 170 mmHg, particularly in older adults, treatment will reduce the statistical risk of a stroke or heart attack, but the balance may be less clear cut for the individual patient. When the diastolic level is between 90 and 100 mmHg, although there is potentially some benefit in drug treatment, the side-effects may outweigh any risk reduction, and the number of patients who have to be treated in order to prevent one stroke or heart attack become very large (see the trial conducted by the Medical Research Council and the IPPPSH and EWPHE trials). Again, stopping smoking reduced the risk more than treating the hypertension does.

When the decision to instigate drug therapy has been made, there is a plethora of drugs available, all of which have their benefits and side-effects. Since patients usually have no symptoms and are on lifelong therapy, it is important to minimize the side-effects of the drugs, or inevitably patients will stop taking the medication, leaving themselves potentially at risk. The drugs used include diuretics (e.g. bendrofluazide), beta-blockers (e.g. atenolol), angiotensin converting enzyme (ACE) inhibitors (e.g. captopril), and calcium antagonists (e.g. nifedipine) (see Chapter 10).

HEART FAILURE

Heart failure is a general term that covers situations in which the heart muscle can no longer cope with the load put upon it. This may be very sudden, such as when a heart valve ruptures, or it may develop more slowly, with many different causes. The underlying cause may predominantly affect the left or the right side of the heart, producing different clinical pictures. Eventually, both sides of the heart are adversely affected as the heart failure reaches its terminal phase (Figure 32.2).

LEFT HEART FAILURE

Contraction of the left atrium and ventricle produce the force (stroke volume) that maintains blood flow around the body. If the heart muscle is diseased or damaged, the output of the heart falls, causing a reduction in the forward flow of blood and also producing back pressure into the lungs. This causes shortness of breath (dyspnoea), which is often acute at night (paroxysmal nocturnal dyspnoea). This occurs because the increased gravitational pressure of lying down increases the pressure in the pulmonary blood vessels, forcing fluid out of the blood vessels into the lung tissue (acute left ventricular failure). The constant lack of forward pressure results in falling blood pressure and poor tissue perfu-

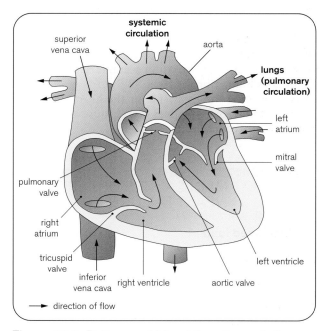

Figure 32.2 Patterns of blood flow through the heart. Diagram of the direction of blood flow through the chambers of the heart.

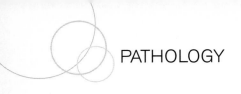

sion, causing weakness, cold extremities, and eventually renal failure as the blood pressure in the renal circulation falls too low to maintain the kidney cells.

The main causes of left heart failure (Box 32.4) include:

- uncontrolled hypertension putting extra strain on the heart muscle;
- coronary atherosclerosis resulting in myocardial infarction and death of myocardial cells; and
- heart muscle diseases (cardiomyopathies).

Left heart failure also results if the aortic or mitral valves are damaged, leading to valvular stenosis, narrowing, or incompetence.

RIGHT HEART FAILURE

Contraction of the right atrium and ventricle maintains the circulation of blood through the lungs, where it is oxygenated before onward circulation around the body by the left atrium and ventricle. If the patient has lung disease which impedes the flow of blood through the lungs, the result is back pressure in the venous circulation, which feeds into the right atrium. This rise in venous pressure causes the characteristic signs of right heart failure – ankle oedema, liver enlargement, and ascites (the accumulation of fluid in the abdomen). The fluid accumulation starts in the ankles because of the added effect of gravity, but if the patient is bedbound, this gravitational effect causes sacral rather than ankle oedema.

The common causes of right heart failure are lung diseases, such as chronic obstructive pulmonary disease, pulmonary hypertension secondary to left heart failure, and lung fibrosis (Box 32.5). Again, damaged heart valves on the right side of the heart – the pulmonary and tricuspid valves – will cause overload of the right heart muscle.

COMBINED HEART FAILURE

As the heart failure worsens, whether left-sided or right-sided, the other chambers become involved. Accordingly, the clinical picture of combined heart failure is of fluid accumulation both peripherally and in the lungs, with a failing cardiac output compromising renal function; renal failure is often the terminal event.

MANAGEMENT OF HEART FAILURE

Acute heart failure presents as pulmonary oedema – fluid exuding from the blood vessels into the alveolar air spaces – and requires urgent treatment with high doses of a loop diuretic, such as frusemide, given intravenously. Maintenance oral diuretics are then needed to keep the problem under control. Recently, ACE inhibitors have been found to be effective in not only helping relieve the symptoms of chronic heart failure, but also in increasing life expectancy.

Digoxin has been in use for 200 years for the treatment of 'dropsy' or oedema. It is still used today, but mainly in atrial fibrillation, when the heart rhythm is abnormal. It may accumulate in the body if the kidneys are not functioning effectively and cause toxic side-effects (see Chapter 13). Patients may also need anticoagulation if they are at increased risk of thrombosis and embolism.

VALVULAR HEART DISEASE

Diseases of the heart valves can be congenital or acquired. In the UK, the commonest cause of acquired valve disease used to be rheumatic fever, which resulted from a streptococcal infection (see Chapter 27). Susceptible patients developed a secondary inflammation of the heart valves, causing long-term structural damage, most often to the mitral valve. Today in the Western world, owing to raised standards of living, rheumatic fever is less prevalent and degenerative diseases of the valves are a more common cause of damage nowadays.

BOX 32.4 MAIN CAUSES OF LEFT HEART FAILURE

Increased load
hypertension
mitral and aortic valve disease
arrhythmias

Myocardial damage
ischaemic heart disease
myocarditis
cardiomyopathies

BOX 32.5 MAIN CAUSES OF RIGHT HEART FAILURE

pulmonary hypertension secondary to left heart failure
pulmonary hypertension secondary to lung disease
pulmonary and tricuspid valve disease
cardiomyopathies

The valves can be affected either by stenosis, in which the valve becomes narrowed and obstructs the blood flow, or by regurgitation or incompetence, in which the valve leaks. Most valve diseases produce characteristic heart murmurs because the flow of blood through them is turbulent and therefore noisy.

MITRAL STENOSIS

The result of mitral stenosis is to obstruct the flow of blood from the left atrium to the left ventricle. This leads to dilatation of the left atrium and subsequently to back pressure in the pulmonary blood vessels – pulmonary hypertension. The patient may be asymptomatic for many years, but an extra strain on the heart, such as exercise or pregnancy, may produce symptoms of left heart failure. The pulmonary hypertension also sometimes leads to haemoptysis (coughing up blood) by causing small vessels in the lung to rupture. Because the left atrium is dilated, the electrical activity of the heart may be disturbed, causing atrial fibrillation, which will exacerbate the heart failure.

Treatment

Once the diagnosis of mitral stenosis has been made on echocardiography, a decision has to be made as to whether the patient requires surgery to the diseased valve. Sometimes, when the problem is discovered by the chance finding of a murmur (e.g. during a routine medical), the degree of stenosis may be very mild, and the patient can be monitored without active intervention. If, however, the stenosis is more severe, it is inevitable that the obstruction will cause permanent damage to the heart and lungs, and surgery is needed. In this situation, the valve needs to be opened up (valvotomy) or replaced if it is heavily calcified or if there is regurgitation as well as stenosis.

MITRAL INCOMPETENCE

Regurgitation of blood through an incompetent mitral valve again overloads the left atrium, resulting in pulmonary hypertension. Because regurgitation produces a low-pressure situation, the effects usually develop more slowly than in mitral stenosis unless there is a sudden rupture of the valve causing a dramatic, sudden increase in left atrial pressure. This sometimes happens as a secondary effect of a myocardial infarction in which the area of heart muscle attached to the valve dies, and the valve can then flap and leak. Slow development of incompetence may result from dilatation of the ventricle caused by heart disease, which overstretches the valve ring and makes the valve leak.

The murmur of mitral regurgitation is distinct from that of mitral stenosis, but since the valve may be stenotic and incompetent at the same time, it must be visualized by echocardiography to evaluate the damage and the haemodynamic effect.

Surgery is less common and is performed later for mitral regurgitation than mitral stenosis, and many patients can be managed medically. If the degree of regurgitation is severe, if regurgitation occurs suddenly, or if the heart failure becomes severe, surgery may then be an option.

AORTIC STENOSIS

Stenosis of the aortic valve causes back pressure in the left ventricle. In the same way as occurs in any other muscle that is exercised, the ventricular muscle initially compensates for this by muscular hypertrophy in order to produce the force required to maintain blood flow through the narrow valve.

The inflow to the coronary arteries is just above the aortic valve, and when the flow through the valve is restricted, the coronary arterial flow is also reduced. This causes ischaemia of the heart muscle, which, because of its increased bulk, requires an increased blood flow, and the patient develops angina. In a patient with aortic stenosis, the onset of angina is a sign that the flow reduction is becoming critical and urgent intervention is required.

The aortic valve usually has three sections, but the congenital abnormality of a bicuspid valve (two leaflets instead of the normal three) is the cause of 50 per cent of the cases of adult aortic stenosis. This is often diagnosed when a systolic murmur is heard on routine examination. The degree of stenosis can be measured and, if it is significant, surgery is required before the myocardium suffers long-term damage.

Stenosis and incompetence of the other valves, the tricuspid and the pulmonary valves, can also occur but are less common.

SUBACUTE BACTERIAL ENDOCARDITIS

Any heart valve that is abnormal is at risk of a potentially fatal complication caused by infection – subacute bacterial endocarditis. Normally, the body's immune system deals perfectly adequately with the transient passages of bacteria in the bloodstream that result from dental work or minor medical procedures such as cystoscopy. However, bacteria are able to establish a focus of infection (known as a vegetation) on damaged heart valves, which can damage the valve further and sometimes be fatal.

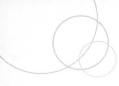

This can be prevented by providing antibiotic cover for these dental and medical procedures. There should be a high index of suspicion of subacute bacterial endocarditis when a patient with heart valve disease develops a fever and anaemia for no obvious cause. If treated in time with high doses of intravenous antibiotics, the infection may be overcome, although the extra damage to the valve may then require surgical intervention.

INVESTIGATIONS FOR HEART DISEASE

THE ELECTROCARDIOGRAM

The electrocardiogram (ECG) is the primary investigation in heart disease because characteristic ECG patterns can be diagnostic. The ECG records the electrical activity of the heart muscle. However, a normal ECG does not exclude heart disease, and it does not predict future events – there have been well-documented cases of people dying from a heart attack hours after a normal ECG has been done! If the myocardial cells are damaged, then the normal electrical pattern is interrupted, and the ECG can be used to diagnose conditions such as myocardial infarction, rhythm disturbances, and pericardial disease (Figure 32.3).

An exercise ECG (or stress ECG) is performed by recording an ECG while the patient is exercising on a treadmill. This will sometimes pick up abnormalities that are not apparent on a resting ECG. For example, exercise may provoke ischaemia, which will cause changes in the ECG, and the patient may develop angina. This is then an indication to investigate the patient further with angiography.

ECHOCARDIOGRAPHY

Echocardiography uses ultrasound waves, which are reflected back by the walls and valves of the heart to give a structural picture. This is the standard investigation for heart valve disease and abnormalities of the muscle such as ventricular hypertrophy. By using Doppler ultrasound, flow rates and pressure gradients can also be measured, and this helps to make management decisions about valve surgery.

CARDIAC CATHETERIZATION

This technique is used extensively in assessing coronary artery disease. It involves the passage of a fine catheter tube down which dye can be squirted to outline the coronary vessels and define stenoses and blockages. If appropriate, angioplasty can be performed at the same time. The catheter, which has a balloon on the tip, is manoeuvred into the narrow segment and the balloon is inflated

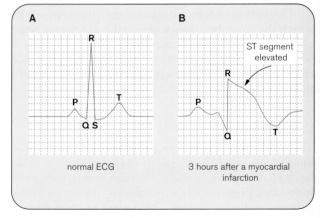

Figure 32.3 ECG patterns. a. Normal ECG. **b.** ECG 3 hours after a myocardial infarction; note that the ST segment is elevated and the T wave is inverted.

to relieve the stenosis. If this is successful, it may avoid or delay coronary artery replacement with grafts.

Cardiac catheterization is also sometimes required to outline congenital abnormalities in children so that corrective heart surgery can be planned.

CONGENITAL HEART DISEASE

Congenital heart disease occurs in approximately eight in 1000 live births and ranges in severity from mild to fatal. Increasingly, heart abnormalities are being diagnosed on antenatal ultrasound, allowing adequate preparations to be made for treatment at delivery. There have even been some cases of the baby receiving surgery before delivery after the diagnosis has been made on a routine antenatal scan.

The known causes of congenital heart disease include intrauterine infections such as rubella, drugs such as alcohol and lithium (see Chapter 12), and various inherited abnormalities.

The abnormality known as a 'hole in the heart' encompasses several different conditions, but in essence means that there is an abnormal connection allowing flow between the left and right heart chambers, either at atrial level (an atrial septal defect) or through the ventricular septum (a ventricular septal defect).

Acyanotic Congenital Heart Disease

The symptoms depend on the size of the communicating hole, and many small septal defects are asymptomatic and are diagnosed only when a murmur is heard on routine examination. Because the pressure is normally higher in the left side of the heart than the right, the direction of flow through the defect is from left to right, so that blood is recirculated through the lungs and is fully oxygenated – hence the term 'acyanotic congenital heart disease'.

Cyanotic Congenital Heart Disease

However, in ventricular septal defects, the continual overload of the right ventricle from the extra blood flow eventually means that the right-sided pressure exceeds the left and the flow reverses. This new right-to-left flow means that the some blood bypasses the lungs and is not oxygenated, causing the patient to be cyanosed – cyanotic congenital heart disease. Clinically, this presents with the characteristic blue-lipped appearance of cyanosis and a sign known as 'clubbing', in which the fingertips are bulbous. (This sign also occurs in other chronic diseases, particularly those affecting the lungs; it is seen in lung cancer as well.) Initially the cyanosis is exertional when the demand for oxygen rises, but as the condition deteriorates, the patient becomes cyanosed at rest.

Fallot's Tetralogy

Fallot's tetralogy is a combination of defects, commonly occurring in children with Down's syndrome, which can be another cause of cyanotic heart disease (Figure 32.4). The four features of Fallot's tetralogy are:

- ventricular septal defect;
- pulmonary stenosis;
- an aorta that over-rides the ventricular septal defect; and
- right ventricular hypertrophy.

Surgical repair is often required for congenital heart disease but it will, if possible, be delayed until the child is older, for technical reasons. The outlook has been transformed over the last 20 years, particularly with the introduction of cardiac bypass, allowing long intricate operations to be performed while still maintaining adequate circulation artificially.

THE CARDIOMYOPATHIES

The heart muscle itself may be diseased. Infection of the heart muscle is known as myocarditis; it can be caused by viruses or, in some tropical countries, by parasites. Viral myocarditis is a rare cause of sudden death and is the reason people are advised not to exercise when suffering from a viral illness. Chronic heart muscle diseases are known as cardiomyopathies; they may result from a variety of causes (e.g. alcohol, cytotoxic drugs such as adriamycin, and systemic diseases such as sarcoidosis). Some are

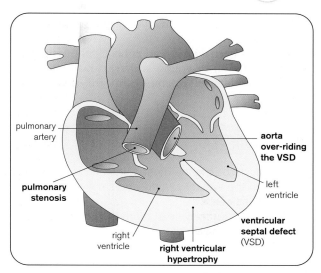

Figure 32.4 Features of Fallot's tetralogy.

inherited but the majority are idiopathic (i.e. the cause is not known).

CONGESTIVE CARDIOMYOPATHY

As the muscle becomes damaged, it becomes dilated and loses its contractile power, resulting in heart failure, both left-sided and right-sided. As the dilatation increases, the valve ring also dilates and there is secondary incompetence of the tricuspid and mitral valves, which in turn worsens the heart failure.

RESTRICTIVE CARDIOMYOPATHY

This type of cardiomyopathy is much less common than congestive cardiomyopathy. It occurs when there is an abnormal infiltration of the heart muscle, such as fibrosis or amyloidosis, in which an abnormal protein accumulates in cells. The muscle becomes stiffer and less compliant, and there may be arrhythmias if the electrical pathways are involved with the infiltration.

HYPERTROPHIC OBSTRUCTIVE CARDIOMYOPATHY

This is sometimes a familial disease and it is a cause of sudden death in young people, particularly during exercise. The myocardium is asymmetrically thickened; the thickening involves the left ventricle and (predominantly) the septal wall. When the heart contracts, this thick wall obstructs the outflow of blood towards the aorta, and this may lead to dizziness and fainting on exercise. The usual cause of death is an arrhythmia

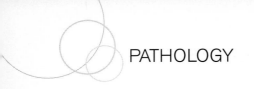

because the electrical pathways are abnormal through the hypertrophic muscle.

There has been widespread publicity about this condition in relation to young athletes, and suggestions that they should have screening echocardiograms, since the condition may be asymptomatic. Recently, the genetic abnormality has been identified in the familial form, allowing screening of patients' relatives to see if they are affected.

KEY POINTS

- Atherosclerosis is the most common cause of death in the Western world, and smoking is the biggest risk factor.
- Total cholesterol levels of more than 5.2 mmol/l are associated with an increased risk of coronary heart disease.
- Familial hypercholesterolaemia dramatically increases the risk of coronary heart disease at an early age.
- Hypertension is asymptomatic until complications occur, and controlling hypertension reduces the risk of atherosclerosis, heart failure, renal disease and stroke.
- Left heart failure causes back pressure in the lungs, producing pulmonary oedema. Right heart failure causes back pressure in the venous system, producing peripheral oedema and hepatomegaly.
- Mitral stenosis causes pulmonary hypertension. Aortic stenosis causes left ventricular hypertrophy and coronary insufficiency.
- The ECG records electrical activity; the echocardiogram demonstrates the structure of the heart, and Doppler ultrasound measures flow rates and pressure gradients.
- The most common form of congenital heart disease is a septal defect. Some types of congenital heart disease are caused by infection or drugs in pregnancy.
- Cardiomyopathies are diseases of the heart muscle. They may result in heart failure.

FURTHER READING

Amery A, Birkenhäger W, Brixko P, *et al*. (1985) Mortality and morbidity results from the European Working Party on High Blood Pressure in the Elderly trial. Lancet i; (8442):1349–54.

Boulton BD, Bashir Y, Ormerod OJ, Gribbin B, Forfar JC (1997) Cardiac catheterisation performed by a clinical nurse specialist. Heart 78:194–7.

Callahan M (1996) The advanced practice nurse in an acute care setting. The nurse practitioner in adult cardiac surgery care. Nurs Clin North Am 31(3):487–93.

Cardiovascular Risk and Risk Factors in a Randomized Trial of Treatment Based on the Beta-Blocker Oxprenolol: The International Prospective Primary Prevention Study in Hypertension (IPPPSH). J Hypertens 1985;3:379–92.

Coronary Heart Disease Statistics. (1997) British Heart Foundation, London.

Dec GW, Fuster V (1994) Idiopathic dilated cardiomyopathy. N Engl J Med 331:1564–75.

Department of Health (1992) The Health of the Nation: a Strategy for Health in England. Her Majesty's Stationery Office, London.

Doll R (1997) One for the heart. BMJ 315:1664–8.

Fourth International Study of Infarct Survival Collaborative Group (1995) A randomised factorial trial assessing early oral captopril, oral mononitrate, and intravenous magnesium sulphate in 58 050 patients with suspected acute myocardial infarction: ISIS-4. Lancet 345:669–85.

Heart Failure (1998). Lancet 352 (Supp 1):1–41.

Jennings K (1994) Acute Cardiac Care: Community and Hospital Management of Myocardial Infarction. Oxford Medical Publications, Oxford.

Julian D, Camm AJ, Fox KM, Hall RJC, Poole-Wilson PA (eds) (1996) Diseases of the Heart, 2nd edition. WB Saunders, London.

Mallon G (1998) An easier guide to ECG. Radcliffe Medical Press, Oxford.

Medical Research Council Working Party (1985) Medical Research Council trial of treatment of mild hypertension: principal results. BMJ 291:97–104.

Medical Research Council's General Practice Research Framework (1998) Thrombosis prevention trial: randomised trial of low-intensity oral anticoagulation with warfarin and low-dose aspirin in the primary prevention of ischaemic heart disease in men at increased risk. Lancet 351:233–41.

Oakley C (1997) Clinical review: aetiology, diagnosis, investigation and management of cardiomyopathies. BMJ 315:1520–4.

O'Brien ET, Beevers DG, Marshall HJ (1995) ABC of Hypertension, 3rd edition. BMJ, London.

Parish S, Collins R, Peto R *et al*. (1995) Cigarette smoking, tar yields, and non-fatal myocardial infarction: 14 000 cases and 32 000 controls in the United Kingdom. BMJ 311:471–7.

Scandinavian Simvastatin Survival Study Group (1994) Randomised trial of cholesterol lowering in 4444 patients with coronary heart disease: the Scandinavian Simvastatin Survival Study (4S). Lancet 344:1383–9.

Stevenson WG (1995) Mechanisms and management of arrhythmias in heart failure. Curr Opin Cardiol 10:274–81.

Tunstall-Pedoe H, Kuulasmaa K, Amouyel, P, *et al*. (1994) Myocardial infarction and coronary deaths in the World Health Organization MONICA project. Registration procedures, event rates, and case-fatality rates in 39 populations from 21 countries in four continents. Circulation 90:583–612.

Wheelock V (1996) Implementing Dietary Guidelines for Healthy Eating. Chapman and Hall, London.

Whelan Y (1997) Cardiac arrest: the skills of the emergency nurse practitioner. Accid Emerg Nurs 5:107–10.

33

DISEASES OF THE RESPIRATORY SYSTEM

LEARNING OBJECTIVES

After studying this chapter students should have a clearer understanding of:
- the pathophysiology of asthma and its precipitating factors
- the aetiology of respiratory malignancies and their prevention
- the pathophysiology of chronic obstructive pulmonary disease and its causes
- the intimate relationship between lung and heart disease

Before reading this chapter, you should have a basic knowledge of:
- the anatomy of the respiratory system, including the bronchial tree and the lobes of the lungs,
- the principles and mechanisms of gas exchange within the alveoli,
- an understanding of the neural and biochemical control of respiration.

ASTHMA

Asthma can be defined as increased responsiveness of the bronchi to various stimuli, resulting in widespread narrowing of the airways that changes in severity, either spontaneously or in response to treatment. This bronchial hyper-reactivity, or 'twitchy airways', characterizes asthma, and immunological mechanisms play an important role in the disease.

Extrinsic Asthma

Asthma can usually be subdivided into extrinsic or intrinsic causes. Extrinsic asthma is usually found in a person who is atopic and may suffer from other allergic diseases, such as hay fever or eczema. There are usually obvious trigger allergens such as pollens or animal fur, which can also be demonstrated on skin prick testing. The asthma often starts early in life, and the patient may have raised eosinophil levels and IgE anti-

bodies to the allergens in the blood. (Eosinophils are polymorphonuclear white cells that are involved in hypersensitivity reactions, and raised levels are a marker of hypersensitivity.) Exposure to the allergen causes a type I hypersensitivity reaction, releasing mast cell histamine and other chemicals that cause inflammation and bronchoconstriction (see also Chapter 26).

Intrinsic Asthma

Intrinsic asthma tends to occur later in life, in patients without a history of atopy. These patients are often less responsive to the standard treatments and their asthma may be more difficult to control.

PATHOPHYSIOLOGY

Two main pathological reactions cause the symptoms of asthma:
- bronchial smooth muscle contraction (bronchoconstriction); and
- inflammation with oedema and excess mucus production by the bronchial lining.

The bronchospasm causes obstruction to air flow, which is worse in expiration and causes wheezing. The mucus produced by inflammation becomes thick and inspissated in the airways, causing more obstruction to the airflow and also trapping air in the alveoli, thereby interfering with gas exchange.

445

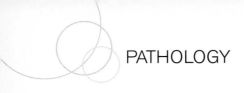

PATHOLOGY

CLINICAL FEATURES

Asthma is a common disease with a rising incidence that is not only due to better diagnosis. Various reasons for the increasing rate have been suggested, including pollution, but none has yet been proven. Asthma affects about 5 per cent of children and 2 per cent of adults in the UK. Although it can be successfully controlled for the vast majority of patients, it cannot be cured and there are still around 2000 deaths a year in the UK. A substantial proportion of children with asthma have a chance of spontaneous improvement with age, but for some it will be a lifelong disease.

Asthma is usually episodic, with the patient suffering attacks that may be provoked by a specific allergen or by non-specific irritants such as smoke, exercise, or cold air.

The typical symptoms of an asthma attack are caused by the inflammatory reaction within the airways. Constriction of the smooth muscle surrounding the bronchioles causes an audible wheeze as the patient tries to force air out of the lungs and also gives rise to the sensation that asthmatics describe of being able to breathe in, but not out. This is often seen on the chest X-ray as overinflation of the lungs. This difficulty in expelling air often leads to persistent coughing as another means of trying to force air out. In children, cough rather than wheeze is often the major symptom, and the cough is often nocturnal.

The inflammation also results in the production of excess mucus. This mucus is thick and sticky and can plug small airways. Its yellow colour can be misleading, suggesting bacterial infection, but this coloration is due to the numerous eosinophils and epithelial cells that are shed into the mucus. This thick mucus also stimulates coughing as the patient tries to clear their airways. Excessive mucus production may continue beyond the acute bronchoconstriction phase and result in more chronic symptoms, when patients are aware that their breathing is not normal even though they are not having an 'asthma attack'.

In an acute asthma attack, the patient is extremely short of breath, usually with a wheeze that is audible to a bystander. The patient often grips on to a chair because this enables the use of the accessory respiratory muscles in addition to the intercostal muscles of the rib cage. As the attack becomes more severe and the bronchioles are more constricted and obstructed by mucus, the wheeze may fade and the ominous 'silent chest' develops. Eventually, the patient is unable to inspire effectively into the overinflated lungs and a respiratory arrest ensues. Even artificial ventilation in a very severe attack may not overcome the very high pressures that exist in the lungs. Using high ventilation pressures may even cause a pneumothorax, in which there is literally a 'blow out' through one of the peripheral alveoli, and air fills the pleural space and restricts lung inflation even further.

PRINCIPLES OF MANAGEMENT

AVOIDANCE OF KNOWN TRIGGERS

Avoidance of known trigger factors, if possible, is crucial. Apart from the allergens already mentioned, there are some well-recognized industrial causes, such as soldering flux, which triggers asthma in susceptible patients in the engineering industry. In the home, the house dust mite is a very common allergen. This mite feeds on house dust, which largely consists of keratin shed from the skin. The mite faeces are dropped in high concentration in bedding and soft furnishings, and allergy to the protein in the droppings can provoke asthma attacks, particularly overnight. Simple measures such as mattress covers, vacuuming the mattress, and wet dusting can reduce the mite population and the frequency and severity of the asthma.

The other principles of management are twofold; to reduce long-term inflammation, and to relieve bronchoconstriction when it occurs (Box 33.1). For both of these purposes, inhaled delivery of the drug to the bronchial tree, rather than as an oral drug, has enabled drugs to be used in minimal doses. This has stimulated advances in the types of inhaler devices available (see Chapter 9).

BRONCHODILATOR THERAPY

Bronchodilators are used for short-term relief of wheezing. They are beta-2-receptor agonists (i.e. they stimulate the beta-receptors that relax the bronchial muscles). Adrenaline and noradrenaline are natural beta-2 agonists but they also stimulate beta-1 receptors in the heart, with potentially serious consequences if they are used therapeutically in high doses. Salbutamol and terbutaline are much more specific for the beta-receptors in the bronchi and are the usual bronchodilators prescribed in the UK.

With a reduction in the bronchoconstriction, the patient gets rapid relief from the distressing symptom of wheezing, but this relief can be short-lived, particularly if the allergen is still present. Patients often rely on these inhalers, using them several times a day to gain quick relief from the symptoms, but this may give a false sense of security as the inflammatory process continues and the situation worsens. In an acute asthma attack, the beta-2 agonist is administered via a nebulizer, which creates a fine mist of the drug, which the patient breathes in through a mask without having to co-ordinate the use of an inhaler.

PROPHYLACTIC TREATMENT
Peak Expiratory Flow Rate Monitoring

If a patient is requiring their bronchodilator more than once a day on a regular basis, they require prophylactic treatment to gain better control. Patients are often unaware of how impaired their breathing is until they gain the benefits of prophylactic treatment. Their improvement can be monitored with a peak expiratory flow rate (PEFR) meter. The PEFR is a simple measure of how fast air can be expelled measured in litres per minute, and is a monitor for airways obstruction. There is a range of normal values for PEFR, based on size, age, and sex, to provide a benchmark for comparison, but more importantly, patients become familiar with their own normal range of PEFR readings. Their PEFR reading will be reduced when the bronchi are obstructed, and it should return to their own normal range when they are using adequate treatment. Patient self-management plans are becoming increasingly important in detecting early deterioration. These plans use PEFR monitoring and give the patient instructions about increasing inhaled treatment and, if necessary, starting oral steroids and seeking medical help. It is hoped that, in the long run, this will reduce hospital admissions and may even prevent some asthma deaths.

Inhaled Corticosteroids and Non-Steroidal Drugs

Prophylactic treatment is either with inhaled corticosteroids or non-steroidal drugs. All have to be used on a daily basis and compliance is the main problem unless the patient fully understands their preventative role. Sodium cromoglycate acts as a mast cell stabilizer to prevent histamine release. It appears to be more effective in young patients, particularly those with exercise-induced asthma.

Inhaled corticosteroids have become the mainstay of prophylactic treatment in asthma (Box 33.1). They work by reducing inflammation and thereby reducing the potential for acute attacks. There were fears of long-term side-effects based mainly on the experience of prolonged use of oral steroids in asthma, which caused adrenal suppression and growth retardation in children. Fortunately, studies have been very reassuring about the low levels of absorption of inhaled steroids, and increasingly, they are used as the maintenance therapy for both adults and children. Oral or intravenous steroids can be lifesaving in an acute asthma attack and fear of side-effects is never a reason to withhold them in these circumstances.

BOX 33.1 Management of chronic asthma

These guidelines are based on the British Thoracic Society guidelines

Step 1
Occasional use of bronchodilator
If bronchodilator therapy is used more than once daily, move to step 2

Step 2
Regular inhaled anti-inflammatory drugs, either sodium cromoglycate or inhaled corticosteroid, twice daily
If asthma is not controlled, move to step 3

Step 3
High-dose inhaled corticosteroid, or low dose inhaled steroid plus long-acting inhaled bronchodilator
If asthma is not controlled, move to step 4

Step 4
High-dose inhaled corticosteroid plus regular bronchodilator. Consider regular nebulized administration and oral theophylline
If asthma is not controlled, move to step 5

Step 5
Regular oral corticosteroid (prednisolone) plus inhaled high-dose steroid plus regular bronchodilator plus long-acting inhaled bronchodilator

STEP UP based on peak expiratory flow rate monitoring and patient's symptoms
STEP DOWN by regular review to achieve lowest step compatible with good control

---

CHRONIC OBSTRUCTIVE PULMONARY DISEASE

The label chronic obstructive pulmonary disease (COPD) has replaced the rather artificial division of chronic bronchitis and emphysema, where clinical features and pathology often overlapped. Chronic bronchitis is a clinical diagnosis of a productive cough for more than 3 months of the year for 2 or more years, and emphysema is a pathological diagnosis made when there is destruction of respiratory tissue

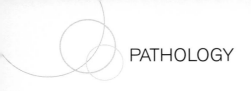

and permanent enlargement of the acini of the lungs the lung unit distal to the terminal bronchiole.

PATHOPHYSIOLOGY

COPD is characterized by the chronic obstruction to air flow in the lungs. In COPD, the amount of air that can be expired in 1 second (the forced expiratory volume or FEV_1) is reduced, and the terminal amount of air at the end of expiration (the residual volume) is increased. The smallest volumes of expired air are associated with the most severe disease.

The chronic bronchitis element of COPD results in hypertrophy of the mucous glands in the bronchi and chronic inflammation and fibrous replacement of muscle in the walls of the bronchioles. The loss of the bronchiolar muscle results in collapse of the bronchioles during expiration, and this, together with the excess mucus, causes airways obstruction. The mucus also encourages the overgrowth of pathogenic bacteria, such as *Haemophilus influenzae*, which cause repeated infections and destruction of lung tissue.

Emphysema results in destruction of lung tissue, mainly in the distal bronchioles. A small group of patients have an inherited deficiency of the $alpha_1$-antitrypsin enzyme, which normally protects the body from the action of its own protein-digesting enzymes. Patients who have inherited this enzyme deficiency develop emphysema at a young age as the lung tissue is destroyed by its own proteolytic enzymes.

Gas transfer is reduced in COPD because the alveoli are reduced in number, particularly in the emphysematous element of the condition. The diffusion capacity of the lung is measured by the transfer of carbon monoxide, which can then be measured in the blood stream. This is the transfer factor (TLCO), which will be reduced in any situation in which oxygen and carbon dioxide cannot diffuse across the alveoli or the alveolar blood supply is impaired.

The major cause of COPD is cigarette smoking, and deaths from COPD can be added to those from lung cancer and atherosclerosis that are caused by smoking.

CLINICAL FEATURES

Shortness of breath (dyspnoea) and a persistent cough are the major symptoms of COPD. As the lung tissue is progressively destroyed, there is decreased oxygenation of the blood with raised carbon dioxide levels, leading to cyanosis. The lung tissue damage also causes changes in the microvasculature and leads to pulmonary hypertension.

Of direct clinical relevance is the respiratory drive that the raised carbon dioxide level causes. Normally, a raised carbon dioxide level stimulates the brain's respiratory centre, but in COPD the centre becomes insensitive to this, and it is the low oxygen levels that stimulate the respiratory effort. If the patient is given a high concentration of oxygen in the belief that it will help their breathing, it raises the oxygen concentration, removing the respiratory drive and possibly precipitating a respiratory arrest. This is why patients with COPD are only given oxygen at 24 per cent concentration, just above the ambient oxygen level of 21 per cent, to preserve the respiratory drive.

MANAGEMENT

The most important element of management is to get the patient to stop smoking to prevent further damage. This will also reduce the ongoing inflammation with excess mucus production with the added complication of repeated infections. Any element of reversible airways obstruction is treated in the same way as asthma, but this may only produce a small effect if any.

The disease can vary in severity, but it often deteriorates with time and the patient becomes more dyspnoeic and cyanosed with a very limited exercise capacity. Patients may require continuous low-dose oxygen to maintain their oxygen levels, as hypoxaemia causes constriction of the blood vessels, making the pulmonary hypertension worse and leading to right heart failure (see Chapter 32).

PULMONARY EMBOLISM

An embolus (impacted material in a blood vessel) in the lung most commonly consists of thrombus, but it may also be made of tumour tissue, amniotic fluid, or air. The embolus has usually travelled from a thrombus in the veins of the legs or pelvis via the inferior vena cava into the right side of the heart and from there into the lung through the pulmonary artery. It causes infarction (tissue death due to ischaemia) of the lung tissue by occluding the supplying arteries as it breaks up and is carried down the arterial tree.

PATHOPHYSIOLOGY

Thrombosis is the formation of a solid mass (thrombus) from blood constituents (red and white blood cells, platelets, and fibrin) within the vascular system, as opposed to clotting, which occurs when blood constituents escape into surrounding tissue or clot in a test tube. A thrombus is composed of layers of aggregated platelets and fibrin, whereas a blood clot is a random collection of fibrin and blood cells (see Chapter 31).

There is a fine balance between normal thrombus formation and dissolution (fibrinolysis), and anything that upsets this balance may predispose to thrombus formation. For example, changes in blood flow (e.g. immobility after surgery or during long journeys) and changes in blood viscosity (e.g. due to polycythaemia – raised red blood cell levels – or thrombocythaemia – raised platelet levels) both make thrombosis more likely.

CLINICAL FEATURES

Any situation in which blood may clot in the legs or pelvis will put the patient at risk of a subsequent pulmonary embolism (PE). This is commonly when the person has been immobile and the normal muscle pump of the calf, which helps to maintain venous return to the heart, has therefore not been working, causing a deep vein thrombosis (DVT). This can happen after surgery when the patient is bed bound, or after a long aircraft or coach journey when the person has not been able to get up and walk around.

A DVT in the leg will usually present as sudden onset of pain and swelling in one calf, although less commonly it occurs in the thigh. A subsequent pulmonary embolus breaking off from this thrombus will cause sudden pain in the chest, shortness of breath and sometimes haemoptysis (coughing up blood). A massive PE, which completely obstructs the pulmonary artery, will cause sudden collapse and often death within a few minutes. A smaller PE may break into smaller pieces and will be carried further out in the arterial tree. As the lung tissue dies through lack of oxygenated blood, the overlying pleura become inflamed and the patient may develop pleuritic pain, which is sharp and worse on breathing and coughing, since the two inflamed layers of pleura grate over each other. This can sometimes be heard through the stethoscope as a pleural rub, which is a clinical sign of pleural inflammation. [A pleural rub may also be heard in other situations, such as pleurisy (infection of the pleura).]

Because the heart must pump harder to overcome the partial obstruction in the pulmonary arteries, there is often tachycardia (raised heart rate) and the patient may become hypoxaemic (low arterial oxygen). This may be clinically obvious as cyanosis, when the patient's lips are blue–grey. As the infarction of the lung segment develops and the tissue dies, an effusion of inflammatory fluid collects at the base of the lung, restricting respiration even further.

Some patients have recurrent multiple pulmonary emboli, sometimes due to an abnormal clotting syndrome, and gradually more and more of the lung tissue dies as more small arteries are obstructed by emboli (Box 33.2). This is normally controllable by long-term

> **BOX 33.2 RISK FACTORS FOR PULMONARY EMBOLISM**
>
> immobility
>   post-operative
>   post-partum
>   prolonged sitting
>
> oral contraceptives
>
> clotting abnormalities
>   thrombocythaemia (increased number of platelets)
>   antithrombin III deficiency
>
> malignancy
>
> pregnancy

anticoagulation with warfarin, but sometimes the infarction continues inexorably destroying lung tissue, and these patients may require lung transplantation to survive (see Chapter 29).

DIAGNOSIS

A chest X-ray is often deceptively normal in PE, particularly in the early stages before pulmonary infarction has developed and there is no effusion to see. The most useful diagnostic test is a ventilation–perfusion (V–Q) scan, in which the patient inhales a radioactive isotope to demonstrate the ventilation pattern of the lung, and an isotope is injected to measure the perfusion of the lung. The two patterns on the scans should match in the normal situation, but when there is a PE, areas of lung without a blood supply will show as missing on the perfusion scan. If there are several emboli there will be multiple filling defects on the scan. However the ventilation scan should be normal in a PE, as there is no obstruction to inhalation. Large mismatched areas on the V–Q scan are highly likely to be due to pulmonary emboli.

TREATMENT

A massive pulmonary embolus is often fatal unless it occurs in or near a hospital and the patient can be rapidly diagnosed and given thrombolytic therapy to

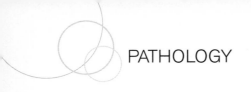
dissolve the clot. Some patients even require an embolectomy (surgical removal of the embolus) with intra-operative cardiac bypass.

Smaller emboli are treated by immediate intravenous heparin and the commencement of oral warfarin as a long-term anticoagulant. Warfarin is usually continued for 3–6 months unless there is chronic embolic disease, in which case it needs to be lifelong.

PREDISPOSING FACTORS AND PREVENTION

Surgical Procedures

Surgical procedures are a common cause of DVT and PE. Thrombi forming in the pelvic veins as the patient sits in bed are clinically silent. When the patient first walks around, the venous return is increased and an embolus may be carried into the pulmonary circulation. Because of this risk, most patients undergoing major surgery are routinely anticoagulated with heparin (usually given subcutaneously) to cover the risk period until they are fully mobile again. Compression stockings are also used; these are graduated in pressure from the ankle upwards to encourage the venous flow back to the heart.

Oral Contraceptives

Oral contraceptives increase the risk of venous thrombosis, especially the third-generation oral contraceptives containing certain progesterones, and these are an added risk factor in surgery. Women should stop the contraceptive pill at least 6 weeks before elective surgery, and emergency surgery should be covered by prophylactic heparin.

Inherited Clotting Abnormalities

Inherited clotting abnormalities such as antithrombin III deficiency predispose to thrombosis and may be an indication for long-term anticoagulation.

Malignancy

Malignancy predisposes to thrombosis, which may be the first presentation of the cancer. In carcinoma of the stomach, superficial thrombophlebitis of the leg veins is known as Trousseau's migratory thrombophlebitis.

Pregnancy, Obesity, and Varicose Veins

These all cause impaired venous return, making DVT more likely.

CARCINOMA OF THE LUNG

Lung cancer is the most common cancer in the UK, killing around 40 000 people a year. Although it occurs more frequently in men than women, the rate in women is increasing, and lung cancer accounts for 1 in 8 of all cancer deaths in women.

AETIOLOGY

Cigarette smoking is the main cause of lung cancer. A heavy smoker has a risk of developing lung cancer that is 20 times higher than a non-smoker's risk. Stopping smoking reduces the risk, and 10 years after stopping the risk is virtually that of a non-smoker. It is still not known which of the thousands of chemicals present in cigarette smoke cause cancer (Figures 33.1 and 33.2). The epithelial cells lining the bronchi of smokers show early changes, known as squamous metaplasia, which can worsen, develop into squamous dysplasia, and finally become carcinoma *in situ*. Metaplasia develops as a response to injury when one differentiated tissue type transforms into another – respiratory to squamous epithelium. Metaplasia is not in itself premalignant but it is a marker of cell damage and may be associated with dysplasia, in which the cells have abnormal nuclei and the potential to become cancerous (see Chapter 5).

Other risk factors for carcinoma of the lung include asbestos (Figure 33.3; also see the section below on pneumoconioses), heavy metal mining, and ionizing radiation.

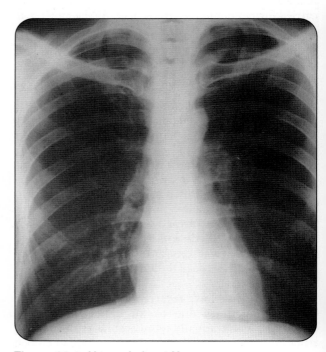

Figure 33.1 Normal chest X-ray.

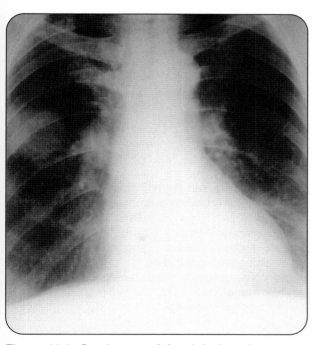

Figure 33.2 Carcinoma of the right lung in a smoker. There is a pleural effusion obscuring the costophrenic angle by the diaphragm.

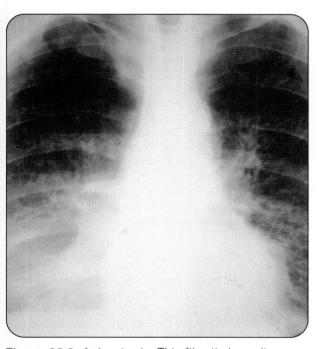

Figure 33.3 Asbestosis. This fibrotic lung disease affects both lungs. In the right lower zone, there is an indistinct, wedge-shaped opacity; this is a carcinoma.

PATHOPHYSIOLOGY

Any cancer can cause disease by local spread and by distant metastases. Squamous cell and small cell (oat cell) tumours are the usual types associated with smoking, while adenocarcinoma tumours are sometimes seen in non-smokers.

Local spread of bronchial carcinoma causes destruction of lung tissue and reduced ventilation capacity. Invasion of blood and lymph vessels allows malignant cells to circulate and establish malignant deposits (metastases) in distant tissues. The lymphatic vessels lead to adjacent lymph nodes, which act as filters and are the commonest site of metastases. The lymph nodes in the lung are commonly involved, as are the nodes in the mediastinum, axillae, and neck. Venous blood from the lungs circulates throughout the body and common sites for metastases are organs with a rich blood supply, such as the liver, brain, bone, kidney, and adrenal glands.

Carcinoma of the lung is often associated with para-neoplastic syndromes, in which there is distant disease in the absence of metastases. These syndromes are thought to be chemically or hormonally mediated and may cause problems such as high blood calcium or cortisol levels, or muscle weakness. Finger clubbing, a common clinical sign in lung cancer, is also thought to be caused in this way.

Staging

The purpose of staging cancers is to try to predict the long-term survival and also to classify appropriate treatments for different stages. The TNM (Tumour Node Metastasis) system is one of several that have been used. For example, $T_1N_1M_0$ means a tumour of less than 3 cm in size that is confined to the lung and that has involvement of the bronchial nodes but no distant metastases (see Chapter 5 for details on the staging of tumours).

CLINICAL FEATURES

The most common lung cancer is a squamous cell carcinoma, which originates within the bronchial wall. Patients may present with haemoptysis (coughing up blood) when the tumour has invaded a blood vessel or with a persistent lung infection when the tumour has blocked the bronchus so that the infection cannot clear. A persistent cough in a smoker or ex-smoker, even without haemoptysis, should prompt a chest X-ray, in which an abnormal shadow may be the first sign of malignancy.

Sometimes the diagnosis is made only when distant metastases have developed. These are commonly in the liver, in which case the patient may present with hepatomegaly (an enlarged liver), or in the brain, in which case the patient may have an epileptic fit. Bony metastases are also common and are sometimes diagnosed when the patient has a pathological fracture.

When lung cancer is associated with paraneoplastic syndromes, the presentation may be confusing. For example, a patient with lung cancer may present with renal colic from a kidney stone that has formed because of high levels of circulating calcium. This in turn is due to high levels of parathyroid hormone, caused not by a disease of the parathyroid glands but by the lung tumour, which is secreting the hormone. This is only discovered as other causes are eliminated (see Chapters 6 and 35). Similarly, a patient may present with the signs and symptoms of myasthenia gravis, a neurological disease characterized by extreme muscle weakness. However, further investigations may reveal a lung cancer as the cause, when it is known as the Eaton–Lambert syndrome. Treating the tumour may relieve the muscle weakness, whereas myasthenia gravis itself requires a different treatment altogether (see Chapter 27).

Other types of lung cancer, such as small cell carcinoma and adenocarcinoma, also often present with cough or haemoptysis, and the histological diagnosis follows later on biopsy.

DIAGNOSIS

The initial investigation to raise suspicions of lung cancer is the chest X-ray, and any abnormal mass or shadowing has to be followed up by a tissue biopsy to confirm malignancy and the histological type. Other disease, including infections, cysts, and benign tumours, may all produce abnormal X-rays and it is crucial to get a tissue diagnosis, not only to give accurate information to the patient, but also to plan treatment, since this varies depending on the tumour (Box 33.3).

A biopsy is usually done endoscopically via a bronchoscope, which is passed through the nose and down into the bronchial tree, from where a biopsy of any abnormal tissue can be taken. If the tumour is very peripheral and the bronchoscope cannot reach far enough, the patient may require an open lung biopsy, which is obviously more invasive and traumatic.

A computerized tomography scan or magnetic resonance imaging is often done to assess the possible spread to lymph nodes within the mediastinum.

TREATMENT

Treatment depends both on the type of tumour and the extent of spread. If the tumour is small and confined to one lobe of the lung without evidence of

---

BOX 33.3 SYMPTOMS AND SIGNS OF LUNG CANCER IN RELATION TO ITS INTRATHORACIC SPREAD

The range of clinical pictures produced by a tumour depends on its site within the chest

peripheral tumour
rib destruction, causing pathological rib fractures
pleural effusion, causing dyspnoea

apical tumour
brachial plexus invasion (Pancoast's tumour), causing pain in the arm
cervical sympathetic nerve involvement (Horner's syndrome), causing constricted pupil, ptosis, and loss of sweating

left hilar tumour
left recurrent laryngeal nerve involvement, causing vocal cord paralysis and a hoarse voice

right paratracheal tumour
superior vena cava obstruction, causing engorgement of the veins of the face and neck

---

metastases, there may be a case for surgical removal of the affected lobe in an attempt to cure the cancer. More commonly, there is spread at the time of diagnosis and treatment is with radiotherapy or chemotherapy or a combination of both. The chances of long-term survival when the tumour has spread are small, although radiotherapy and chemotherapy may prolong life.

Lung Metastases

The lungs are a very common site for metastases from other primary cancers. A solitary lung metastasis from a renal carcinoma is not uncommon and occasionally can be removed surgically. Usually metastatic spread to the lungs represents a significant deterioration in the cancer control, and the treatment is with chemotherapy and is usually palliative rather than curative. One exception to this is in testicular teratoma, in which a young man with a testicular tumour may have lung metastases at presentation. This disease is very sensitive to chemotherapy and there is a good chance of long-term survival even when the disease has spread to the lungs.

PULMONARY FIBROSIS

Pulmonary fibrosis results from damage to the lung tissue, which can be due to a number of factors, including infection, autoimmune disease, and occupational exposure (Box 33.4). The pneumoconioses (e.g. asbestosis and silicosis) are a group of diseases caused by inorganic dust inhalation, which results in fibrosis (Figures 33.4 and 33.5). Extrinsic allergic alveolitis is another occupational lung disease, in which the inhaled material is organic and may provoke an allergic reaction, which ultimately results in lung fibrosis. Farmer's lung and bird fancier's lung are examples of extrinsic allergic alveolitis (see Chapter 26).

It is important that these occupational diseases are recognized and diagnosed, since there are compensation payments available for these patients.

COAL WORKER'S PNEUMOCONIOSIS

Prolonged inhalation of coal dust causes lung damage in 12 per cent of all miners, though up to 50 per cent of anthracite miners with over 20 years of exposure

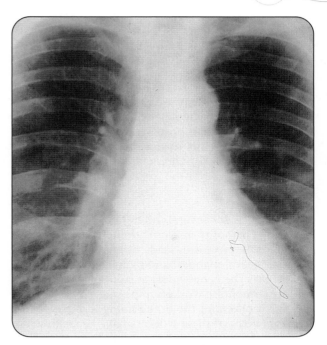

Figure 33.4 Left-sided pleural plaques in asbestosis.

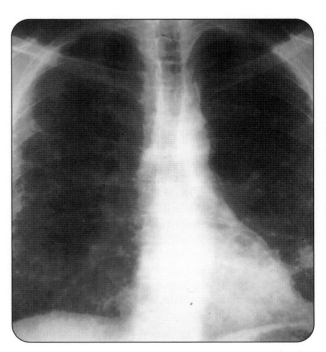

Figure 33.5 Fibrosing alveolitis. This is a cause of pulmonary fibrosis, and it can be seen in both lung fields. This chest X-ray also shows a carcinoma of the lung in the left zone.

BOX 33.4 CAUSES OF PULMONARY FIBROSIS

inhalation of dust or chemicals
mineral dusts (e.g. coal dust, asbestos, silica)
organic dusts (e.g. moulds, avian proteins)
chemicals (e.g. chlorine)

poisons
drugs (e.g. bleomycin)
paraquat
radiation pneumonitis

systemic disease
rheumatoid arthritis
systemic sclerosis
ankylosing spondylitis

unknown cause
cryptogenic fibrosing alveolitis
sarcoidosis

will develop lung fibrosis. Initially, small, black nodules (less than 1.5 mm in diameter) develop in the lung tissue; this is known as simple pneumoconiosis. About 15 per cent of patients develop progressive massive fibrosis, in which the nodules enlarge and may cavitate, along with widespread pulmonary fibrosis.

The miner with simple pneumoconiosis may have no symptoms but, in the progressive form, the lung tissue destruction leads to dyspnoea and pulmonary hypertension with right heart failure (see Chapter 32).

ASBESTOSIS

Asbestos includes several different types of silicates, including chrysolite and crocidolite (blue asbestos). Inhaling asbestos fibres leads to massive pulmonary fibrosis, pleural plaques, and malignancy of the lung and pleura. The people most at risk of asbestos exposure are demolition workers, pipe laggers, boiler makers, and workers in the brake-lining industry. More recently, wives of these workers have been shown to be at risk if they washed their husband's work clothes, which were contaminated with fibres. People living around old asbestos factories are also being diagnosed with asbestos-related lung diseases many years later.

Asbestosis is a progressive disease of fibrosis, involving lung and pleural tissue eventually leading to heart and lung failure. Malignancy, either bronchial carcinoma or mesotheliana, often supervenes as the ultimate cause of death.

The most common malignancy associated with asbestos is lung cancer of the squamous or adenocarcinoma cell type, and smokers who are exposed to asbestos are at particularly high risk. There is also a risk of malignancy of the pleura, mesothelioma, associated with asbestos exposure often 20 to 30 years before.

SILICOSIS

Silicosis results from the inhalation of silica particles, which are a hazard in mining, quarrying, sandblasting and the pottery industry. Again pulmonary fibrosis is the long-term result for some patients, although there is also an acute syndrome with rapid progression and death within a few weeks after short exposure. Sufferers from silicosis are also at increased risk of developing tuberculosis.

EXTRINSIC ALLERGIC ALVEOLITIS

When organic dusts are inhaled, the antigens may provoke antibody formation; if a chronic allergic reaction persists in the lung, fibrosis is the result. In farmer's lung, various fungi in mouldy hay act as antigens; in bird fancier's lung and rat handler's lung, the antigen is a protein found in the animal droppings. Initially, the patient may have an acute illness, with fever, cough, and dyspnoea, which settles until there is further exposure to the antigen. Antibodies to the fungus or protein can often be identified in the patient's serum and this is often very helpful in making the diagnosis (see also Chapter 26).

RESPIRATORY INFECTIONS

Viral upper respiratory tract infections are the most frequent reason for patients attending their general practitioner. They seldom require specific treatment. Lower respiratory tract infections, such as pneumonia, may be both bacterial and viral and may require specific antibiotic treatment. The term 'pneumonia' is used when the lung tissue is infected, whereas 'acute bronchitis' indicates infection of the tracheobronchial tree.

MICROBIOLOGY OF PNEUMONIA

The commonest pneumonia acquired in the community is pneumococcal pneumonia, caused by the bacterium *Streptococcus pneumoniae*. Other bacterial causes are *Haemophilus influenzae*, which usually affects those with pre-existing lung disease, and *Legionella pneumophila*, which can occur in epidemics and is usually acquired from contaminated water in air-conditioning systems or showers.

Viral, chlamydial, and rickettsial pneumonias are less common and are often accompanied by other viral symptoms such as arthralgia (joint pain), myalgia (muscle pain), and headaches.

CLINICAL FEATURES

Most pneumonias present with cough, dyspnoea, and fever; there is also sometimes chest pain, which may be pleuritic in nature – if the pleural covering of the lung is inflamed, it will grate against the pleural layer lining the rib cage, and the patient experiences a sharp, localized, pleuritic pain on inspiration. Sometimes this inflamed area of pleura can be detected through the stethoscope, when a pleural rub (a rough creaking sound on inspiration) is heard. Air entry is reduced on auscultation and, in the case of lobar pneumonia, the chest X-ray shows an area of increased shadowing following the anatomical margins of the lobe (Figure 33.6).

Bacterial pneumonia and bronchitis often lead to the production of purulent sputum, which can be cultured in the laboratory to identify the infecting organ-

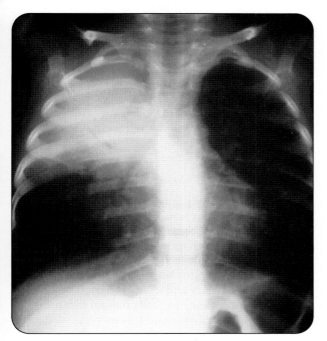

Figure 33.6 Right upper lobe consolidation in lobar pneumonia. There is no loss of lung volume, and air can be seen in the bronchi (air bronchogram) within consolidated tissue.

ism. The sputum is often blood stained owing to the intense inflammatory process. Antibiotics may need to be given by injection to achieve satisfactory blood levels to kill the organisms.

The organisms that commonly cause viral and viral-like pneumonias are:

- the measles virus;
- the chickenpox virus;
- the influenza virus;
- respiratory syncytial virus;
- adenoviruses;
- *Mycoplasma pneumoniae*; and
- *Chlamydia* species (e.g. in psittacosis)

Antibiotics are ineffective in viral pneumonias and only supportive treatment can be given (see Chapter 19).

TUBERCULOSIS

Tuberculosis was a disease that was diminishing until recently, having been a major killer throughout the 19th and early 20th centuries. However, the rates of infection are rising and it is becoming a major public health issue once more. It is still a very common cause of death in the developing world.

PATHOPHYSIOLOGY

The organism which causes tuberculosis, *Mycobacterium tuberculosis*, causes focal inflammation in the lung when it is inhaled by a non-immune person. There is also inflammation of the associated lymph nodes at the same time. The infection usually heals by scarring, and further development of the disease depends on the individual patient's immune response.

Patients who have been infected and who subsequently develop any degree of immunosuppression may become re-infected without being able to mount an adequate immune response, and other areas of the lung become infected or the disease may spread to other organs. Patients who are particularly at risk are those on immunosuppressant drugs (e.g. transplant patients), those with immunodeficiencies (e.g. acquired immunodeficiency syndrome), and those with other diseases (e.g. diabetes mellitus or silicosis). Poor general health and poor nutrition, such as occur in people who misuse alcohol and in people who are homeless, also predispose to tuberculosis.

DIAGNOSIS

Tuberculosis is sometimes detected on a routine X-ray, since many patients will not have any symptoms. This was the rationale behind mass screening X-rays when the disease was common, but the pick-up rate became so low that screening was no longer worthwhile. The symptoms, if any, include a persistent cough, sometimes haemoptysis, weight loss, and night sweats. The organism is very difficult to grow in culture in the laboratory, taking 6–8 weeks.

TREATMENT

A combination of antituberculous drugs must be used to overcome problems of drug resistance. Worryingly, there are strains of tuberculosis currently emerging that are multi-drug resistant, and this is a major problem for the future. The four most commonly used drugs at present are rifampicin, isoniazid, pyrizinamide, and ethambutol.

Another major problem with treatment is compliance. The course of therapy lasts at least 9 months and patients frequently drop out. In the USA, there are programmes in which outreach workers visit patients every day to ensure that they comply with treatment, since one of the causes of increasing drug resistance is poor compliance leading to incomplete treatment courses.

PREVENTION

Social conditions of hygiene and nutrition play a major part in reducing the transmission of tuberculosis as well

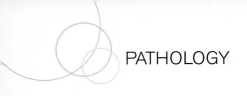

as contact tracing when a case is diagnosed. The Bacille Calmette-Guérin (BCG) immunization gives a mild primary infection and a large element of protection, although not complete protection, against tuberculosis.

CYSTIC FIBROSIS

Cystic fibrosis is the most common genetic disease in Caucasians. The autosomal-recessive gene is carried by about 1 in 20 of the Caucasian population. For the disease to be manifest, the individual must inherit a defective gene from each parent, and the incidence is about 1 in 2000 live births. Each parent who carries one defective gene is known as a carrier. Therefore, when both parents are carriers, each pregnancy has:
- a 1 in 4 chance of producing a child with cystic fibrosis;
- a 1 in 2 chance of producing a child who is a carrier;
- a 1 in 4 chance of producing a child with a normal gene complement.

The disease is rare in Asian and black populations.

PATHOPHYSIOLOGY

The genetic defect is carried on chromosome 7 and is related to a protein that controls the flow of water, and sodium and chloride levels in the cells of the sweat ducts. The mucus-secreting glands in the lungs, pancreas, liver, bowel, and genital tract are abnormal and the ducts become blocked. The defect in the lung causes problems with local defence mechanisms, making the patient vulnerable to repeated bacterial infections and permanent damage to the lung tissue. In the gut, the abnormal pancreatic secretions lead to malabsorption and a high incidence of diabetes mellitus in adult patients.

CLINICAL FEATURES

Suspicions of cystic fibrosis are usually raised in the neonatal period when the child fails to thrive and gain weight or starts to develop repeated chest infections that are slow to respond to treatment (Box 33.5). Newborn babies may present with meconium ileus when meconium, the bowel material that is usually passed when a child is first born, is extremely thick and sticky, and the bowel becomes partially obstructed. If the child is straining to pass the meconium, the rectal mucosa may prolapse through the anus. The malabsorption problem presents as diarrhoea often with very pale stools owing to the high content of fat (steatorrhoea), and the child fails to gain weight.

As the child gets older, there may be continuing problems, with repeated lung infections leading to bronchiectasis (areas of lung destroyed by infection and acting as reservoirs of bacterial colonization and pus). The abnormal cells in the liver may lead to signs of chronic liver damage and cirrhosis, with hepatomegaly (an enlarged liver). Because the cell abnormality also occurs in the genital tract, patients are often infertile, and nearly all male patients have maldevelopment of the vas deferens.

DIAGNOSIS

Once suspicions have been raised, the diagnosis is usually made on a sweat test. The sodium concentration of the sweat is measured; in cystic fibrosis this is found to be abnormally high (greater than 70 mmol/l in children). Prenatal diagnosis is now possible with genetic testing, and some pilot screening programmes have been introduced to try and identify carriers before they undertake a pregnancy so that prenatal diagnosis can be done if requested (see also Chapter 7).

MANAGEMENT

Management of the patient with cystic fibrosis is currently supportive, although research is very active in the field of genetic manipulation with a view to reversing the underlying cellular abnormality.

The respiratory problems are managed with intensive

BOX 33.5 CLINICAL SIGNS OF CYSTIC FIBROSIS

neonatal period
meconium ileus
failure to thrive
rectal prolapse
recurrent respiratory infections

infancy and childhood
bronchiectasis
malabsorption
cirrhosis
portal hypertension

adulthood
bronchiectasis and lung tissue destruction
right heart failure
cirrhosis and portal hypertension, causing oesophageal varices and splenomegaly
infertility

chest physiotherapy, which patients and their parents are taught to administer at home, and antibiotic therapy, which is sometimes administered by nebulizer to try to increase its effectiveness. The infecting organisms are sometimes difficult to eradicate and may become resistant to many of the standard antibiotics.

Oral pancreatic supplements are used as substitutes for the defective pancreatic digestive enzymes, and diabetes mellitus is treated with insulin injections (see Chapter 35).

Patients used to die in childhood, usually from overwhelming respiratory infections, but as management has improved so more are surviving into adulthood. Lung transplants are one possible mode of treatment for patients with cystic fibrosis (see Chapter 29).

RESPIRATORY FAILURE AND VENTILATION

The definition of respiratory failure is based on arterial oxygen and carbon dioxide levels. If the arterial oxygen tension (paO$_2$) is below 8 kPa (normal range 11–13 kPa) or if the arterial carbon dioxide tension (paCO$_2$) is above 6.6 kPa (normal range 4.6–6 kPa) when the patient is breathing air at sea level, then they are said to be in respiratory failure (Box 33.6). This may result from:
- a ventilation problem in which the patient cannot inhale enough oxygen or exhale enough carbon dioxide (e.g. airways obstruction or paralysis of the respiratory muscles); or
- a failure of the gas exchange of oxygen and carbon dioxide (e.g. pulmonary oedema or pulmonary fibrosis)

PRINCIPLES OF MANAGEMENT

The airway must be clear and, if necessary, access must be obtained via a tracheostomy. The oxygen tension of the inspired air can be increased via a mask to try to achieve higher arterial oxygen levels. If the carbon dioxide levels continue to rise, a decision may have to be made to ventilate the patient artificially.

Artificial Ventilation

The ventilator provides the power to force the oxygen mixture into the patient's lungs. If there is a high tissue resistance, such as in the tight bronchoconstriction of an acute asthma attack, high pressures of ventilation may be needed to overcome it. Most artificially ventilated patients are deeply sedated and some are given drugs to paralyse them, and all the ventilatory effort is provided by the machine – controlled mandatory ventilation. However, the ventilator can

> ### BOX 33.6 CAUSES OF RESPIRATORY FAILURE
>
> abnormalities of gas exchange
> acute asthma
> pulmonary oedema
> pulmonary fibrosis
> chronic obstructive pulmonary disease
> pneumonia
>
> abnormalities of ventilation
> neural causes
> cerebral trauma
> drugs
> cervical spinal cord damage
> poliomyelitis
> motor neurone disease
> thoracic cage causes
> chest injury
> thoracic surgery
> kyphoscoliosis
> lung causes
> airway obstruction
> bronchiectasis

also act as a support for the patient's own respiratory efforts in synchronized intermittent mandatory ventilation. This is a specialized field of medicine with rapid advances in techniques and technology (see Person-Centred Study: Adult Respiratory Distress Syndrome).

There can be serious complications with artificial ventilation. The high pressure required to achieve ventilation may cause pressure damage to the lung – barotrauma. Pneumothorax and surgical emphysema may occur when air leaks into the pleural space or the soft tissues. There are also all the other complications of the critically ill, immobile patient, such as pressure sores, DVT, and infection.

Withdrawing artificial ventilation can be another very difficult area. Sedation is withdrawn and the patient is weaned off the ventilator. Patients who have only been ventilated for a short time and whose acute problem has been treated can usually be withdrawn with no problems. However, there are some situations in which withdrawal of ventilation results in deterioration of the arterial blood gases and the patient lapses back in to respiratory failure. This then presents a major dilemma about ongoing treatment with long-term ventilation.

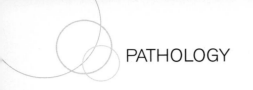

PERSON-CENTRED STUDY: ADULT RESPIRATORY DISTRESS SYNDROME

A serious motorbike accident resulted in Andrew's admission to the intensive care unit of his local hospital. He had fractured both legs and had suffered a head injury as well. He required surgery to his fractures to insert intramedullary nails in both femurs and he had multiple blood transfusions both before and after the surgery. He was artificially ventilated, and over the next few hours the pressures required to inflate his lungs increased (i.e. his lungs became stiffer). At the same time the gas exchange deteriorated, with lower oxygen tensions and raised carbon dioxide tensions. A chest X-ray showed widespread infiltration, confirming the diagnosis of adult respiratory distress syndrome (ARDS).

ARDS results from 'leaky' capillaries that allow fluid and blood cells to accumulate in the alveoli, thereby compromising ventilation and gas exchange. The underlying mechanism of capillary endothelial damage may result from a variety of serious factors, including trauma, septicaemia, drug overdoses, and inhaled toxins.

In addition to artificial ventilation, there were three mainstays of Andrew's treatment; first, to try to maintain his fluid balance so as not to overload the lungs any further yet maintain perfusion in other vital organs such as the brain and kidneys; second, to give him very high concentrations of inspired oxygen to improve gas exchange, though this cannot be maintained for too long since a high inspired oxygen concentration causes pulmonary damage in itself; and third to treat infection with intravenous, broad-spectrum antibiotics.

Sadly, despite all these efforts, Andrew died 48 hours later having developed acute renal failure as well as ARDS. The overall mortality of ARDS is 50–70 per cent, and supervening renal failure makes survival very unusual.

KEY POINTS

- Asthma is characterized by bronchial hyper-reactivity and inflammation. The incidence of asthma is rising due to a variety of possible factors. Inhaled bronchodilators and corticosteroids form the basis for treatment.
- Smoking is a primary risk factor for chronic obstructive pulmonary disease. The progressive destruction of the lung tissue leads to pulmonary hypertension and right heart failure.
- A pulmonary embolus usually originates from a deep vein thrombosis in the leg or pelvic veins. Most post-operative pulmonary emboli can be prevented by anticoagulation with heparin, early mobilization, and compression stockings.
- Smoking causes lung cancer, with a rising death rate in women. Lung cancer frequently metastasizes to the liver, brain, and bone, and may cause paraneoplastic syndromes by abnormal secretion of hormones.

- Pulmonary fibrosis destroys lung tissue and causes secondary heart failure. Asbestos exposure causes lung and pleural fibrosis, lung cancer and malignant mesothelioma. Pneumoconioses are caused by the inhalation of inorganic dusts, whereas organic dust inhalation leads to extrinsic allergic alveolitis.
- Most upper respiratory tract infections are viral. *Streptococcus pneumoniae* and *Haemophilus influenzae* are the usual infective agents in bacterial pneumonia. The incidence of tuberculosis is rising and multiple drug resistance is emerging.
- Cystic fibrosis is an inherited disease caused by an abnormal autosomal-recessive gene. Screening is now available to determine carrier status.
- Respiratory failure is the inability to maintain normal arterial oxygen and carbon dioxide levels. Artificial ventilation can overcome short-term ventilatory failure, but there can be significant long-term problems.

Chest X-rays reproduced with kind permission of Dr. C. George, Consultant Radiologist, Epsom General Hospital. Epsom, UK.

FURTHER READING

The British Guidelines on Asthma Management (1997) 1995 Review and Position Statement. Thorax 52: Supp 1.

Cross JJ, Kemp PM, Flower CD (1997) Diagnostic imaging in pulmonary embolic disease. Br J Hosp Med 58:93–6.

Davis CL (1997) ABC of palliative care: breathlessness, cough and other respiratory problems. BMJ 315:931–4.

Farrell PM, Kosorok MR, Laxova A, *et al.* (1997) Nutritional benefits of neonatal screening for cystic fibrosis. Wisconsin Cystic Fibrosis Neonatal Screening Study Group. N Engl J Med 337:963–9.

Greenberger PA (1997) Immunologic aspects of lung diseases and cystic fibrosis. JAMA 278:1924–30.

Hackshaw AK, Law MR, Wald NJ (1997) The accumulated evidence on lung cancer and environmental tobacco smoke. BMJ 315:980–8.

Haire WD (1998) Vena caval filters for the prevention of pulmonary embolism. N Engl J Med 338:463–4.

Hudson LD (1998) Protective ventilation for patients with acute respiratory distress syndrome. N Engl J Med 338:385–7.

Rees J, Price JF (1999) ABC of Asthma 4th ed (in press). BMJ Books, London.

Roche N, Huchon GJ (1997) Current issues in the management of chronic obstructive pulmonary diseases. Respirology 2:215–29.

Rosenstein BJ, Zeitlin PL (1997) Cystic fibrosis. Lancet 351:277–82.

Souhami RL, Moxham J (1997) Textbook of Medicine, 3rd edition. Churchill Livingstone, Edinburgh.

Van Schayck CP (1996) Primary and Secondary Care Respiratory Specialists Working Group. Diagnosis of asthma and chronic obstructive pulmonary disease in general practice. Br J Gen Pract 46:193–7.

Xu X, Rijcken B, Schouten JP, Weiss ST (1997) Airways responsiveness and development and remission of chronic respiratory symptoms in adults. Lancet 350:1431–4.

Wagner GR (1997) Asbestosis and silicosis. Lancet 349:1311–15.

Weg JG, Anzueto A, Balk RA, *et al.* (1998) The relation of pneumothorax and other air leaks to mortality in the acute respiratory distress syndrome. N Engl J Med 338(6):341–6.

Yang SP, Luh KT, Yang PC (1996) New developments in diagnosis and management of lung cancer. Respirology 1:39–47.

34

DISEASES OF THE GUT, LIVER, AND BILIARY TRACT

LEARNING OBJECTIVES

After studying this chapter students should have a clearer understanding of:
- the current theories and principles of management of peptic ulceration
- inflammatory bowel disease and diarrhoeal diseases
- the different bowel malignancies and their presentation and incidence
- the causes of jaundice and the principles of management of liver failure
- the different types of hepatitis and their routes of transmission, and preventative measures

You should have a basic understanding of the anatomy and physiology of the gastrointestinal tract and the liver and biliary tract.

INTRODUCTION

Disorders of the gastrointestinal tract, liver, and biliary tracts are significant health problems in developing countries and Western society. This chapter describes the techniques used to investigate these anatomical structures and the more common disorders encountered in clinical practice.

INVESTIGATIONS OF THE GASTROINTESTINAL TRACT AND LIVER

Visualization of the gastrointestinal tract is achieved by either inserting a fibreoptic endoscope into the tract or by radiology. Endoscopy can examine the upper gastro-oesophageal tract. Colonoscopy is used for inspecting the lower gastrointestinal tract.

IMAGING TECHNIQUES

A plain abdominal X-ray may reveal gallstones in the gall bladder, an enlarged organ such as the spleen displacing air-filled loops of bowel, or fluid levels in the bowel signifying obstruction of the gastrointestinal tract. Free gas under the diaphragm suggests intestinal perforation, either from an ulcer (benign or malignant) or diverticular disease of the colon.

Barium examinations enable a more detailed inspection of the gastrointestinal anatomy by using a radio-opaque substance. The substance can either be swallowed by the patient (i.e. a barium swallow or barium meal) or injected into the colon from the rectum (i.e. a barium enema). A double-contrast radiological image is visible when the gut mucosa has a thin barium coating. This coating is achieved by also giving the patient effervescents to distend the stomach or air to distend the colon. Accordingly, these techniques will reveal strictures or ulcers in the oesophagus, eroding ulcers, or protruding tumours in the stomach or intestine, as well as the features of inflammatory disease of the small and large bowel.

Ultrasound is particularly helpful in investigation of liver diseases, and it will reveal the presence of liver abscesses, tumours, gallstones, and an enlarged or inflamed gall bladder as well as abnormalities of the hepatic biliary and vascular systems.

Computerized tomography (CT) scans of the abdomen are also valuable in the investigation of hepatic lesions and assist in the diagnosis of cirrhosis and other diffuse pathological changes in the liver. CT scan is probably the preferred method for investigating pancreatic disease. Magnetic resonance imaging (MRI) is valuable as a complementary imaging method to CT scanning, and is important in the diagnosis and assessment of colonic and rectal tumours, as well as recurrent colorectal cancer.

ENDOSCOPY

Endoscopic examinations may also be used as part of a therapeutic intervention (e.g. the injection of bleeding oesophageal varices), to obtain tissue for histological examination, and to perform intracavity ultrasound, sometimes called endoscopic sonography. There is now growing experience in performing abdominal operations, such as splenectomy, or cholecystectomy, using a laparoscope. (See Chapter 6 for information on laboratory investigations of the gut and liver.)

PEPTIC DISEASE

The stomach acts as a reservoir for food and initiates digestion by secreting enzymes. The gastric cells in the lining of the stomach also secrete hydrochloric acid, which provides the optimum pH for the enzyme action, and intrinsic factor, a polypeptide required for the absorption of vitamin B12 (see Chapters 27 and 31). However, in some circumstances, the acidic environment may damage the mucosal lining of the stomach and the duodenum. This produces inflammatory changes (gastritis and duodenitis) and gives rise to symptoms of dyspepsia (indigestion), which refers to upper abdominal discomfort experienced after meals, sometimes accompanied by nausea.

OESOPHAGITIS

Weakness or relaxation of the gastro-oesophageal sphincter may lead to reflux of the acid contents of the stomach up into the oesophagus, causing oesophagitis (irritation or even ulceration of the oesophageal lining). Oesophagitis gives rise to the symptoms of heartburn – pain (often described as 'burning' pain) and discomfort just behind the sternum coming on after food, particularly at night. Herniation of the upper part of the stomach through the diaphragm (i.e. hiatus hernia), facilitates the reflux of acid into the oesophagus, and reflux oesophagitis and hiatus hernia often co-exist.

GASTRITIS

Gastritis may cause a range of symptoms, from none at all to dyspepsia, to sudden haemorrhage from gastric erosions. The distinction between peptic ulceration and the so-called 'non-ulcer dyspepsia' is based on the findings at endoscopy. Thus, patients with typical 'dyspeptic' symptoms who have signs of inflammation on biopsy but no frank ulceration are classified as having non-ulcer dyspepsia. A diagnostic problem arises because the symptoms of non-ulcer dyspepsia may be due to reflux oesophagitis or irritable bowel syndrome.

PEPTIC ULCERATION

Peptic ulceration is ulceration of the gastric or duodenal mucosa. It presents with upper abdominal pain, usually after eating. Studies that have evaluated its pathogenesis have identify personality variables, such as anxiety, conflict, and stress, as having a positive correlation with peptic ulcer disease. However, in the past few years, infection with *Helicobacter pylori* has been recognized as being a major factor in the causation of both gastritis and duodenal ulceration. This Gram-negative bacterium lives in the mucus overlying the gastric epithelial cells and is mainly transmitted by the faeco-oral route. *Helicobacter pylori* is now considered to be the most common cause of chronic gastritis. It is also found in up to 95 per cent of patients with duodenal ulcers. Important evidence that *Helicobacter pylori* infection is causally linked to peptic ulcer disease has been provided by the finding that successful treatment of the infection speeds up the healing of the peptic ulcer.

Another important risk factor for the development of peptic ulceration is the habitual use of non-steroidal anti-inflammatory drugs. These drugs, which include aspirin and many of the drugs prescribed for arthritic complaints, such as ibuprofen, are thought to cause direct damage to the mucosa and to inhibit prostaglandin synthesis (see Chapter 10). Management of dyspepsia includes the use of antacids or of drugs that reduce the acid secretion in the stomach (e.g. omeprazole). If infection with *Helicobacter pylori* is demonstrated, antibiotic treatment to eradicate the bacteria may speed up the resolution of the condition. The regimen is triple therapy with a bismuth compound, tetracycline, and metronidazole; this is successful in more than 80 per cent of cases.

The most significant complication of duodenal ulcer disease is haemorrhage. Erosion of a blood vessel at the base of the ulcer can cause haemorrhage, which may be catastrophic. Upper gastrointestinal haemorrhage is a common presentation of peptic ulceration, though it can also be caused by gastritis. Altered blood in the stool may be found; this is termed melaena, and is characterized by black stools with a characteristic odour. Blood in the stomach may also be vomited up (haematemesis), where the appearance is described typically as 'coffee grounds'. Chronic blood loss may lead to an iron-deficient anaemia, and the patient presents with symptoms of anaemia without a history of any blood loss (see Chapter 31).

GASTROINTESTINAL HAEMORRHAGE

The gastrointestinal tract is usually divided into the upper and lower tract, the anatomical boundary being the junction of the duodenum and jejunum. Bleeding from the upper tract typically presents as haematemesis or melaena (see above), and bleeding from the lower tract presents as frank blood per rectum. Gastrointestinal haemorrhage may present as acute, chronic, or intermittent episodes of bleeding.

When a patient presents with an acute massive bleed, the main priority in the clinical management is to stabilize blood pressure and intravascular volume. Any large amounts of blood in the stomach should be evacuated by nasogastric suction. In an upper gastrointestinal bleed, endoscopy to diagnose the site of bleeding should be performed as soon as is feasible. With lower gastrointestinal bleeds a colonoscopy may be necessary, but if this is unsuccessful, an angiogram is performed. This involves cannulating the femoral vein and injecting contrast into the vessel. The bleeding spot should show up as a leak of contrast outside the vascular system. Angiography should be done as soon as possible, since active bleeding provides a better opportunity for demonstrating the site of blood loss. In some instances, angiography allows therapeutic intervention, such as embolization of the bleeding vessel. Various strategies are available for the management of gastrointestinal haemorrhaging. For example, inserting a tube with inflatable balloons to compress bleeding varices in the oesophagus and upper stomach (Sengstaken tube) is still a common option. Endoscopic methods include the injecting of bleeding varices, or using lasers to 'burn' out peptic ulcers.

IRRITABLE BOWEL SYNDROME

The irritable bowel syndrome is a functional bowel disorder with episodes of abdominal pain, disordered defaecation, and abdominal distension. Although there is a high prevalence of irritable bowel syndrome in Western countries, it also occurs in other parts of the world, including the Far East and southern European countries. The pathogenesis of irritable bowel syndrome remains a mystery, although disordered gut motility, certain foods, inflammation, and stress have all been implicated.

The criteria for diagnosis of irritable bowel syndrome have been drawn up by an international working team (Box 34.1). One of the problems of diagnosing this condition is that the diagnosis rests solely on symptoms. Care must be taken to exclude structural bowel disease. For diagnosis, sigmoidoscopy findings, the full blood count, and the erythrocyte sedimentation rate (ESR) should all be normal. Despite the high prevalence of this disorder (as established by questionnaires), only a small proportion of people consult their doctor. The reason for the consultation may be an important clue to management. For example, the patient may have a fear of cancer, have had recent stressful or emotional life events, have had previous physical or sexual abuse, or have anxiety or depression. Constipation should be managed with a high-fibre diet, perhaps together with an osmotic laxative such as magnesium sulphate or lactulose. Antispasmodics such as mebeverine may give some relief. Peppermint oil may be useful in patients with constipation and bloating. Diarrhoea can be managed with loperamide. It is important to remember that around one-third of patients will get better whatever medication is prescribed and that reassurance and a caring attitude are equally important. Dyspeptic symptoms may respond to metoclopramide or antacids, and anxiolytic or antidepressant drugs may help some patients.

DIARRHOEAL DISEASES

Diarrhoea implies that the daily volume of stool is greater than normal (300 cm^2 in the UK) and has a

---

> ### BOX 34.1 SYMPTOM CRITERIA FOR IRRITABLE BOWEL SYNDROME
>
> At least 3 months of:
> Abdominal pain or discomfort that is:
> • relieved with defaecation; and/or
> • associated with change in frequency of stool; and/or
> • associated with a change in consistency of stool, and
>
> Two or more of the following:
> • altered stool frequency;
> • altered stool consistency;
> • sensation of straining or urgency;
> • passage of mucus;
> • bloating or feeling of abdominal distension.

more fluid consistency than normal. The additional features include an increased frequency of bowel motions, and sometimes there may be urgency or even incontinence. The major factor that determines the volume and consistency of the stool is colonic motility, which is under the influence of neurological factors and endogenous chemical messengers released by the gut (notably glucagon and vasoactive intestinal peptide). Even with normal colonic function, excess unabsorbed dietary material may lead to diarrhoea. It is useful to divide diarrhoea and its causes into acute and chronic (Box 34.2).

GASTROENTERITIS

Gastroenteritis is a self-limiting infection within the lumen of the gastrointestinal tract. It results in diarrhoea and abdominal pain, which come on suddenly, often with vomiting. Virus infections are the most common cause, particularly in outbreaks in the winter months. Bacteria may invade the gut mucosa or may exert their effects through toxins. Infections of the gastrointestinal tract are most frequently acquired by eating contaminated food; however, person-to-person transmission is also possible. Travellers from industrialized countries visiting developing areas of the world are most at risk.

The most common bacterial organisms are *Escherichia coli* and *Shigella sonnei* (Box 34.3). *Salmonella* species and *Campylobacter* species continue to contaminate

chicken flocks. Water in swimming pools may become contaminated by the faeces of young children; cysts of *Giardia lamblia* and *Cryptosporidium* species can survive in chlorinated water for long periods of time. The incubation period depends on the organism.

Bloody diarrhoea is more likely to be due to *Shigella* species or *Campylobacter* species, and vomiting is characteristic of infection with *Bacillus cereus*. Systemic features, such as fever, headache and muscle pains, are common in *Shigella*, *Campylobacter*, or *Yersinia enterocolitica* infections. Symptoms usually subside after 24–96 hours (see Chapters 16 and 17). The very young, the elderly, and the immunosuppressed are particularly vulnerable and may go on to develop septicaemia, with a high mortality.

Persistent diarrhoea may be due to secondary lactase deficiency, a viral infection (especially in children), infection with *Giardia lamblia*, or the unmasking of inflammatory bowel disease. Patients who have recovered from an episode of gastroenteritis caused by *Salmonella* species may continue to excrete the organism in the stool, and hence are asymptomatic but infectious carriers (see Chapter 20).

BOX 34.2 CAUSES OF DIARRHOEA

Acute diarrhoea
- infections (gastroenteritis, dysentery, giardiasis, amoebiasis)
- food poisoning
- drug induced diarrhoea
- laxatives
- ischaemic colitis
- travellers' diarrhoea
- overflow incontinence

Chronic diarrhoea
- irritable bowel syndrome
- diverticular disease
- carcinoma of the colon
- inflammatory bowel disease (ulcerative colitis, Crohn's disease)
- malabsorption
- hyperthyroidism

BOX 34.3 COMMON CAUSES OF ACUTE GASTROENTERITIS

Bacterial pathogens
Salmonella species
Shigella species
Campylobacter species
Yersinia enterocolitica
Clostridium perfringens
Clostridium difficile *
Escherichia coli *
Staphylococcus aureus *
Bacillus cereus *
Vibrio cholerae *
Vibrio parahaemolyticus *
Clostridium botulinum *

Viral pathogens
rotavirus
Norwalk agent
echovirus

Other agents
Giardia lamblia
Cryptosporidium species
alcohol

* action is through production of a toxin

Some patients with gastroenteritis may develop symptoms related to organs outside the gut, such as a reactive arthritis affecting mainly large joints. This may be accompanied by conjunctivitis and orogenital ulceration (Reiter's syndrome), particularly following an infection with *Yersinia enterocolitica* or *Campylobacter* species. Erythema nodosum is also seen after these particular infections.

Uncomplicated gastroenteritis does not require further investigations and is generally managed with fluid replacement to correct any problems of dehydration, and resting the gut for 24–48 hours. Investigation is indicated:

- in older adults;
- if more than one person is affected;
- if symptoms persist for more than 4 days;
- if there is associated bleeding;
- if there are non-gastrointestinal features (see above); or
- if gastroenteritis occurs in a residential home.

Antibiotics are not usually needed to treat an acute episode of gastroenteritis. If they are needed, however, ciprofloxacin may be used to treat *Salmonella* septicaemia, haemorrhagic colitis caused by *Escherichia coli* infection, *Shigella* or *Campylobacter* infection. *Giardia lamblia* is treated with tinidazole. *Clostridium difficile*, which can cause pseudomembranous colitis, is treated with metronidazole or vancomycin (see also Chapter 19).

Some infections, including *Giardia lamblia*, *Escherichia coli*, and some viruses may cause damage to mucosal cells, which may progress to a condition called partial villous atrophy. In this condition, the intestinal villi are shortened and there is an inflammatory cell infiltrate in the lamina propria.

OTHER GASTROINTESTINAL INFECTIONS
Intestinal Tuberculosis

This is caused by *Mycobacterium tuberculosis* or *Mycobacterium bovis*, which are acquired either by ingestion or via blood-borne spread. It is more common in individuals from the Indian subcontinent, Africa, South America, or south-east Asia. Patients have recurrent abdominal pain, fever, weight loss, or diarrhoea. Some develop tuberculous peritonitis with ascites. Many have a strongly positive Mantoux test (see Chapter 26); microbiological culture of biopsy specimens is necessary in order to determine antibiotic sensitivities. Treatment is with quadruple therapy (isoniazid, rifampicin, pyrazinamide, and ethambutol for 2 months, followed by isoniazid and rifampicin for 4 months).

Typhoid

Typhoid fever (caused by *Salmonella typhi*) and paratyphoid fever (caused by *Salmonella paratyphi*) still occur in the UK. Patients develop fever with headache, and a period of constipation precedes the diarrhoea. The characteristic faint 'rose spots' rash is often missed. Untreated cases may suffer complications such as haemorrhage and bowel perforation. Treatment is with chloramphenicol; however, resistant strains may need treatment with ciprofloxacin.

Amoebiasis

This is common in the tropics and subtropics, and amoebic dysentery has a similar presentation to ulcerative colitis (see below). Occasionally, hepatic cysts may form; these may rupture into the pleural, peritoneal, or pericardial cavities. Diagnosis is made on finding the amoebae in fresh, warm stools. Amoebiasis is treated with metronidazole.

Schistosomiasis

This infection is endemic in Africa, Asia, and South America. The parasite schistosoma has an animal vector, the fresh-water snail. Most infections are asymptomatic but some patients may develop a skin rash or an acute illness with fevers, shakes, diarrhoea, cough, and hepatosplenomegaly.

Other parasites, apart from amoeba and schistosoma, that may infect the gut include *Strongyloides stercoralis*, *Trichuris trichuria*, *Enterobius vermicularis* (threadworm), *Ascaris lumbricoides* (roundworm), and *Trichinella spiralis*.

INFLAMMATORY BOWEL DISEASE

The term 'inflammatory bowel disease' is widely accepted as referring to two distinctive disorders, ulcerative colitis and Crohn's disease. Other conditions involving inflammation of the colon, such as dysentery or diverticulitis, are excluded.

CROHN'S DISEASE

Crohn's disease affects around 40 in 100 000 of the population. The incidence has increased markedly since the 1950s but has now reached a plateau. The disease usually presents in the second and third decade of life and is more common in smokers. A number of studies have suggested that *in utero* exposure to viral infections such as measles is an influential risk factor. Genetic factors are important, as evidenced by clustering within families and ethnic groups, although no strong evidence of an HLA linkage has been found.

PATHOLOGY

The pathological manifestation of Crohn's disease is one of chronic inflammation that affects the whole thickness of the gut lining (i.e. it is transmural), and hence there is a tendency to form fistulae or strictures. The disease may affect any part of the gastrointestinal tract, often in a discontinuous fashion. The sites most frequently affected are the terminal ileum and the proximal colon. The rectum is not often involved, although the perianal region is, and this can give rise to fistulae and abscesses which are very difficult to treat.

Clinical Features

Patients have symptoms of diarrhoea, abdominal pain, and weight loss; severe diarrhoea suggests colonic disease. Fever, malaise, and anorexia occur during acute exacerbations of the disease. Up to one-third of patients with colonic disease have symptoms outside the gut, such as inflammation and arthritic pain in the sacroiliac joints and fatty liver (see also Chapter 39).

Investigative Findings

Typical radiological features include strictures, fistulae, 'rose-thorn ulcers', and a 'cobblestone' appearance of the diseased mucosa (Figure 34.1). The diagnosis is made on the symptoms, biopsy of affected mucosa (a significant proportion have microscopic granulomas; see also Chapter 26), and radiological examination of the bowel. Patients are often anaemic with or without iron deficiency, with a high ESR and elevated platelet count (as a response to blood loss) during exacerbations of the disease.

Treatment

Mild attacks are treated with oral corticosteroids, which can usually be withdrawn carefully once the symptoms have settled. In patients in whom steroid withdrawal is difficult, sulphasalazine or mesalazine may be tried. Patients with perianal disease may benefit from antibiotics such as metronidazole and ciprofloxacin.

In severe attacks, patients are very ill, with vomiting, fever, abdominal pain, and tachycardia. They should be admitted to hospital to be given intravenous fluids, hydrocortisone, and antibiotics. Fluids may be allowed by mouth, but no solid foods are allowed. Once symptoms are subsiding, feeding may be restarted, together with oral prednisolone. Response should be monitored by symptoms and signs (bowel frequency, pain, anorexia, fever, tachycardia, abdominal tenderness) and blood tests, including ESR and C-reactive protein. Once appetite has returned and abdominal tenderness resolves, patients can be discharged home on a reducing dose of steroids.

Failure to respond may be due to complications, such as fistulae, abscesses, perforation, or intestinal obstruction from strictures; it may be an indication for surgery. Up to 80 per cent of patients have an operation at some stage of their disease, which may be performed for any of the conditions mentioned above. A limited resection of the affected bowel may be required for symptomatic disease that remains unresponsive to medical treatment. Intravenous hydrocortisone should be given to cover the operation and the postoperative period until the patient is eating and drinking; after this, a decreasing dose of oral prednisolone is prescribed. Local surgery for perianal fistulae, abscesses, or ulcers should be avoided because recurrences are common.

ULCERATIVE COLITIS

Ulcerative colitis is an inflammatory disease that affects the mucosa of the colon. Symptoms are typically cyclic, with relapse followed by periods of remission. Ulcerative colitis is twice as common as Crohn's disease, affecting up to 80 per 100 000 of the population. Most patients present between the ages of 15 and 30 years, and there is a second peak incidence at around 60 years. There are familial associations, and 15 per cent of patients have a family member with either Crohn's disease or ulcerative colitis. The disease is twice as common in non-smokers.

Clinical Features

Patients present with bloody diarrhoea, usually with mucus; cramping abdominal discomfort is common. Severe persistent pain suggests a different diagnosis. In an acute attack, there may be fever, malaise and abdominal tenderness. Up to 20 per cent of patients

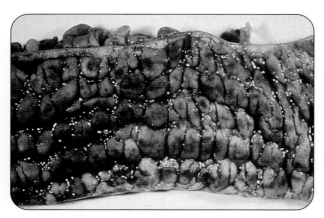

Figure 34.1 Cobblestone appearance of the intestinal mucosa in Crohn's disease. This is a typical feature of the disease. ©Medical Illustration, Addenbrooke's NHS Trust, Cambridge, UK.

have symptoms relating to organs outside the gut. Primary sclerosing cholangitis affects about 2 per cent of patients, and arthritis in large joints is a well-known association.

Complications of ulcerative colitis include toxic dilatation of the colon, which may lead to perforation, severe haemorrhage, and colonic carcinoma.

Investigative Findings

Sigmoidoscopy reveals diffuse mucosal changes; the biopsy specimen shows inflammatory infiltrate, glandular disruption, and crypt abscesses. Typical radiological findings are a granular mucosa, loss of haustra (the transverse indentations in the colon), and pseudopolyps. Blood tests may show anaemia, raised white cell count, and a raised ESR or C-reactive protein, which are all indicative of severe disease. In addition, such patients are likely to have a low serum albumin and potassium levels owing to the chronic loss of protein and electrolytes in the colon.

Treatment

The principles of management in ulcerative colitis are prompt treatment of acute attacks, maintenance therapy to prevent relapses, selection of patients for colectomy, and early detection of colorectal carcinoma. Mild-to-moderate acute attacks are treated with oral corticosteroids, together with corticosteroid enemas and sulphasalazine (or mesalazine).

Patients with severe attacks should be admitted to hospital for surgical assessment and radiological monitoring. Plain abdominal X-rays may have to be performed daily in order to detect dilatation and perforation. These patients require intravenous steroids in the form of hydrocortisone, as well as rectal steroids, which can be given as hydrocortisone in normal saline, dripped through an intravenous giving set into the rectum. Oral intake should be restricted to sips of fluid only, with intravenous fluids given for hydration and potassium replacement. Daily blood tests are required to monitor the full blood count and electrolytes. Patients who deteriorate or fail to respond after a week should be considered for a colectomy. This is an operation in which the colon is resected and the ileum is anastomosed to the rectal stump (an ileorectal anastomosis).

Proctitis (disease which is confined to the sigmoid colon and rectum) is treated with local steroids and sulphasalazine, but it may be difficult to treat even when oral steroids are used.

The rate of acute attacks (relapses) can be reduced by sulphasalazine (and mesalazine or olsalazine are just as effective) and such treatment should be continued for life. The risk of colorectal cancer increases with the extent and duration of disease, but it is still low, with a cumulative probability of 3 per cent at 15 years and 5 per cent at 20 years. Disease that is confined to the colon distal to the splenic flexure is not associated with an increased risk of cancer, and one study suggests that the risk of developing colorectal carcinoma is similar whether patients have extensive colitis or just left-sided disease.

MALABSORPTION

Malabsorption can be caused by abnormal digestion, mucosal disease, or structural abnormalities of the gastrointestinal tract. Patients may present with diarrhoea, weight loss, lassitude, or abdominal discomfort. Stool may be bulky and chalky, with oil globules that float after flushing; this is called steatorrhoea and is due to inadequate digestion of fat. It occurs in pancreatic disease and in obstructive jaundice. Malabsorption can occur without diarrhoea, such as in coeliac disease (gluten-sensitive enteropathy) or bacterial overgrowth (Box 34.4).

Coeliac Disease (Gluten-Sensitive Enteropathy)

Coeliac disease, also called gluten-sensitive enteropathy, is defined as villous atrophy (flattened villi) of the small intestine that resolves when gluten is withdrawn from the diet. Gluten is a protein derived from wheat, rye, and barley but not from oats, maize, or rice. The toxic substance is alpha-gliadin; however the mechanism that leads to the characteristic pathological features of the villi is unclear (Figures 34.2 and 34.3). The diagnosis is made on jejunal biopsy and treatment is with a gluten-free diet.

BOX 34.4 CAUSES OF MALABSORPTION

coeliac disease (gluten-sensitive enteropathy)
chronic pancreatitis
cirrhosis
Crohn's disease
biliary obstruction
post infection
tropical sprue
parasites
bacterial overgrowth
drugs (e.g. cholestyramine)
short bowel syndrome
pancreatic cancer

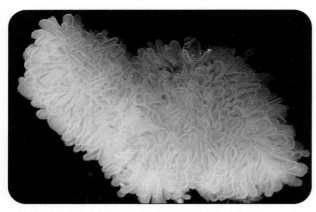

Figure 34.2 Section of healthy jejunum with evidence of villi. ©Medical Illustration, Addenbrooke's NHS Trust, Cambridge, UK.

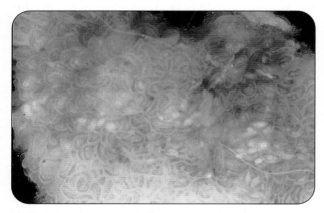

Figure 34.3 Typical flattened villi found in coeliac disease (gluten-sensitive enteropathy). ©Medical Illustration, Addenbrooke's NHS Trust, Cambridge, UK.

Coeliac disease may present at any age, and it is usually diagnosed as failure to thrive in infancy, slow growth in childhood, or nutritional deficiencies in adulthood. Patients may have aphthous ulcers, and hyposplenism is common. Nutritional deficiencies give rise to many of the classical clinical features. Folate deficiency leads to a megaloblastic anaemia, while vitamin D deficiency leads to bone pain and muscle weakness (myopathy). Coeliac disease is also associated with non-intestinal clinical features including dermatitis herpetiformis (a characteristic, intensely itchy skin rash on the elbows and buttocks). Diabetes, thyrotoxicosis, and arthritis are also found in association with coeliac disease. A small proportion (less than 5 per cent) of patients develop non-Hodgkin's lymphoma of the small intestine.

Tropical Sprue

Tropical sprue is the term given to a post-infective malabsorption syndrome that occurs in adults living in India, Asia and Central America. Following an acute attack of diarrhoea, mucosal damage leads to secondary bacterial overgrowth and secondary lactase deficiency. Treatment is with tetracycline.

Giardiasis is another common cause of malabsorption.

INVESTIGATION OF DIARRHOEA

Stool samples should be sent to the microbiology department (see Chapter 17). These should be examined by microscopy for *Giardia lamblia* (and other parasites and ova if the patient has been abroad). In immunodeficient patients, the presence of cysts of *Cryptosporidium* should also be looked for (see Chapter 18). Culture for *Salmonella, Shigella, Campylobacter and Yersinia* species should be carried out. Patients who have recently been on antibiotics may have *Clostridium difficile* infection; this is diagnosed by an assay for the toxin. During outbreaks, or in young children, electron microscopy is used to detect viruses.

A number of patients with Crohn's disease will have microscopic changes even when the mucosa looks normal on sigmoidoscopy. A barium enema in older patients with chronic or relapsing diarrhoea is important to exclude carcinoma. Haematological blood tests may reveal an anaemia; a microcytic anaemia suggesting iron deficiency may be due to carcinoma or inflammatory bowel disease. A macrocytosis may be due to folate deficiency in coeliac disease (see Chapter 31) or Crohn's disease affecting the distal ileum.

High serum levels of C-reactive protein is indicative of inflammatory bowel disease or carcinoma. Severe or intractable diarrhoea leads to loss of potassium, because of the sodium–potassium pump in the epithelial cells of the colon. Hence, potassium and other electrolyte levels should be checked. Albumin levels may also be low because of loss in the gut.

Hyperthyroidism is a cause of diarrhoea (conversely patients who are hypothyroid complain of constipation) and so thyroid function should also be checked (see Chapter 6).

PANCREATIC DISEASE

The pancreas contains two kinds of tissue – the exocrine glandular tissue, which secretes enzymes, and the endocrine glandular tissue, which secretes insulin and glucagon. Pancreatic enzymes include lipases and phospholipases, which break down lipids; amylase, which breaks down carbohydrates; and the precursors trypsinogens, chymotrypsinogens, elastases, and carboxypeptidases, which are broken down to their active forms in the duodenum and digest protein. The pancreas also produces several important messengers, such as secretin (which acts to induce secretion of bicarbonate and fluid) and cholecystokinin, which induces the secretion of enzymes. Insulin is also important in stimulating secretion of enzymes from the exocrine pancreas (see Chapter 35).

ACUTE PANCREATITIS

This condition occurs suddenly, and the well-recognised causes are alcohol misuse and disease of the biliary tract (usually obstruction by gallstones), although the cause cannot be identified in more than half the cases. The major clinical feature is pain in the epigastrium radiating to the back and sometimes to the left shoulder tip. Patients complain of nausea, and they may vomit. In severe cases, there is fever, shallow breathing, and delirium. The abdomen is tender and rigid, and, in severe cases, there is paralytic ileus (i.e. bowel motility ceases), and dilated loops of bowel are seen on abdominal X-ray. The patient may be hypoxic; indeed, complications include pulmonary oedema and the adult respiratory distress syndrome (see Chapter 33), which has a high mortality. Blood tests reveal a high serum amylase level.

Management of acute pancreatitis is aimed at treating symptoms of shock with fluids, and with blood transfusion and fresh frozen plasma if there is evidence of bleeding. Serum electrolyte levels should be monitored, and low calcium and magnesium levels need to be corrected. Nasogastric suction is applied until nausea and vomiting have stopped. Opiate analgesia may be needed for pain relief.

If there is any doubt of the diagnosis, then a laparotomy should be performed. Recent studies have shown that high-dose-bolus contrast-enhanced CT scanning allows an accurate assessment of the extent of pancreatic necrosis, and hence the rational timing of surgical intervention. Pancreatitis may be caused by gallstones obstructing the outlet of the pancreatic duct. An endoscopic procedure (endoscopic retrograde cholangiopancreatography) may be used to relieve the obstruction. This should be performed early in the attack.

CHRONIC PANCREATITIS

In chronic pancreatitis, there is gradual destruction of the exocrine tissue of the pancreas by an inflammatory process such that regeneration and recovery of function is not possible. Inflammation is followed by fibrosis, and calcification may occur. The most common identifiable cause is chronic alcohol misuse, although the causative mechanisms remain unclear. In the tropics, malnutrition is a recognized cause.

The majority of patients with chronic pancreatitis experience episodes of pain, which may be exacerbated by food, and is of the same nature and distribution as in acute pancreatitis. Weight loss occurs and there may be mild jaundice. Some degree of glucose intolerance is common, but patients generally do not suffer from primary diabetes mellitus. A characteristic clinical feature is steatorrhoea; malabsorption of protein, fat-soluble vitamins and vitamin B12 may also occur.

Medical management includes adequate analgesia and enzyme replacement therapy. Alcohol is forbidden. Surgery is occasionally needed to relieve obstruction of the biliary tree by the fibrotic head of the pancreas. Partial pancreatectomy may be of value to improve the drainage of any residual normal glandular tissue; it may also relieve pain and halt the progression of the disease.

CANCER OF THE PANCREAS

The incidence of pancreatic cancer is increasing in the Western world but the only factor that has been confirmed to be associated with this disease is tobacco smoking. Patients usually present at around 60–70 years of age with weight loss, anorexia, pain, and sometimes jaundice if the tumour is in the head of the pancreas. Painless obstructive jaundice should always alert one to the suspicion of pancreatic carcinoma. Advanced disease is said to be associated with recurrent venous thrombosis.

Many patients are incurable at diagnosis and management is usually directed at relieving symptoms. Jaundice may be relieved by the insertion of a stent using an endoscopic technique. However, if this fails or if there is evidence of duodenal obstruction, surgery may be necessary to bypass the obstruction. Pain relief is very important; therefore opiate analgesics should be introduced early (see also Chapter 14). Local radiotherapy may relieve intractable pain. In carefully selected patients, surgery to resect the tumour may have a mortality of less than 10 per cent, provided that it is done by experienced surgeons. In these patients, survival after surgery may be improved by the use of postoperative radiotherapy and chemotherapy with 5-fluorouracil.

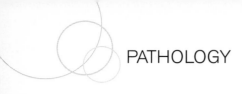

PATHOLOGY

MALIGNANCIES OF THE GASTROINTESTINAL TRACT

COLORECTAL CANCER

Colorectal cancer is one of the most common malignancies in the Western world.

Some rare, inherited syndromes predispose to colorectal cancer; for example, familial adenomatous polyposis. In this condition, multiple polyps develop in the colon from adolescence onwards. These polyps have a tendency to undergo malignant change, and colorectal cancer usually develops by the age of 45 years. Patients with familial adenomatous polyposis who do not develop colorectal cancer because they have had a prophylactic total colectomy are at risk of developing other malignancies such as duodenal and extra-intestinal tumours. Similarly, hereditary non-polyposis colorectal cancer is a dominantly inherited predisposition to colorectal cancer, though these patients do not have an increased number of polyps in their colon. This syndrome is thought to account for up to 5 per cent of all colonic cancers, whereas familial adenomatous polyposis accounts for 1 per cent. Apart from these two inherited syndromes which have well-characterized pedigrees, there is also evidence of familial clustering of colorectal cancer. For instance, a first-degree relative of a patient with colorectal cancer is at more than twice the risk of developing the disease than the rest of the population.

Clinical Features

Epidemiological studies suggest that the Western diet has a major influence on the risk of developing colon cancer (i.e. a high consumption of animal fat, together with a low intake of dietary fibre). Typical symptoms of the disease are blood loss in the stool, a change in bowel habit, anorexia, weight loss, and abdominal pain. Some patients present as an emergency, with intestinal obstruction or even bowel perforation. Left-sided tumours are more likely to present with changes in bowel habit and obstruction, whereas right-sided tumours (which are less common) may present with iron deficiency anaemia (from chronic blood loss) or an abdominal mass (from a caecal tumour).

Diagnostic Findings

The diagnosis is usually made on barium enema or by colonoscopy, which is useful because it allows histological diagnosis before surgery. Investigations to determine the presence of metastases are essential. These include an ultrasound of the liver, a chest X-ray, liver function tests, and a full blood count. Definitive management of colorectal cancer is surgical, and the prognosis is closely related to the stage of disease.

The staging of colorectal cancer is based on Duke's original classification of rectal tumours and depends on the findings at laparotomy as well as on the histology of resected or biopsied lymph nodes (Box 34.5). Most patients have a successful resection of the tumour, but sometimes the disease is so far advanced that surgery is not an option. These patients are managed with a combination of chemotherapeutic agents – trials so far have shown some benefit from a combination of 5-fluorouracil and folinic acid. Improved results may be achieved with the treatment of liver metastases by administering chemotherapy directly into the hepatic artery, although some degree of systemic chemotherapy is also needed.

In patients with Stage B and Stage C disease, surgical resection is often followed with chemotherapy or radiotherapy or both in order to prevent recurrence of the tumour; this is termed adjuvant therapy. Although recurrence of colonic cancer is usually in the form of liver metastases, rectal tumours tend to recur locally. Combined radiotherapy and chemotherapy may offer some advantage, and trials are in progress to assess the benefits of combined therapy and of chemotherapy alone.

LIVER AND BILIARY TRACT DISORDERS

JAUNDICE

Bilirubin Metabolism and the Causes of Jaundice

Jaundice is the yellow coloration of the tissues that is caused by the accumulation of bilirubin. It is most evident in the skin, the mucous membranes, and the sclera. Bilirubin is formed from the breakdown of

---

BOX 34.5 STAGING OF COLORECTAL CANCER (DUKE'S CLASSIFICATION) AND SURVIVAL RATES

Stage A (survival over 95 per cent at 5 years) tumour confined to the intestinal wall
no spread beyond muscularis mucosa or lymph nodes

Stage B (survival about 70 per cent at 5 years) tumour spread beyond muscularis mucosa
no lymph node involvement

Stage C (survival less than 50 per cent at 5 years) tumour spread to lymph nodes

compounds containing haem, the major one being haemoglobin although the metabolism of other haem-containing proteins (i.e. myoglobin and the cytochromes) also contribute to bilirubin in the bloodstream. Bilirubin in the plasma is 'unconjugated' and is transported tightly bound to albumin. In the liver, bilirubin is conjugated with glucuronic acid to a water-soluble form, which is then excreted in the bile. In the intestine, bacteria metabolize bilirubin to urobilinogen, which is absorbed and passes into the hepatic portal circulation, where most of it is extracted by the liver and re-excreted in the bile, although a small amount enters the systemic circulation and is excreted in the urine. Both urobilinogen and conjugated bilirubin are excreted in the urine. Figure 34.4 shows the pathways of bilirubin metabolism.

Therefore, jaundice may be caused by :

- excessive production of bilirubin, such as occurs in the haemolytic anaemias (pre-hepatic jaundice);
- reduced uptake or conjugation by the liver cells (hepatic jaundice); or
- reduced excretion of conjugated bilirubin in the biliary system (cholestatic jaundice) (Box 34.6).

BOX 34.6 CLASSIFICATION OF THE CAUSES OF JAUNDICE

Type of jaundice	Cause
pre-hepatic jaundice	haemolysis
hepatic jaundice	hepatitis (viral or alcoholic) cirrhosis
cholestatic jaundice	gallstones cancer of the bile ducts or pancreas

---

Clinical Features

The clinical features of the jaundice patient depend on the underlying cause. Jaundice due to haemolysis is usually mild, and the only symptoms may be related to the degree of anaemia. Cholestatic jaundice has a gradual onset and is often accompanied by skin itching; in severe cases, patients may have a greenish tinge to the skin. In acute hepatitis, anorexia and nausea accompany the jaundice, which can develop rapidly – in a day or so. A history of weight loss may suggest cancer of the pancreas, while severe intermittent right-sided abdominal pain together with fevers and rigors may suggest biliary colic and cholangitis associated with gallstones. In alcoholics, signs of cirrhosis may be present.

GALLSTONE DISEASE

Gallstones can be of 3 types:

- cholesterol stones;
- black, composed mainly of bilirubin; or
- brown, composed of calcium bilirubinate.

Most gallstones encountered in the Western world are cholesterol stones. The gall bladder holds and concentrates bile, which is injected into the intestine during a meal. It is generally assumed that the inefficient emptying of the gall bladder increases the likelihood of gallstone formation. Several other factors are also thought to play a role, including obesity, a low-fibre diet, and cirrhosis. Women, particularly those who have had several pregnancies, are more likely to develop gallstones, perhaps because of the incomplete emptying of the gall bladder in late pregnancy.

The majority of gallstones remain in the gall bladder and are only discovered incidentally on radiographic examination. If a gallstone becomes impact-

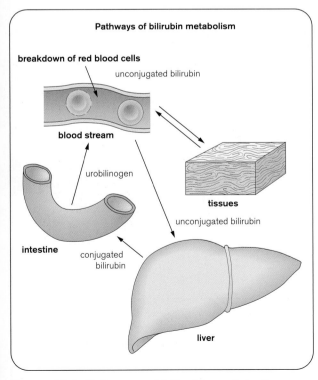

Figure 34.4 Pathways of bilirubin metabolism.

ed at the entrance to the cystic duct, the gall bladder may become inflamed and the contents infected; this is known as cholecystitis. It may resolve spontaneously as the gallstone disimpacts.

In acute cholecystitis, the patient is sweaty and unwell, with pain in the upper right abdomen. A fever indicates bacterial infection, while jaundice suggests a gallstone in the common bile duct.

Treatment includes bed rest, intravenous fluids, pain relief, and antibiotics. In patients who suffer recurrent attacks, urgent cholecystectomy may be required to remove the gall bladder and cystic duct. In the past few years, controlled trials have shown that laparoscopic cholecystectomy (i.e. performed through a flexible scope inserted into the abdominal cavity through a small incision) is better than the traditional 'open' cholecystectomy in terms of reducing the number of post-operative hospital days, causing fewer post-operative complications, and allowing a faster return to normal activities.

Gallstones may also obstruct the common bile duct and cause bacterial infection of the stagnant bile, commonly with *Escherichia coli*. This is called cholangitis, and patients are very ill with fevers, rigors, and right-sided abdominal pain. Gallstones may also obstruct the ampulla of Vater, causing acute or chronic pancreatitis (Figure 34.5).

VIRAL HEPATITIS

Viral hepatitis may be caused by one of the five major hepatotrophic viruses (hepatitis A, B, C, D, or E) or by other viruses, such as the Epstein–Barr virus or cytomegalovirus, which typically cause a more generalized infection.

Hepatitis A

Hepatitis A virus is spread via the faeco-oral route and is therefore associated with overcrowding, poor hygiene, and poor sanitation. Hepatitis A is endemic

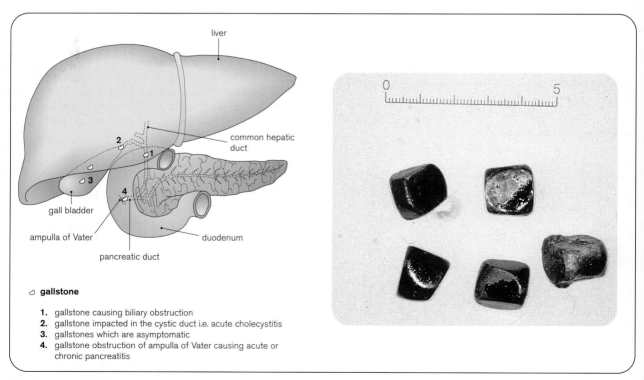

○ **gallstone**

1. gallstone causing biliary obstruction
2. gallstone impacted in the cystic duct i.e. acute cholecystitis
3. gallstones which are asymptomatic
4. gallstone obstruction of ampulla of Vater causing acute or chronic pancreatitis

Figure 34.5 Gallstones. (a) Sites within the biliary tree where gallstones commonly lodge include the common hepatic duct below the cystic duct, the cystic duct (as in acute cholecystitis, the gall bladder (where gallstones are asymptomatic), and the ampulla of Vater (which causes acute or chronic pancreatitis). (b) Gallstones retrieved from a patient. (By kind permission of Mr M Knight, Consultant Surgeon, St. George's Hospital Healthcare Trust, London, UK.)

in developing countries, where infection is generally acquired by the age of 5 years. In more developed countries, such as those in Europe, the mean age of infection is higher. Infection usually causes antibodies against the virus to develop, and these can be detected in the serum (see Chapters 17 and 24). Therefore, the prevalence of antibodies to hepatitis A virus in a population is a measure of both the infection rate and the immunity to the virus in the community. In many developed countries, only 5–10 per cent of young adults have serum antibodies to hepatitis A virus.

Infections in infants and young children often pass unnoticed, whereas older patients have a more severe disease. Some patients have relapses following an initial recovery from the illness; these relapses are characterized by jaundice, fever, weight loss, and diarrhoea. However, these patients do not develop chronic hepatitis.

Prophylaxis for travellers can be achieved by passive immunization with human immunoglobulin or active immunization with an inactivated form of the virus, which has a very high immune response rate (see Chapters 21 and 23).

Hepatitis B

Hepatitis B virus is a double-stranded deoxyribonucleic acid (DNA) virus. It can cause acute or chronic hepatitis, and hepatitis B is also an important risk factor for liver cancer (hepatocellular carcinoma). The virus is transmitted by the parenteral route (e.g. blood transfusion, intravenous drug use), by intimate contact (e.g. sexual contact), or by vertical transmission from mother to neonate. Several antigenic components of the virus have been characterized:

- the outer envelope component of the virus – the hepatitis B surface antigen (HBsAg);
- the inner nucleocapsid core – the hepatitis B core antigen (HBcAg); and
- a further product of the HBV genome (HBeAg).

When a person is infected with hepatitis B virus, the first markers to appear in the serum HBeAg, which appears 4–6 weeks after infection and is then detectable for 6 weeks or so. The HBsAg appears later and persists for longer. HBcAg cannot be demonstrated in circulating blood, but the antibody to this antigen (anti-HBc) is detectable, and it, together with serum HBsAg, is one of the diagnostic indicators of acute hepatitis B. Typical biochemical features include raised levels of hepatic enzymes, particularly alanine aminotransferase; serum bilirubin levels increase with severity of the infection. The DNA of hepatitis B virus can also be demonstrated during an acute infection using Southern blotting (see Chapter 7). Following infection with hepatitis B, a person develops immunity to the virus, characterized by antibodies to both HBsAg and HBcAg.

Carrier status

Persistence of HBsAg after 6 months indicates a carrier status. While only 10 per cent of adults contracting hepatitis B will become carriers, more than 75 per cent of those acquiring the infection in early childhood will do so. Hepatitis B carriers are usually healthy, but they have the potential to transmit the disease. Such 'healthy' carriers may have minimal histological evidence of liver damage, and only 1–2 per cent develop chronic disease. Similarly, patients who experience an acute attack seldom go on to develop chronic disease.

Fulminant hepatitis

Acute hepatitis B usually resolves, with eradication of infected hepatocytes, cessation of viral replication, and regeneration of the damaged liver. A small proportion of patients develop 'fulminant' hepatitis, in which mortality is high and often the only chance of survival is to undergo liver transplantation (see Chapter 29).

Chronic hepatitis B

The majority of cases of chronic hepatitis caused by hepatitis B occur in patients who have no history of an acute illness with jaundice. Chronic infection is more common in people who are immunosuppressed (e.g. kidney transplant patients, patients infected with human immunodeficiency virus) and in those who acquire the infection in childhood in areas of the world where there is a high incidence of the disease, such as Africa and the Far East. Chronic hepatitis B is also more prevalent in males. It is usually a silent disease, though patients may become ill suddenly with fatigue, jaundice and increased circulating liver enzymes. Hepatitis B virus DNA and HBeAg is present in the serum of these patients. A small proportion of patients with chronic hepatitis B develop cirrhosis or hepatocellular carcinoma.

Immunization

Passive immunization against hepatitis B using hyperimmune serum globulin is effective prophylaxis if it is administered within hours of infection. Hepatitis vaccine should always be given as well, particularly if the person is at risk of re-infection. This applies to the at-risk groups (health care professionals, prison workers, and the sexual contacts of those with acute hepatitis B).

Treatment

Most cases of acute hepatitis B will resolve; there is no evidence that antiviral therapy either accelerates the healing process, or prevents the development of chronic disease.

Alpha-interferon is used to treat chronic hepatitis. It works by enhancing the immune response to the virus. Side-effects include flu-like symptoms, with headache, muscle aches, and depression (see Chapter 25).

About 30–40 per cent of patients respond to treatment but many remain carriers (i.e. HBsAg-positive), and a small number will relapse. Liver transplantation can be offered to treat patients with chronic hepatitis, but the main drawback is the re-infection of the engrafted liver, particularly if the patient has detectable hepatitis B virus DNA at the time of transplantation (see Chapter 29). Recurrent hepatitis in such patients has an accelerated course, with nearly 50 per cent mortality at 3 years. High doses of hyperimmune globulin are used to prevent re-infection and are effective in some of these patients but have to be given over a long period.

Hepatitis C

Hepatitis C virus is a single-stranded ribonucleic acid virus. Although the nucleotide sequence has been known for some time, viral particles have not been demonstrated. Therefore, in the absence of a suitable known antigen, it is difficult to develop specific diagnostic tests for the presence of anti-hepatitis C antibody. Infection with hepatitis C virus is most commonly seen after transfusion of blood products. However, in many countries, such as Japan and in Africa, there is community-acquired transmission. In the UK, certain groups of patients have a high prevalence of hepatitis C, including those with thalassaemia (who receive repeated blood transfusion) and those with haemophilia (who are exposed to contaminated commercially prepared blood products such as factor VIII).

Hepatitis C infection may manifest as an acute hepatitis, but this is less common than with hepatitis B. Conversely, the risk of chronic hepatitis is much higher than for hepatitis B, with about 50 per cent of patients developing chronic hepatitis.

Acute hepatitis C infection is usually mild, and only 25 per cent of cases develop jaundice. Chronic hepatitis C is usually a slowly progressive disease in which about 20 per cent of patients develop cirrhosis, and there is the risk of hepatocellular carcinoma. The diagnosis of chronic hepatitis C is made by detecting antibodies to hepatitis C virus, although, as mentioned above, the specificity of the tests is not high, hence there are false positive results. The major clinical features of chronic hepatitis are fatigue and raised circulating levels of liver enzymes.

Treatment of patients with acute hepatitis C is aimed at preventing the progression to the chronic form of the disease. Cytokine therapy with alpha-interferon and beta-interferon have been used – in one series, 50 per cent of patients responded after 6 months of treatment

with alpha-interferon; however, half of these patients relapsed soon after stopping treatment. Ribavirin, a synthetic guanosine nucleotide analogue, has been used with some success in many viral diseases (see also Chapter 19). It can be taken orally, in contrast to the interferons, which are administered by intramuscular injection. Ribavirin may be effective when used in conjunction with alpha-interferon. Patients who develop cirrhosis are candidates for liver transplantation, although the majority of patients will get recurrent disease. It is not yet known if hepatitis C in transplanted patients has a higher rate of progression to cirrhosis and hepatocellular carcinoma than in nontransplanted patients.

CHRONIC HEPATITIS

Chronic hepatitis is defined as a chronic inflammatory process in the liver that persists for more than 6 months. The end-stage of this process is cirrhosis, in which the normal architecture of the liver is destroyed, leaving nodules interspersed with fibrous bands of tissue. Broadly speaking, there are three groups of patients who develop chronic hepatitis: those with hepatitis B infection, those with chronic hepatitis C infection, and those who develop an autoimmune disease associated with autoantibodies in the serum (see Chapter 27). Of these, the last has the worst prognosis, with 60 per cent of sufferers dead in 5 years.

Patients typically present with fatigue; some may have jaundice, an enlarged spleen, or (rarely) an enlarged liver. Biochemical tests may reveal a mild elevation of serum bilirubin, increased liver enzymes, and raised gamma-globulin levels (see Chapter 6).

Management depends on whether tests for HBsAg and anti-hepatitis C virus are positive or negative. A liver biopsy is essential to confirm the diagnosis, to assess the activity of the disease, and to provide histological evidence of the presence or absence of cirrhosis. The histology may also help in identifying a possible cause, and it may be used to follow the response to treatment.

Chronic Active Autoimmune Hepatitis

This is a form of hepatitis associated with raised circulating levels of gamma-globulin and a spectrum of autoimmune antibodies:

- antinuclear antibody (diffuse type), found in 80 per cent of patients;
- smooth muscle antibody, found in 70 per cent of patients; and
- liver–kidney microsomal type 1 antibody, an antibody that is mainly directed against cytochrome P450, a mitochondrial enzyme.

This disorder is prevalent in females aged between 10 and 20 years, who present feeling generally unwell with jaundice; menstrual disturbances are also common. Spider naevi (a type of vascular lesion) are found on the face, neck, and arms. There is often evidence of splenomegaly, and in the early stages the liver is also enlarged and feels firm and smooth on examination. In the later stages, the liver shrinks and becomes impalpable, and there is free fluid in the abdomen (ascites). Other features are swelling (oedema) of the limbs, caused by lack of albumin production by the liver, and hepatic encephalopathy, caused by toxic substances of intestinal origin (which are normally removed by the liver) reaching the brain.

Chronic autoimmune active hepatitis is associated with other autoimmune conditions, such as Hashimoto's thyroiditis and autoimmune haemolytic anaemia (see Chapters 27 and 35). Patients may also have fevers, arthritic pains in large joints, and skin rashes such as acne.

Biochemical tests show a raised serum bilirubin, very high gamma-globulin levels, and high circulating liver-specific enzymes. These parameters reflect damage to the liver cells (see Chapter 6). The liver is also the major site of synthesis of many of the plasma proteins, including albumin and many coagulation factors. While serum albumin falls only in the later stages of the disease (causing oedema), impaired synthesis of coagulation proteins (as evidenced by a prolonged prothrombin time (see Chapter 31) is present even in the early stages.

Corticosteroid therapy is effective in prolonging life in severe chronic active hepatitis. Prednisolone is used, and it may be continued for many years, sometimes for life. Complications of treatment include moon face, acne, obesity, and excess hair (see also Chapter 35). In the later stages of the disease, cirrhosis develops, and liver transplantation must be considered.

CIRRHOSIS

In cirrhosis, the normal histological structures of the liver are replaced by nodules surrounded by fibrous tissue. The diagnosis can be made by direct visualization, for example at laparotomy, or by laparoscopy or radiological investigations (e.g. ultrasound, CT scanning). Cirrhosis may occur as the result of a variety of conditions in which the liver cells are damaged (Box 34.7).

In western Europe, the most common identified causes are alcohol misuse, hepatitis B, and hepatitis C. Patients with cirrhosis have evidence of liver failure [jaundice, ascites, encephalopathy, raised circulating levels of aminotranfersases, and a prolonged

> **BOX 34.7 CAUSES OF CIRRHOSIS**
>
> viral hepatitis
> alcohol misuse
> iron overload
> cholestasis
> drugs (e.g. methotrexate)
> cardiac failure
> cryptogenic (i.e. cause unknown)

prothrombin time (see Chapter 6)]. The severe disruption of the liver architecture means that the portal venous blood flow within the liver is obstructed. This gives rise to portal hypertension and the development of an extensive collateral circulation. Diversion of blood to the spleen leads to splenic enlargement, and blood diverted through the para-umbilical vein opens up superficial collateral vessels around the umbilicus, termed Medusa's head.

The major clinical significance of portal hypertension is formation of varices in the gastro-oesophageal circulation. These may bleed, causing upper gastrointestinal haemorrhage. Hepatic cirrhosis is the most common cause of portal hypertension, which frequently presents as vomiting of blood (haematemesis) from bleeding gastro-oesophageal varices. Blood from bleeding varices may also be lost in the stool, causing melaena.

Other clinical features that may be associated with cirrhosis are chronic relapsing pancreatitis, steatorrhoea (caused by the reduction in bile secretion from the damaged liver), gallstones, and primary liver cancer (hepatocellular carcinoma). Bacterial infections are common owing to the shunting of blood past the phagocytic cells in the mononuclear phagocytic system of the liver. Many patients are asymptomatic in the early stages, and the condition may be discovered only at routine examination or blood tests. These patients have what is termed 'compensated cirrhosis', which may last for some years or may progress more rapidly to liver failure. The course of the disease is very variable, and liver function tests do not correlate with the severity of portal hypertension.

Decompensated cirrhosis occurs when the clinical effects of liver failure become evident. Patients have increasing weakness, muscle wasting, ascites, and jaundice. Mild persistent fever may be due to Gram-negative bacteraemia or to cytokines such as tumour necrosis factor (see Chapter 25). There is general dilatation of peripheral vessels, which causes increased blood flow in the skin; this leads to flushed extremities, the characteristic red 'liver palms' and bounding pulses. Release of vasodilators from the failing liver is thought to be important in producing these changes. Spider naevi are found in the upper trunk; these consist of a raised central arteriole with many small vessels radiating from it. Skin pigmentation and clubbing of the fingers may be present. Shunting of blood through retrovenous fistulae in the lungs leads to a reduced oxygen saturation and cyanosis in about one-third of patients with decompensated cirrhosis. Hepatic encephalopathy is manifested as sleep disorders, personality changes, and intellectual deterioration; it may progress to confusion, drowsiness, and coma. These symptoms may worsen suddenly following gastrointestinal haemorrhage, owing to the increased amount of nitrogen absorbed into the circulation from the blood in the gastrointestinal system.

The prognosis varies depending on the underlying cause. Hepatic encephalopathy, haemorrhage, prolonged prothrombin time, hepatitis B, and hepatocellular carcinoma are factors associated with a worse prognosis. Severe persistent jaundice and ascites indicate a poor outlook.

The management of a patient with compensated cirrhosis includes avoidance of alcohol and a balanced diet containing 1g of protein/kg of body weight per day. The onset of encephalopathy requires protein restriction in the diet. This disorder arises because the diseased liver can not effectively convert nitrogenous waste into urea, and therefore ammonia, which is toxic, is produced. The development of ascites and oedema is managed with diuretics and dietary sodium restriction. Therapeutic manoeuvres directed at reducing or switching off collagen synthesis (which leads to fibrosis) include the use of colchicine, and anti-inflammatory drugs such as corticosteroids. Liver transplantation is an option for carefully selected patients.

ALCOHOLIC LIVER DISEASE

The incidence of cirrhosis among alcoholics at postmortem examination is 10–20 per cent; therefore, it seems that some people have a predisposition to develop alcoholic cirrhosis. Alcohol is metabolized by the liver to acetaldehyde, a toxic substance that is thought to be responsible for many of the features of acute alcoholic hepatitis (e.g. membrane damage and cell necrosis). Further metabolism of acetaldehyde to acetyl coenzyme A and acetate generates increased hepatocyte levels of the reduced form of nicotinamide adenine dinucleotide (NADH) compared to nicotinamide adenine dinucleotide (NAD). This has several metabolic consequences, including increased formation of fat and collagen in the liver (see Chapter 2).

Morphological changes in alcoholic liver disease range from fatty liver to alcoholic hepatitis to cirrhosis. The patient with a fatty liver has a smooth, enlarged, firm liver edge and mild elevation of blood liver enzymes. Acute alcoholic hepatitis can follow an episode of heavy drinking, and in its most severe form, presents with anorexia, vomiting, jaundice and pyrexia. The patient has an enlarged and tender liver and is very unwell. Diarrhoea is due to decreased excretion of bile salts, pancreatic insufficiency, and a direct toxic effect of alcohol on the intestinal mucosa. Blood tests show raised levels of liver enzymes; elevated bilirubin levels and prolonged prothrombin times are associated with more severe disease. White blood counts are raised (leukocytosis) and platelet count and function will be reduced. The mortality in patients with acute alcoholic hepatitis varies from 20–40 per cent, and recovery may take several months.

Alcoholic cirrhosis presents like other forms of cirrhosis, and there may not be any preceding episode of alcoholic hepatitis. The prognosis in alcoholic cirrhosis is generally better than in other forms of cirrhosis. An ability to abstain from further drinking increases survival, whereas continued heavy drinking is associated with a poor prognosis. Treatment of patients is directed at the complications, notably portal hypertension, encephalopathy, and ascites.

The selection of alcoholics for liver transplantation is a controversial issue, but the results of transplantation in this group of patients are as good as in any other group of patients with cirrhosis, with a greater than 60 per cent survival at 2 years.

KEY POINTS

- Visualization of the gastrointestinal tract is achieved by inserting a fibreoptic endoscope into the tract (endoscopy, colonoscopy) and by barium examinations (in which barium is swallowed as a barium meal or injected into the colon as a barium enema).
- Weakness or relaxation of the gastro-oesophageal sphincter may lead to reflux of acid contents of the stomach up into the oesophagus, causing irritation or even ulceration of the oesophageal lining; i.e. reflux oesophagitis.
- The most significant cause of peptic ulcers is infection with *Helicobacter pylori*, which is treatable with antibiotics.
- Bleeding from the upper gastrointestinal tract typically presents as haematemesis or melaena.
- The irritable bowel syndrome is a functional bowel disorder with episodes of abdominal pain, disordered defaecation, and abdominal distension. Disordered gut motility, certain foods, inflammation, and stress have all been implicated in the pathogenesis.
- Inflammatory bowel disease is widely accepted as referring to two distinctive disorders, ulcerative colitis and Crohn's disease, in which virus infections, and familial associations are among some of the risk factors.

- The best-recognized causes of acute pancreatitis are alcohol misuse and disease of the biliary tract.
- In chronic pancreatitis, there is gradual destruction of the exocrine tissue of the pancreas. The common identifiable cause is chronic alcohol misuse.
- The incidence of pancreatic cancer is increasing in the Western world and the main risk factor identified is tobacco smoking. Patients usually present at about 60–70 years of age with weight loss, anorexia, pain, and sometimes jaundice if the tumour is in the head of the pancreas.
- Epidemiological studies suggest a major risk factor for colorectal cancer is the Western diet (i.e. high animal fat with a low intake of dietary fibre); there are also rare, inherited syndromes.
- Jaundice may be caused by excessive production of bilirubin as occurs in haemolytic anaemias (pre-hepatic jaundice), by reduced uptake or conjugation by the liver cells (hepatic jaundice), or by reduced excretion of conjugated bilirubin in the biliary system (cholestatic jaundice).
- Viral hepatitis may be caused by one of the five major hepatotrophic viruses (hepatitis A, B, C, D, and E) or by other viruses such as the Epstein–Barr virus or cytomegalovirus.

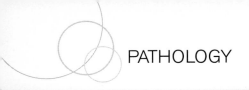

**Aldoori WH, Giovannucci EL, Stampfer MJ, *et al.* (1997) A prospective study of alcohol, smoking, caffeine, and the risk of duodenal ulcers in men. Epidemiology 8:420–4.

Allan RN, Hodgson HJF (1992) Inflammatory bowel disease. In: Pounder RE (ed) Recent Advances in Gastroenterology. Churchill Livingstone, London.

Aspinall R, Taylor-Robinson S (1999) Gastroenterology: Colour Atlas and Text (in press). Mosby International, London.

Baines MJ (1997) ABC of palliative care: nausea, vomiting and intestinal obstruction. BMJ 315:1148–50.

Brenner H, Rothenbacher D, Bode G, Adler G (1997) Relation of smoking, alcohol and coffee consumption to active *Helicobacter pylori* infection. BMJ 315:1489–92.

Di Bisceglie AM (1998) Hepatitis C. Lancet 351:351–5.

Dolan M, Hughes N (1997) Hepatitis C: a bloody business. Nurs Times 93:71–2.

Dunlop MG (1997) Colorectal cancer. BMJ 314:1882–5.

Ekbom A, Daszak P, Kraaz W, Wakefield AJ (1996) Crohn's disease after *in-utero* measles virus exposure. Lancet 348:515–17.

Haddock G, Carter DC (1990) Aetiology of pancreatic cancer. Br J Surg 77:1159–66.

Kay J (1997) Vital signs: spotting liver disease in babies and children. Prof Care Mother Child 7:41–2.

Lefton HB, Pilcham J, Harmatz A (1996) Colon cancer screening and the evaluation and follow-up of colonic polyps. Prim Care 23(3):515–23.

Lennard-Jones JE, Melville DM, Morson BC, Ritchie JK, Williams CB (1990) Precancer and cancer in extensive ulcerative colitis: findings among 401 patients over 22 years. Gut 31:800–6.

National Institute of Health Consensus Conference (1994) *Helicobacter pylori* in peptic ulcer disease. JAMA 272:65–9.

Neoptolemos JP (1992) Pancreatic disease. In: Pounder RE (ed) Recent Advances in Gastroenterology. Churchill Livingstone, Edinburgh.

Norman J (1998) The role of cytokines in the pathogenesis of acute pancreatitis. Am J Surg 175:76–83.

Plevris JN, Hayes PC (1997) Investigation and management of acute diarrhoea. Br J Hosp Med 56:569–73.

Shaw B (1996) Primary care for women. Management and treatment of gastrointestinal disorders. J Nurs Midwifery 41:155–72.

Thomas HJW (1992) Colorectal oncology. In: Pounder RE (ed) Recent Advances in Gastroenterology. Churchill Livingstone, London.

DISEASES OF THE ENDOCRINE SYSTEM

Before reading this chapter, you should have an understanding of:
- the names and functions of endocrine organs
- homeostatic control by endocrine hormones.

THE ENDOCRINE SYSTEM

The endocrine system is made up of several glands located in different areas of the body. They are ductless glands and produce hormones, which are released directly into the circulation in order to be dispersed and influence their target tissues and organs. The classical endocrine glands are listed in Table 35.1. Many hormones are also produced by organs that have not been primarily or traditionally regarded as endocrine organs. These include:
- the hypothalamus, which produces hormones that control the release of hormones by other tissues and glands, including corticotrophin releasing hormone, thyrotrophin releasing hormone, and the gonadotrophin releasing hormones that regulate production of pituitary hormones (Figure 35.1);
- the kidney, which produces erythropoietin, the growth factor that regulates red blood cell production;
- the gastrointestinal tract, which produces gastrin and cholecystokinin; and

- the liver, which produces insulin-like growth factor. Hormones may be synthesized from a number of different sources – for example, from:
- single amino acids, as with the amines (e.g. noradrenaline, adrenaline, and the thyroid hormones);
- peptides or proteins (e.g. growth hormone);
- cholesterol, which is obtained from the diet but is also manufactured by the liver for use in the production of steroid hormones (e.g. the gonadal and adrenal hormones) as well as for the endogenous synthesis of vitamin D.

In order to exert its actions, each hormone must bind to a specific receptor. Such receptors may be located on the cell membrane of the target organ, as is the case for protein hormone receptors, or intracellularly in the cytosol or the nucleus, as is the case for steroid hormone receptors.

DIABETES MELLITUS

CLASSIFICATION AND AETIOLOGY
Diabetes mellitus results from the relative or absolute lack of insulin. It is characterized by the consequent metabolic disturbances, the most notable of which is hyperglycaemia.

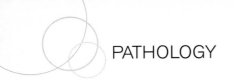

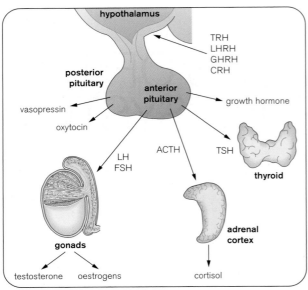

Figure 35.1 Hormones released by the hypothalamus and pituitary glands. The influence of these hormones on other endocrine glands is shown.

Insulin-Dependent Diabetes Mellitus

Broadly speaking, insulin-dependent diabetes (type 1 diabetes) refers to an autoimmune disease, which progresses eventually to a complete failure of insulin production by the islet cells of the pancreas. Histologically, there is an aggressive infiltration of mononuclear cells into these islets in patients with advanced disease, and anti-islet cell antibodies may be found in the serum. Patients present in childhood or early adulthood, hence the old term 'juvenile onset' diabetes. Insulin-dependent diabetes has a genetic base, and there is an association with HLA-DR3 and -DR4 (see also Chapter 24).

Non-Insulin-Dependent Diabetes Mellitus

Non-insulin-dependent diabetes (type 2 diabetes), a more heterogeneous category of disease, usually presents later in life. It includes elderly, non-obese patients who can often be easily maintained on non-insulin therapy, as well as the obese patients who have 'insulin insensitivity'. It remains unclear whether the primary abnormality is one of defective insulin secretion or one of resistance of peripheral tissues to the effects of insulin. Non-insulin-dependent diabetes has a strong familial association.

Classical Endocrine Glands and Related Hormones

Gland	Hormone(s)
pituitary (anterior lobe)	luteinizing hormone (LH), follicle stimulating hormone (FSH), prolactin, growth hormone, adrenocorticotrophin (ACTH), thyroid-stimulating hormone (TSH)
pituitary (posterior lobe)	antidiuretic hormone (vasopressin), oxytocin
thyroid	thyroxine, tri-iodothyronine, calcitonin
parathyroid	parathyroid hormone (PTH)
adrenal cortex	cortisol, aldosterone, dehydroepiandosterone, androstenedione
adrenal medulla	adrenaline, noradrenaline
testis	testosterone, oestradiol, androstenedione
ovary	oestradiol, progesterone, testosterone, androstenedione
placenta	human chorionic gonadotrophin (hCG), progesterone, oestrogens
pancreas	insulin, glucagon, somatostatin, pancreatic polypeptide, gastrin, vasoactive intestinal peptide (VIP)

Table 35.1 Endocrine glands and their hormones.

Other Types of Diabetes Mellitus

Diabetes can also develop as a result of pancreatic damage (e.g. in chronic alcoholic pancreatitis or in iron overload).

Pregnant women are occasionally identified as having gestational diabetes from the results from a urine analysis performed at the antenatal clinic (see also Chapter 6). This condition is regarded as a form of impaired glucose tolerance resulting from the altered hormonal and metabolic state of pregnancy, including the presence of hormones with anti-insulin effects (e.g. prolactin). Some of these patients develop diabetes in later life, but most go into remission once they are no longer pregnant.

A secondary form of diabetes mellitus may develop where there is an excess of hormones which have an anti-insulin effect. Such conditions may arise with Cushing's syndrome, in which there is excess cortisol. This is also a complication to be aware of in patients prescribed long-term corticosteroid therapy. Likewise diabetes can occur with acromegaly, in which there is an excessive secretion of growth hormone (see below).

METABOLIC DISTURBANCES

The endocrine pancreas produces insulin and glucagon, the hormones responsible for regulating fuel metabolism. Insulin is responsible for the anabolic phase of fuel metabolism, which typically begins with food ingestion and lasts several hours. In this phase, caloric intake exceeds demands and energy storage takes place – glycogen synthesis occurs in liver and muscle, fatty acid synthesis and triglyceride formation occur in the hepatocytes, and protein synthesis is initiated (see Chapter 2).

There is no backup hormone for insulin, whereas the catabolic functions of glucagon are also exhibited by other hormones such as adrenaline, noradrenaline, cortisol, and growth hormone. These hormones oppose the actions of insulin and protect the body from hypoglycaemia, stimulating glycogen breakdown, gluconeogenesis, and fatty acid oxidation by the liver, which produces ketones, a source of fuel that can be utilized by the brain when glucose levels are low. Proteolysis occurs in muscle, supplying amino acids for gluconeogenesis.

Insulin and glucagon release are normally well co-ordinated in order to keep plasma glucose levels within a certain range. Release of each hormone is regulated by the other as well as by plasma glucose levels .

Insulin deficiency and unbalanced glucagon secretion therefore leads to elevated plasma glucose levels, owing to uncontrolled glycogen breakdown and overproduction of glucose by the liver. Ketone production and triglyceride breakdown leads to a loss of adipose tissue. Plasma levels of glucose will rise until the non-insulin-dependent mechanisms for removal of glucose are overcome; this leads to an overspill into the urine with glycosuria and a resultant osmotic diuresis. Hence polydipsia and polyuria are some of the prominent, characteristic features of uncontrolled diabetes. Hyperglycaemia and ketoacidosis result, and the latter can be life-threatening. Prolonged deficiency of insulin results in skeletal muscle breakdown and, with loss of fat stores, there is weight loss even though the person has a good appetite.

In non-insulin-dependent diabetes, there is resistance of peripheral tissues to the effects of insulin, leading to the unopposed actions of glucagon. This is sometimes referred to as a relative insulin deficiency, or insulin resistance. In these patients, ketoacidosis rarely develops, but severe hyperglycaemia may lead to massive loss of body fluids through the kidney. The water deficit that results raises plasma osmotic pressure from normal levels of 280–300 mOsmol/l to as high as 400–500 mOsmol/l. In this situation, patients can go into a hyperosmolar, non-ketotic diabetic coma, which has a high mortality.

CLINICAL FEATURES

Insulin-Dependent Diabetes Mellitus

Insulin-dependent diabetes commonly presents in childhood and early adulthood. Peak incidence occurs during the winter, with a short history of an acute illness characterized by polyuria, polydipsia, and weight loss. Skin or genitourinary infections are common. The onset of ketoacidosis is marked by anorexia, vomiting, and abdominal pain, followed by signs of dehydration and impaired consciousness. In older patients, the history might be longer, with weight loss and recurrent candidal infections being common features.

Non-Insulin-Dependent Diabetes Mellitus

People with non-insulin-dependent diabetes may present with polyuria, polydipsia, weight loss, and genitourinary infections, but the onset of symptoms is more insidious (see Person-Centred Study: The Presentation of Non-Insulin-Dependent Diabetes Mellitus). In these patients, who are generally older than the patients with insulin-dependent diabetes, other pathological manifestations may occur, the most notable being major vessel disease, such as angina or myocardial infarction.

MANAGEMENT

The aims of management of the diabetic patient have evolved over the years, and today they include the control of blood glucose levels and the prevention of microvascular and macrovascular complications, the attainment of a normal duration and quality of life. To this end, metabolic targets have been set up, which

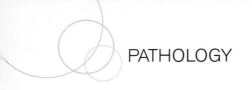

include not just glucose levels but also serum lipid concentrations.

The successful management of diabetes is largely delivered by the patients themselves, but they must be well educated about their disorder and highly motivated. Dietary management, which is the key to the treatment of the disease, regular monitoring of blood glucose levels, and administration of appropriate amounts of insulin several times a day are all key features for the adequate control of this condition – all of which intimately involves the patient. Unpredictable events, such as illness (e.g. influenza) alter insulin requirements, emphasizing the need for patient education and understanding of the disease. Other areas of management that should be targeted include nutrition, foot care, and self-monitoring; an enlightened approach is needed by patients so that they are able to appreciate why these must become part of their everyday existence (Box 35.1).

Diet

The primary aim of management is the reduction of high blood glucose concentrations, although not only carbohydrate intake needs to be controlled. Obesity increases the requirement for insulin delivery from the pancreas, and hence control of overall energy intake is important. Previously, patients with diabetes were prescribed a low-carbohydrate diet, and therefore much of their calorific intake was derived from other sources like fat. However, it has subsequently been realized that these patient are at high risk of major arterial disease, and therefore it is important to control the amount and types of fat that they consume. Hence, patients with diabetes are encouraged to select a diet that is rich in complex carbohydrates (e.g. wholemeal bread, high-fibre cereals, fruit, and vegetables). Foods containing great amounts of free sugar (sucrose and

glucose) are rapidly absorbed and result in a massive glucose load in the circulation; these foods should be avoided. Thus, the carbohydrate intake should be regulated to include a certain amount of dietary fibre, which slows down absorption and helps to prevent large surges in blood glucose level following a meal.

Advice regarding fat intake for diabetics is generally much the same as for non-diabetics, with a view to reducing the risk of cardiovascular disease. Dietary requirements vary according to the circumstances of the patient; for example, during illness carbohydrate intake needs to be maintained, particularly if there is a fever.

In cases of diabetic nephropathy, a dietary restriction of protein and electrolytes is generally required.

Drugs

The largest group of drugs used in the treatment of non-insulin-dependent diabetes is the sulphonylureas (e.g. chlorpropamide, glibenclamide, tolbutamide), which are considered to act by increasing secretion of

BOX 35.2 MANAGEMENT OF KETOACIDOSIS

- Restore adequate circulation with normal saline – give up to 4 l of fluid in the first 3 hours, then 500 ml every 2–4 hours until signs of dehydration disappear.
- Start an insulin infusion with a bolus of 6 IU, then 6 IU hourly.
- Frequently monitor the pulse, blood pressure, respiration, and state of consciousness.
- Take arterial blood for analysis of blood gases.
- Monitor potassium levels and give potassium as necessary – plasma potassium will fall as the glucose level does in response to treatment.
- Catheterize the patient to monitor urine output.
- Screen the patient for infection, including collecting a mid-stream urine sample and blood for cultures; start antibiotics if there is any suspicion of infection.
- In unconscious patients, aspirate the stomach contents with a nasogastric tube.
- Monitor the patient for cardiac arrhythmias (e.g. as occur in hypokalaemia) with a continuous ECG display.

insulin by the islet cells. Some problems encountered with the sulphonylureas include hypoglycaemia, fluid retention, and alcohol intolerance. The other group of drugs commonly used are the biguanides, which act by inhibiting hepatic gluconeogenesis – metformin is the most widely used of these.

Insulin

Insulin preparations may be short acting (e.g. Actrapid), intermediate acting (e.g. Lente), or long acting (e.g. isophane). Insulin is extracted from a number of different sources, including pigs and cattle; a human recombinant form of insulin is also available.

A number of problems may be encountered with insulin therapy. When treatment has been obtained from a non-human sources, anti-insulin antibodies may be raised because the patient's immune system perceives it as foreign. In addition, lipoatrophy may be found at the injection site (owing to immunological reactions to components of insulin). From another perspective, patients of certain religious beliefs may be unwilling to accept insulin from a non-human source (e.g. strict adherents of Hinduism cannot use bovine insulin; orthodox Jews cannot use porcine insulin).

Hypoglycaemia is another possible complication. This is an invariable side-effect in patients with no endogenous insulin secretion who attempt very tight control of blood glucose levels. Many patients quickly learn to recognize the symptoms of hypoglycaemia, which include sweating, unsteadiness, and headaches; however, hypoglycaemia may also present with fitting or even coma.

Insulin is generally given as subcutaneous injections which may be self-administered or given by a carer (e.g. a parent or health care professional). Multiple,

twice-daily or thrice-daily regimens are prescribed to suit the patient's needs. A twice-daily pattern of administration is the most common, and a mixture of short-acting and either long-acting or intermediate-acting insulin is generally used.

Other causes of coma in diabetic patients must be borne in mind; these include hyperglycaemic ketoacidosis, uraemic coma, and lactic acidosis (Box 35.2) (see also Chapter 6).

COMPLICATIONS

These are sometimes referred to as late tissue damage. Broadly speaking, they can be divided into those caused by microvascular disease and those caused by macrovascular disease. In the former group are the classical retinopathy, nephropathy, and neuropathy generally ascribed to small-vessel disease in the retinas, glomeruli, and nerves respectively. Macrovascular complications in diabetes include ischaemic heart disease, hypertension, and peripheral vascular disease.

There are also complications that do not appear to be directly related to any kind of vascular problem, such as damage to the fetus in poorly controlled pregnant mothers and chronic pyelonephritis, which results in renal failure.

The pathological and biochemical mechanisms that lead to the various types of tissue injury in diabetes remain poorly understood. Suggested mechanisms include vascular leakage, abnormal attachment of some of the excess glucose molecules to plasma proteins, and abnormal platelet function. The risk of developing these complications is greater in patients whose glucose levels are poorly controlled, though well-controlled diabetics can still develop these complications.

It seems that susceptibility is governed to some extent by the length of time that the patient has had diabetes.

Diabetic Eye Disease

Diabetic eye disease particularly affects patients with insulin-dependent diabetes. Abnormalities in the retinal vessels lead to reduced blood flow as well as capillary leakage and microaneurysm formation (background retinopathy). Retinal haemorrhages, protein exudates ('hard exudates'), and areas of focal ischaemia ('cotton wool spots') may occur. The next phase involves the formation of new, abnormal vessels (proliferative retinopathy). These vessels tend to cause recurrent vitreous haemorrhage and progressive visual loss. Finally, fibrosis occurs, and the retraction of fibrous tissue leads to retinal detachment. Hard exudates may form around the macula, leading to blindness.

Cataracts are also common in diabetic patients, particularly the older adults with non-insulin-dependent diabetes, who tend to develop the exudative form of diabetic eye disease. Insulin-dependent diabetics are more prone to develop proliferative retinopathy (see Figure 35.2).

Diabetic Renal Disease

Around one-third of patients with diabetes are likely to develop diabetic renal disease. Abnormalities of the basement membrane lining the renal capillaries lead to the leakage of protein (microalbuminuria), which can be detected at an early stage with immunological tests. The loss of larger amounts of protein can be detected with reagent strips. The period of time it takes for a patient to progress from intermittent albuminuria to renal failure is variable, but the average is about 5 years. Patients have no symptoms early in diabetic renal disease, but as renal failure progresses, patients become fatigued, glucose control becomes more difficult, and some patients develop ankle swelling (oedema) if there is excessive loss of albumin in the urine. Both insulin-dependent and non-insulin dependent diabetics are at risk of developing diabetic renal disease. Diabetic nephropathy is often accompanied by hypertension.

Renal failure is managed with dialysis, and renal transplantation is an option for patients who are otherwise healthy (i.e. who do not suffer with cardiac disease) (see Chapter 29).

Diabetic Neuropathy

Diabetic neuropathy may affect the sensory, motor, or autonomic nerves. Distal sensory neuropathy is the most common form, but most patients are asymptomatic. It is usually symmetrical and the feet are most often affected. Typically, patients complain of a numbness or heaviness in the soles of the feet. Motor neuropathy is rare; in a form called diabetic amyotrophy, there is wasting and weakness, mainly affecting the thigh muscles. Myalgia may be troublesome; severely painful diabetic neuropathy also occurs, affecting mainly the feet. Autonomic neuropathy manifests as erectile dysfunction in men and bladder dysfunction, leading to recurrent urinary tract infections and possibly urinary retention. Diabetic diarrhoea may arise where the gut is affected; postural hypotension and sweating disorders are other possible manifestations.

Arteriosclerosis

All people with diabetes have an increased tendency to develop arteriosclerosis in the large and medium arteries, with the coronary and leg vessels particularly likely to be affected. Myocardial infarction probably accounts for more deaths than any other diabetes-related health problem. Diabetic patients experiencing a myocardial infarct have a poorer prognosis than non-diabetics. In the periphery, the femoral arteries are most often diseased, causing ischaemic pain on walking (intermittent claudication) and in extreme cases, the need for amputation. Cerebrovascular events and hypertension also occur more frequently in diabetics than in non-diabetic.

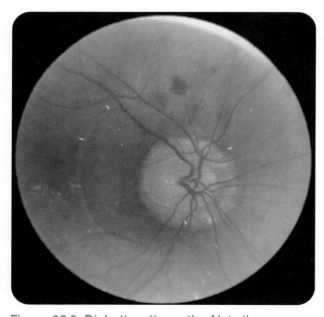

Figure 35.2 Diabetic retinopathy. Note the microaneurysms and soft exudates in the retina, which cause deterioration of vision. (© Medical Illustration., Addenbrooke's NHS Trust, Cambridge, UK.)

The Diabetic Foot

Foot and ankle ulcers constitute one of the most common problems in patients with diabetes, particularly those with non-insulin-dependent diabetes. It is multifactorial in origin. Vessel disease, peripheral neuropathy, poorly controlled diabetes, poor hygiene, and poor eyesight (which is common in people with diabetes) are some of the factors that lead to foot ulceration. Foot problems in diabetic patients account for more hospital bed occupancy than any of the other medical complications of this disease. Superficial infected ulcers are more common than the classical neuropathic ulcer (due to loss of sensation) or the ischaemic ulcer (due to impaired blood supply) (see Figure 35.3). Fulminant infection and the spread of gangrene may require amputation.

PREVENTION OF COMPLICATIONS AND SPECIAL PROBLEMS

Patients with diabetes should be screened regularly for eye disease and for microalbuminuria. It is generally held that good metabolic control is essential to the prevention, or the delay of onset, of microvascular complications. Good dietary habits and well-controlled diabetes reduce serum cholesterol levels and the risk of major vessel disease. Risk factors such as smoking should also be discouraged.

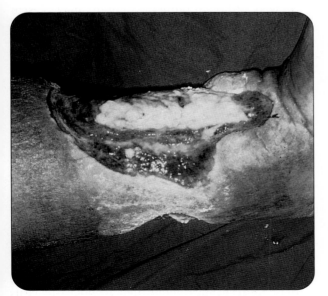

Figure 35.3 Diabetic leg ulcer. (© Medical Illustration,. Addenbrooke's NHS Trust, Cambridge, UK.)

Pregnancy

Diabetes during pregnancy carries risks both to the mother and the fetus. The pregnant diabetic woman is at higher risk of ketoacidosis, pre-eclampsia, hypertension, and urinary tract infections. Poor metabolic control in early pregnancy can lead to growth retardation of the fetus and congenital malformations. In the third trimester of pregnancy, poorly controlled diabetes may lead to large but immature babies who are at risk of respiratory distress syndrome. The large baby of a diabetic mother is thought to be the result of hyperstimulation of the fetal pancreas, and this tendency to hyperinsulin secretion may lead to hypoglycaemia in neonatal life. Patients should receive pre-pregnancy counselling, and they should be closely monitored during pregnancy. Many patients with diabetes who were not previously on insulin will require insulin during pregnancy, and insulin doses will need to rise as the pregnancy progresses.

Surgery

Many diabetic patients require surgery at some time. Anaesthesia elicits a stress response, and the surgery itself invariably provokes a major catabolic response, leading to the release of cortisol, noradrenaline, and growth hormone. All of these reactions have the capacity to induce severe hyperglycaemia and ketoacidosis in the diabetic patient. Thus, an insulin-dependent diabetic patient undergoing surgery should be admitted to hospital at least 2 days before the surgery in order to be stabilized on short-acting and intermediate-acting insulins. On the day of surgery, the morning dose of insulin and breakfast is generally omitted, and blood glucose is controlled by an intravenous infusion of insulin, glucose, and potassium. Blood glucose and electrolytes must be checked regularly during surgery, and again at the end of the operation.

At present, patients with insulin-dependent diabetes need a regular, injectable source of insulin in order to survive. However, new preparations of insulin have been developed that can be given orally, although these are still at the stage of clinical trials. Another treatment strategy being explored is the transplant of fetally derived pancreatic islet tissue into the kidney capsule of patients with diabetes. This transplanted tissue would act as a source of insulin. However, the use of fetal tissue is highly controversial, and data so far have been mainly based on procedures in rodents.

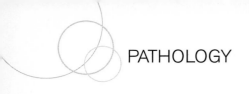

PATHOLOGY

HYPOTHALAMUS AND PITUITARY

The pituitary gland is situated in the pituitary fossa, a saddle-shaped, bony cavity at the base of the brain. It comprises a posterior lobe, which arises from the neural tissue of the forebrain, and an anterior lobe, which develops from the oropharynx. The secretory functions of the pituitary gland are largely controlled by the hypothalamus, which is situated above it and connected to it by a stalk. This stalk carries nerve fibres to the posterior pituitary and blood vessels to the anterior pituitary.

There are two groups of nuclei in the hypothalamus; one group in the anterior hypothalamus contains neurones that synthesize vasopressin (antidiuretic hormone, or ADH) and oxytocin. These are carried down the nerve axons in the stalk, to be stored and released in the posterior pituitary. The second set of nuclei in the hypothalamus are neurones that respond to stimulation from many areas of the brain. These nuclei secrete hormones (see Table 35.1), which travel along the vessels in the pituitary stalk to reach the anterior pituitary gland, where they regulate the secretion of hormones from the anterior pituitary gland (see Figure 35.1).

ANTERIOR PITUITARY HORMONES

The anterior pituitary gland synthesizes and releases trophic hormones into the circulation, which act on target organs to induce the secretion of other hormones:
- thyroid-stimulating hormone (TSH) acts on the thyroid gland to stimulate the release of the thyroid hormones, thyroxine (T_4) and tri-iodothyronine (T_3);
- adrenocorticotrophic hormone (ACTH) acts on the adrenal cortex to stimulate release of glucocorticoids; and
- luteinizing hormone (LH) and follicle-stimulating hormone (FSH) act on the gonads to stimulate production of testosterone and oestrogens, and are essential for pubertal development.

Other hormones produced by the pituitary include growth hormone and prolactin. The synthesis and secretion of the anterior pituitary hormones are controlled by regulatory hormones produced by the hypothalamus and carried in the hypophyseal venous system down to the pituitary gland. Many of these are given the name of 'releasing hormones' – thyrotrophin-releasing hormone, growth hormone-releasing hormone, corticotrophin-releasing hormone, and gonadotrophin-releasing hormone. Negative regulatory mechanisms also operate, either from the hypothalamus or from the levels of hormones released by target organs in the body. For example, dopamine produced by the hypothalamus inhibits prolactin secretion, while high levels of circulating cortisol produced by the adrenal gland suppress the release of ACTH from the pituitary. The positive and negative regulatory mechanisms highly complex, but are highly significant when considering the clinical implications of excessive production or decreased production of any one of these hormones.

POSTERIOR PITUITARY HORMONES

Antidiuretic hormone and oxytocin are synthesized in nerve cell bodies in the hypothalamus and carried down the axons to be released in the posterior pituitary gland (see Figure 35.1).

PITUITARY TUMOURS

Tumours arising in the pituitary gland can have profound effects on endocrine function, either by increasing or suppressing normal hormone production. For example, an excess of growth hormone released by patients with a pituitary tumour leads to acromegaly. Similarly, infertility may arise when there is a prolactinoma, one of the more common forms of pituitary tumours, because of the resultant secretion of excess prolactin, which causes hypogonadism. Chromophobe tumours may arise, but most of them are non-functioning and simply lead to anterior pituitary failure (see also Chapter 5).

Indeed, although pituitary tumours may present with the clinical features of hormone excess or lack of production, some patients present with headaches or with symptoms caused by compression of the optic chiasm by upward extension of the tumour. The optic nerves cross at the optic chiasm, with the fibres from the nasal retina being the most vulnerable; hence, patients classically lose vision in the outer parts of their visual field on both sides. Occasionally, pituitary tumours extend downward into the sphenoid sinus and cause leakage of cerebrospinal fluid through the nose (cerebrospinal fluid rhinorrhoea).

Acromegaly

Acromegaly is caused by a tumour of the pituitary that secretes excessive amounts of growth hormone. Patients present late in the natural history of the condition; hence an X-ray of the skull will often show an enlarged pituitary fossa. Computerized tomography scanning is useful for revealing tumours that are not easily visualized on conventional X-ray. However, the enlarged hands and feet that occur in acromegaly are one of several clinical features that can help to confirm the diagnosis. Growth hormone acts on peripheral tissues to stimulate the growth of both soft tissue and bone through its effects on protein, fat, and carbohydrate metabolism. Excess secretion leads to gigantism or acromegaly (and absence leads to dwarfism). In acromegaly, there is overgrowth of cancellous bone, leading to a protruding jaw and coarsening of facial features with thickened lips, tongue, and nose and enlarged head circumference. In addition, ovarian function may be influenced by growth hormone levels, and therefore women may present with amenorrhoea. Other problems include hypertension and impaired cardiac function, arthritis, headache, and visual field defects. Secondary diabetes occurs in up to 20 per cent of acromegaly patients. Untreated patients have a reduced life expectancy and an increased risk of death from cardiovascular and cerebrovascular events.

Diagnosis is made on the elevated levels of growth hormone in the serum. A glucose tolerance test may also be useful. Treatment is aimed at eliminating the tumour or at least at reducing its effects by using drugs such as bromocriptine and somatostatin, which inhibit growth hormone production. Surgery or radiation to the pituitary are the major treatment options, with bromocriptine used as an adjunct.

Hyperprolactinaemia

Prolactinomas are tumours of the pituitary that secrete prolactin. Large tumours are called macroprolactinomas; smaller one are called microprolactinomas. Microprolactinomas are more common and do not often progress to become large tumours. Hyperprolactinaemia causes galactorrhoea (secretion of milk from the breasts), irregularities in the menstrual cycle and infertility in women, and impotence in men. In addition to prolactin-secreting tumours of the pituitary, hypersecretion of prolactin can also be due to pregnancy, hypothyroidism, or drugs. Diagnosis is made on elevated serum prolactin levels.

Drugs that stimulate dopamine receptors, such as bromocriptine and dopamine itself, are able to suppress prolactin secretion. Bromocriptine remains the treatment of choice, since even large prolactinomas will shrink in response to treatment with this drug (see also Chapter 37).

Diabetes Insipidus

Diabetes insipidus is caused by a deficiency in antidiuretic hormone (ADH) activity. It is characterized by polyuria and polydipsia, because patients are unable to concentrate urine and hence to conserve water. The condition may be precipitated by a lack of production of ADH (cranial diabetes insipidus) or because the kidneys are unresponsive to the hormone (nephrogenic

diabetes insipidus). The former may be caused by head injury, trauma, or by surgery. The diagnosis is made on the basis of a high plasma osmolality, in conjunction with a low urine osmolality. Treatment is with a synthetic analogue of ADH, deamino-dys-*d*-arginine vasopressin (DDAVP), which is given by intranasal spray.

TESTS OF PITUITARY FUNCTION

Assays for serum or plasma concentrations of hormones are immunologically based – that is, the amount of specific antibody that binds the hormone is quantified, either by radioactive assay or by enzymatic means. A radioimmunoassay measures the degree to which the hormone in the patient's serum or plasma competes with radiolabelled hormone for binding to a specific antibody. The more hormone there is, the less radioactivity will be detected bound to the antibody. In an enzyme-linked immunoassay, the specific antibody is conjugated to an enzyme and then quantified by measuring the amount of conversion of a coloured substrate (see also Chapter 24). In addition to measuring steady-state serum levels of hormones, many tests of endocrine function are aimed at assessing the ability of the body to respond to stress or a pharmacological stimulus. Such tests are termed dynamic tests of endocrine function and are often very useful.

Dynamic Test of Endocrine Function

The diagnosis of Cushing's syndrome is made by:
- demonstrating loss of the normal regulation of ACTH production by the anterior pituitary using an adrenal suppression test (see Chapter 6).
- This distinguishes between Cushing's syndrome caused by an overactive adrenal gland and the presence of an ACTH-secreting tumour either in the pituitary gland or in some other tissue such as lung.

The insulin or hypoglycaemia stress test evaluates the ability of the body to respond to insulin-induced hypoglycaemia by increasing plasma levels of cortisol.
- This response is dependent on the ability of the anterior pituitary to respond by secreting ACTH.
- Failure to respond appropriately to this test suggests an inadequate production of ACTH, which could be due to prolonged suppression caused by an autonomous source of cortisol, as may occur with an adrenal tumour, for example.

In the investigation of adrenocortical failure, synacthen (a synthetic analogue of ACTH) is administered. This stimulates cortisol secretion.

- If an increase in plasma cortisol is not detected in response to a synacthen test, this indicates reduced function of the adrenal cortex.
- A glucose tolerance test assesses the ability of the pituitary to suppress production of growth hormone, which opposes the actions of insulin (see also Chapter 6).
- Loss of this regulatory response may be due to a growth-hormone-producing tumour causing acromegaly.

ADRENAL DISEASE

The adrenal glands are found on the upper pole of each kidney, and the adrenal cortex is the major source of steroid hormones in the body. The steroid hormones can be divided into:

- the glucocorticoids;
- the mineralocorticoids; and
- the sex hormones.

Glucocorticoids stimulate gluconeogenesis and protein breakdown, and hence excess glucocorticoids may lead to diabetes mellitus and a catabolic state, whereas a deficiency may lead to hypoglycaemia. Another important action of glucocorticoids, and one that is much exploited in clinical medicine, is immunosuppression (see Chapter 29).

Mineralocorticoids, such as aldosterone, act to increase sodium retention in the kidneys, with concomitant potassium loss.

Androgen secretion from the adrenal cortex is not clinically significant except in rare states of overproduction, such as congenital adrenal hyperplasia.

ADDISON'S DISEASE

This is a rare but life-threatening condition caused by lack of glucocorticoid production by the adrenal cortex. It gives rise to adrenal insufficiency, which may present acutely or insidiously. Historically, the commonest cause was tuberculosis, but these days it is invariably found because there has either been autoimmune destruction of the adrenal gland or because corticosteroid therapy has been abruptly withdrawn.

Acute adrenal insufficiency presents as shock, with hypotension and dehydration. Chronic adrenal insufficiency presents as lassitude, weakness, vomiting, diarrhoea, weight loss, thirst, and polyuria. Patients may develop the classical bronzed pigmentation owing to uncontrolled pituitary secretion of ACTH, which has some melanocyte-stimulating

activity. Acute adrenal insufficiency is a medical emergency and should be treated with hydrocortisone and rehydration.

CUSHING'S SYNDROME

Hypersecretion of adrenocorticoids is most often due to excessive pituitary secretion of ACTH (Cushing's syndrome). However, it may rarely be due to hypersecretion by an adrenal adenoma or carcinoma (most commonly found in children) or by an ectopic source of ACTH, such as a bronchial carcinoma (ectopic ACTH syndrome). However, the syndrome of excess cortisol often occurs as a complication of steroid therapy (Figure 35.4).

The altered apearance produced by the condition causes much morbidity, as do the metabolic distur-

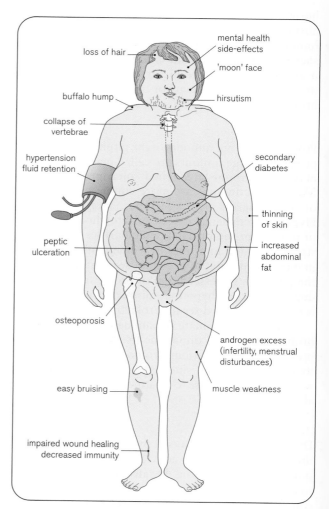

Figure 35.4 Clinical features of Cushing's syndrome.

bances, muscle weakness, hypertension, back pain associated with osteoporosis, and adverse mental health effects. Frank peptic ulceration and subsequent bleeding may develop. In females, the increased androgen secretion as a consequence of the increased production of all adrenocorticohormones may lead to hirsutism (especially excessive facial hair). When an ACTH-secreting tumour is the cause, patients may have increased skin pigmentation, which is really the response of the melanocytes to ACTH (see also Addison's disease).

The differential diagnosis of Cushing's syndrome is made on specific tests of adrenal and pituitary function. For example, ACTH levels in the plasma are virtually undetectable in patients with adrenal tumours. If the dexamethasone suppression test is performed using high-dose dexamethasone, patients with ectopic ACTH secretion do not respond, but those with pituitary disease (Cushing's disease) will demonstrate some response (see also Chapter 6).

Treatment of Cushing's syndrome involves surgical removal of the adrenal gland, or pituitary secreting tumour, where possible. Metyrapone acts to block the synthesis of cortisol, but it is seldom effective on its own but given as an adjunct to surgery.

THYROID DISEASE

The thyroid gland develops in the first month of embryonic life. In the adult it consists of two lobes joined by an isthmus that lies in front of the trachea. Thyroid hormones are essential for normal growth and development. There are two major hormones produced by the thyroid gland: thyroxine (T_4) and tri-iodothyronine (T_3), which is the most active form of the hormone. The synthesis and release of thyroid hormones is under the regulation of the pituitary and hypothalamus (see above).

The major cause of thyroid disease world-wide is iodine deficiency, which leads to an enlargement of the thyroid gland, termed goitre (Figure 35.5), and hypothyroidism. Severe thyroid deficiency in infancy is called congenital hypothyroidism, and growth retardation, neurological impairment, and intellectual impairment result if the disorder is not effectively treated. A blood spot test (similar to the Guthrie test for phenylketonuria) may be performed on newborn infants. The specimen of blood is used to estimate the blood level of thyroid-stimulating hormone, which is raised in infants with congenital hypothyroidism. The adverse effects of this disorder can be prevented by starting the thyroxine therapy in early infancy.

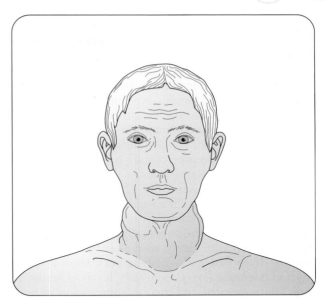

Figure 35.5 A large goitre.

In non-iodine deficient areas, the most common cause of thyroid dysfunction is autoimmune thyroid disease, which can give rise to either excessive or diminished production of thyroid hormones (see Chapter 27).

GOITRE

The thyroid gland enlarges physiologically during puberty and pregnancy. Other causes of enlargement of the thyroid gland include autoimmune disease (accompanied by either hypothyroidism or hyperthyroidism). Goitre is endemic in parts of Asia, Africa, and South America, where it is caused by a nutritional deficiency of iodine (e.g. low levels of iodine in water and the crops).

Nodules and cysts may also form in the thyroid. These are usually benign, as is a thyroid adenoma (i.e. a non-malignant growth of the glandular tissue of the thyroid). Thyroid cancers include lymphomas and carcinomas. They may be treated surgically with or without a dose of radioactive iodine.

HYPERTHYROIDISM

Hyperthyroidism affects some 2 per cent of women and is ten times more common in women than in men. In young women, it is usually due to Graves' disease, in which autoantibodies directed against thyroid cells initially stimulate production and secretion of thyroid hormones but the disease eventually evolves into a state of hypothyroidism due to damage to the thyroid cells.

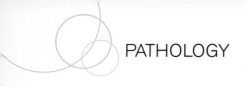

Graves' disease is associated with a smooth diffuse goitre (see Chapter 27). In older women, hyperthyroidism is more often due to a multinodular goitre.

Symptoms are due to an increased metabolic rate and increased protein catabolism, and include restlessness, irritability, fatigue, heat intolerance, palpitations, and sleeplessness. Weight loss in the face of increased food intake is common, as are frequent bowel actions, a fine tremor of the hands, and eyelid retraction, giving the impression of staring eyes. Some women may suffer from amenorrhoea.

Thyrotoxic crisis is rare but it has a significant mortality. It is characterized by a sudden surge in the release of thyroid hormones, causing arrhythmias, cardiac failure, hyperpyrexia, and eventually coma. It may arise as a result of major stress, such as surgery. The diagnosis of thyrotoxicosis is made an evaluation of serum thyroid hormone levels. Generally, levels of serum T_4 and T_3 are elevated and there is suppression of pituitary production of TSH.

Treatment of hyperthyroidism is aimed at removal or destruction of glandular tissue or suppression of thyroid hormone synthesis with drugs. Surgical removal of part of the thyroid carries the risk of damage to the parathyroid glands, which are situated nearby. Radioactive iodine (^{131}Iodine) destroys thyroid cells and is effective treatment in older patients past childbearing years. Anti-thyroid drugs include carbimazole and propylthiouracil; these inhibit the synthesis of thyroid hormones.

HYPOTHYROIDISM

As mentioned above, this commonly results from iodine deficiency in many parts of the world, but it may also arise as one end of the spectrum of autoimmune thyroid disease. Regrettably, previous surgery or radioactive iodine therapy for hyperthyroidism can result in a hypothyroid state.

Hypothyroidism generally affects older women, who present with a long history of general fatigue, slowing of mental and physical activity, intolerance to cold, constipation, and weight gain. Mental health features are not uncommon (e.g. depression, psychosis, and dementia). In fact, this disorder was named myxoedema madness, and it was responsible for the institutionalization of a large number of patients in mental hospital in the 19th century.

Patients may also suffer from menorrhagia, anaemia, and cardiac failure. Patients with primary hypothyroidism (i.e. hypothyroidism that is due to primary failure of the thyroid gland) have a low T_4 level together with an elevated level of TSH. The serum TSH is often used to screen for hypothyroidism and to monitor the adequacy of replacement therapy. Treatment with thyroxine replacement therapy should be commenced in small doses, and with care, particularly in older adult patients. With adequate replacement, the TSH level should return to within the normal range. Occasionally, hypothyroidism may result from pituitary disease or pituitary surgery, in which case the TSH is low at diagnosis.

PARATHYROID DISEASE AND CALCIUM METABOLISM

Parathyroid hormone is produced by the four parathyroid glands, which are situated at the upper and lower poles of the thyroid gland. Parathyroid hormone (PTH) acts primarily on the kidneys to increase calcium absorption and on bone to increase calcium resorption. Therefore it has the effect of raising serum calcium levels. Secretion of PTH is regulated by the serum calcium.

Calcitonin is another calcium-regulating hormone. It is made by the thyroid C-cells and is released in response to high plasma calcium levels. It inhibits bone resorption by osteoclasts and promotes the renal excretion of calcium. Therefore it has the effect of lowering serum calcium levels.

HYPERCALCAEMIA

The commonest causes of hypercalcaemia are malignancy and primary hyperparathyroidism. Mild hypercalcaemia is more likely to be due to hyperparathyroidism, whereas a vastly elevated calcium level is likely to be due to malignancy. For instance, hypercalcaemia may be seen in carcinoma of the lung and myeloma, where the tumour cells produce a substance that stimulates bone resorption and calcium release. This may also occur with malignancies of the breast, ovary, and prostate when there are multiple secondary bony metastases. Myeloma has also been characteristically associated with hypercalcaemia.

Primary hyperparathyroidism is much more common in women. It is usually due to an adenoma of one of the parathyroid glands. Rarely, is it associated with hyperplasia of the glands, such as in multiple endocrine neoplasia with associated pancreatic, thyroid, and pituitary tumours (see Chapters 3 and 5). Other rare causes of hypercalcaemia include sarcoidosis and severe thyrotoxicosis.

Patients with hypercalcaemia may experience symptoms of lethargy, constipation, polyuria and thirst, nausea, vomiting, and dehydration. In severe cases, renal failure and coma may result. This demands prompt rehydration with close attention to cardiac status. Calcium-lowering drugs, such as disodium etidronate and the biphosphonates, are also useful. In patients with malignant hypercalcaemia, oral steroid therapy may be useful. Primary hyperparathyroidism may be treated with surgery, but this carries the risk of post-operative hypocalcaemia.

KEY POINTS

- Diabetes mellitus is a condition that results from the relative or absolute lack of insulin.
- Insulin-dependent diabetes commonly presents in childhood and early adulthood and is considered to be an autoimmune disease that progresses to a complete failure of insulin production by the islet cells.
- Non-insulin-dependent diabetes presents with polyuria, polydipsia, weight loss, and genitourinary infections. In these patients, who are generally older, other pathological manifestations occur, the most notable being major vessel disease, such as angina or myocardial infarction.
- Complications of diabetes mellitus may be microvascular, generally ascribed to small-vessel disease in the retinas, glomeruli, and nerves, and retinopathy, nephropathy, and neuropathy.
- The macrovascular complications in diabetes include ischaemic heart disease, hypertension, and peripheral vascular disease.
- The successful management of diabetes is largely delivered by the patients – dietary management, regular monitoring of blood glucose levels, and administration of appropriate amounts of insulin or oral hypoglycaemic drugs.
- Tumours arising in the pituitary gland may have profound effects on endocrine function.

Although they may present with the clinical features of hormone excess or deficiency, some patients present with headaches or with visual disturbances.
- Addison's disease is a rare but life-threatening condition caused by lack of glucocorticoid production by the adrenal cortex.
- Cushing's syndrome is provoked by excess cortisol, and it may present as a complication of steroid therapy. The symptoms include muscle weakness, hypertension, back pain associated with osteoporosis. Frank peptic ulceration and bleeding may also develop.
- Hyperthyroidism causes an increased metabolic rate and protein catabolism. The symptoms include restlessness, weight loss, tremor, irritability, fatigue, heat intolerance, palpitations, and sleeplessness.
- Hypothyroidism generally affects older women, who present with a long history of general fatigue, slowing of mental and physical activity, weight gain, intolerance to cold, and constipation. Features such as depression and psychosis are not uncommon.
- The commonest causes of hypercalcaemia are malignancy and primary hyperparathyroidism, the latter being more common in women.

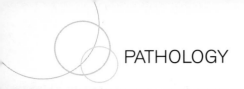

PATHOLOGY

FURTHER READING

Ahmed SF, Barnes ND, Hughes IA (1997) Initial evaluation of congenital hypothyroidism: a survey of general paediatricians in East Anglia. Arch Dis Child 77:339–41.

Anonymous (1997) Report of the expert committee on the diagnosis and classification of diabetes mellitus Diabetes Care 7:1183–97.

Baars J, Van den Broeck J, le Cessie S, Massa G, Wit JM (1998) Body mass index in growth hormone deficient children before and during growth hormone treatment. Horm Res 49:39–45.

Boehm S, Schlenk EA, Funnell MM, Powers H, Ronis DL (1997) Predictors of adherence to nutrition recommendations in people with non-insulin-dependent diabetes mellitus. Diabetes Educ 23:157–65.

Dattani M, Brook CG (1996) Outcomes of neonatal screening for congenital hypothyroidism. Curr Opin Pediatr 8:389–95.

Dussault JH (1997) Childhood primary hypothyroidism and endemic cretinism. Curr Ther Endocrinol Metab 6:107–9.

Hiatt JR, Hiatt N (1997) The conquest of Addison's disease. Am J Surg 174:280–3.

Hunter SK, Wang Y, Weiner CP, Niebyl J (1997) Encapsulated beta-islet cells as a bioartificial pancreas to treat insulin-dependent diabetes during pregnancy. Am J Obstet Gynecol 177:746–52.

Jarrett RJ Soares J de A, Dornhorstt A, Bread RW (1997) A case for screening for gestational diabetes. BMJ 315:735–9.

Low PA, Suarez GA (1995) Diabetic neuropathies. Baillieres Clin Neurol 4:401–25.

Lowes L, Davis R (1997) Minimizing hospitalization: children with newly diagnosed diabetes. Br J Nurs 6:28–33.

Ogilvy-Stuart AL (1995) Endocrinology of the neonate Br J Hosp Med 54:207–11.

Persily CA (1996)Relationships between the perceived impact of gestational diabetes mellitus and treatment adherence. J Obstet Gynecol Neonatal Nurs 25:601–7.

Reavley A, Fisher AD, Owen D, Creed FH, Davis JR (1997) Psychological distress in patients with hyperprolactinaemia. Clin Endocrinol (Oxf) 47:343–8.

Souhami RL, Moxham J (1997) Textbook of Medicine, 3rd edition. Churchill Livingstone, London.

Trump D, Farren B, Wooding C, et al. (1996) Clinical studies of multiple endocrine neoplasia type 1. Q J Med 89:653–69.

van der Lely AJ, de Herder WW, Lamberts SW (1997) A risk–benefit assessment of octreotide in the treatment of acromegaly. Drug Saf 17:317–24.

Walsh JP, Pullan PT (1997) Hyperprolactinaemia in males: a heterogeneous disorder. Aust N Z J Med 27:385–90.

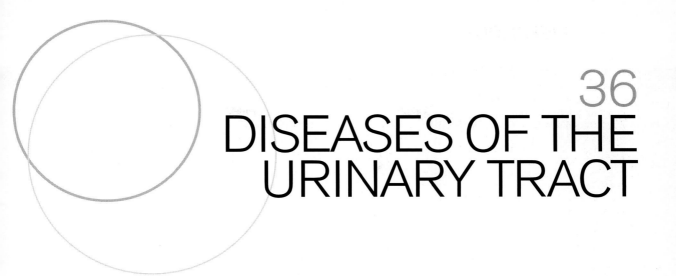

36
DISEASES OF THE
URINARY TRACT

LEARNING OBJECTIVES

After studying this chapter students should have a clearer understanding of:
• the common causes of infections of the urinary tract and the possible consequences
• the different tumours of the renal tract and their prognoses
• the pathophysiology of renal failure and the principles of management including dialysis
• the importance of the kidney in the role of excretion, including the excretion of drugs

Before reading this chapter you should have a basic understanding of:
• the anatomy of the urinary tract, including the kidneys, ureters, and bladder;
• the physiology of kidney function as an organ of excretion and hormone secretion,
• the role of the kidney in maintaining homeostasis.

URINARY TRACT INFECTIONS

Urinary tract infections (UTIs) may involve any part of the renal tract, from the kidney itself in pyelonephritis down to the more common infections of the bladder (cystitis).

PREDISPOSING FACTORS
Predisposing factors include:
• female sex – lower UTIs are very common in women, who have a shorter urethra than men, which increases the risk of ascending infection by bacteria from the gut (e.g. coliform bacteria);
• anatomical abnormality – a bladder diverticulum (an outpouching of the bladder) allows urine to collect and stagnate, increasing the risk of infection;
• vesicoureteric reflux – normally the urine in the bladder is prevented from refluxing back up the ureters

by valves, but if this mechanism is incompetent, the urine is forced up the ureters during micturition, which may lead to pyelonephritis (Figure 36.1);
• pregnancy – the relaxant effect of the hormones of pregnancy causes dilatation of the ureters with stasis of urine flow, increasing the risk of infection;
• diabetes mellitus – the risk of UTI is higher in patients with secondary damage to the bladder nerves due to the diabetes;
• calculi – stones developing anywhere in the renal tract can first present with UTI or with blood in the urine (haematuria), and the infection often recurs until the stone is dealt with;
• catheters – a foreign body in the bladder increases the likelihood of bacteria being present in the normally sterile urine. However, the presence of bacteria in this situation does not necessarily mean that patients require antibiotics unless they are systemically unwell.

CLINICAL FEATURES
Cystitis
Infection confined to the bladder is the most common form of UTI and presents with dysuria (painful stinging and burning) on micturition, frequency of micturition (sometimes every few minutes), cloudy urine, and sometimes haematuria (blood in the urine). Some patients have a fever and abdominal pain as well.

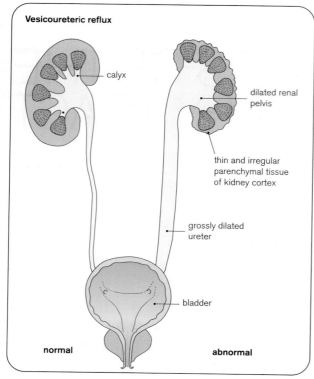

Vesicoureteric reflux

- calyx
- dilated renal pelvis
- thin and irregular parenchymal tissue of kidney cortex
- grossly dilated ureter
- bladder

normal   abnormal

Figure 36.1 Vesicoureteric reflux. Normal structure of the ureter and kidney compared with effects of persistent vesicoureteric reflux, which causes dilatation of the collecting system and destruction of the functioning renal tissue.

Acute Pyelonephritis

This is usually caused by ascending infection following on from cystitis, although the symptoms may be localized to the kidney. Patients are often unwell with pyrexia, loin pain, vomiting, and sometimes dysuria and haematuria.

Urinary Tract Infections in Children

Children with a UTI are often generally unwell, with a fever but no other obvious focus of infection, such as tonsillitis or ear infections. There should be a high index of suspicion for urinary infection and a low threshold for collecting a urine sample for culture, since it is important for future management to prove the presence of infection.

Vesicoureteric reflux predisposes to UTI and chronic pyelonephritis, which may cause long-term renal damage. This is particularly true in children; hence any UTI in a child is investigated after treatment. Surgery to the bladder and ureters can correct the reflux and prevent chronic pyelonephritis, which in turn can be a cause of chronic renal failure requiring dialysis and transplantation. Reflux is sometimes diagnosed *in utero* and the newborn child is treated with prophylactic antibiotics while being investigated; surgery may then be performed if required.

INVESTIGATIONS

Midstream Urine

Microscopy and culture of a midstream urine sample is the most important investigation (see Chapter 17). Taking the midstream portion of the sample reduces the likelihood of bacterial skin contaminants in the sample. The urine is examined microscopically for the presence of red and white blood cells, which are often increased in a UTI. The normal result is less than 10 red or white blood cells per high-power field.

The urine is then cultured on agar jelly laboratory plates to identify the infecting organism. The plate also contains antibiotic discs to specify the sensitivity of the bacteria to treatment. This has become increasingly important since some bacteria are becoming resistant to standard antibiotics. The whole process takes at least 48 hours and often treatment is started empirically and changed if the antibiotic chosen proves not to be the correct one.

The usual organisms are those found in the gut, including coliforms, *Enterococcus* species, *Proteus* species, and *Klebsiella* species. More rarely, though particularly if there is an underlying cause for the UTI, *Pseudomonas aeruginosa* is isolated (see Chapter 16).

Imaging

Investigating the underlying cause may involve an ultrasound of the renal tract, which can detect the presence of calculi and dilatation of the renal pelvis and ureters. Intravenous urography (IVU) gives a picture of the excreting function of the kidney. An intravenous injection of a dye is given; the dye is excreted by the kidney, thereby outlining the kidneys, ureters, and bladder on X-ray and so demonstrating any obstruction or lack of excretion.

Cystoscopy

Checking the bladder requires a cystoscopy, in which a flexible scope with a fibreoptic light source is passed through the urethra into the bladder and a visual inspection made, particularly to look for tumours and stones. Occasionally, recurrent UTIs are associated with the presence of a bladder tumour; this may be seen as a filling defect in the bladder on the IVU, and a cystoscopy is then required to examine the mass and take tissue biopsies (see Chapter 6).

MANAGEMENT

A high fluid intake is important to relieve symptoms by diluting the urine concentration. Low-grade infections may not require antibiotic therapy, and changing the pH of the urine with mixtures such as potassium citrate sometimes makes the urine unfavourable to bacterial multiplication and survival.

If an antibiotic is required, the one most frequently prescribed for UTIs is trimethoprim, followed by amoxycillin, although resistance to the latter is increasing. A 3-day course is usually long enough for a simple bladder infection, but acute pyelonephritis may require intravenous antibiotics and fluids, particularly if the patient is repeatedly vomiting.

CHRONIC PYELONEPHRITIS

Chronic pyelonephritis is a common cause of renal failure and is diagnosed on IVU appearances and histologically. There is unilateral or bilateral scarring of the kidney tissue, producing an irregular outline to the normally smooth kidney. The renal papillae are flattened, giving a characteristic 'clubbed' appearance on the IVU. Histologically, there is scarring and fibrosis, with atrophy of the renal tubules. There is also inflammation and thickening of the collecting system.

PATHOGENESIS

Originally, chronic pyelonephritis was thought to be due to repeated episodes of acute pyelonephritis leading to scarring and tissue destruction. However, it is now clear that it may develop in the absence of infection and may progress without further infection.

There are two conditions that are clearly associated with chronic pyelonephritis – vesicoureteric reflux and urinary obstruction – but the exact mechanism of injury is not yet identified.

Vesicoureteric reflux is frequently associated with chronic pyelonephritis. Although reflux of infected urine is particularly harmful, even in the absence of infection, the reflux itself seems to produce repeated insults to the renal tissue leading to scarring.

Obstruction to the renal tract is another association with chronic pyelonephritis. It is often due to structural abnormalities of the bladder. Chronic pyelonephritis developing in the absence of reflux and obstruction may occur, and there is often no obvious explanation.

CLINICAL FEATURES AND MANAGEMENT

Patients often first present after they have developed chronic renal failure. Rarely, chronic pyelonephritis is discovered when a patient is found to be hypertensive and further investigations show that there is abnormal renal function causing the hypertension (see Chapter 32).

By this time, surgery for reflux is rarely useful, and this is why it is so important to identify reflux in childhood before scarring has occurred. Occasionally if a kidney is grossly infected and has minimal function, it is removed to reduce the risk of spread of infection.

Patients with chronic pyelonephritis who develop chronic renal failure require dialysis with a view to transplantation if a suitable match can be found.

URINARY CALCULI

Urinary stone formation is probably as old as humanity, and they have been found in human remains at archaeological digs of graves. One of the most famous victims was Samuel Pepys, who describes his sufferings in his diary. The incidence is about four times higher in men than women, and the stones may form recurrently or occur in isolation.

TYPES OF STONES

The most common chemical constituents of urinary stones are pure calcium oxalate (35 per cent) or a mixture of calcium oxalate and hydroxapatite (45 per cent). Magnesium ammonium phosphate stones, which often contain calcium phosphate as well, usually develop in association with infection. Rarer chemical types are uric acid and cystine stones.

PATHOGENESIS

The urinary system is the main route of excretion, and waste chemicals are carried in solution in the urine, often at a relatively high concentration. If the concentration of a chemical rises too high, the chemical may precipitate out and start to form a stone. There are some natural protective chemicals such as citrate and magnesium in the urine, that reduce the precipitation rate, and deficiencies of these predispose to stone formation.

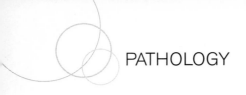

PATHOLOGY

Calcium Stones

Abnormally high levels of calcium may occur in the urine alone (hypercalciuria) or be secondary to high levels in the serum (hypercalcaemia). Hypercalcaemia may be caused by high levels of parathyroid hormone, which controls the blood concentration of calcium and is secreted by the parathyroid glands, which lie on the back of the thyroid gland in the neck (see Chapter 35). If a small benign tumour (adenoma) develops in one of these glands, excess amounts of parathyroid hormone may be secreted, causing the blood calcium level to rise. Urinary calcium stones may be the first sign of disease. Malignant disease may also cause hypercalcaemia; this is particularly common in cancer of the breast and lung.

An isolated rise in the amount of calcium in the urine is much more common than hypercalcaemia. This can be caused by vitamin D intoxication, sometimes from over-enthusiastic use of vitamin pills, when too much calcium is absorbed from the gut and has to be excreted. Some drugs, such as long-term frusemide, also cause high calcium levels in the urine. Often, however, no specific cause can be identified, and this is known as idiopathic hypercalciuria.

Uric Acid Stones

Uric acid stones form when there are high levels of uric acid in the blood (hyperuricaemia). Hyperuricaemia may also manifest as acute gout where the uric acid crystallizes in the joint fluid, causing acute pain and swelling (see Chapter 39). Uric acid is the breakdown product of purine bases, the majority of which come from the recycling of nucleotides, though a small proportion comes from dietary sources. Older age, male sex, excess weight and genetic predisposition all contribute to the risk of developing hyperuricaemia. Some rare enzyme deficiencies also cause raised levels.

Another special situation occurs when there is rapid cell breakdown, producing a high load of nucleoprotein to be excreted (e.g. in the treatment of leukaemia with chemotherapy). Prophylactic treatment is often given to prevent acute gout or renal stone formation in this situation.

Cystine Stones

Cystine stones form when there is an inherited enzyme deficiency that causes raised levels of cystine in the urine. Uric acid and cystine stones are relatively radiolucent, which means that they are not easily seen on a plain X-ray.

CLINICAL FEATURES

The most frequent presentation is an attack of renal or ureteric colic. This occurs when the stone moves into the ureter and the muscular wall starts to contract to try and move the obstruction down towards the bladder. This produces the characteristic pain of colic, which occurs in waves of intense pain. There is usually no tenderness on palpation, but the muscular contraction is said to be the nearest that men get to experiencing the pain of childbirth! The pain radiates into the groin and in men is often referred to the testis on the same side or even to the tip of the penis.

If the stone is small enough, the ureteric contraction may move it down into the bladder, when the pain ceases. The patient may then spontaneously pass the stone during micturition, and it is helpful to retrieve the stone by asking the patient to pass urine through a sieve so that it can be sent for chemical analysis. The stone may remain in the bladder and gradually enlarge, acting as a focus for bacteria and causing recurrent infections. There is usually blood in the urine at the time of the passage of the stone because it damages the lining epithelium.

Very occasionally, the stone may completely obstruct the ureter and create an acute build up of back pressure, causing damage to the kidney. This is an acute surgical emergency requiring relief of the pressure, which can be done in a variety of ways depending on where the stone is situated (see below).

DIAGNOSIS AND ACUTE MANAGEMENT

The history of renal colic is very characteristic and treatment is often required before the diagnosis is formally made because of the extreme pain that the patient is suffering. Analgesia is the first priority. Intramuscular pethidine used to be given, but parenteral diclofenac, a non-steroidal anti-inflammatory drug, has now been demonstrated to be more effective.

Once the pain has been relieved, the patient requires a plain abdominal X-ray – most stones are radio-opaque and will be fairly obvious. However, if the stone is small or overlies another radio-opaque structure such as bone, or if the stone is radiolucent, the patient will require an IVU. As the dye outlines the kidney pelvis and ureters, the stone will appear as a filling defect, and this will also identify the position at which it has become lodged.

A high fluid intake is important and the patient may require hospital admission for intravenous fluid administration and repeated parenteral analgesia if the attack does not subside. If the stone is not moving, it can be removed endoscopically through the bladder if it is at the lower end of the ureter. Lithotripsy, in which external ultrasound is directed at the stone to shatter it into fragments that the patient can then pass naturally in the urine, is sometimes used. This is more usually done in between acute attacks when residual stones are identifiable in the renal pelvis. Rarely, an open operation is required to remove the stone; this is indicated only if there is complete obstruction of the ureter.

LONG-TERM MANAGEMENT

Once the acute phase has been dealt with, it is important to investigate and correct, if possible, any underlying cause to prevent new stones forming. Chemical analysis of the stone may be helpful in identifying the abnormality, but otherwise screening for blood and urine calcium levels and uric acid levels, and checking drug therapy will identify most treatable causes.

If the calcium levels are high, a high fluid intake is a sensible precaution particularly when the person is likely to be sweating, and the person should not use vitamin D supplements or calcium tablets.

Underlying causes of hypercalcaemia need treating if possible (see Chapter 6), and removal of a parathyroid adenoma will solve the problem in the long term. If the high calcium level is due to malignancy, this may not be curable, but it can sometimes be controlled with chemotherapy.

For uric acid stones, allopurinol is a prophylactic drug that reduces the level of uric acid in the blood and reduces the incidence both of stone formation and acute gout.

RENAL FAILURE

Renal failure is a general term applied when the kidney function is severely compromised, and the excretory capacity of the kidneys is seriously reduced. The symptoms and signs vary depending on whether the problem has arisen suddenly, as in acute renal failure (ARF), or more slowly, as in chronic renal failure (CRF). The underlying causes are many and varied and may result from inherited disease, trauma, infection, or autoimmune disease (see Chapter 27).

ACUTE RENAL FAILURE

In ARF, the reduction in renal function occurs over a few hours or days, and the most common presenting sign is a reduced volume of urine. Less then 500 ml per 24 hours is defined as oliguria, and the patient may go on to become anuric, when they do not produce any urine at all.

The standard measure of renal excretory function is the glomerular filtration rate (GFR), which is measured by the rate at which a natural breakdown product, creatinine, is excreted (creatinine clearance rate). Creatinine levels rise when the GFR falls, and the higher the serum

levels of creatinine, the poorer the excretory capacity of the kidney (see Chapter 6). The causes of ARF are usually divided into pre-renal, renal and postrenal factors (Box 36.1).

Pre-renal causes

The underlying problem is a reduction in blood flow through the kidney from a low cardiac output, which in turn causes intense vasoconstriction and a reduced GFR. If this can be corrected by quickly restoring blood flow, this type of renal failure is reversible because the kidney is structurally normal. However, if the vasoconstriction persists for too long, there is ischaemic damage to the kidney (acute tubular necrosis), which is permanent.

Renal causes

Renal disease leading to ARF may be isolated to the kidney itself (e.g. acute glomerulonephritis) or be part of a multisystem disease (e.g. systemic lupus erythematosus). The kidney is also the site of action of some toxic chemicals, such as ethylene glycol (the chemical component of antifreeze) or heavy metals. Diseases of the glomeruli, the filtration system of the kidney, are often immunological (see Chapter 27). Acute glomerulonephritis may be caused by an abnormal immune response to a streptococcal throat infection, in which

---

BOX 36.1 CAUSES OF ACUTE RENAL FAILURE

Pre-renal causes
- shock (e.g. sepsis, haemorrhage, fluid loss as in burns, cardiogenic shock)
- reduced blood flow (e.g. renal artery stenosis)

Renal causes
- acute tubular damage (e.g. tubular necrosis)
- acute glomerular damage (e.g. glomerulonephritis)
- nephrotoxins (e.g. drugs, chemicals)
- vascular disease (e.g. disseminated intravascular coagulation)

Postrenal causes
- obstruction (e.g. bilateral stones, pelvic malignancy, retroperitoneal ureter compression as may be caused by a lymphoma)

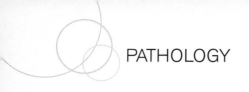
antigen–antibody complexes accumulate in the glomeruli and damage them (see Person-Centred Study: Acute Glomerulonephritis).

Postrenal causes

Any total obstruction to the drainage system of the kidneys causes back pressure and damage to the renal tissue. If the obstruction is quickly relieved, no permanent damage is done, but when the pressure is not easily reduced (e.g. in pelvic malignancy), renal failure often occurs.

Management

The identification and reversal of underlying causes are the most important elements of the management, since this may prevent progression to permanent renal damage.

Fluid balance

As the body has temporarily lost its homeostatic mechanism for fluid balance, it is crucial that fluid intake and output are carefully monitored. Fluid overload causes peripheral oedema and compromises cardiac function, leading to pulmonary oedema. Under-replacement of fluid worsens the kidney perfusion and exacerbates the renal injury. Daily weighing of the patient helps in the monitoring, along with fluid balance charts.

Sodium–potassium levels

The renal damage leads to a loss of control of sodium and potassium balance, which is crucial to sustaining life. High or low levels of potassium cause cardiac arrhythmias and sudden death, so stringent monitoring and control are critical.

Short-term dialysis

This may be necessary to maintain the body's biochemistry in a stable state while the kidney recovers. It can be performed by haemodialysis or peritoneal dialysis (see Chapter 1) and it can usually be withdrawn as the renal function improves.

PERSON-CENTRED STUDY: ACUTE GLOMERULONEPHRITIS

Jared, who was 10 years old, was a healthy boy who occasionally developed sore throats like all other children. This time, his sore throat lasted a few days and then improved as usual, but about 3 weeks later he suddenly started passing blood in the urine. His mother also noticed that he was passing only a very small volume of urine. He began to look puffy around the eyes and developed some ankle swelling.

He was admitted to hospital, where he was also found to have high blood pressure and protein in the urine. Blood tests showed that he had high levels of urea and creatinine, and that the sodium–potassium levels in his blood were abnormal. A renal biopsy confirmed that Jared had acute glomerulonephritis. The timing in relation to his sore throat suggested that he had post-streptococcal glomerulonephritis, and this was confirmed on further blood tests, which showed that there were antistreptolysin O antibodies (see also Chapter 17).

The underlying problem is an abnormal immune response to infection with streptococci. The bacterial antigens trigger the formation of antibodies which combine to form antigen–antibody immune complexes, and these complexes circulate in the blood. These are deposited in the glomerular capillaries and trigger many inflammatory chemical mediators, which damage the blood vessels, leading to leakage of blood cells and protein. The glomeruli do not function properly and cannot excrete waste products or control the body's fluid balance and blood pressure. This produces the signs and symptoms of the acute nephritic syndrome, which can also be caused by other infections, such as malaria.

During the time that Jared's kidneys were not functioning properly, his fluid balance was strictly monitored – all his drinks were carefully measured and all his output of urine collected (Table 36.1). His blood pressure was only mildly raised, which was fortunate, for children are very susceptible to hypertensive encephalopathy (brain damage as a result of hypertension). He had daily blood tests to check on the levels of urea and creatinine, in case he required temporary haemodialysis if the levels became too high.

Jared's renal function slowly recovered, but as it is estimated that up to 30 per cent of the patients with acute glomerulonephritis develop chronic renal disease in later life, he will continue to be monitored over the next few years.

CHRONIC RENAL FAILURE

There are many different causes of CRF (Box 36.2), of which one of the most common in the UK is the diabetic nephropathy of diabetes mellitus. The progressive damage to the microvasculature in the glomeruli caused by the diabetes leads to CRF, and many patients with diabetes require long-term dialysis. Some causes of CRF are hereditary, such as polycystic kidney disease, which is inherited as an autosomal-dominant gene. The renal tissue is gradually reduced by the formation of cysts and the patient develops chronic renal failure. Any episode of acute renal failure that does not fully resolve can also lead to chronic renal failure.

Clinical Features

Chronic renal failure presents as the uraemic syndrome, signs and symptoms of which develop when renal excretory function is severely reduced and the GFR is 20 per cent or less of normal. The kidney is important not only as an organ of excretion; it also has a very important role in hormone production. The clinical features of the uraemic syndrome are caused by lack of excretion of accumulated waste products and impaired hormone control. The effects are seen throughout the body, in every system (Box 36.3).

Anaemia

Most patients with renal failure are anaemic for several reasons. The kidney is the site of production of erythropoietin, a hormone that has a regulating effect on erythropoiesis (the production of red blood cells) (see Chapter 31). The diseased kidney produces less erythropoietin and the patient becomes anaemic. Furthermore, the accumulating toxins directly suppress the bone marrow production of red blood cells, and the red blood cells also have a shorter life span than normal. Platelet function is also abnormal in renal failure, and therefore patients have a faulty clotting system, causing increased blood loss and a worsening of the anaemia.

Recombinant erythropoietin replacement is now possible by regular injection. At the moment this is very expensive, but it has proved its worth in improved quality of life and reduced need for blood transfusions.

The cardiovascular system

Chronic renal failure leads to hyperlipidaemia (see Chapter 32) with arterial disease as a result. In turn, this means that patients with CRF have an increased incidence of coronary artery disease and myocardial infarction.

Hypertension is a sign in its own right of renal disease. The kidney is the site of the renin–angiotensin system, which controls blood pressure, and kidney damage disrupts this feedback loop, causing hypertension. Renal disease is one of the causes of secondary hypertension. Conversely, severe hypertension may lead to renal damage by inducing vascular changes in the kidney tissue. Hypertension is also a risk factor for coronary artery disease (in addition to the lipid abnormalities described above), and it also puts patients at increased risk of stroke.

Cardiomyopathy (heart muscle damage) and pericarditis (inflammation of the pericardial sac) are also common in uraemia, and are not fully reversible by dialysis.

Renal osteodystrophy

The kidney has a dual role in the control of bone metabolism. It converts vitamin D to its active form, which in turn controls bone mineralization and calcium absorption. Reduced levels of vitamin D lead to renal osteomalacia, in which the bone is not properly mineralized.

The kidney is also the site of action of parathyroid hormone, produced by the parathyroid glands and involved in calcium–phosphate balance. As the GFR falls, the kidney retains more phosphate, with a reciprocal fall in calcium. The body responds by producing more parathyroid hormone to raise the level of calcium, but this increasing level of parathyroid hormone damages the bone by accelerating bone resorption to maintain the calcium levels (secondary hyperparathyroidism). This leads to bone pain, bone deformity, and pathological fractures.

> **BOX 36.2 CAUSES OF CHRONIC RENAL FAILURE**
>
> - diabetic nephropathy
> - chronic obstruction or reflux (e.g. stones, vesicoureteric reflux, pelvic or retroperitoneal fibrosis or malignancy)
> - chronic pyelonephritis
> - polycystic kidney disease
> - glomerular disease (e.g. glomerulonephritis, multisystem disease such as systemic lupus erythematosus, toxins such as gold, penicillamine)
> - tubular disease (e.g. metabolic diseases such as gout, drugs such as phenacetin, multisystem diseases such as sarcoidosis)
> - vascular causes (e.g. renal artery stenosis, vasculitis, hypertension)

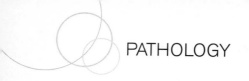

BOX 36.3 CLINICAL FEATURES OF URAEMIC SYNDROME

General
fatigue, lethargy
anorexia, nausea, vomiting

Skin
pallor and sallow complexion
pruritus, leading to scratch marks
brownish line in the nails

Haematological system
anaemia, caused by reduced erythropoietin production
thrombocytopenia, leading to bruising

Cardiovascular system
hypertension, because of the effects on the renin–angiotensin system
coronary heart disease (angina, myocardial infarction)
hyperlipidaemia
oedema, both peripheral and pulmonary
hypotension from disturbed fluid balance
pericarditis
cardiomyopathy

Neurological system
peripheral neuropathy
convulsions
muscular twitching
dementia

Metabolic changes
renal osteodystrophy (low calcium/high phosphate, due to lack of response to parathyroid hormone and impaired vitamin D metabolism thirst/polyuria in CRF – loss of concentrating capacity)

BOX 36.4 DIETARY MANAGEMENT OF CHRONIC RENAL FAILURE

Aims
Maintain adequate nutritional status with respect to energy and nitrogen balance
Prevent toxicity caused by the accumulation of electrolytes and metabolites in body fluids (e.g. hyperkalaemia, uraemia)
Avert hypertension, oedema, renal osteodystrophy, and stunted growth (in children)
Slow down the progress of the renal failure in order to delay the need for dialysis

Dietary advice
Adequate calorific intake of diet to maintain a stable body weight in adults and growth in children.
Reduced saturated fat intake to prevent hyperlipidaemia
Controlled protein intake to prevent excess urea production
Restricted intake of foods that are high in sodium and potassium, and no added salt to food at the table to avert electrolyte imbalances (see Chapter 6)
Daily fluid allowance calculated as:
Volume of urinary output of the previous day plus 500 ml (obligatory loss)
Foods with a high water content to be counted as part of the allowance as well as the volume of fluid consumed as drinks
Nutritional supplements as required (e.g. iron, calcium, zinc, water-soluble vitamins, vitamin D analogue) to prevent micronutrient deficiencies and disorders such as renal osteodystrophy

---

The nervous system
Uraemic toxins may affect both the central and peripheral nervous systems. There is a general dysfunctional effect on global brain function that may eventually lead to a clinical picture of dementia. Some patients have fits, motor weakness, and tremors.

Management
Maintaining the patient with CRF means paying meticulous attention to control of the problems outlined above. However, in the long term, the patient will reach end-stage renal failure and will require dialysis and consideration of transplantation (see Box 36.4).

DIALYSIS

The underlying principle of dialysis is that the patient's blood flows on one side of a selectively permeable membrane, allowing waste products to diffuse down a concentration gradient into the dialysate fluid flowing on the other side of the membrane. Dialysis can be provided in two forms – haemodialysis and peritoneal dialysis (Figure 36.2).

HAEMODIALYSIS

The first successful haemodialysis machine was developed in Nazi-occupied Holland in 1944. It consisted of 30 m of cellophane tube wound round a large cylinder. This rotated in a drum containing the dialysing fluid, which was a weak solution of salts. The first patient treated with the machine was a 29-year-old woman whose blood urea was kept stable for 26 days using this technique.

In haemodialysis, the selectively permeable membrane is synthetic and the dialysate is a similar fluid to extracellular fluid so that chemicals like urea, which are present only in plasma (not in extracellular fluid) will diffuse out. In order to create sufficient blood flow, an arteriovenous fistula is created in the patient's forearm and this is cannulated to allow the blood to flow through the dialysis machine. The flow rate is about 250 ml/minute through the machine. After flowing through the machine the blood is returned to the patient through another cannula. To maintain adequate excretion, the patient usually needs three sessions a week, each lasting 4 hours.

Some patients have a special room at home fitted out for haemodialysis, while others travel to hospital units to have their dialysis. Whichever way it is done, it is extremely time consuming, and patients' lives revolve around dialysing.

PERITONEAL DIALYSIS

Peritoneal dialysis depends on the same principles, but instead of a synthetic membrane, the dialysate is placed in the abdominal cavity and, as the blood flows through the vessels of the peritoneum, the same exchange process occurs, with the peritoneal tissue acting as the selectively permeable membrane. The dialysate fluid is introduced and removed through a flexible tube in the abdominal wall.

Continuous ambulatory peritoneal dialysis (CAPD) is used by many patients at home and they exchange the fluid three or four times a day. Again, this occupies a good deal of time and energy in maintaining the discipline of treatment (see Person-Centred Study in Chapter 1).

COMPLICATIONS OF DIALYSIS

The main drawback to dialysis is that it replaces only a limited part of normal kidney function, and even this it does very slowly. The normal creatinine clearance rate by the kidney is approximately 100 ml/minute, but dialysis clears only about 6–7 ml/min. The normal kidney is very sophisticated in retaining and excreting different chemicals at different rates, and the dialysis membrane is a very crude substitute (Box 36.5).

Dialysis cannot replace the endocrine function of the kidney, so many of the problems such as anaemia and bone disease are still present.

There are often technical problems with the process of dialysis. Fluid overload can cause problems with pulmonary oedema, and volume depletion can lead to postural hypotension and fainting. Infection is a particular complication of peritoneal dialysis, and peritonitis is a serious problem requiring hospital admission and intravenous antibiotics. There have been trials of putting antibiotics into the dialysate fluid but this has not been entirely successful either.

Venous access can become impossible after several years of haemodialysis, when fistulae thrombose and the surgeons run out of accessible vessels to create new fistulae.

Psychologically, patients often find it very difficult to cope with the physical dependence on dialysis and the very restricted life that they have to lead, particularly with limitations on their diet and fluids. They are often dependent on relatives for support, both financial and emotional, and this may lead to serious strains on the family. Many patients are waiting for the chance of kidney transplantation and the uncertainty of this long wait can be very difficult to cope with.

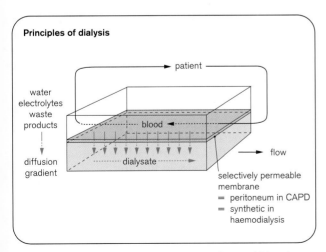

Figure 36.2 Principles of dialysis. Arterial blood from the uraemic patient flows on one side of the selectively permeable membrane, and waste products diffuse down a concentration gradient into the dialysate fluid, which is then discarded.

PATHOLOGY

BOX 36.5 PROBLEMS OF DIALYSIS

General
- time consuming
- restrictive
- expensive
- only limited treatment of symptoms of renal failure

Haemodialysis
- risk of infection (septicaemia, hepatitis B, human immunodeficiency virus)
- fluid balance – excess retention or loss of water
- dietary restrictions on protein and fluid intake
- machine failure (e.g. blood leaks, air embolus)
- circulatory access (fistula infection, thrombosis)
- haemorrhage from heparin
- cardiac arrhythmias, caused by electrolyte imbalance
- myocardial infarction and stroke, caused by hypertension and hyperlipidaemia
- psychiatric problems (e.g. depression, dementia)
- repeated self-needling required
- space at home required

Peritoneal dialysis
- peritonitis
- protein loss, leading to malnutrition
- abdominal or inguinal hernias from raised intra-abdominal pressure
- hydrothorax and compromised respiratory function
- storage space for dialysate fluids required
- catheter problems
- outflow failure when omentum blocks catheter holes

RENAL TRANSPLANTATION

Dialysis represented a great step forward in the management of chronic renal failure, which up till its development had been a fatal disease. However the advent of transplantation has transformed the chances of these patients. The successfully transplanted kidney takes over all the functions of the kidney, including its endocrine and homeostatic functions.

IMMUNOLOGY

Attempts at transplantation occurred in the 18th and 19th centuries, but the major problem has always been that of immunological rejection. In the early 1950s, cortisone was available and was beginning to be used to try to reduce the rates of rejection. In 1954, transplantation between identical twins was performed in Boston and the transplanted patient survived for 8 years before dying of a myocardial infarction. This proved that transplantation could be successful if the incompatibility and rejection problems could be overcome.

Various techniques were used to try to reduce rejection rates, such as total body irradiation, and patients sometimes died of the complications of the treatment instead. Immunosuppressive drugs were seen as the way forward and gradually better drugs were developed. Azathioprine and 6-mercaptopurine along with prednisolone were some of the first drugs to be used. In the 1970s cyclosporin was developed from two strains of fungus; it proved to be a successful immunosuppressant and continues to be used today, although ironically it also has directly toxic effects on the kidney. The search continues for better drugs with fewer side-effects.

Organ Rejection
Hyperacute rejection
Hyperacute rejection occurs within minutes or hours of transplantation, and the kidney becomes mottled and swollen. This very rapid rejection is due to the action of pre-formed antibodies from a previous transplant or multiple blood transfusions.

Acute rejection
Acute rejection is the most common type of reaction. More than 50 per cent of the recipients will experience some form of rejection episode, of which more than 75 per cent are of the acute type. The patient develops a fever, the graft kidney swells, and the urine output falls. The treatment is a short course of high-dose corticosteroids.

An acute accelerated rejection may occur within a few days to a few weeks of the transplant. It presents with deteriorating renal function, weight gain caused by oedema, and fever. This type of reaction does not usually respond to immunosuppressant drugs.

Chronic rejection
Chronic rejection occurs in most allografts to some degree, and manifests itself as gradually decreasing renal function over many years. It is a major cause of graft loss. The mechanism is poorly understood, but it is thought to be a reaction against the arterial endothelium.

The diagnosis of rejection episodes usually requires a fine needle biopsy to get histological evidence of an immune reaction (Box 36.6).

BOX 36.6 PROBLEMS OF TRANSPLANTATION

Organ supply
- shortage of cadaver organs
- compatibility
- living donors are at some risk

Rejection
- acute early rejection
- chronic rejection

Immunosuppression
- increased risk of infection
- bacterial (e.g. pneumococcal septicaemia)
- viral (e.g. warts, molluscum contagiosum, herpes)
- fungal (e.g. aspergillosis)
- increased risk of malignancy
- skin (e.g. squamous cell carcinoma)

Drug toxicity
- azathioprine may cause marrow suppression
- cyclosporin may cause nephrotoxicity, platelet suppression
- prednisolone may cause osteoporosis

Psychological
- guilt about donor
- 'sword of Damocles' feeling about rejection

Social
- finding employment if previously on dialysis and on long-term sick leave
- life insurance and mortgage problems
- long-term drug therapy and side-effects

The kidney has to match the recipient immunologically as far as possible so as to reduce the risk of rejection. Histocompatibility antigens and blood group are matched and the best matching recipient chosen from the waiting list. Certain ethnic groups are disadvantaged by this, since the pool of donors is predominantly Caucasian, and the chances of a successful match for an Asian or Afro-Caribbean patient are much smaller. There has been a drive to encourage these groups to carry donor cards but some religious cultures preclude organ donation (see Chapter 29).

Kidneys from living related donors stand a better chance of success, but obviously there is a certain risk to the donor, both in terms of the operation to remove the kidney, and in the future if any problems develop with the sole remaining kidney.

About 80 per cent of cadaver grafts survive for 2 years or more, and living donor rates of survival are even better. Most graft rejection occurs early and can be controlled with immunosuppressive therapy; therefore many patients are now living with grafts that are between 15 and 20 years old.

TRANSPLANTATION SURGERY

The cadaver donor kidney is at great risk of ischaemic damage, both just before death and just after circulatory arrest. Ventilating the patient and ensuring the prevention of hypotension are protective, and rapid uniform cooling reduces metabolic activity by hypothermia, which again delays deterioration.

The transplanted kidney is placed in the iliac fossa and the blood vessels are anastomosed to the iliac vessels. The ureter is implanted into the bladder. The diseased kidneys are not usually removed unless they are causing problems (e.g. infection).

URINARY TRACT TUMOURS

Malignancies in the bladder, ureters, and pelvis of the kidney are all of one cell type, the transitional cell, which lines the collecting system of the urinary tract. Malignant tumours of the kidney substance are epithelial cell tumours, and almost all are adenocarcinomas. These tumours are common in the UK, and the incidence increases with age. In England and Wales in 1995, there were just over 4800 deaths from bladder cancer and over 2600 deaths from renal tumours.

ORGAN SUPPLY

The donor kidneys are either from unrelated cadavers or from living relatives. The supplies of cadaver kidneys are very limited and there is always a long waiting list. The main sources are from victims of intracerebral haemorrhage or cerebral trauma. Brain death is confirmed according to strict protocols; the patient must be brain-stem dead and dependent on a ventilator. Drugs and hypothermia must be excluded and the absence of cranial reflexes (such as the corneal, gag, and oculogyric reflexes) must be confirmed. The medical suitability of the donor must be checked and permission sought to use the patient's organs.

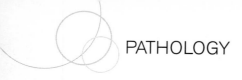

PATHOLOGY

RENAL ADENOCARCINOMA

Clinical Features

This tumour, which arises from the renal tubules, is twice as common in men as in women and is associated with cigarette smoking. The most frequently presenting symptom is haematuria (blood in the urine), a symptom that always requires investigation on first presentation. The patient may also have pain in the loin at the site of the kidney, and sometimes a kidney mass is palpable.

Sometimes the cancer presents with a metastasis in the lung, found when a chest X-ray is done for a persistent cough. Bony metastases may cause pathological fractures.

The kidney has endocrine functions, and malignancy can sometimes cause abnormalities of hormone secretion. Excessive erythropoietin may cause polycythaemia (excessive red blood cell count) and disruption to the control of calcium metabolism may cause hypercalcaemia, with symptoms such as abdominal pain, bone pain, and formation of renal stones. Sometimes, the patient may present with an unexplained pyrexia as the only symptom.

Staging and management

The prognosis of renal adenocarcinoma depends on the degree of spread at the time of diagnosis. If the cancer is small, has not breached the renal capsule, and has not extended into the renal vein, the 10-year survival rate is about 50 per cent after radical surgery. If the tumour has invaded the capsule, this rate is reduced to around 5 per cent. Occasionally, there is a solitary lung metastasis at the time of the original kidney resection. Some patients have had a good outcome after resection of the metastasis as well. As always, initial staging is very important so that unhelpful surgery is avoided in the presence of extensive tumour spread (see Chapters 5 and 6).

Chemotherapy so far has not proved very helpful. Radiotherapy has a limited role in post-operative treatment when the tumour extends through the capsule.

TRANSITIONAL CELL CARCINOMA

Aetiology

Cigarette smoking has been shown to be an important risk factor for bladder cancer. Another chemical risk factor is exposure to beta-naphthylamine, which is present in the aniline dye industry. A carcinogenic metabolite is excreted into the urine, directly affecting the transitional cells (see Chapter 5). Workers in the rubber industry are also at increased risk (Box 36.7).

However, world-wide, the greatest risk factor for bladder cancer is infection with the fluke *Schistosoma*

> ### BOX 36.7 RISK FACTORS FOR BLADDER CANCER
>
> - cigarette smoking
> - parasitic infections
> - occupational exposure
>   painters and decorators
>   leather workers
>   dental technicians
>   dry cleaners
>   mechanics and lorry drivers
>   paper manufacturers
> - chemical exposure
>   aniline dyes
>   beta-naphthylamine
>   xenylamine
>   benzidine

---

haematobium which causes schistosomiasis. The flukes are excreted by freshwater snails and then burrow into the skin of people wading or swimming in the water. Maturation of the worms occurs in the pelvic veins and eggs are laid in the bladder wall causing a chronic granulomatous inflammation predisposing to malignant change. The life cycle continues when infected urine contaminates freshwater lakes and rivers and the eggs are ingested by snails. The species that affects the bladder is endemic in India and the Middle East.

Clinical Features, Staging, and Management

The first presentation of transitional cell carcinoma is usually painless haematuria, although there may be urinary frequency and back pain as well. Diagnosis is by cystoscopy and biopsy, which also allows small polypoid growths to be removed at the same time.

Seventy per cent of bladder tumours are either non-infiltrating or only infiltrate the submucosa, and for these patients with early tumours, treatment is by repeat

---

> ### BOX 36.8 STAGING OF BLADDER CARCINOMA
>
> | | |
> |---|---|
> | Ta | confined to the mucosa |
> | T1 | invading the submucosa only |
> | T2 | invading superficial muscle |
> | T3 | invading deep muscle |
> | T4 | spreading beyond the bladder |

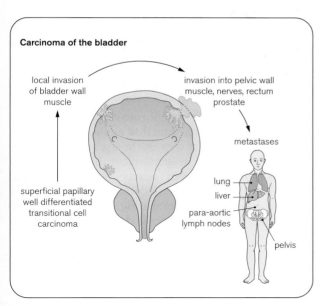

Figure 36.3 Carcinoma of the bladder. The stages of progressive and invasive bladder carcinoma with metastases.

cystoscopies with removal of any new foci of disease and diathermy of the surrounding tissue. If the tumour is well differentiated, there is an 80 per cent 5-year survival rate, but this falls to 40 per cent in undifferentiated tumours. Treatment by instilling chemotherapeutic drugs, such as mitomycin, into the bladder has become established as an adjuvant treatment (Box 36.8 and Figure 36.3).

Once the tumour has started to invade the muscle wall, more radical surgery or radiotherapy is required. If technically possible, a partial cystectomy is done, but sometimes a total cystectomy is necessary and a substitute bladder is created using an ileal conduit (an isolated loop of ileum) into which the ureters can be implanted. One end of the conduit is brought out onto the abdominal wall to drain into a urostomy bag.

Radical radiotherapy has proved to be effective in treating the tumour but it may have other long-term side-effects such as radiation cystitis, in which the bladder becomes very shrunken. The overall 5-year survival rate once the muscle layer has been invaded is less than 30 per cent.

NEPHROBLASTOMA (WILM'S TUMOUR)

This is the second most common abdominal tumour occurring in childhood, although even so it is very rare. It originates in the kidney but arises from embryological remnants in the abdominal cavity. Patients usually present under the age of 4 years with a large abdominal mass. It typically metastasizes to the lung and, less commonly, to bone. Combined treatment with surgery, radiotherapy, and chemotherapy gives a 90 per cent survival at 5 years post-surgery; it used to be uniformly fatal. Bone metastases indicate a poorer prognosis.

URINARY INCONTINENCE

NORMAL MICTURITION AND CONTINENCE

Urinary continence depends on a combination of conscious control and reflex control, plus a normal intact bladder and urethra. Micturition occurs when the bladder pressure is greater than the urethral pressure. The detrusor muscle of the bladder is normally relaxed as the bladder fills and the outlet tone is high to prevent outflow. When the bladder is full, the detrusor muscle contracts and the outlet relaxes simultaneously, allowing voiding. This is co-ordinated by a micturition centre in the brain stem, which is under voluntary control by the cerebral cortex.

HISTORY AND INVESTIGATION

Interruption of any of these controls or a reduction of bladder capacity may lead to incontinence. Investigation of the cause includes a neurological assessment as well as a general medical history. Any cause of polyuria and frequency (e.g. urinary tract infection or diabetes mellitus) may tip the balance and cause incontinence in a patient who has impaired control from other causes.

Urodynamic studies are an objective method of measuring flow rate to assess outflow obstruction. Renal ultrasound or an IVU will demonstrate the anatomy, including any sites of obstruction or congenital malformations.

Stress Incontinence

Stress incontinence occurs when the intra-abdominal pressure is raised by coughing or sneezing, and the person leaks a small volume of urine. This is due to muscular laxity around the bladder outlet. It is seen almost invariably in women who have had children. Weakened pelvic floor muscles reduce the closure of the bladder outlet. Strengthening these muscles by specific exercises may improve mild cases, but sometimes surgery is necessary to improve the bladder outlet closure.

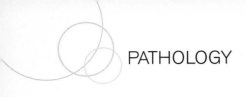

Urge Incontinence

This is a very common problem, in which, once patients are aware of the need to void their bladder, they have to do so almost immediately despite trying to control the urge. The bladder will often empty a large volume of urine rather than just leaking a small quantity. Sometimes there is an identifiable cause such as local bladder irritation from a tumour. Urge incontinence may also be due to a failure of central inhibition in neurological diseases such as multiple sclerosis or brain tumours. However, often there is no detectable cause, particularly in women, and it is labelled 'bladder instability'.

The underlying cause, if one is identified, needs to be treated if possible, but otherwise drugs with anticholinergic activity, such as tricyclics may help the symptoms.

Reflex Incontinence

When spinal cord control is lost above the sacral level, the bladder voids reflexly without warning. The neural control is disturbed and the detrusor muscle may be at high resting tone, with a closed outlet, creating a high pressure situation in which there may be back pressure causing renal damage. Keeping the bladder emptied becomes very important, and catheterization, either continuous or intermittent, is often used.

DRUGS AND THE KIDNEY

The kidney is a major organ of excretion, not only for natural waste products but also for drugs. Therefore any change in renal function may dramatically alter the way in which a drug acts. The kidney's concentrating powers also mean that it is exposed to high levels of some drugs as it excretes them, which can be toxic to the renal tissue during the process (Box 36.9).

REDUCED DRUG EXCRETION

Reduced excretion of a drug usually means that the drug accumulates in the body and serum levels rise. It is often necessary to reduce the dose in anticipation of this effect, and some dose regimens encompass this. Older adult patients often have mildly compromised renal function and are particularly vulnerable to this problem (see Chapters 12 and 40).

A typical example is digoxin, which is very toxic if it accumulates to high serum levels and may even lead to death by causing arrhythmias.

NEPHROTOXICITY

Some drugs are directly nephrotoxic, and their toxicity is increased if renal function is already impaired. An example of this is seen in the use of aminoglycoside antibiotics such as gentamicin. It is excreted by the kidney and the dose is reduced in impaired renal function, but serum levels need to be checked to ensure that the drug is not accumulating. If it does accumulate, it may cause further renal damage and deafness.

BOX 36.9 DRUG-INDUCED RENAL DISEASE

Drugs causing acute renal failure
amphotericin B, cephaloridine – high doses directly toxic
penicillin – hypersensitivity reaction
sulphonamides – crystal formation causing obstruction
X-ray contrast media
aminoglycoside antibiotics (e.g. gentamicin)

Drugs causing nephrotic syndrome (protein leakage)
penicillamine (used in rheumatoid arthritis)
gold (used in rheumatoid arthritis)

Drugs causing interstitial nephropathy and tubular damage
diuretics (e.g. frusemide, thiazides)
non-steroidal anti-inflammatory drugs
lithium carbonate
tetracyclines

Drugs causing retroperitoneal fibrosis
methysergide (used in migraine)
practolol (a beta-blocker) – an antihypertensive withdrawn because of this reaction
methyldopa (used in hypertension)

Many drugs can cause renal damage, and the use of non-steroidal anti-inflammatory drugs have been implicated in the development of renal failure in some patients (see Chapter 13).

REDUCED EFFICACY

Sometimes the drug has to pass through the kidney to be activated. If the renal function is reduced, the amount of active drug is also reduced. This can be seen when vitamin D is given therapeutically for osteomalacia – it cannot be converted to its active form when there is severe renal disease. Diuretics are another example of reduced efficacy when the kidney is damaged and their effect on the renal cells is reduced. Much higher doses may be needed to produce the same effect.

KEY POINTS

- Infections may affect any part of the urinary tract from the kidney (pyelonephritis) to the bladder (cystitis). Predisposing factors include vesicoureteric reflux, pregnancy, anatomical abnormalities, diabetes, and female sex.
- Investigations of a UTI may entail microbiological culture of the urine, ultrasound of the renal tract, intravenous urography, and cystoscopy.
- Urinary stones form when there is precipitation of crystals from an abnormally high urinary concentration of substances such as calcium, uric acid, or cystine.
- Acute renal failure usually presents with oliguria or anuria. It may be reversible if the underlying cause is treatable. It is managed by fluid and dietary restrictions and dialysis if necessary.
- Chronic renal failure presents with the uraemic syndrome, resulting from the failure of excretion of toxic waste products, and deficiencies of hormone production and homeostatic control caused by the failing kidney.
- Dialysis relies on the diffusion of substances across a selectively permeable membrane from the patient's blood into the dialysate fluid. In haemodialysis, the membrane is synthetic, whereas in peritoneal dialysis the peritoneum acts as the membrane.
- Cigarette smoking is a risk factor for adenocarcinoma of the kidney and transitional cell carcinoma of the bladder. Other carcinogens active on the bladder urothelium are the chemical beta-naphthylamine and chronic infection with the helminthic parasite, *Schistosoma haematobium*.
- Urinary continence depends on a combination of conscious and reflex control, with an intact autonomic nervous system, spinal cord, brain stem, and cortex acting on a normal bladder and urethra.

FURTHER READING

Chisholm GD, Fair WR (1989) The Scientific Foundations of Urology, 3rd edition. Butterworth Heinenann Medical Books, Oxford and Year Book Medical Publishers, Chicago. Chapters 11,12,13 Renal Failure, Transplantation, Hypertension.

Dawson C, Whitfield H (1996) ABC of urology. Introduction to Urology. BMJ 312:623–5.

Dawson C, Whitfield H (1996) ABC of urology. Urological evaluation. BMJ 312:695–8.

Dawson C, Whitfield H (1996) ABC of urology. Urological malignancy III: renal and testicular carcinoma. BMJ 312:1146–8.

Dawson C, Whitfield H (1996) ABC of urology. Urinary stone disease. BMJ 312:1219–21.

Fanci A, Braunwald E, Isselbacher KJ, *et al.* (eds) (1997) Harrison's Principles of Internal Medicine 14th edition, McGraw–Hill, New York.

Fellner SK, Follman D, Dasgupta DS, Ward C, Spencer J,

Rizowy C (1996) Ischemic heart disease in patients with end-stage renal disease. Adv Ren Replace Ther 3:240–9.

Gibson R (1997)Management of the critically ill pediatric patient with acute renal failure. Crit Care Nurs Q 20:22–5.

Ikizler TA, Hakim RM (1996) Nutrition in end stage renal disease. Kidney Int 50:346–57.

Massy ZA, Ma JZ, Louis TA, Kasiske BL (1995) Lipid lowering therapy in patients with renal disease. Kidney Int 48(1):188–98.

Ormandy P (1997) Dialysis (Part 2): haemodialysis (continuing education credit). Nurs Stand 11:48–54.

Souhami RL, Moxham J (1997) Textbook of Medicine, 3rd edition. Churchill Livingstone, London.

Walker R (1997) Recent advances: general management of end stage renal failure. BMJ 315:1429–32.

Whitfield HN, Hendry WF (eds) (1985) Textbook of Genito-Urinary Surgery, volumes I and II. Churchill Livingstone, Edinburgh.

DISEASES OF THE REPRODUCTIVE TRACT

Before reading this chapter you should have a basic understanding of:
- the anatomy and structure of the male and female reproductive organs,
- the physiology of the menstrual cycle and conception,
- the physiology of spermatogenesis and oogenesis.

DISEASES OF THE BREAST

The major symptoms and signs of breast disease are lumps, pain, and nipple discharge. All of these can be caused by breast cancer but are more commonly due to benign breast disease. It is important that the symptoms are properly managed to avoid unnecessary investigation and morbidity.

DIAGNOSTIC INVESTIGATIONS

Mammography

Mammography is an X-ray of the breast. It requires the breast to be compressed between two plates, and two views are taken to facilitate the most accurate interpretation. An abnormal mammogram may show distortion of the normal tissue architecture or deposits of microcalcification. Because the breast tissue is very dense in younger women, interpreting mammograms in those under 35 years can be very difficult, and a higher dose of X-ray is required to obtain a good image. Therefore, mammography is rarely indicated in this age group.

Ultrasound

Ultrasonography may be helpful in detecting fluid filled cysts, and it can be used in the younger age group. However, it is more subjective and less specific than mammography.

Fine Needle Aspiration Cytology

Fine needle aspiration cytology is a technique in which cells are withdrawn from a breast lump by a needle and syringe, smeared on a slide, and then examined by a cytologist. The cells are graded for abnormality, from grade I to grade V. Grade V smears are diagnostic of malignancy and grade IV are highly suspicious.

Stereotactic Cytology

This is a technique that combines mammography and cytology. A localizing wire is inserted into the suspicious lesion under X-ray control so that it can be accurately located for aspiration or excision biopsy. This is particularly important for small lesions, which may be impalpable and invisible to the naked eye.

Excision or Incision Biopsy

Excision or incision biopsy is the removal of tissue at open operation for histopathological diagnosis. This is described further in the section on breast cancer (see below).

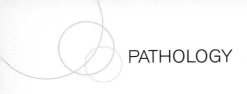

PATHOLOGY

BENIGN BREAST DISEASE
Fibroadenoma
Fibroadenomas are benign growths arising from a breast lobule. They usually present as painless breast lumps. They occur more frequently in young women – 60 per cent of breast lumps in women aged under 20 years are fibroadenomas. Overall, they account for approximately 12 per cent of all palpable breast masses. They are less common over the age of 40 years.

Clinical features and diagnosis
The lump is often in the upper, outer quadrant of the breast, where there is the most breast tissue. They are well circumscribed and mobile, and they are not attached to adjoining tissue. Sometimes they are multiple. Diagnosis may be made by a combination of clinical examination, mammography or ultrasound, and fine needle aspiration cytology.

Management
If the diagnosis is certain, particularly in a young woman, it can be a reasonable option to leave the fibroadenoma alone. It appears that up to 20 per cent may spontaneously resolve, and many get smaller with time. If there is any doubt over the diagnosis or if the woman is particularly concerned, the lump is removed by excision biopsy. However, this can mean an imbalance in the size of the breasts, particularly if the fibroadenomas are multiple or recurrent. In women over 40, when the risk of breast cancer is higher, many surgeons would excise the lump to confirm the histology.

Breast cancer does not arise more commonly in a fibroadenoma than any other part of the breast.

Nodular and Cystic Disease of the Breast
This previously used to be known as fibrocystic disease of the breast. It mainly occurs as part of normal breast involution with age.

Focal nodularity
Focal nodularity is the most frequent cause of a breast lump under the age of 50 years, and it accounts for 70 per cent of breast lumps under the age of 40 years. The breast tissue develops areas of fibrosis, increased glandularity, and small cysts, which are then palpable as a nodular area. Diagnosis again is by a combination of clinical examination, mammography or ultrasound, and fine needle aspiration cytology. Only rarely, when there is doubt as to the diagnosis, is biopsy needed.

Cystic disease
Cystic disease is common in the perimenopausal phase and is unusual after the menopause. This suggests a strong hormonal influence, as does the fact that it is often bilateral and responds to endocrine treatment. The lump may appear quite suddenly and it may be painful. It is smooth, not tethered, and sometimes fluctuant. Cysts more often occur in the left breast than right, the same pattern as is seen in breast cancer. Diagnostic investigations should include a mammogram, since 1–3 per cent of these women will have an incidental carcinoma. The cyst is then aspirated to remove the fluid. This may need repeating if the cyst refills.

Patients with cystic breast disease are between 1.5 and 4 times more likely to develop breast cancer than women in the general population; those with multiple and bilateral cysts, and those with cysts that keep refilling are at particular risk.

Sclerosing Adenosis and Epithelial Hyperplasia
Sclerosing adenosis
Sclerosing adenosis occurs in involution of the breast tissue and leads to dense areas of fibrosis, which can produce architectural distortion on mammography and may require excision biopsy to ensure that no malignancy is present.

Epithelial hyperplasia
Epithelial hyperplasia occurs when there is proliferation of the cells lining the ductules. As well as increasing in number, the cells are sometimes atypical, and these women have an increased risk of cancer of about four or five times that of the general population.

CARCINOMA OF THE BREAST

EPIDEMIOLOGY AND RISK FACTORS
Breast cancer is the most common malignancy in women world-wide, with more than 500 000 new cases per year. In England and Wales, more than 12 000 women die of breast cancer each year, and it is the leading cause of death in women between the ages of 40 and 50 (Box 37.1). The UK has the highest incidence and mortality of breast cancer in the world.

Risk Factors
Age
The incidence increases with age, doubling every 10 years until the menopause. There is a slight downward trend during the menopause, but the incidence rises again in the post menopausal years although at a reduced rate.

Geography
The incidence in Japan is much lower than the UK, and migrants from high to low incidence areas acquire the local risk in two generations. This means that environmental factors as well as genetic risk are important.

BOX 37.1 DEATHS FROM CANCER OF THE REPRODUCTIVE SYSTEM IN ENGLAND AND WALES IN 1995

Breast cancer	12 509
Cervical cancer	1329
Ovarian cancer	3879
Prostate cancer	8848
Testicular cancer	83

(Figures from the Office for National Statistics – Census Population and Health Group)

Age at menarche and menopause

Starting to menstruate early or having a late menopause significantly increases the risk.

Pregnancy

Having a late first pregnancy or never being pregnant increases the risk, although interestingly, being over 35 at first pregnancy confers a higher risk than never being pregnant at all.

Family history

Possibly up to 10 per cent of breast cancer is due to genetic predisposition, and two genes, BRCA 1 and BRCA 2, have been identified (see Chapter 7). A woman's risk is doubled if she has a mother, sister, or aunt who had the disease before 50 years of age, and the risk is between four and six times higher if two first-degree relatives have had breast cancer.

Oral contraception

No consistent risk has been demonstrated although prolonged use of oral contraceptives before the first pregnancy appears to increase the risk.

Hormone replacement therapy

Current research shows that hormone replacement therapy (HRT) taken for 5 years, increases the risk of developing breast cancer from 45 per 1000 women in non-users to 47 per 1000 women taking HRT. After 15 years of HRT, the extra number of breast cancers rises to 57 per 1000 women.

CLINICAL FEATURES

The most frequent presentation of a breast cancer is a lump in the breast, which may be found by the patient or during a routine examination. The lump is usually painless and feels firm and it may be fixed to the surrounding tissue. There may be enlargement of the axillary lymph nodes if there has been spread before presentation. Very occasionally, patients present with an acutely inflamed lump that appears to be a breast abscess but on biopsy turns out to be an inflammatory carcinoma.

Other less common presentations are with a scaling rash of the nipple, which can be ductal carcinoma extending to the skin, or nipple retraction or inversion with no palpable lump.

Mastalgia (generalized breast pain) is very rarely a symptom of breast cancer.

DIAGNOSIS

The diagnostic techniques of clinical examination, mammography, and fine needle aspiration cytology are used initially to obtain a tissue diagnosis, although sometimes an open biopsy is required. If cancer is diagnosed, the patient needs to be staged so that a definitive management plan can be made. Staging includes the size of the tumour and the presence of lymph node spread and any distant metastases.

For smaller tumours with no clinical evidence of distant spread, definitive surgery is excision of the lump or mastectomy, along with axillary lymph node sampling to establish whether there has been spread. There is no clinical benefit in excising large, fixed tumours with metastases, since these can be better managed by chemotherapy and local radiotherapy.

PATHOLOGY

Breast cancer arises in the terminal duct lobular unit, and it has distinctive cell types on histology. The two most common types of breast cancer are ductal and lobular, both of which can be present as:

• carcinoma *in situ* (carcinoma confined to the duct without invasion of the basement membrane); or
• invasive carcinoma, in which the tumour has invaded the surrounding breast tissue (Figure 37.1).

The commonest form of breast cancer is invasive ductal carcinoma, which accounts for about 85 per cent of the cases. Breast cancer may be bilateral, particularly the lobular type, and investigations are required when the patient first presents in order to establish whether there is a second tumour in the other breast. The cancer can also be multifocal and, in this situation, a mastectomy rather than lumpectomy is required in order to clear the tumour and reduce the risk of local recurrence.

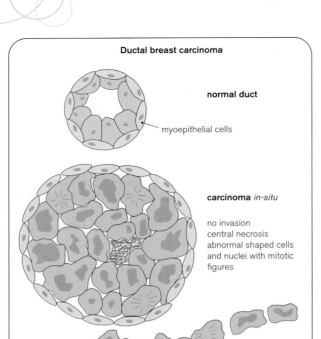

Ductal breast carcinoma

normal duct

myoepithelial cells

carcinoma *in-situ*

no invasion
central necrosis
abnormal shaped cells
and nuclei with mitotic
figures

invasive carcinoma

malignant cells invading
surrounding stroma
central necrosis

Figure 37.1 Ductal breast carcinoma. The stages of development of ductal breast carcinoma from the *in-situ* stage, in which there is an intact basement membrane and no invasion, to invasive cancer with stromal invasion.

BOX 37.2 NOTTINGHAM PROGNOSTIC INDEX FOR BREAST CANCER

The Nottingham prognostic
index = (0.2 × size) + lymph node stage + grade

Lymph node stage
score
lymph node stage 1 — no nodes involved
lymph node stage 2 — 1–3 nodes involved
lymph node stage 3 — 4 or more nodes involved

Histological grade
score
histological grade 1 — I low grade (relatively well differentiated)
histological grade 2 — II medium grade (moderately differentiated)
histological grade 3 — III high grade (poorly differentiated)

Scores
<3.4 = good; 3.4–5.4 = moderate;
>5.4 = poor

TREATMENT

There is still no clear-cut absolute 'best' way of treating breast cancer. Because it presents at many different stages and because there are other variables (such as being premenopausal or postmenopausal), there is still debate as to when patients should receive radiotherapy or chemotherapy and what type of surgery is appropriate. Trials are ongoing but it can be difficult to recruit patients in a proper randomized fashion if they have clear ideas about their treatment and refuse to join a trial.

In brief, surgery is indicated for removal of the lump and for axillary lymph node sampling. A lumpectomy may be performed, in which case the rest of the breast is preserved, but a mastectomy may be required if the cancer is multifocal (Box 37.3). Post-operative radiotherapy is often used for axillary node irradiation, and increasingly younger women, even those with negative lymph nodes, are being offered chemotherapy. Combinations of these treatment modalities vary from country to country and between cancer centres in the UK, but there is an increasing trend towards standardizing treatment to try to achieve better survival rates.

Breast cancer is a hormone-dependent tumour with varying degrees of response to oestrogen level

---

Occasionally, a breast lump turns out to be a secondary deposit from elsewhere, and sometimes lymphoma presents as a breast lump.

The tumour is graded pathologically by size and cellular differentiation, which, together with lymph node status gives a prognostic index (Box 37.2). In the Nottingham Index, a combination of these factors categorizes women as having a good, moderate, or poor prognostic index, with 10-year survival rates of about 65 per cent, 55 per cent and 35 per cent respectively. oThe aim of adjuvant treatment is to improve these survival rates (e.g. combination chemotherapy in premenopausal, node-positive women achieves an overall 10 per cent increase in survival).

BOX 37.3 SURGICAL OPTIONS IN BREAST CANCER

Breast conservation
single clinical and mammographic lesion
tumour less than 4 cm in diameter
no sign of local advancement, extensive nodal
involvement, or metastases

Mastectomy
patient preference for mastectomy
clinical or mammographic evidence of
multifocal disease

manipulation. The best-known endocrine therapy used in breast cancer is tamoxifen, which is effective in both pre- and postmenopausal women (see Chapter 10). In premenopausal women, oophorectomy confers the same benefits as combination chemotherapy.

Treatment for advanced breast cancer is symptomatic, particularly for metastases, which tend to be in bone, liver, and brain. Such metastases may cause pathological fractures, hepatomegaly and jaundice, and fits. Sometimes, the tumour itself ulcerates through the skin and local radiotherapy or even surgery may make the patient more comfortable.

SCREENING PROGRAMMES

In order to be worthwhile, screening should detect a disease in a presymptomatic phase, enabling early treatment, which improves the outcome of the disease. The ideal screening test should be harmless, cheap, and easy to perform and should produce standardized, repeatable results, with no false-positive or false-negative results. The mammographic screening programme introduced to reduce mortality from breast cancer certainly fails on many of these criteria, but is the best available test at the moment.

The problems with mammography as a screening tool are that:
- it is expensive;
- it requires high levels of technical expertise and equipment;
- it is not 100 per cent specific or sensitive (especially in younger women); and
- it exposes the patient to radiation.

There have been many trials throughout the world to try to quantify the benefit of mammographic screening,

and for women aged over 50 years, there is an average reduction in mortality of 29 per cent over 12 years of follow-up. Cancers detected on screening tend to be smaller and node-negative, which tends towards a better prognosis.

The current UK screening programme runs for women between 50 and 65 years at 3-yearly intervals. Women over 65 can continue to be screened at their own request. Cancers may develop between screenings, and the rate of this is higher in the third year, suggesting that the interval between mammograms should be 2 years rather than 3 years.

The mammogram is examined for distortions in architecture and the presence of microcalcification, which may be associated with malignancy. This is then further investigated with fine needle aspiration cytology and with biopsy if necessary.

Initial figures from the UK screening programme appear to confirm increased survival rates, but more needs to be done to encourage women to attend.

CARCINOMA OF THE CERVIX

EPIDEMIOLOGY

In 1988, 4940 new cases of invasive cervical cancer were registered in the UK, making it the eighth most common cancer in women, and over 18 000 women were registered with carcinoma *in situ*. In 1995, 1329 women in England and Wales died of cervical cancer (see Box 37.1). Over the past 20 years the mortality in women aged 45 years and over has fallen significantly. In the 1970s and 1980s there was an increase in mortality in women aged between 40 and 44 years, but this has now been reversed, possibly because of increased screening in the last decade.

Risk Factors
Number of sexual partners
There is a linear relationship between the number of sexual partners and the likelihood of developing cervical abnormalities.

Sexually transmitted infection
Strong evidence now links certain strains of the genital wart virus, human papilloma virus types 16 and 18, with invasive cervical cancer (see Chapter 5).

Occupation and social class
Cervical cancer is more common in the north of the UK than in the south and in urban rather than rural areas. It is five times more prevalent in social class V than in the professional classes.

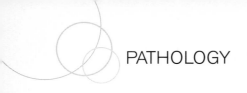

Smoking
Smoking is a major independent risk factor for cervical cancer.

PATHOLOGY

Squamous cell carcinoma of the cervix arises in the epithelial covering of the cervix, particularly in the transformation zone, which lies between two different types of epithelium – squamous epithelium, which forms keratin, and columnar epithelium, which lines the cervical canal and produces mucus.

Invasive cancer is usually preceded by dysplasia of the squamous epithelium, which may be mild, moderate, or severe. Dysplasia (abnormality of development) describes cervical epithelium with atypical cells, which are irregularly sized and shaped and have enlarged, abnormal nuclei (dyskaryosis) with frequent mitoses (see Chapters 3 and 5). An overall grading system, cervical intraepithelial neoplasia (CIN), has superseded terms such as dysplasia and dyskaryosis. CIN has three grades (I, II, and III), relating to the thickness of the epithelium that is occupied by neoplastic cells (Box 37.4 and Figure 37.2).

The progression of CIN to cervical cancer is not linear and inevitable. In 1978, 60 women who had positive smears but missed follow-up were traced 2 years later. Of these 60 women, seven had by then developed clinically diagnosed carcinoma of the cervix. The other 53 underwent further smears – three had invasive carcinoma, three had microinvasive carcinoma, and 20 still had dysplasia. However, 18 of the original 60 women (30 per cent) had a normal smear (i.e. there had been spontaneous regression of the dysplasia). All the women with spontaneous regression were under the age of 40 at the time of the original smear.

Women who have had a negative smear can develop cervical carcinoma. This may be due to sampling error or the rapid development of the cancer between smear tests. However, it is worth noting that in a study in the Grampian region of Scotland, 73 per cent of the women diagnosed with invasive cancer had never had a smear.

CLINICAL FEATURES

Invasive cervical cancer may be asymptomatic and detected only on a routine cervical smear test and subsequent biopsy. The most common symptom, if there is one, is irregular spotting or bleeding (intermenstrual bleeding) or a persistent offensive vaginal discharge. The bleeding may follow intercourse – postcoital bleeding. On vaginal examination, the tumour may appear as an ulcer on the cervix, or as a cauliflower-like growth.

> ### BOX 37.4 CERVICAL INTRAEPITHELIAL NEOPLASIA (CIN)
>
> **CIN I**
> undifferentiated cells in the basal third or less of the epithelium
>
> **CIN II**
> undifferentiated cells occupy between one-third and two-thirds of the epithelium
>
> **CIN III**
> undifferentiated cells occupy more than two-thirds of the epithelium

If the cancer is not detected early, the tumour may invade locally, involving the bladder, the sacral nerve plexus, and the rectum, and it may cause obstruction of the ureters, leading to renal failure. There may also be lymphatic spread to the iliac lymph nodes and, rarely, metastatic spread via the bloodstream to the ovaries, brain, bones, or lungs, producing the symptoms and signs of any tumour in those sites.

SCREENING, DIAGNOSIS, AND MANAGEMENT

The cervical cancer screening programme in the UK has been quite haphazard, but from 1988 it has been more successfully organized by running a recall system via Health Authorities. Since 1990, general practitioners have been set payment-related targets for smear uptake, which has increased coverage levels even further. The Department of Health guidelines still operate around a 5-year recall, but many Health Authorities recall women on a 3-yearly cycle.

A cervical smear is taken by gently scraping a wooden spatula around the cervical os, under direct vision, to ensure that the transformation zone is properly sampled. The cells are then transferred to a glass slide and covered with preservative fluid. In the laboratory, the cells are stained and examined under the microscope by cytologists. New ways of computerizing this cellular analysis are already under trial since it is a very time-consuming and tedious task for laboratory technicians, and one that is subject to human error (Box 37.5).

If a minor abnormality is detected, the smear is repeated after 6 months. If the abnormality persists, the patient is referred to the hospital for colposcopy. The colposcope

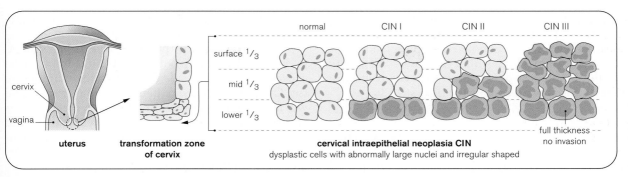

Figure 37.2 Cervical cytology sampling. Cervical intraepithelial neoplasia (CIN) grades I, II, and III are shown and compared to normal cervical cytology. The higher the grade of CIN, the more dysplastic the cells. Dysplastic cells are enlarged and irregular in shape and have abnormal nuclei and mitoses.

is a microscope that is used to obtain a direct microscopic view of the cervical cells in their original anatomical position. If cell abnormalities are found, a biopsy is taken to establish the proportion of the epithelium that is involved so that it can be graded. If treatment is required, a laser is usually used to destroy the area of abnormal cells, and the epithelium heals over the subsequent weeks.

If the biopsy shows invasive carcinoma, the woman requires radiotherapy or surgery or chemotherapy, or a combination of all three. Radiotherapy involves a radioactive implant such as caesium in the cavity of the uterus and external radiotherapy to cover the adjacent tissues. Complications of radiotherapy include radiation diarrhoea and cystitis and, sometimes, late fibrosis of the bowel and bladder. Ovarian function is reduced, often inducing an early menopause.

Surgery, which is sometimes used as a first-line treatment option, involves a Wertheim hysterectomy, in which the uterus and cervix, the upper half of the vagina, the Fallopian tubes and usually the ovaries, and the broad ligaments are removed. Possible complications of surgery include bladder and ureter damage, which may cause long-term renal problems. At the moment, there is no clear evidence to suggest that one treatment mode is better than the others in terms of survival.

Overall survival rates range from a 5-year survival rate of 99–100 per cent for precancerous lesions to a 7 per cent 5-year survival when there is distant spread.

DISEASES OF THE OVARY

The ovary has a very important endocrine function, and any abnormality of this can lead to significant problems with conception, menstruation, and the menopause. Cysts and tumours of the ovaries are quite common but they do not often interfere with the endocrine function; sometimes patients present with an abdominal mass or abdominal pain.

BENIGN OVARIAN CYSTS
Follicular Cysts
Follicular cysts are the most common type of benign ovarian cysts. They are often small and resolve spontaneously, but ones that persist and enlarge may need laparoscopic drainage. Polycystic ovarian disease is a syndrome in which the ovaries are enlarged by multiple small follicular cysts; the patients have infrequent menstruation and are often infertile. They may also be hirsute, obese, and suffer from acne owing to a relative excess of testosterone.

Endometriosis
Endometriosis may also lead to ovarian cysts. This is a condition of unknown cause, in which endometrial

Result of test	Mean %
normal	92.9
borderline changes	3.4
dyskaryosis	
mild	2.1
moderate	0.9
severe	0.6
possible invasive carcinoma	0.1
possible glandular neoplasia	0.1
inadequate for assessment	6.3

BOX 37.5 CERVICAL SMEAR TEST RESULTS IN ENGLAND (1991-92)

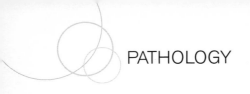

tissue, identical to the lining layer of the uterus, develops outside the uterus, and responds to the normal menstrual cycle. The endometrial deposits may be in the ovary, or anywhere within the abdominal cavity, and the blood lost at the time of menstruation is trapped, forming an endometriotic cyst.

Other Benign Cysts

Other benign cysts include mucinous cysts and serous cysts. These may grow extremely large, and malignancy can be excluded only on histological examination.

MALIGNANT OVARIAN TUMOURS

Most ovarian tumours arise from the epithelium covering the ovary, which is modified peritoneal tissue. About 5 per cent of mucinous cysts turn out to be malignant. The malignant serous tumour is the most common variety of primary ovarian cancer detected, and it is bilateral in 50 per cent of cases. The malignant cells disseminate throughout the abdominal cavity early in the course of the disease, causing metastatic peritoneal seedlings and ascites.

The overall death rate for all primary ovarian cancer in the UK is approximately 4000 deaths per year, far exceeding the death rate of cervical cancer (see Box 37.1).

Clinical Features

Ovarian tumours present more commonly in older women. Unfortunately the disease has often already spread by the time the diagnosis is made. Patients may be free of symptoms and the diagnosis is sometimes made when a pelvic mass is felt on routine pelvic examination while taking a routine cervical smear. Sometimes, the patient may notice her abdominal girth expanding because of ascites and the ovarian mass, or she may experience abdominal pain owing to pressure. Sometimes the tumour obstructs venous or lymph return from the leg, causing leg oedema. Very occasionally, the tumour may secrete an excess of hormones, such as testosterone, causing a virilizing effect, with hirsutism and acne.

Ultrasound, in particular vaginal ultrasound, helps to characterize the tumour as fluid-filled or solid, the latter being more likely to be malignant. However, the definitive diagnosis has to be made histologically after removal of the tumour. Open abdominal surgery is sometimes preceded by laparoscopy to assess the tumour and the extent of the disease. However, even if the tumour is widespread, debulking the tumour mass may improve the effectiveness of subsequent chemotherapy. As the tumour may be bilateral, there is often a need for both ovaries to be removed, and

sometimes for a hysterectomy as well. This is a specialist field of gynaecological surgery.

The introduction of platinum-based chemotherapy regimes has improved survival rates for ovarian cancer, although the side-effects may be quite severe (see Chapter 10). Some tumours are radiosensitive and will respond to radiotherapy. However, the overall 5-year survival rates for tumours that have spread beyond the ovary is about 10 per cent, while early diagnosis when the tumour is confined to the ovary gives survival rates of 90–95 per cent. This has led to trials of screening tests to establish their effectiveness. Ovarian cancer does have a familial trend, and regular ultrasound screening of those with affected relatives may lead to earlier diagnosis. A blood marker for malignancy, CA-125 (ovarian tumour antigen), may also be helpful, but it is too non-specific to be used as a full-scale screening test.

The problem of late diagnosis has also raised the question of whether women who are having a hysterectomy for other reasons, such as uterine fibroids, should have the ovaries removed as well. The rationale for this is to remove the potential site of ovarian cancer before it arises, based on the knowledge that ovarian function can be maintained by hormone replacement therapy after bilateral oophorectomy. However, the choice lies with the woman at the time of surgery, and some prefer to keep their ovaries and take their chances of developing ovarian cancer in later life.

DISEASES OF THE UTERUS

BENIGN FIBROMYOMA

The most common tumour of the uterus is the benign fibromyoma, more generally known as a fibroid. The tumour is composed of muscle and fibrous tissue and starts growing within the muscular wall of the uterus. The muscle fibres are whorled and encapsulated, and the tumours may be multiple.

The most familiar symptom is of heavy menstruation (menorrhagia), especially if the tumours have grown in to the endometrial cavity, increasing the area of endometrial tissue to be shed at menstruation. The patient may also be aware of an abdominal mass – it is not uncommon for the uterus to be enlarged to the size of a 20-week pregnancy. The enlarged uterus may cause pressure effects on the bladder and obstruct the outflow of urine.

The tumours are hormone dependent, and tend to increase in size throughout the woman's menstrual life. Once the menopause occurs, the tumours often start to shrink, although if the women receives HRT growth

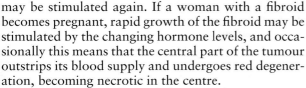

may be stimulated again. If a woman with a fibroid becomes pregnant, rapid growth of the fibroid may be stimulated by the changing hormone levels, and occasionally this means that the central part of the tumour outstrips its blood supply and undergoes red degeneration, becoming necrotic in the centre.

Diagnosis is usually made by clinical examination, although it needs to be confirmed on ultrasound scanning, since it may be difficult to differentiate an ovarian cyst from a fibroid on clinical grounds alone.

The management of fibromyomas depends on the symptoms and the woman's own choice. Occasionally, a fibroid may be contributing to problems with conception. In this situation, removal of the tumour alone (myomectomy) is indicated, although this can be quite a difficult operation, and a subsequent pregnancy has to be closely monitored because there is a risk of uterine rupture along the line of the scar.

Women who have completed their family may choose not to have surgery if the symptoms are not too bad, but if they are becoming anaemic from menorrhagia or there are pressure symptoms, they may choose to undergo hysterectomy. The ovaries may be conserved or removed, depending on the assessed risk of ovarian cancer for the individual. Women who have chosen to retain their ovaries at the time of hysterectomy often undergo the menopause earlier than women who have not had a hysterectomy, although the reason for this is not clear.

Very exceptionally, a fibromyoma may contain a malignant sarcomatous element – this is so rare that it does not usually influence the decision to operate or not. Malignant change is usually heralded by pain or a sudden rapid growth in size.

ENDOMETRIAL CARCINOMA

The endometrial lining of the uterus can be the site of development of an adenocarcinoma. Patients are characteristically postmenopausal, about half are nulliparous, and many are obese. There is also thought to be an association with diabetes mellitus. It is much less common than cancer of the breast or ovary.

Endometrial carcinoma is another hormone-dependent tumour and it is thought to be associated with an excess of oestrogen. Evidence for this comes partly from the finding that women who were given oestrogen for menopausal symptoms are at greatly increased risk of developing endometrial cancer. However, this risk may be removed by adding at least 12 days of progesterone to the treatment so as to stop the unopposed stimulation of the endometrium by oestrogen and the possible malignant transformation that this may cause. This is why it is so important for women

with an intact uterus who are being treated with HRT to take both oestrogen and progesterone.

Endometrial carcinoma usually presents with postmenopausal bleeding. This is difficult to define since periods can become very sparse when the woman enters the climacteric, but it is generally accepted as bleeding more than 1 year after the last period. However, if the tumour does develop before the menopause, it may cause irregular bleeding, which should always be investigated.

A tissue sample of the endometrial tissue is needed for investigation and diagnosis. Dilatation and curettage used to be the standard method for this, but direct hysteroscopy, in which an endoscope is introduced through the cervix into the endometrial cavity, has started to replace this. It is also possible to obtain a sample without anaesthetic in the out-patient department by using a very narrow suction device, although this may fail to sample adequately.

Combination therapy is the usual treatment, with a total abdominal hysterectomy and a bilateral salpingo-oophorectomy (removal of the Fallopian tubes and ovaries) either preceded or followed by radiotherapy. Endocrine therapy with high doses of progesterone has been found to contain metastatic disease and it sometimes induces temporary remission. If the tumour is confined to the uterus and the woman undergoes total hysterectomy, the 5-year survival is around 80 per cent; even if there are macroscopic ovarian metastases, the survival rate may still be 40 per cent. The addition of radiotherapy improves survival rates by between 5 and 10 per cent.

THE MENOPAUSE

The climacteric is the counterpart of puberty and refers to the transitional phase when the reproductive organs involute as ovarian function diminishes. This may take 1–5 years, whereas the menopause refers to the cessation of menstruation, which may precede cessation of ovarian function by several months or even years. The average age of menopause in the UK is 51 years; with a range of 45 to 52 years.

Waning ovarian function causes the breast tissue to shrink owing to atrophy of the breast glandular tissue, leaving predominantly fatty tissue. The pituitary stimulation of the ovary continues but the ovary fails to respond. This leads to raised levels of pituitary follicle-stimulating hormone (FSH) and luteinizing hormone (LH) accompanied by low levels of circulating oestrogen. The lack of oestrogen causes local tissue changes in the vagina (atrophic vaginitis) and around the urethra, causing urinary frequency and dysuria.

Systemic symptoms typically include vasomotor instability (hot flushes), joint pains, and skin changes. Longer-term effects of reduced oestrogen include loss of bone mass, leading to osteoporosis in vulnerable women, and an increased risk of coronary heart disease, from which premenopausal women seem to be relatively protected by oestrogen (Figure 37.3) (see Chapters 32, 39, and 40).

HORMONE REPLACEMENT THERAPY

HRT can be used with two aims in mind:
- the relief of menopausal symptoms; and
- the prevention of conditions induced by oestrogen deficiency, such as osteoporosis.

If a woman has had a hysterectomy, HRT can be with oestrogen alone, but if she has an intact uterus, progesterone must be given as well to prevent the risk of endometrial carcinoma (see above).

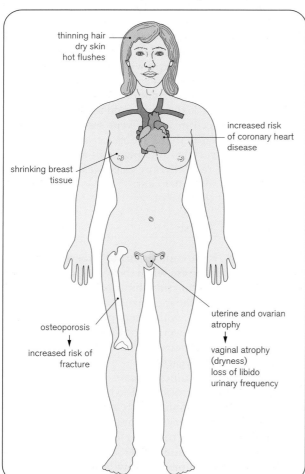

Figure 37.3 The effects of lack of oestrogen on body tissues in the menopause.

thinning hair
dry skin
hot flushes

increased risk of coronary heart disease

shrinking breast tissue

osteoporosis
↓
increased risk of fracture

uterine and ovarian atrophy
↓
vaginal atrophy (dryness)
loss of libido
urinary frequency

The risk of osteoporotic fractures is almost halved by HRT, but bone loss is only prevented while the HRT continues to be taken. Some studies have shown that coronary heart disease and stroke risk are also reduced and there has been a recent suggestion that Alzheimer's disease is less common in women who have taken HRT.

However, there is evidence that HRT use for longer than 10 years increases the risk of breast cancer by up to 1.5 times (see breast cancer), though if a breast tumour does develop, it seems to have a better prognosis. There is also a two- to four-fold increased risk of thromboembolism in HRT users, but even this increase produces only a very small overall risk.

Oestrogens may be administered orally or by implant, topical gel, or patch, and locally as vaginal creams, pessaries, or tablets. Women who have not had a hysterectomy may take the progesterone cyclically, to produce a regular bleed, or continuously, which will sometimes lead to amenorrhoea, although the younger the woman, the more likely she is to have irregular bleeding on the continuous regime. There is also a synthetic steroid, tibolone, based on natural oestrogens, which usually produces an amenorrhoeic cycle and relieves menopausal symptoms, as well as being licensed for the prevention of osteoporosis.

The question of how long to take HRT is a difficult one, given that prolonged use appears to increase the risk of breast cancer but the protective effect on the bones is only there during current use. Often a woman will try stopping treatment, sometimes because they want to stop the cyclical bleeding, but will start again because the symptoms return.

INFERTILITY

Infertility is a problem affecting approximately 10 per cent of couples at some point. It is a huge topic in its own right and this section provides a brief overview of the causes and some of the treatment options.

FEMALE INFERTILITY

There are a number of causes of female infertility.

Ovulatory Failure

Ovulatory failure can be total or – more commonly – sporadic. Ovulation depends on the correct sequence of pituitary and ovarian hormones to stimulate the growth of the follicle containing the oocyte and then the surge of LH to cause the release of the oocyte. Oestrogen and progesterone produced by the ovary are responsible for the developing and maturing endometrium, which is necessary for the successful

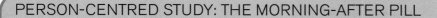

Lisa was in an agitated state when she came into the surgery. 'I was really stupid last night – I need the morning-after pill.' Dr Barton asked her when her last period had been and found out that she was at day 14 of her cycle. This is the time of ovulation, so it put Lisa at high risk of pregnancy, and since she was within the 72-hour time limit since unprotected intercourse, postcoital contraception was appropriate.

'How does it work?' asked Lisa. 'The high levels of oestrogen and progesterone, equivalent to a week's worth of oral contraceptive pills taken in the space of 12 hours, change the lining of the uterus so that the egg is unlikely to implant. It is about 95 per cent successful in preventing pregnancy,' answered Dr Barton.

'My friend was fitted with a coil instead, because she has had a thrombosis in the past' commented Lisa. 'Yes, that can be an alternative, particularly if you want to keep the coil as a long-term method of contraception. It too works by stopping the egg from implanting and works up to 5 days after intercourse. We need to decide which method of

contraception would be suitable for you for the future, as you cannot rely on repeated doses of the postcoital pill,' replied Dr Barton.

'I want to go back on the pill' said Lisa firmly. 'I'm not going through this worry again!' She had been on a low-dose combined oral contraceptive, which contains oestrogen and progesterone, in the past. This works on the ovarian hormonal feedback loop to prevent ovulation. The other type of oral contraceptive, the so-called mini-pill, contains only progesterone. This does not inhibit ovulation, and it works by making the cervical mucus unfavourable to sperm penetration. It has to be taken reliably every 24 hours and is not as effective a means of contraception as the combined version.

After examining Lisa, Dr Barton carefully explained how to take the postcoital pill, ensuring that she understood the risk of pregnancy. She then explained how to begin the combined pill when her next period had properly started. She arranged to see Lisa the following month, and Lisa departed, obviously relieved and much calmer than on her arrival.

implantation of a fertilized ovum. Any failure of the hormone cycle will lead to ovulatory failure, as will abnormal levels of some other hormones, such as thyroxine and prolactin.

Blockage of the Fallopian Tubes

Tubal blockage obstructs the passage of the oocyte once it has been released from the ovary. The most common cause of blockage is pelvic infection. Chlamydial infection is one of the common causes. It is often sexually acquired and it may be asymptomatic. Chlamydia can be eradicated by treatment with tetracycline antibiotics. Less frequently, these days, gonorrhoea may also cause pelvic infection. Occasionally, peritonitis from acute appendicitis leads to tubal scarring.

Endometriosis

Endometriosis (see above) causes tissue damage where the deposits of endometrial tissue happen to develop and cyclically bleed. This can lead to tubal scarring or sometimes irregular ovulation.

MALE INFERTILITY

The production of sperm is dependent on a complex sequence of hormonal influences on the seminiferous tubules. Semen analysis (Box 37.6) is a very important initial investigation for a couple with infertility.

Causes of male infertility include damage to the testicular tissue from infections such as mumps, chemotherapy, or congenital abnormalities such as undescended testicles or an absent vas deferens (which

BOX 37.6 NORMAL SEMEN ANALYSIS

semen volume > 1.5 ml
sperm concentration > 20 million/ml
motility > 70 per cent of spermatozoa
motile grade > 2 (0 = no movement; 4 = excellent forward movement)
normal morphology > 60 per cent of spermatozoa
fructose present in semen

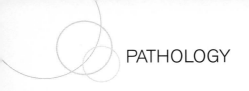
is found in up to 2 per cent of infertile men). A varicocoele (varicosities of the plexus of veins around the testis) is found in about 40 per cent of men referred for subfertility. It is thought that the increased blood flow may raise the testicular temperature, which is known to reduce sperm production, and ligation of the varicocoele may correct the problem.

Some other causes include sperm with abnormal motility or morphology which do not seem to penetrate the oocyte successfully. There are also situations in which antibodies in the woman's cervical mucus are hostile to the sperm.

INVESTIGATIONS

It is important to establish whether each case of infertility is primary infertility for the couple (i.e. neither partner has achieved a previous pregnancy) or whether it is secondary infertility (i.e. either partner has achieved a pregnancy in the past, even if the pregnancy did not survive to term).

Successful ovulation may be checked by measuring the surge of LH at the time of ovulation, and commercial kits for home use are available so that sexual intercourse can be optimally timed. The peak rise in serum progesterone on the seventh day after ovulation (usually Day 21 of the menstrual cycle) may also be measured to provide this information (Figure 37.4). Other hormone abnormalities may also be detected on basic screening blood tests. Most of these abnormalities can be corrected (e.g. hypothyroidism can be treated with oral thyroxine).

Tubal patency may be checked by hysterosalpingography, in which a cannula is inserted through the cervix and a radio-opaque dye squirted through it. The dye can be detected on pelvic X-ray, and it outlines the uterine cavity and tubes and demonstrates any anatomical abnormality, such as fibroids or tubal obstruction. This dye procedure is sometimes combined with laparoscopy, when the pelvic organs can be directly inspected, in particular looking for evidence of endometriosis.

Semen analysis may reveal a low total sperm count or abnormal shapes or motility. Sometimes a postcoital test is done, in which samples are taken from the vagina after intercourse and examined under the microscope. Normally, the sperm are very actively moving through the cervical mucus, and any delay here may be due to agglutinating and immobilizing antibodies in the mucus (see Chapter 27).

TREATMENT

Ovulatory failure can often be corrected by the use of drug clomiphene on a cyclical basis. This is both an

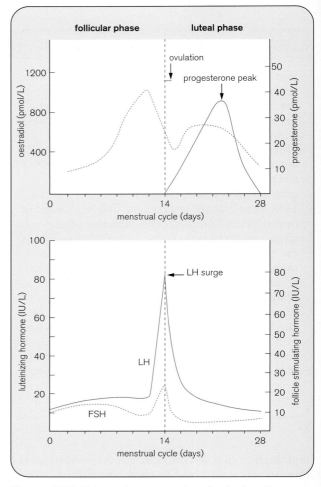

Figure 37.4 Serum hormone levels during the menstrual cycle. The graphs show an ovulatory cycle of 28 days.

oestrogenic and an anti-oestrogenic agent; it stimulates the release of FSH and LH and often promotes ovulation. The rate of twin pregnancies is increased with this drug, but higher multiple pregnancies are rare just on treatment with clomiphene. The drug is given for the first 5 days of the menstrual cycle and repeated cyclically until pregnancy is achieved or six cycles have been completed.

Tubal obstruction is more difficult to deal with. Surgical division of scars and adhesions is sometimes successful; however, rather than undergoing prolonged attempts at tubal surgery, these patients tend to progress to a form of *in-vitro* fertilization (IVF), in which the tube is bypassed altogether. Even when there is evidence of a patent Fallopian tube, some couples remain childless for reasons that are not always known. Then an alternative form of assisted reproduction may be offered – gamete intra-fallopian transfer (GIFT). In this technique, the oocyte and sperm are retrieved, then introduced for possible fertilization in the Fallopian tube rather than cultured in a 'test tube'. There is a higher rate of conception with GIFT than with conventional IVF.

Treatment of sperm abnormalities is limited, although tamoxifen has sometimes successfully been used in men with low sperm counts. Artificial insemination with donor sperm has allowed couples to achieve a pregnancy when the primary problem lies with the quality or quantity of sperm.

There has been a tremendous expansion in IVF techniques since the original 'test-tube' baby, Louise Brown, was born in 1978, and an individual sperm can now be injected into an ovum to achieve fertilization. However, the overall success rate of these techniques is still quite low, with even the best units achieving less than 20 per cent live birth rates; this is also heavily dependent on other factors, such as the age of the patient and the number of previous attempts.

Control of laboratories and units dealing with the research and administration of these techniques falls under the regulation of the Human Fertility and Embryology Authority, which licenses the units.

DISEASES OF THE MALE REPRODUCTIVE TRACT

DISEASES OF THE PROSTATE

Prostatic diseases largely affects men over the age of 50. By far the most common problem is that of benign prostatic hypertrophy and, by the age of 80, most men have some symptoms. However, prostatic cancer is now the second most common cause of death from cancer in men in northern Europe, and as the population ages the numbers are gradually rising.

Benign Prostatic Hypertrophy

The symptoms of benign prostatic hypertrophy (BPH) are mainly due to obstruction of the urine outflow from the bladder. The man experiences hesitancy, a poor or intermittent flow, and incomplete bladder emptying with terminal dribble. Sometimes, there are also symptoms of bladder irritation, such as frequency, urgency, incontinence, and nocturia.

Examination of the patient sometimes reveals an enlarged bladder, which may be as large as a 4-month pregnancy. This gradual distension of the bladder is painless, but it may cause back pressure on the kidneys, finally leading to chronic renal failure (see Chapter 36). The prostate can be examined rectally and often feels enlarged but (usually) smooth. If the prostate feels hard, craggy, or irregular, prostatic cancer is much more likely than BPH.

Investigations include urine culture to exclude infection, measurement of urinary flow rate and residual urine volume, and serum urea and electrolytes to check renal function. A further blood test, prostate specific antigen, is also usually done, since this can be a marker of prostate cancer, although it may also be raised in BPH, infections of the prostate, and with increasing age. Transrectal ultrasound and needle biopsy of suspicious areas in the prostate is often performed to exclude malignancy.

Management of BPH is broadly either with drug therapy or surgery. For those with only mild-to-moderate symptoms or those who are unfit for surgery, drugs such as finasteride, which blocks the testosterone effect on the prostate, or drugs that relax smooth muscle may well be all that is required to manage the situation.

Transurethral resection of the prostate (TURP) is still considered the mainstay of treatment for significant disease. It involves resection of the prostatic lobes with a cutting diathermy introduced via the urethra. Complications include heavy post-operative bleeding, retrograde ejaculation in more than 50 per cent of men, and occasionally incontinence and impotence. Laser ablation of the prostate may have fewer complications, but it provides no tissue for histological analysis and it is quite common for small foci of cancer to be unexpectedly found in the chippings of a patient thought only to have BPH. Other techniques include putting a metal stent in the prostate to open the urethra, balloon dilatation, and microwave treatment.

Carcinoma of the Prostate

The incidence of prostatic cancer is rising by 3 per cent per year, and the use of the prostatic specific antigen blood test has probably increased the diagnosis of early, symptomless tumours. However, the natural history of prostatic cancer is unpredictable in that although it may be an aggressive tumour with metastatic spread, it is also well known that at routine post-mortem, one-third of men over the age of 75 have foci of prostatic cancer. These tiny tumours are undetectable by current methods and have not caused any problems to the patient. There is a real dilemma about screening and early diagnosis, since any treatment may cause serious morbidity and death, yet the patient may never develop significant disease from the original cancer (Figure 37.5).

Symptoms of prostate cancer are very similar to those of BPH, which is why malignancy needs to be excluded when BPH is suspected. Sometimes, the patient presents with symptoms from metastases, which are usually bony, and severe back pain due to vertebral collapse may be the first problem.

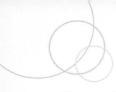

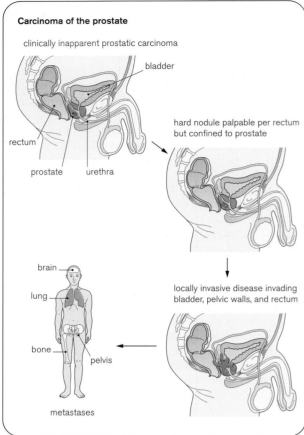

Carcinoma of the prostate

clinically inapparent prostatic carcinoma

bladder

rectum

prostate   urethra

hard nodule palpable per rectum
but confined to prostate

brain

lung

locally invasive disease invading
bladder, pelvic walls, and rectum

bone

pelvis

metastases

Figure 37.5 Carcinoma of the prostate. The stages of progressive and invasive prostatic carcinoma with metastases.

Management of cancer that is localized to the prostate and does not breach the capsule is either with radiotherapy or hormonal therapy. Radiotherapy causes a high rate of impotence, but 15-year disease-free survival rates of 85 per cent have been achieved. In younger patients, the option of radical prostatectomy can be considered. This involves major surgery with potential complications of incontinence and impotence, but it may produce longer disease-free survival rates.

Hormonal therapies are based on suppressing testosterone production or blocking its action. This can be achieved by bilateral orchidectomy (castration), but anti-testosterone drugs, such as cyproterone or goserelin, are usually more acceptable. If the patient has metastases, the hormonal therapies may help to contain metastatic symptoms as well. Chronic renal failure due to obstruction (see Chapter 36) may be the cause of death in the terminal phase of prostatic cancer.

DISEASES OF THE TESTIS
Undescended Testes (Cryptorchidism)

In the embryo, the testes develop from specialized tissue in the abdominal cavity; during the gestation period they migrate caudally until, by the time of birth, both testes should be in the scrotum. Sometimes the testis may only partly descend and be found in the inguinal canal (ectopic testis), or they may not descend at all and remain in the abdominal cavity (undescended testis).

If the testis is not fully descended by puberty, it is unlikely that normal sperm production will occur. There is also a significant risk of malignancy in a maldescended testis, which appears to be reduced if the testis is surgically placed in the scrotum. It is for this reason that boys who do not have both testes in the scrotum by the age of 5 or 6 years undergo surgery. If technically possible, the aberrant testis is pulled down into the scrotum and fixed there, but if the testis is in the abdomen, it is removed to prevent the future risk of malignant change.

Torsion of the Testis

If the testis twists on the spermatic cord, the vascular supply may be occluded. If this is not urgently corrected surgically, the testis will infarct and die. This is why it is so important not to miss an acute torsion of the testis. It usually occurs in children or adolescents, and they present with a sudden pain in the testis, which is usually red, very painful to touch, and swollen. Occasionally the main site of the pain is in the abdomen, where the supplying nerve originates, and this may lead to confusion over the diagnosis.

The differential diagnosis includes infection of the testis or epididymis, but if the diagnosis is uncertain, it is safer to operate within the 6-hour time limit, since delay causes irreversible tissue damage. If the testis is viable, it is untwisted and fixed to prevent further episodes of torsion.

Testicular Tumours

Testicular tumours are increasing in incidence, but the numbers are still small overall and the cause of the rise is not certain. They occur in young men from their mid-teens to their 30s, with the incidence falling off over the age of 40. The different cell types of testicular tumours depend on the abnormal development of the germ cells which would normally produce sperm. This abnormal differentiation can produce seminomas, teratomas, yolk-sac tumours, or choriocarcinomas.

Nearly all testicular tumours present as a lump in the testis, which may be painless or painful. The tumour is staged (Box 37.7); an important part of this process is the measurement of specific tumour markers in the blood, such as alpha-fetoprotein and beta-human chorionic gonadotrophin. The response of the tumour marker levels to treatment is a good indicator of overall treatment success.

Seminomas are extremely radiosensitive, and orchidectomy and radiotherapy in Stage I disease gives 95 per cent cure rates. Even in Stage II disease, in which regional lymph nodes are involved, radiotherapy produces very good long-term results. Combination chemotherapy with platinum agents is necessary for more advanced stages of disease.

Non-seminomatous tumours, including teratomas are usually treated by orchidectomy, with chemotherapy for the more advanced tumours. Stage I tumours are being managed by surveillance of tumour markers and computerized tomography scans, with chemotherapy being introduced later if necessary.

The successful treatment regimes of testicular tumours have revolutionized survival rates – these used to be rapidly fatal tumours before the introduction of platinum-based chemotherapy.

BOX 37.7 STAGING OF TESTICULAR TUMOURS

Stage I
tumour confined to the testis

Stage II
involvement of lymph nodes below the diaphragm

Stage III
involvement of lymph nodes above the diaphragm

Stage IV
tumour spread to lungs and liver

KEY POINTS

- Benign breast disease tends to occur in younger women, with the incidence of breast cancer rising with age. The prognosis of breast cancer depends on the size of the original tumour, the cell differentiation, and whether the cancer has spread to lymph nodes.
- The death rate from cancer of the cervix is declining in the UK. Abnormalities on screening cervical smears can spontaneously regress without treatment.
- Ovarian cysts are common and only a small minority are malignant, but approximately 4000 women die each year in the UK from ovarian cancer. The incidence rises with age, and ovarian cancers usually present late. There is a familial trend to ovarian cancer.
- Hormone replacement therapy treats symptoms of oestrogen deficiency as well as preventing the long-term effects, such as osteoporosis. There is small but definite increased risk of breast cancer after more than 5 years' treatment with oestrogen.
- Infertility investigations focus on ovulatory problems, abnormalities in sperm production, and functional and mechanical obstruction to fertilization. Treatment is targeted at the underlying cause, and there are now many different techniques available to achieve conception, although overall live birth rates are still relatively low with *in vitro* fertilization.
- Prostatic cancer may be asymptomatic and is sometimes discovered coincidentally, or it may be aggressive and fatal. At present, no screening test can differentiate between the spectrum of disease, and since radical treatments can produce significant morbidity, there is controversy over the current management of asymptomatic disease.

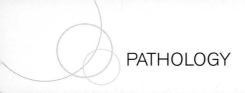

PATHOLOGY

FURTHER READING

Alberg AJ, Helzlsouer KJ (1997) Epidemiology, prevention and early detection of breast cancer. Curr Opin Oncol 9:505–11.

Balen A (1997) Anovulatory infertility and ovulation induction. Policy and Practice Subcommittee of the British Fertility Society. Hum Reprod 12 (Suppl):83–7.

Collaborative Group on Hormonal Factors in Breast Cancer. Beral V breasr cancer and hormone replacement therapy: collaborative reanalysis of data from 51 epidemiological studies of 52705 women with breast cancer and 108411 women without breast cancer. Lancet 1997; 350:1047–59.

Cresswell JL, Barker DJ, Osmond C, Egger P, Phillips DI, Fraser RB (1997) Fetal growth, length of gestation, and polycystic ovaries in adult life. Lancet 350:1131–5.

Dawson C, Whitfield H (1996) ABC of urology. Subfertility and male sexual dysfunction. BMJ. 312(7035): 902–905.

Dawson C, Whitfield H (1996) ABC of urology. Urological malignancy I: prostate cancer. BMJ 312:1032–4.

Dixon JM, Sainsbury JRC (1998) Handbook of Diseases of the Breast, 2nd edition. Churchill Livingstone, Edinburgh.

Dixon JM (ed) (1995) ABC of Breast Diseases. BMJ Publishing, London.

Early Breast Trialist' Collaborative Group (1992) Systemic treatment of early breast cancer by hormonal, cytotoxic or immune therapy: 133 randomised trials involving 31,000 recurrences and 24,000 deaths among 75,000 women. Lancet 339:1–15.

Jeffcoate S (1987) Principles of Gynaecology, 5th Edition [revised by Tindall VR]. Butterworth, London.

Kavanagh AM, Broom DH (1997) Women's understanding of abnormal cervical smear test results: a qualitative interview study. BMJ 314:1388–91.

Kinlen LJ, Spriggs AI (1978) Women with positive cervical smears but without surgical intervention. A follow-up study. Lancet 2:463–5.

Macgregor JE, Moss SM, Parkin DM, Day NE (1985) A case-control study of cervical cancer screening in north east Scotland. BMJ 290:1543–6.

Leslie NS, Roche BG (1997) The effectiveness of the breast self-examination facilitation shield. Oncol Nurs Forum 24:1759–65.

Marantides D (1997) Management of polycystic ovary syndrome. Nurse Pract 22:34–8.

McPherson A (ed) (1993) Women's Problems in General Practice, 3rd edition. Oxford University Press, Oxford.

O'Rourke ME, Germino BB (1998) Prostate cancer treatment decisions: a focus group exploration. Oncol Nurs Forum 25:97–104.

Parker L (1997) Causes of testicular cancer. Lancet 350:827–8.

Posner T, Vessey M (1997) Prevention of cervical cancer: the patient's view. King's Fund, London.

Price EH, Little HK, Grant ECG, Steel CM (1997) Women need to be warned about dangers of hormone replacement therapy. BMJ 314:376–7.

Recent Advances in Surgery. Johnson Ed Johnson CD, Taylor I (1994) Vol 17 Chapter 7 Harries SA Prognostic Factors in Early Breast Cancer p.105–120.

Salvesen HB, Akslen LA, Iversen T, Iversen OE (1997) Recurrence of endometrial carcinoma and the value of routine follow up. Br J Obstet Gynaecol 104:1302–7.

Samarel N (1997) Therapeutic touch, dialogue, and women's experiences in breast cancer surgery. Holist Nurs Pract 12:62–70.

Todd JH, Dowle C, Williams M *et al*. (1987) Confirmation of a prognostic index in primary breast cancer. Br J Cancer 56:489–492.

Whooley MA, Grady D, Cummings SR (1997) Postmenopausal hormone therapy and mortality. N Engl J Med 337:1389–90.

38

DISORDERS OF THE CENTRAL NERVOUS SYSTEM

LEARNING OBJECTIVES

After studying this chapter students should have a clearer understanding of:
- the clinical features of meningoencephalitis
- the pathophysiology of stroke and the principles of management
- the causes of epilepsy and the basis of management
- the pathophysiology of spinal cord injury, the clinical picture, and the principles of management

Before reading this chapter you should have an understanding of:
- the basic anatomy of the brain and spinal cord
- the structure and function of the peripheral nerves.

INTRODUCTION

The central nervous system comprises the brain and the spinal cord; the peripheral nervous system consists of all the nerve fibres which run from the brain and spinal cord to all parts of the body. The brain is made up of the forebrain (cerebrum and diencephalon), the brain stem (medulla oblongata, pons and midbrain), and the cerebellum. The cerebrum is made up of the left and right cerebral hemispheres, and the diencephalon consists of the hypothalamus and the thalamus.

The cerebral cortex is responsible for integrating information from all parts of the nervous system, for cognitive function, for the control of states of arousal and attention, and for the fine tuning of all motor activity. Much of the information is relayed via the thalamus. The hypothalamus controls endocrine functions (see Chapter 35).

The cerebellum is largely concerned with co-ordinating movements and the learning of motor skills, including balance, posture, and speech. The brain stem contains bundles of nerve fibres that run from the cerebrum and the cerebellum down to the spinal cord, and it contains nuclei concerned with cardiovascular and respiratory functions, wakefulness, and the control of eye movement. The brain stem also contains nuclei of the cranial nerve, which control the muscles and glands of the head and some of the upper parts of the body; sensory information is also relayed from these areas.

The meninges are three membranes (the dura mater, the arachnoid, and the pia mater) that cover the soft neural tissue of the brain. Cerebrospinal fluid (CSF) fills the space between two of the membranes, the arachnoid and the pia mater, and thus acts to cushion the brain against impact on the skull. The CSF originates from the choroid plexuses, which are ventricles (cavities) in the brain. They contain CSF and lie at the boundary between the blood stream and the ventricles (Figure 38.1).

Nervous tissue comprises nerve cells (neurones) and supporting glial cells. Neurones generate electrical signals, which are passed along the axons (also called the nerve fibres). Dendrites are branched processes with which a neurone communicates with other neurones. Electrical signals are transmitted by a neurone by way of chemical messengers (neurotransmitters) which are released at the ends of nerve fibres. There are two main types of glial cell – the oligodendroglia, which produce the myelin sheath that encloses long nerve fibres, thus enabling the rapid transmission of electrical signals

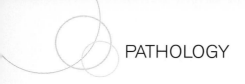

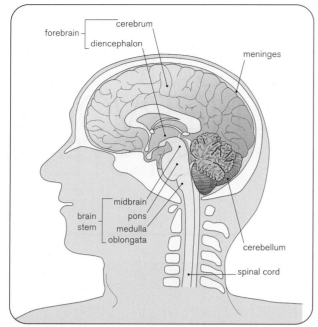

Figure 38.1 The central nervous system.
Diagrammatic representation of the brain and associated tissues.

over long distances, and the astrocytes, which regulate the composition of the extracellular fluid and have a controlling influence on neural development and metabolism.

INVESTIGATING THE CENTRAL NERVOUS SYSTEM

Although a careful history and examination of the patient often yields the diagnosis of a neurological disorder, certain investigations are indispensable as confirmation i.e. a differential diagnosis (see Chapter 6). The recent advances in radiology have made it possible to diagnose the nature and site of intracranial pathology more rapidly.

Electroencephalography

The electroencephalogram (EEG) records the electrical activity of the brain through electrodes placed on the scalp. The record obtained is influenced by age, the level of consciousness, and the emotional state. An EEG may reveal a focus for abnormal electrical activity in epilepsy, but one should be aware that some people with epilepsy have a normal EEG. The EEG is abnormal when there is diffuse cerebral pathology (e.g. in Alzheimer's disease) and in metabolic disturbances,

such as hepatic encephalopathy (see Chapter 34).

Computerized Tomography

Computerized tomography (CT) scanning is an essential tool in the diagnosis and localization of intracranial pathology, such as tumours, haematomas, and abscesses, as well as in the investigation of diffuse changes.

Cerebral Angiography

Cerebral angiography enables the visualization of the cerebral circulation and is useful in demonstrating vascular malformations and aneurysms. This procedure is done by cannulating either the carotid or the vertebral artery and injecting contrast medium, which can be visualized on X-ray.

Magnetic Resonance Imaging

Magnetic resonance imaging (MRI) uses radio-frequency radiation in the presence of a magnetic field to obtain images of the brain and spinal cord. It is particularly useful for demonstrating the lesions of multiple sclerosis, and for revealing lesions of the brain stem and spinal cord.

Nerve Conduction Studies

Conduction in the sensory and motor nerves can be examined by using surface electrodes to record the time of arrival and the amplitude of an electrical impulse generated by a stimulus of a known magnitude. Such studies can also be applied to the optic nerves by placing electrodes over the scalp and recording the signal generated by stimuli in the visual field. These are called visual evoked potentials and are particularly helpful in the investigation of suspected multiple sclerosis.

VASCULAR DISORDERS

STROKE
Presentation and Diagnosis

A stroke (also called a cerebrovascular accident) is a rapidly developing loss of cerebral function which is vascular in origin. It may be focal or global. The clinical severity varies widely from full recovery in a few days through permanent disability to death. A stroke may result from occlusion of an artery supplying the brain, the rupture of an aneurysm (leading to intracranial haemorrhage) or other vascular malformations or diseases.

The most common pathological cause of ischaemic stroke is atheroma complicated by thrombus (see Chapter 32) or embolism, which leads to cerebral ischaemia and infarction. The next most common cause of ischaemic stroke is disease affecting the small penetrating arteries of the brain (microatheroma), which, when occluded, cause lacunar infarcts (infarction in tiny areas of the brain). Patients with lacunar infarcts often have hypertension. Another cause of ischaemic stroke is embolism from the heart, such as might occur in bacterial endocarditis or a mural thrombus.

The so-called vasculitic disorders are multisystem disorders that, during their course, may be complicated by ischaemic stroke, intracranial haemorrhage, or (more commonly) a generalized ischaemic encephalopathy. Giant cell arteritis is the most common vasculitic cause of stroke. Systemic lupus erythematosus (see Chapter 27) is more likely to cause a generalized encephalopathy than focal ischaemia.

Haematological disorders, including polycythaemia, essential thrombocythaemia, and sickle cell disease may, rarely, cause thrombotic stroke; leukaemia is more commonly a cause of intracranial haemorrhage. Patients with inherited abnormalities of the coagulation system (see Chapter 31), such as protein C or S deficiency or Factor V Leiden, are also at risk of thrombotic stroke.

Intracranial haemorrhage may occur into the subarachnoid space (subarachnoid haemorrhage), within the brain (primary intracerebral haemorrhage) (see Figure 38.2), or more rarely, into the ventricles or subdural space. Ruptured aneurysm is the most frequent cause of a subarachnoid haemorrhage, and the incidence increases with age. Primary intracranial haemorrhage is generally due to hypertensive vascular disease or vascular malformations.

With a stroke, there is often a clear history of focal brain dysfunction that started suddenly or is first noticed on waking; sometimes, though, the onset of symptoms is more gradual or stepwise. A typical presentation may involve:

- weakness of one side of the body or face (hemiparesis), with or without sensory loss, together with loss of the left or right side of the visual field (homonymous hemianopia);
- the side of the body affected being opposite to the side of the lesion;
- features such as slurred speech, and an altered level or quality of consciousness, which, if present, may 'evolve' over a few hours.

A more slowly developing clinical picture of cerebral dysfunction may suggest an intracranial tumour, and a chronic subdural haematoma is often accompanied by drowsiness, headache, and confusion, together with a history of head injury in the preceding few weeks.

The site of the lesion may be established with the aid of CT scan or MRI, although a clue is often gleaned from simple clinical examination. The CT scan can be normal shortly after onset of a cerebral infarct, while intracerebral haemorrhage can be seen immediately on CT. MRI is more sensitive for infarction than CT is, but it is less specific, so that although many more lesions are shown, it can be difficult to decide which is relevant to the current symptoms. An angiogram of the cerebral vessels may provide evidence of a vascular malformation or aneurysm that can be removed, or obliterated, surgically. This is really only possible in young patients who have had a mild stroke or are recovering well from a more major stroke. Some ischaemic strokes are due to atheromatous disease of one of the carotid arteries, which can be revealed on carotid angiography, and is treatable by endarterectomy.

Management

The prognosis for cerebral infarction (10 per cent mortality) is better than for intracranial haemorrhage (50 per cent mortality). However, the general approach to management is similar for both types of stroke. Initial management is aimed at confirmation of diagnosis and correction of treatable causes (e.g. cardiogenic embolism, vascular malformation). The evacuation of haematomas remains controversial, but it may be of benefit if there is delayed deterioration. Unless the patient is expected to die very rapidly, it is important to reduce early mortality and later disability by the following measures:

- maintaining pulmonary, cardiovascular, fluid and electrolyte, and nutritional homeostasis;
- avoiding, or recognizing, and treating systemic complications; and
- minimizing further neurological deterioration.

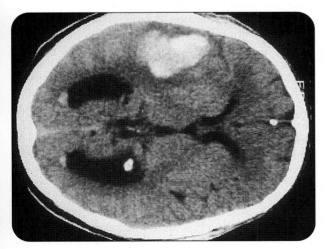

Figure 38.2 Computerized tomography (CT) scan of intracranial haemorrhage. (By permission of Dr A Valentine, Royal Free Hospital School of Medicine, London, UK.)

If the stroke causes more than mild disability, then good nursing care is essential to ensure that:
- the patient is comfortable;
- the airway is well maintained; and
- swallowing is safe.

If there is any difficulty in swallowing, fluids must be given by a nasogastric tube or even intravenously. The patient should be kept well nourished and toileted, kept clean, and turned regularly to reduce the risk of pressure sores. After a severe stroke, there is often a stress response (i.e. raised blood pressure, mild fever, hyperglycaemia and even glycosuria) but this normally subsides spontaneously in a few days. The most frequently observed complications of acute stroke include pneumonia, venous thromboembolism, urinary tract infection, pressure sores, cardiac arrhythmias, muscle contractures, mood disorders, and fits.

The majority of patients who survive the first month after stroke will improve, and some of them get back to their previous level of function. The rate of recovery of all impairments is maximal in the first few weeks, and probably stops at 6–12 months after the stroke. Later improvement in functional abilities, particularly social activities, is likely to be due to minimizing handicap rather than to further recovery of physical impairments. Impaired quality of life is very common, even when patients appear to be little disabled. Immediately after the onset of stroke, it is difficult to predict the prognosis for eventual recovery. However, by about 2 weeks after the stroke, when it becomes clear that the patient is likely to survive, the following are indictors for a good prognosis:
- urinary continence;
- young age;
- rapid improvement;
- good perceptual abilities; and
- no cognitive disorder.

Important goals for rehabilitation are to maximize the patient's role fulfilment and independence in his environment within the limitations imposed by his pathology and resources, and to help the patient make the best adaptation to any differences between roles achieved and roles desired. A multidisciplinary team is needed to provide help and support, including nurses, physiotherapists, occupational therapists, speech therapists, voluntary workers, doctors (including neurologists and general physicians), social workers, chiropodists, home helps, meals-on-wheels services and the local housing department. The carers also need support and counselling. Careful planning should set out realistic short-term, medium-term, and long-term goals to be agreed by the rehabilitation team, patient, and carers.

TRANSIENT ISCHAEMIC ATTACKS

A transient ischaemic attack(TIA) is an acute loss of focal cerebral, or monocular function, which lasts less than 24 hours and which, after appropriate investigation, is presumed to be due to thrombotic or embolic vascular disease. The pathological causes of a TIA are essentially the same as for ischaemic stroke, and about 15 per cent of patients having a first stroke have had earlier TIAs.

Motor symptoms are the most common features, with weakness or clumsiness of a limb often described, confusingly, by the patient, as a 'dead' feeling. Sensory impairment (such as numbness or tingling) slurred speech, visual loss in one eye (sometimes described as a 'shutter coming down') are all common. Loss of consciousness is extremely rare. The symptoms can sometimes allow attacks to be categorized into those due to vascular disease in the territory supplied by the carotid artery (80 per cent) and those due to vascular disease in the territory supplied by the vertebrobasilar arteries (20 per cent). The pathology is usually arterial stenosis; occasionally it is embolism.

MULTI-INFARCT DEMENTIA

This is deterioration in a person with a previously normal intellect and memory caused by repeated clinical or subclinical episodes of cerebral ischaemia, infarction, or haemorrhage. The decline in cerebral function is gradual.

MIGRAINE

Migraine is defined as a spasmodic disorder involving a visual or tactile aura (or both) associated with nausea and vomiting and unilateral headache. This is very common, affecting up to 10 per cent of the population, and there is a familial association. The first attack often occurs around puberty, and in adults it is twice as common in females. Attacks are more frequent at the time of menstruation and may recede during pregnancy. Dietary precipitants that have been implicated include cheese, chocolate, caffeine, and alcohol. Recent evidence has also implicated infection with *Heliobacter pylori* since eradication of the bacteria has been shown to result in a significant reduction in intensity, duration and frequency of migraine attacks.

Spasm of the arteries within the internal carotid territory is thought to give rise to the aura, and the subsequent dilatation in the distribution of the external carotid artery is considered to be responsible for the headache. Migraine sufferers should be advised to avoid excessive physical or mental fatigue and any known dietary precipitants. Drugs are used, both for treatment and for prophylaxis. Many attacks can be controlled by simple analgesics such as aspirin or paracetamol. Ergotamine constricts vessels, and is used in combination with an anti-emetic in preparations such as Migril and Cafergot. The $5HT_1$ agonist drugs (e.g. sumatriptan, naratriptan, zolmitriptan) may be prescribed for patients who do not respond to simple analgesics taken with or without anti-emetics (see also Chapter 10).

INFECTIONS

Infections of the nervous system are commonly caused by bacteria or viruses, and may be either generalized or localized. Examples of localized infections include acute poliomyelitis, shingles (caused by herpes zoster), and cold sores (caused by herpes simplex).

ACUTE MENINGOENCEPHALITIS

This is an acute inflammatory illness affecting the meninges (meningitis) and brain tissue (encephalitis), although sometimes the features of one will predominate. Bacterial meningitis is a medical emergency. In neonates, the causative organisms are commonly *Escherichia coli* and group B streptococci, whereas in later life meningococcus, pneumococcus, and *Haemophilus influenzae* are the important causative pathogens. Meningococcal meningitis often occurs in association with septicaemia and presents with fever, headache, purpuric rash, rapidly progressive shock, deterioration in conscious level, and neck stiffness (see also Box 38.1). Many viral infections, including mumps, measles, and chickenpox, are accompanied by a mild, self-limiting meningoencephalitis. Herpes simplex virus encephalitis is the most serious of these, and it can occur at any age. Brain swelling is common, reflecting damage to brain tissue, and survivors are often left with neurological deficits such as epilepsy or intellectual impairment.

The diagnosis of acute meningoencephalitis is made on the findings in the CSF obtained by lumbar puncture, which is done after a CT scan has been performed to exclude a cerebral abscess or mass lesion. Increased amounts of protein and white blood cells are typically found, and the causative micro-organism may be cultured from the CSF.

The treatment consists of intravenous antibiotics (e.g. benzylpenicillin for meningococcus) or antiviral agents (e.g. acyclovir for herpes simplex virus and varicella–zoster virus) and general supportive measures for patients with depressed conscious levels or neurological deficits (see Chapters 16, 17, and 18). Prophylactic measures include the immunization programmes for

---

> ### BOX 38.1 CLINICAL FEATURES OF ACUTE MENINGOENCEPHALITIS
>
> headache
> photophobia
> neck stiffness
> confusion
> drowsiness or coma
> disorientation
> vomiting
> fever

---

measles, mumps, polio, and, during outbreaks of meningococcal meningitis, against the particular meningococcal strain responsible (see Chapter 21).

SPECIFIC VIRAL NEUROLOGICAL INFECTIONS

Poliomyelitis

This is an acute infection that is transmitted by the oral route and is associated with overcrowding and poor sanitation. In endemic areas, most children have serological evidence of infection by the age of 5 years. The disease is asymptomatic in most people, but about 5 per cent have a minor illness. Only 1–2 per cent develop neurological disease, and these people have symptoms of paralysis, which occur about 2 weeks after contracting the virus and are often preceded by fever, headache, and vomiting. The virus is thought to spread to the nervous tissue via the bloodstream. Many patients have a mild paralysis and recover completely. A minority have severe and life-threatening paralysis involving the muscles of respiration and swallowing. Adults are more likely to develop severe paralytic disease than children, particularly in non-endemic areas.

Subacute Sclerosing Panencephalitis

This is due to persistence of the measles virus in the central nervous system, and it occurs in children. Why this develops in only a very small minority of people who get measles is unclear, although most children who do develop subacute sclerosing panencephalitis have had measles at a very early age.

The onset is gradual and may occur several years after measles infection. Symptoms include loss of energy and interest, leading to clumsiness and movement disorders. Some children progress to rigidity, spasticity, and death; others are left with a disability.

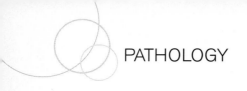
Progressive Multifocal Leukoencephalopathy

This occurs as a result of opportunistic viral infection in immunocompromised patients. Slow viruses are so called because the clinical disease occurs several years, sometimes decades, after the infection is thought to have been contracted.

Tetanus

Tetanus is caused by contamination of wounds by microbial spores of *Clostridium tetani*. These spores are found in animal faeces, and thus tetanus is more likely to occur in wounds inflicted by thorns, twigs, and garden or farm implements.

The damage is caused by the toxin produced by the bacterium, which invades the lower segments of the motor nerve pathways from the central nervous system. The affected nerves generate repeated electric impulses, causing the innervated muscles to contract in spasm. The muscles most often affected are the cheek muscles that open the mouth (i.e. the masseters), causing the characteristic trismus or 'lockjaw'. Eventually the neck and back muscles are also affected, and death may result if the respiratory muscles are also involved.

The best management is by preventative immunization, and most developed countries now have an active immunization programme. Any patient with a wound should have a booster immunization unless he or she has been immunized within the last 5 years.

Treatment of an acute infection with human antitoxin is effective only against toxin in the blood stream, not once it has reached the nervous system. A course of antibiotics active against *Clostridium tetani* (penicillin or tetracycline) should be given. Severe cases of tetanus in which there are problems swallowing may need to be managed by sedation, paralysis, and artificial respiration in an appropriate hospital unit.

NEUROLOGICAL TUMOURS

PATHOLOGY AND DIAGNOSIS

These may be benign or malignant. Benign tumours include meningiomas, which arise from the meninges, benign gliomas, pituitary adenomas, and acoustic neuromas. Common malignant tumours are primary malignant gliomas (which, unfortunately, occur more often than the benign gliomas) and secondary metastatic carcinomas (e.g. from a primary tumour in the lung).

The growth of the tumour mass within the brain produces compression of vital structures and obstruction of CSF flow. An expanding mass lesion within a cerebral hemisphere, for example, exerts pressure on inferior structures, compressing the midbrain and pushing the brain stem downwards so that the lower parts of the cerebellum and medulla oblongata become impacted at the foramen magnum (see Figure 38.3).

The clinical picture may be rapidly evolving and consists of a depression in conscious level, dilatation of the pupil on the affected side, and altered respiration if the medulla is compressed. Some of the symptoms of raised intracranial pressure include headache and vomiting and blurring or loss of vision. Other clinical features of a brain tumour are epilepsy and an evolving focal neurological deficit. Epilepsy is not generally caused by tumours, but the onset of epilepsy in adulthood should suggest the possibility of a brain tumour. The nature of focal neurological deficits depends on the site of the tumour, and a careful study of a patient's symptoms and signs will often reveal the possible site of a lesion. These can be confirmed on CT scanning and MRI. CT scanning will also reveal the amount of cerebral oedema present, while MRI scan can provide a better definition of lesions at the base of the skull. In general, neurological deficits caused by a brain tumour evolve over time, whereas those caused by a stroke occur abruptly, although there are always exceptions to this rule.

MANAGEMENT

Raised intracranial pressure is treated with a corticosteroid (dexamethasone), which serves to relieve clinical symptoms. It also reduces brain swelling, which means that neurosurgical procedures can be performed with less risks to the patient. Surgical measures include biopsy of the lesion to establish a histological diagnosis, and partial or complete removal of a tumour. However, such intervention may be limited by the possibility of damage to vital structures and the postoperative neurological deficits which may occur. Radiotherapy may be used to treat middle-grade gliomas, metastatic carcinoma, and pituitary adenomas. Epilepsy should be controlled by anticonvulsants. Chemotherapy is rarely effective except in the case of a lymphoma.

The outlook for patients with benign tumours is generally good, although residual neurological deficits after surgical removal or radiotherapy is not uncommon. Unfortunately, the outlook for the more common malignant tumours is poor, with only a small percentage of patients surviving over 2 years and considerable morbidity during the survival period.

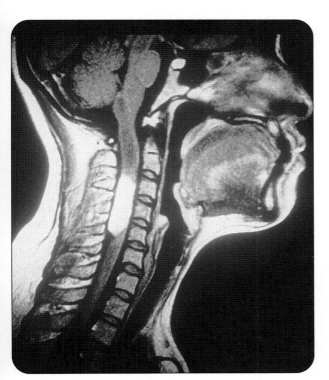

Figure 38.3 Magnetic resonance imaging (MRI) scan of enhanced spots, which are typical lesions in multiple sclerosis. (By permission of Dr A Valentine, Royal Free Hospital School of Medicine, London, UK.)

EPILEPSY

The term 'epilepsy' describes a condition in which periods of neurological dysfunction occur as the result of abnormal electrical activity in the brain. Such neurological disturbances may produce a variety of clinical phenomena, but the person is normal between attacks.

Grand Mal Epilepsy

The common major form of epilepsy is grand mal fit, in which sudden violent movements are followed by coma. It is often accompanied by incontinence. After regaining consciousness, patients may be confused, drowsy, and experience headaches.

Petit Mal Epilepsy

In contrast, a petit mal attack has a sudden onset but seldom lasts more than 10 seconds. It usually ends abruptly. The patient is observed to stop whatever he or she is doing and to become unresponsive to verbal or physical stimuli.

Temporal Lobe Epilepsy

Temporal lobe epilepsy is the most common form of focal epilepsy, in which the epileptogenic lesion is located in one of the temporal lobes. In this type of epilepsy, the patient reports characteristic sensations of taste and smell as part of the aura leading up to an attack. Then the attack itself may consist of convulsive movements, affecting predominantly one part of the body.

Febrile Convulsions

Febrile convulsions occurring in young children under the age of 5 years during febrile illnesses are transient and not uncommon. Only a small percentage of these children go on to have epileptic attacks that are not associated with fever.

CAUSES

Primary generalized, or idiopathic, epilepsy, may be familial. Focal epilepsy suggests the presence of intracranial pathology, and this could be trauma to the brain, either at birth or later in life, previous meningoencephalitis, cerebral infarction or haemorrhage, or a result of neurosurgery. Occasionally, biochemical upsets such as alcohol or drug withdrawal, hypoglycaemia, or drugs themselves (see below) may be the cause of epileptic seizures. Epilepsy may also be one of the first sign of a brain tumour.

MANAGEMENT OF EPILEPSY

In most cases, epilepsy can be controlled by drugs, but these have side-effects, and the optimum dose has to be established for each patient. Anticonvulsant drugs are usually continued for at least 2 years, after which gradual withdrawal of treatment may be possible. Febrile convulsions in children are managed with rectal diazepam and measures to reduce the temperature, which include tepid sponging and paracetamol.

Until satisfactory control of epileptic fits has been achieved, patients may have to make adjustments to their lifestyle and activities. For example, patients who have had more than one attack of epilepsy must stop driving until they have had 2 years without fits. Patients with photosensitive epilepsy should avoid video games and discos with fast-flashing lights.

TRAUMA

HEAD INJURY

Head injuries may occur in road traffic accidents, at the workplace, and in sports; as a consequence, they often happen in young people. Up to 50 per cent of head injuries present in people below the age of 20 years. Sudden, violent movement of the brain within the skull can damage nerve fibres and brain tissue, as well as small blood vessels, leading to small haemorrhages. Such damage to the brain leads to brain swelling, the consequences of which are discussed above.

Careful neurological observations must be carried out and recorded on a neurological chart. This includes an assessment of the patient's state of consciousness using the Glasgow Coma Scale, as well as eye, motor, and verbal responses. Indicators of brain stem function are also noted – these are pupil size and reactivity, blood pressure, pulse, respiratory rate, and temperature. General supportive care during and after the period of unconsciousness is important. Deteriorating neurological signs may signify an expanding haematoma, which will require surgical removal.

The severity of the head injury and its sequelae depend on a number of factors including the duration of coma and whether there is a skull fracture or any other possible complications, such as meningitis or epilepsy. A postconcussion syndrome may accompany a minor concussive head injury; the patient has a headache, impaired concentration, fatigue, and anxiety.

Chronic subdural haematomas typically occur in older adults following an insignificant head injury. They are due to slow bleeding into the subdural space. With time (often 2 weeks or more), the blood clot causes increased pressure on the brain, leading to drowsiness, confusion, and an unsteady gait.

SPINAL INJURY

The clinical consequences of an injury to the spinal cord depend on the level of the injury and how extensive it is. The nerve fibres from the motor cortex run down along the lateral column of the cord, while sensory fibres run up along the posterior and anterolateral column. A complete lesion affecting all parts of the cord at any one level will therefore give rise to loss of sensory and motor function on both sides below the level of the lesion. Most lesions are incomplete, however, and will therefore lead to weakness rather than paralysis and to impaired sensation rather than complete sensory loss. Bladder, bowel, and sexual function are controlled by autonomic nerves that travel in the central anterior part of the spinal cord, and they may be affected by injuries to this part of the cord.

Causes of spinal cord injury include trauma, involvement by cancer (usually from the breast, prostate, or lung), and prolapsed intervertebral discs. Neurosurgical intervention, if appropriate, should be carried out as soon as possible, since damage to the nervous system is generally irreversible. A number of patients survive with a permanent degree of paralysis, and their care and management requires the help of nurses, physiotherapists, dietitians, occupational therapists, urologists, neurologists, psychologists, and friends and family (Box 38.2).

MOVEMENT DISORDERS

PARKINSON'S DISEASE

This disorder was first described in the early 19th century by the physician, James Parkinson, who called it the 'shaking palsy'. It is relatively common and usually has an onset in later adulthood (those over 50 years). It occurs world-wide and is perhaps more frequently seen in men than women.

The pathological cause is degeneration of the pigmented nuclei (substantia nigra) in the brain stem. These nerve cells, which use dopamine as a neurotransmitter, project to the caudate nucleus and the putamen. As a consequence, there is a depletion of dopamine in the area of the brain that contains the basal nuclei. The disease is progressive, and by the time it is manifest clinically, there is greater than 75 per cent neuronal loss in the affected area.

Typical early symptoms are tremor and rigidity. Patients complain of being unable to 'get going' (i.e. to initiate a motor activity, such as walking). Their

---

BOX 38.2 CARE OF THE PARALYSED PATIENT AFTER THE ACUTE STAGES

- education regarding the functions that are lost
- teaching of wheelchair skills
- physiotherapy and drugs to reduce spasticity
- care of skin where there is sensory loss
- bladder management, (e.g. self-catheterization)
- bowel management with diet and laxatives
- sexual counselling
- psychological care and family support
- home and car adaptation
- employment (when possible)
- recreational activity
- financial and legal advice
- respite care for relatives and carers

posture is stiff and there is a tendency to fall. The face is typically mask-like, and the voice monotonous. Handwriting becomes small and untidy, and everyday tasks that involve small rapid movements, such as getting dressed or peeling vegetables, become difficult. The disease usually progresses in a step-wise fashion but at a variable rate.

The mainstay of treatment is with levodopa (L-dopa). This is converted into dopamine in the brain, thus restoring the stores of dopamine in the basal ganglia. The amount of L-dopa reaching the brain can be maximized if it is given with carbidopa, a drug that inhibits the metabolism of L-dopa outside the brain. Although therapy with these drugs can lead to a dramatic lessening of symptoms, they do not alter the course of the disease, and many patients who initially respond to them lose the benefit of the drugs after 3–5 years. Depression is common in Parkinson's disease, and unfortunately the drugs used in the treatment of this disease may in themselves cause confusion and delirium.

New developments in treatment include brain surgery, in which specific areas of the brain are destroyed to try to control the tremor. Another experimental advance has been the transplantation of fetal tissue into the brain to try and replace the missing cells and their dopamine (see Chapter 29). However the use of fetal tissue is the subject of a continuing ethical debate.

A parkinsonian disorder may develop in patients on neuroleptic drugs, such as those used in the treatment of schizophrenia. This so-called drug-induced parkinsonism remits spontaneously over a period of time once the 'offending' drug is withdrawn.

INVOLUNTARY MOVEMENTS

The most common involuntary movements are tremors, the most prevalent of which is a physiological tremor. A physiological tremor is increased by stress, alcohol, anxiety states, and thyrotoxicosis (see Chapter 35). Other causes of tremor include the rest tremor of Parkinson's disease and an intention tremor, which indicates pathology in the brain stem, such as multiple sclerosis or a tumour.

Chorea consists of a series of jerky and irregular movements which can be caused by reaction to a streptococcal infection (St Vitus's dance, which is rare today), or a tumour.

Huntington's Disease

This is a rare, dominantly inherited disease that comes on in middle life. It is characterized by chorea and dementia (see Chapter 7). First described by George Huntington in the late 19th century, this disorder is inherited as an autosomal dominant trait which has an onset in middle life, between the ages of 30 and 50 years, often, tragically, by the time the patient has had children. The children of a person with Huntington's disease have a 50 per cent chance of having the disease.

Pathological changes include shrinking of the cerebral cortex with loss of nerve cells. Early signs include personality changes, and unsteadiness of gait. As the disease progresses, constant choreiform movements distort and make impossible all daily motor activities, and dementia becomes more pronounced. Finally the patient becomes bed-ridden and emaciated, and death ensues some 10 years after the onset of the disease. Although the causative gene has now been identified, it is not known how the product of the gene is involved in the pathogenesis of this disorder.

DEGENERATIVE NEUROLOGICAL CONDITIONS

DEMYELINATING DISEASES

These are a group of disorders in which the myelin sheaths that enclose some axons are destroyed, while the neurones and axons themselves are left intact.

Multiple Sclerosis

In multiple sclerosis, characteristic plaques of demyelination occur in nerves in the central nervous system, including the optic nerves. In the early stages of the disease process, the axons appear intact and there is proliferation of astrocytes, which produce increased amounts of glial fibrils. Later in the disease, these cells shrink, leading to glial scarring, and axons are also destroyed.

Multiple sclerosis often starts in adolescence or young adulthood. Typically, there are episodic acute attacks of demyelination, with quiescent periods in between (i.e. attacks followed by remission). Patients may present with numbness or weakness of an upper or lower limb; such symptoms may be due to plaques in the spinal cord. The optic nerves are frequently involved, and patients may present with blurred vision and pain around the eye. Plaques in the brain stem give rise to vertigo, double vision, and nystagmus. These acute symptoms generally improve; however with subsequent attacks, there is increasing disability. Vision may become permanently impaired, and walking may become gradually more difficult. Early attacks may go undiagnosed, since patients may appear to make a full recovery and be free of symptoms for more than a year.

The clinical course is extremely variable. Patients presenting initially with visual symptoms are more likely to have a more benign course, while others experience crippling disability after the first attack. A less common form of the disorder is the progressive form, in which there is a gradual deterioration without the acute relapsing and remitting symptoms. The diagnosis is made on a history of relapsing disease and symptoms and signs compatible with multiple lesions in characteristic sites (Figure 38.4).

Examination of the eyes may reveal pallor in the temporal half of the optic disc, while response to sensory or visual evoked electrical stimuli are often abnormal. Frequently an abnormal response may be detected in an area of the central nervous system that is not clinically involved in the disease. Examination of the CSF may show raised levels of immunoglobulin, with the characteristic oligoclonal pattern of bands on electrophoresis (see Chapter 27). MRI now provides a sensitive marker of the extent and progress of the pathological process.

Current therapeutic approaches to multiple sclerosis are based on the hypothesis that this is an autoimmune disease (in which the central nervous system is the target organ) that occurs in genetically susceptible people. High doses of corticosteroids given intravenously in an acute attack will often speed recovery from that particular attack, but whether the overall degree of recovery is improved or the final outcome is altered remains uncertain. Multiple-centre clinical trials have demonstrated that interferon-beta-1a is able to decrease the rate of formation of new lesions and thus reduce the relapse rate in patients with the relapsing–remitting form of the disease. Unfortunately, not all patients with the progressive form of the disease respond to interferon-beta, and other means of immune suppression (such as azathioprine, methotrexate, and cyclosporin) are of only moderate benefit (see also Chapter 29). The chronic progressive disability gives rise to many psychological, sexual and social problems, which require a multi- disciplinary approach to management.

Motor Neurone Disease

In motor neurone disease (also known as amyotrophic lateral sclerosis) there is degeneration of motor neurones in the spinal cord, cortex, and somatic motor cranial nerves. Muscle atrophy and thus progressive spastic paraparesis follows; and symptoms of dysphonia, dysphagia, and muscle cramps are common. In most cases intellect and memory remain intact, and dementia is rare. Bowel and bladder functions are also not generally affected, and neither are the senses (i.e. hearing, sight, taste, smell, and touch).

Motor neurone disease mostly presents in middle life (between the ages of 40 and 60 years), and survival from the onset of symptoms is around 5 years. There are no specific diagnostic tests, but a range of tests are used to exclude other conditions. An electromyograph may be performed to measure electrical activity in muscle. Riluzole may be given as therapy, although no treatment has been shown to alter the progress of the disease dramatically.

Acute Disseminated Encephalomyelitis

This is an acute demyelinating illness that typically follows infection with chickenpox or measles, or smallpox vaccination. It more commonly affects children than adults. The illness comes on abruptly with fever, vomiting, and headache. The child may become increasingly drowsy and have convulsions. Some children recover completely; others are left with a disability (e.g. hemiparesis or epilepsy).

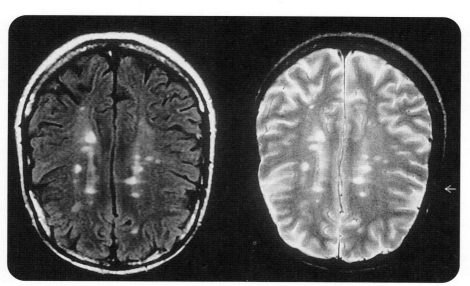

Figure 38.4 Magnetic resonance imaging (MRI) scan of glioma in the spinal cord at the level of the brain stem. (By permission of Dr A Valentine, Royal Free Hospital School of Medicine, London, UK.)

DEMENTIA

Alzheimer's Disease

This is the most common cause of pre-senile dementia. Pathologically, there is extensive loss of neurones in the cerebral cortex and the basal nuclei. This leads to dilatation of the ventricles and the surface of the cerebrum looks shrunken as a consequence. Neurofibrillary tangles are found among the degenerating nerve cells, but the significance of this characteristic feature is not known.

By definition, Alzheimer's disease starts before the age of 65, but it is rare in people below 45 years of age. The disease comes on insidiously, with loss of memory, a decline in initiative, and failing intellectual performance. Patients are often distressingly aware of these deficits. Progression occurs to a virtually helpless state with little or no spontaneous speech.

Pick's Disease and Other Causes of Dementia

Pick's disease is a rare cause of pre-senile dementia. It is relentlessly progressive to death in 5–10 years.

Dementia can also occur as a result of vascular disease, and as part of diseases such as Parkinson's disease, Huntington's disease, and Creutzfelt–Jakob disease.

Creutzfelt–Jakob Disease (CJD)

Creutzfelt–Jakob disease (CJD) is a neurodegenerative disorder that leads to a slow and progressive dementia. It is caused by a prion, an infectious agent that is not killed by the usual sterilization technique; therefore there is the very slight risk of cross-infection with prion-contaminated surgical instruments. In addition, CJD has been transmitted between patients in corneal grafts, and it has occurred in people given growth hormone therapy from cadaver-derived human pituitary glands. There is no longer a risk of CJD from growth hormone therapy, since recombinant growth hormone is now used (i.e. growth hormone synthesized by a genetically manipulated micro-organism (see also Chapter 7)).

The recent epidemic of the similar disease found in cattle, bovine spongiform encephalopathy (BSE), has been a matter of grave concern to the general public, farmers, and the Government, because of its possible transmission to humans. Therefore, in 1990, surveillance of CJD cases in the UK was established to ascertain whether there were any changes in the epidemiology of the disease. A new variant of CJD seems to have emerged; it presents in younger people and differs from the sporadic form previously found in that behavioural changes are seen in the new variant but the characteristic EEG pattern of CJD are not.

Neuropathological examination confirms the diagnosis with the spongiform changes presented. It has been proposed that the rise in the number of cases of CJD (both in young and older adults) is probably more due to improved diagnostic verification of disease, highlighted by the BSE crisis, than to a real increase caused by a sudden epidemic.

KEY POINTS

- A stroke (also called a cerebrovascular accident) is a rapidly developing loss of cerebral function. It may result from occlusion of an artery supplying the brain, the rupture of an aneurysm (leading to intracranial haemorrhage), or other vascular malformations and diseases.
- The clinical severity varies widely, from full recovery in a few days, through permanent disability, to death. Good nursing care is essential to ensure that the patient is comfortable, the airway is well maintained, and swallowing is safe.
- Migraine is defined as a spasmodic disorder involving a visual or tactile aura (or both) associated with nausea and vomiting and unilateral headache. Dietary precipitants that have been implicated include cheese, chocolate, caffeine, and alcohol.
- The diagnosis of acute meningoencephalitis is made on the findings in cerebrospinal fluid (CSF) obtained by lumbar puncture. Clinical features include headache, photophobia, neck stiffness, confusion, fever, and vomiting.
- Tetanus is caused by contamination of wounds by microbial spores of *Clostridium tetani* found in animal faeces, thorns, twigs, and implements or tools in a garden or on a farm. Neurological effects are the result of bacterial toxin invading motor nerve pathways and causing muscular spasm. Treatments include prophylactic immunization and a course of antibiotics active against *Clostridium tetani* (penicillin or tetracycline).
- Tumours of the central nervous system may be benign or malignant. The growth of the tumour mass within the brain produces compression of vital structures, obstruction of CSF flow, and a rise in intracranial pressure. Other clinical features are epilepsy and an evolving focal neurological deficit.
- Epilepsy describes a condition in which periods of neurological dysfunction occur as the result of abnormal electrical activity in the brain.
- Parkinson's disease is degeneration of the pigmented nuclei (substantia nigra) in the brain stem of patients. There is a depletion of dopamine in the basal nuclei, and the mainstay of treatment is with levodopa (L-dopa).
- Alzheimer's disease is the most common cause of pre-senile dementia. The disease comes on insidiously, with loss of memory, a decline in initiative, and failing intellectual performance. Patients are often distressingly aware of these deficits.
- Creutzfelt–Jakob disease is a neurodegenerative disorder that leads to a slow and progressive dementia. It is caused by an infectious agent called a prion, which is not killed by the usual sterilization techniques.

FURTHER READING

Acute treatment of migraine: new products. (1997) MeReC Bull 8:37–40.

Bahn MM, Oser AB, Cross DT 3rd (1996) CT and MRI of stroke. J Magn Reson Imaging 6:833–45.

Brown P, Preece MA, Will RG (1992) 'Friendly fire' in medicine: hormones, homografts, and Creutzfeldt–Jakob disease. Lancet 340:24–7.

Campion K (1997) Multiple sclerosis. Professional issues. Nurs Times 93:57–60.

Crawford JG (1996) Alzheimer's disease risk factors as related to cerebral blood flow. Med Hypotheses 46:367–77.

Duncan JS (1997) Imaging and epilepsy. Brain 120:339–77.

Fisher M (1994) Clinical Atlas of Cerebrovascular Disorders. Mosby–Year Book Europe, London.

Gasbarrini A, DeLuca A, Fiore G et al. (1998) Beneficial effects of Helicobacter pylori eradication on migraine. Hepatogastroenterology 45(21): 765–70.

Hudak CM, Gallo BM, Morton BG (1997) Critical Care Nursing, 7th edition. JB Lippincott, Philadelphia.

Hughes RAC (1997) Neurological investigations. BMJ Publishing, London

Jennett B, Lindsay KW (1993) An Introduction to Neurosurgery. Butterworth-Heinmann, Oxford.

Kent MA (1996)The ethical arguments concerning the artificial ventilation of patients with motor neurone disease. Nurs Ethics 3:317–28.

Koroshetz WJ, Moskowitz MA (1996) Emerging treatments for stroke in humans. Trends Pharmacol Sci. 17(6):227–33.

Lewis J (1994) The Migraine Handbook. The Definitive Guide to the Causes, Symptoms and Treatments. Vermilon, London.

Martyn CN (1997) Infection in childhood and neurological diseases in adult life. Br Med Bull 53:24–39.

Mayeux R, Saunders AM, Shea S, et al. (1998) Utility of the apolipoprotein E genotype in the diagnosis of Alzheimer's disease. N Engl J Med 338:506–11.

Miller CM (1997) The lived experience of relapsing multiple sclerosis: a phenomenological study. J Neurosci Nurs 29:294–304.

Moussa B, Youdim H, Riederer P (1997) Understanding Parkinson's disease. Sci Am 276:38–53.

Ojemann GA (1997) Treatment of temporal lobe epilepsy. Annu Rev Med 48:317–28.

Richardson M (1996) Bacterial meningitis. Br J Hosp Med 55:685–8.

Robinson RG (1997) Neuropsychiatric consequences of stroke. Annu Rev Med 48:217–29.

Rudick RA, Cohen JA, Weinstock-Guttman B, Kinkel RP, Ransohoff RM (1997) Drug therapy of multiple sclerosis. N Engl J Med 337:1604–11.

Welch KM, Lewis D (1997) Migraine and epilepsy. Neurol Clin 15:107–14.

Wildrick D (1997) Intraventricular hemorrhage and long-term outcome in the premature infant. J Neurosci Nurs 29:281–9.

Will RG, Ironside JW, Zeilder M, et al. (1996) A new variant of Creutzfeldt–Jakob disease in the UK. Lancet 347: 921–5.

Wilson EA. Brodie MJ (1996) New antiepileptic drugs. Baillieres Clin Neurol 5:723–47.

Wright R, Jordan C (1997) Videofluoroscopic evaluation of dysphagia in motor neurone disease with modified barium swallow. Palliat Med 11:44–8.

BONE AND JOINT DISORDERS

For a broader understanding of this chapter, you would be advised to have:
- a basic knowledge of the anatomy of the skeleton,
- the functional performance of joints, and
- the relationship of muscles, bones, ligaments, and tendons.
- For more information, read Chapters 1, 2, 6, and 27.

INTRODUCTION

Rheumatologists deal with disorders of the locomotor system. The diagnosis and treatment of locomotor disorders makes up 20–30 per cent of a general practitioner's work. The most common problems are a variety of soft tissue syndromes, some of which are caused by injury, others by ageing, and others by causes that have not been identified. Many of these disorders are self-limiting. The most important type of arthritis in terms of prevalence and potential for disability is osteoarthritis (OA). It is a disease whose cause is in part genetic; it is also in part due to ageing processes in the joint. Attempts by the affected cartilage and bone to repair themselves are also involved. OA is usually treated by a general practitioner, but it is referred to a rheumatologist for differential diagnosis or when surgery is being considered. Although rheumatologists do not perform surgery, they are often in a good posi-tion to make sure that all other therapeutic alterna-tives have been tried first and that the patient is fit for the operation.

The most common inflammatory arthritic condi-tion is rheumatoid arthritis (RA). In RA, an autoim-mune mechanism is involved in the disease process (see Chapter 27). Although the main impact of RA is on the joints, other organs may also be affected since it is a systemic disorder. RA is usually managed by a hospital-based specialist team and requires careful use of drugs and other measures to minimize pain and reduce the risk of progressive joint damage. This specialist team should ideally include a rheumatolo-gist, a specialist nurse, a physiotherapist, a podiatrist, an occupational therapist, and, often, a social work-er and psychologist.

There is a group of inflammatory arthritic condi-tions, often called seronegative spondarthritis, that are genetically linked and associated with a variety of non-arthritic diseases such as psoriasis, ulcerative colitis, and iritis.

Acute monoarthritis may be due to injury (acute haemarthrosis), to crystals, such as urate (gout) or calcium pyrophosphate (pseudogout), or to a vari-ety of infective agents. Septic arthritis is a rare dis-order but a significant and potentially fatal cause of arthritis.

In this chapter the more frequently encountered disorders of the locomotor system are discussed in

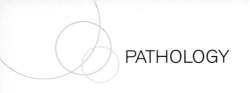

relation to their causes, symptoms, and investigations to confirm the diagnosis, and possible therapies (Table 39.1).

OBSERVATION OF SYMPTOMS AND COMMUNICATION WITH THE PATIENT

It is important to recognize when specialist referral is needed. For example, a podiatrist may be the first health care professional to see patients with arthritis who have painful feet and needs to know when to refer them on. Similarly, the physiotherapist may see patients with spinal pain and must know that, if the disease manifestations or signs suggest a serious underlying diagnosis, these patients need specialist review. A practice nurse should be able to recognize when patients complaining of worsening symptoms from their joints or spine need to be seen by their general practitioner. The nurse specialist in a rheumatology team is trained to deal with patients and to recognize when their disease is getting out of control or when they are developing side-effects from their drugs. All these roles will be better performed if the practitioner has a good basic knowledge of the diseases and their management.

The chronic course of many locomotor diseases means that those who deal with such patients must be skilled in caring and communication. Therefore, healthcare professionals dealing with patients suffering from rheumatic disorders need to:

- listen to the patient explaining the symptoms and recognize the likely diagnosis;
- have a basic understanding of the functions of the locomotor system and how problems present, and understand how the diagnostic tests are used to make a more accurate diagnosis; and
- be able to explain the diagnosis, the likely problems that may arise, the outlook, and the type of treatment that has been prescribed.

Although there is often no traditional 'cure', there is always something that can be done to relieve symptoms. Patients attending rheumatology units are remarkable for their ability to cope with chronic ill health and disability, but it is important to recognize when their coping strategies are beginning to falter and more active intervention is needed. The aim of all who deal with people with rheumatic diseases should be to help them lead as normal a life as possible, despite their disease.

Common Words and Phrases in Rheumatology

Word or phrase	Meaning
arthralgia	joint pain without swelling
arthritis	joint inflammation with swelling and pain
monarthritis	arthritis affecting a single joint
polyarthritis	arthritis affecting many joints
pauciarthritis	arthritis affecting between two and four joints
seropositive arthritis	arthritis in which serum rheumatoid factor antibodies (usually IgM) have been detected
seronegative	arthritis in which serum rheumatoid factor antibodies (usually IgM) have not been detected
spondylosis	spinal changes that worsen with age and that are mainly caused by intervertebral disc degeneration
spondylitis	an inflammatory process affecting the spine (most commonly ankylosing spondylitis)
rheumatism	a word that is best avoided because it is non-specific; it means any form of muscular pain; in the past it meant rheumatic fever and was feared for this reason
early morning stiffness	typical stiffness of the joints or spine that persists from 30 minutes to several hours in patients with inflammatory arthritis or spondylitis

Table 39.1 Common terms used in rheumatology clinics.

TALKING TO PATIENTS WITH RHEUMATIC DISEASES

Be sympathetic when dealing with patients in pain and allow them time to tell their story, but play an active role in the process in order to draw out and develop important details. Psychological and social problems often worsen people's ability to cope with pain and disability – they may have had a problem for a long time but then some other life event motivates them to consult a doctor or other practitioner. For example, chronic back pain may only become a worry to the patient when a friend with similar symptoms has been diagnosed with malignant secondary deposits. Similarly, a painful joint may be more worrying when they are under pressure at work. Family stresses and strains often exacerbate neck pain and headaches, and tension is a common cause of muscular pain (see Chapter 14). When patients have a self-limiting problem and are otherwise well, it is usually enough to provide reassurance as they wait for the pain to settle and to offer advice about over-the-counter medication and physical measures, such as rest, splints or supports, or physiotherapy. However, when they have rheumatic symptoms and are ill, they should be reviewed by the general practitioner and sometimes by a specialist.

QUESTIONNAIRES IN THE ASSESSMENT OF PATIENTS WITH RHEUMATIC DISEASES

Patients are often helped by being asked to answer simple written questions about their symptoms, disability, or mood. The questions act as a stimulus for them to recall problems that they might have forgotten or that they did not think were important. Specially designed questionnaires are available and have the advantage of being a measurable and a reasonably objective means of assessing change in symptoms over time (see Chapter 14). They provide helpful information in addition to that obtained from the medical examination (Box 39.1) and laboratory investigations. Some of the questionnaires are simple (e.g. the Health Assessment Questionnaire); others are longer and more complicated (e.g. the Arthritis Impact Measurement Scale) or pose broader questions in order to allow rheumatic diseases to be compared with other diseases with regard to their impact on health, day-to-day activity, and mood.

INVESTIGATIONS

Many people with spinal pain, soft tissue rheumatism, or OA do not require investigation because the diagnosis is clear from the medical history and examination. Laboratory tests help both to make a diagnosis

> ## BOX 39.1 EXAMINING THE JOINTS AND SPINE IN RHEUMATIC DISORDERS
>
> **Look**
> for deformity, swelling, change in the overlying skin, or wasted muscles
>
> **Watch**
> the patient move and look for movement affected by pain, movement causing pain, and loss of range of movement
>
> **Feel**
> for tenderness, warmth (suggesting inflammation) or swelling, which may be caused by fluid ('fluctuant' swelling), inflamed synovium ('firm' or 'boggy' swelling) or bone ('hard' swelling)
>
> **Move**
> the joint, feeling for grating (crepitus), instability, abnormal range of movement, muscle weakness, or spasm; the range of joint and spinal movement can be measured in degrees
>
> **Functional assessment**
> to describe the way in which activities of daily living are affected (e.g. difficulty combing hair, zipping a skirt or doing up a bra, putting on socks)

and to exclude other conditions (see Chapter 6). The fact that investigations are undertaken is generally reassuring for the patient, but this is not a sufficient reason for carrying them out. Tests play an important role in monitoring the effects of the disease and drugs on the individual patient.

LABORATORY TESTS
Haematology

A full blood count may reveal:

- anaemia of chronic inflammatory diseases, a normochromic and normocytic anaemia caused by circulating inflammatory cytokines affecting the bone marrow;
- iron deficiency anaemia, a hypochromic and microcytic anaemia, which may be due to gastrointestinal bleeding induced by non-steroidal anti-inflammatory drugs (NSAIDs) (see Chapters 10 and 31);

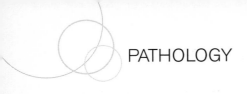

- a neutrophilia (high white cell count), which suggests bacterial infection but also occurs with corticosteroid treatment;
- a raised platelet count, which occurs in chronic inflammatory diseases;
- a low neutrophil or platelet count, which may be due to drug-induced bone marrow suppression.

Erythrocyte sedimentation rate (ESR) and C-reactive protein (CRP) measure acute phase reactants, which are bioactive substances produced by the liver in response to circulating inflammatory cytokines. They are non-specific but are not seen in OA.

Biochemistry
A raised alkaline phosphatase level may indicate liver or bone disease. Liver enzymes rise with drug-induced toxicity. A raised serum urate suggests gout but it sometimes occurs in people who have no symptoms and may not need treatment (see Chapter 6).

Immunology
Serum autoantibody levels (see Chapters 24 and 27) are also measured. This may reveal:
- rheumatoid factors; and
- antinuclear antibodies.

Rheumatoid factors (RF) are autoantibodies against the Fc portion of immunoglobulin. They are not diagnostic of RA. High titres in early disease suggest a poor prognosis. RF are detected in other autoimmune rheumatic disorders, in chronic infections, and in asymptomatic older people.

Antinuclear antibodies (ANA) are antibodies to a variety of specific antigens that lie inside the cell nucleus. They are detected by indirect immunofluorescent staining techniques. ANA is a screening test for systemic lupus erythematosus (see Chapters 24, and 27), which cannot be diagnosed unless ANA are present. Low titres of ANA may also occur in RA and chronic infections and in healthy people, especially older adults. Antibodies against double-stranded deoxyribonucleic acid are diagnostic of active systemic lupus erythematosus and indicate a poor prognosis. They are negative in mild or inactive disease.

IMAGING TECHNIQUES
X-rays
X-rays use low doses of radiation. They are only necessary in certain situations and should not be done unless the findings are likely to change the management plan or assist in the diagnosis. They reveal great detail about bony anatomy and some details of soft tissues.

Ultrasound
Ultrasound is used for imaging periarticular structures, soft tissue swellings, and tendons and as a means of guiding injections and biopsies.

Magnetic Resonance Imaging
Magnetic resonance imaging uses radio waves to obtain information which is then manipulated by computer to produce images of planes (or slices) through a structure. It is used for imaging bone and soft tissues.

Computerized Axial Tomography
Computerized axial tomography (CT) uses X-irradiation and computes images of planes (or slices) through bone and other structures.

Bone Scintigraphy
Bone scintigraphy (bone scanning) requires prior injection of a tiny dose of a radioactive substance (usually technetium-99) to visualize bone. The pattern of emitted radiation reveals changes in blood flow and bone metabolism caused by inflammation, infection, or malignancy. It is usually performed in combination with a more anatomically accurate imaging technique.

DEXA (Dual Emission X-ray Absorbtiometry) Scanning
DEXA scanning measures bone density using very low doses of X-rays. It is useful for screening in people who are at risk of osteoporosis and subsequently to monitor for the effects of its treatment.

JOINT ASPIRATION AND INJECTION
Patients are often worried about joint or soft tissue injections because they fear that they will be painful or carry a risk of complications. In preparing them for the procedure, the following points are helpful:
- Local anaesthetic is used. After the initial needle prick and stinging sensation, the procedure is virtually pain free.
- In some circumstances the procedure is diagnostic (e.g. looking for crystals in gout or pseudogout, or for bacteria if joint infection is suspected).
- A corticosteroid injection reduces pain and swelling. Corticosteroids used in this way do not cause the common and widely feared side-effects such as weight increase, moon face, hair loss, osteoporosis, and cataracts (see Chapter 35).
- A brief flare of pain for a day or two after the injection may occur. If it lasts any longer, the patient should be asked to telephone the rheumatology unit or their general practitioner for advice.
- Resting the joint for about 24 hours after the injection improves the benefit. For weight-bearing joints,

this will entail walking as little as possible for a day or so.

Synovial Fluid Examination

The fluid should be examined in the syringe. It is clear, yellow, and viscous in OA but runny and varies between translucent and cloudy in RA and other types of inflammatory arthritis. The degree of cloudiness reflects the number of inflammatory cells in the fluid. Very cloudy or purulent fluid may indicate infection or a crystal arthritis. Polarized light microscopy with a red filter distinguishes gout (negatively birefringent, needle shaped crystals of sodium urate) from pseudogout (weakly positively birefringent crystals of calcium pyrophosphate). Microbiological culture and Gram staining are undertaken in suspected septic arthritis and whenever the fluid is very cloudy (see Chapters 16 and 17).

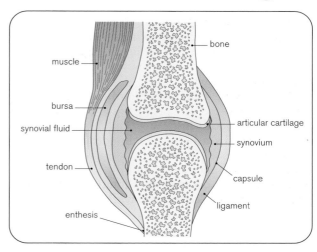

Figure 39.1 Typical elements of a synovial joint.

SYNOVIAL JOINTS

Synovial joints have a cavity (Figure 39.1). Other joints, such as the intervertebral discs and the pubic symphysis, do not. Normal synovium encloses joints, bursae, and tendon sheaths and is a thin, highly vascular tissue with a surface layer of macrophages and fibroblast-like cells that secrete hyaluronan. The surface is usually permeable to proteins and crystalloids but lacks macroscopic gaps so that normal joint fluid is retained in the joint. Glycoproteins in the fluid keep the friction between the cartilaginous surfaces low.

Epiphyseal bone abuts joints and has a light framework of mineralized collagen struts or trabeculae enclosed in a thin coating of tough, cortical bone. It is protected from pressure by the overlying hyaline cartilage. In OA the hyaline cartilage is worn away and the epiphysis may collapse or fracture.

Chondrocytes are embedded in the cartilage and secrete the collagen and proteoglycans. Hyaline cartilage is avascular and nutrients diffuse from the synovial fluid. Hyaline cartilage comprises a meshwork of type II collagen, which encloses giant aggregates (clumps) of proteoglycan. This structure retains water under tension and intermittent loading pressure encourages movement of water, minerals and nutrients between the cartilage and the synovial fluid.

Ligaments and tendons stabilize joints. Some people have more elastic ligaments and are hypermobile, others are stiffer. Tendons transmit muscle power to bones and need to be inelastic.

OSTEOARTHRITIS

Established OA is defined as a condition of synovial joints characterized by cartilage loss and evidence of an accompanying periarticular bone response. It is the most common joint problem in humans and an important cause of pain, disability, and handicap. It occurs with a similar prevalence in a wide variety of ethnic groups, although OA of the hip is less common in black and Oriental people than in Caucasians. Symptomatic OA is less frequent than radiologically detected OA; in other words, radiological evidence of OA does not always cause symptoms. The prevalence of OA increases with age and varies between the sexes, with a female preponderance.

OA is the result of active, sometimes inflammatory processes in the joint, rather than simply the inevitable end result of trauma and ageing. An attempt at repairing the joint and cartilage is involved but the process is abnormal. OA is rarely reversible. Normally, cartilage degradation by wear and its production by chondrocytes are balanced. Early in OA the cartilage becomes fissured and the collagen matrix breaks down. Chondrocytes die and disordered repair occurs. Cartilage loss exposes the underlying bone to abnormal stresses and it develops microfractures and cysts. The bone becomes abnormally dense (sclerosis).

Outgrowths of bone develop around the joint margin (osteophytes). These changes can be seen on X-rays but need to be interpreted clinically, because severe changes may produce little pain but minimal changes may be associated with severe pain (Figure 39.2). Pain may sometimes be due to a joint effusion, which is usually cool and not inflamed.

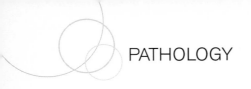
Primary and Secondary Osteoarthritis

The term primary OA is used when no underlying cause is known. Secondary OA is related to such predisposing factors as:

- joint damage due to:
    - chronic inflammatory arthritis;
    - gout;
    - septic arthritis;
- metabolic diseases (e.g. chondrocalcinosis or acromegaly);
- haemophilias; and
- mechanical factors (e.g. after injuries such as fractures or meniscal or cruciate tears).

CLINICAL FEATURES

The symptoms of OA vary according to the joint or joints affected and the severity of the disease. It may be asymptomatic. Sometimes the pain arises from ligaments or other structures around the joint. In weight-bearing joints, the pain is worse when walking and standing and the joint is stiff or painful for a few minutes after a period of immobility in a chair or in bed – this is called jelling. This contrasts with the prolonged pain and stiffness in the morning of inflammatory arthritis. Deformity may develop as the joint damage increases, and this often adds to the disability.

Patterns of Osteoarthritis

Nodal osteoarthritis

Nodal OA is familial, occurs more commonly in women, and produces pain and bony swelling of the distal interphalangeal joints, the proximal interphalangeal joints, and the first carpometacarpal joints of the hand in late middle age (Figure 39.3). Although unsightly, it is rarely disabling.

Generalized osteoarthritis

Generalized OA is seen in some people with nodal OA; it affects the knees, the first metatarsophalangeal joints, and the hip joints.

Erosive osteoarthritis

Erosive OA is rare and disabling. It affects the hands.

Osteoarthritis of the hip

Hip OA usually results from wear of the superior, weight-bearing surface of the femoral head and adjacent acetabulum. It is more common in men. Total hip replacement is a highly effective means of treatment.

Osteoarthritis of the knee

Knee OA is generally bilateral and is associated with nodal OA in older women. It frequently leads to a varus (bow-legged) deformity.

Crystal-associated osteoarthritis

Crystal-associated OA occurs when there is calcium pyrophosphate deposition in the cartilage (chondrocalcinosis).

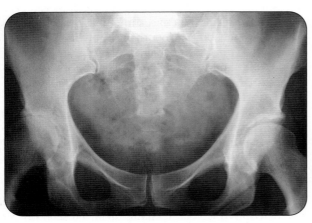

Figure 39.2 Normal joint (left) and osteoarthritic joint (right). The X-ray of the osteoarthritic joint shows loss of joint space, subarticular sclerosis, and osteophyte formation.

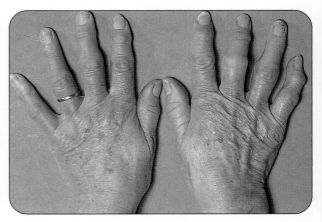

Figure 39.3 Nodal osteoarthritis of the hand. Note the typical Heberden's nodes at the distal interphalangeal joints and the Bouchard's nodes at the proximal interphalangeal joints of most fingers. The thumbs are adducted owing to osteoarthritis of the first carpometacarpal joint.

TREATMENT

OA cannot be cured but much can be done to help. Educating people with OA about its causes and likely effects reduces pain, distress, and disability. Booklets and self-help programmes are available. Diet helps weight loss and reduces pressure through weight-bearing joints. Maintaining muscle strength and joint movement by regular non-weight bearing exercise, taught by a physiotherapist, helps maintain normal activities. Locally applied creams (rubefacients) are sometimes helpful and do no harm. Pain and joint stiffness should be treated on a 'when necessary' basis, first with simple or compound analgesics, occasionally with NSAIDs (see Chapters 10 and 14). Intra-articular corticosteroid injections may be helpful if there is a joint effusion.

Surgical procedures are used only in severe disease, but total joint replacement of hip or knee is highly successful in most people and helps those who might otherwise have been wheelchair-bound to get back to normal mobility. The risks of such surgery are few but important (loosening due to failure of the cement–bone interface, or infection), and the risks and the expected outcome need to be carefully discussed with the patient, preferably with a relative or friend present, before surgery is undertaken.

INFLAMMATORY ARTHRITIS

The predominant feature of inflammatory arthritis is synovial inflammation. The pain and stiffness of inflammatory arthritis are typically worse in the morning and after rest. This early morning exacerbation often lasts several hours, in contrast to the much shorter jelling that occurs after rest in OA. Inflammatory markers (the ESR and CRP) are raised in inflammatory arthritis, and there is often a normochromic, normocytic anaemia of chronic disease – these are not found in OA. Inflammatory arthritis of more than 6–12 weeks' duration requires a specialist rheumatology opinion (Table 39.2).

RHEUMATOID ARTHRITIS

The term 'rheumatoid arthritis' describes a chronic, symmetrical polyarthritis of unexplained cause. There are several forms of the disease – transient, remitting, episodic, chronic progressive, and rapidly progressive. In the early stages it is not always easy to predict the type or prognosis; a high titre of rheumatoid factors indicates a generally worse prognosis (see Chapter 27). RA affects 1–3 per cent of the population and is a significant cause of disability and mortality. It most commonly starts in young adults (30–50 years) but it can

---

Classification of Inflammatory Arthritis

Acute synovitis may be caused by injury, crystals (gout or pseudogout), direct infection (septic arthritis), or immune complexes in postinfective reactive arthritis (rheumatic fever or Lyme disease)

The pattern of joint involvement is important – monarthritis, pauciarticular arthritis (two to four joints) or polyarthritis

Rheumatoid-pattern synovitis is usually peripheral, symmetrical and involves multiple joints; there is an an association with HLA-D, and rheumatoid factors are also found in the serum of 70% of patients (see also Chapters 24 and 27)

Rheumatoid variants (also called seronegative spondarthritis) are more commonly asymmetrical and predominantly affect the large joints of the lower limb; again a link with HLA has been shown (with HLA-B), but they are not associated with the presence of rheumatoid factors in the joint or serum

Diseases such as psoriasis, ulcerative colitis, Crohn's disease, and ankylosing spondylitis are associated with seronegative-pattern arthritis

Table 39.2 Classification of inflammatory arthritis.

---

present at any age. Three times more women are affected than men before the age of menopause, but when RA starts after age 50, men and women are equally affected. It is seen world-wide. Twin studies confirm that heredity plays a role in between 15 and 30 per cent of cases.

PATHOLOGY

RA causes chronic synovitis. A typical feature is the production of rheumatoid factors (RF) by plasma cells that have infiltrated the synovium. The initiating factor for this is not known. These RF are autoantibodies that can self-associate (bind together) to form immune complexes, and these probably cause the chronic persistent inflammation.

The synovium is palpably thickened owing to proliferation of synovial lining cells, infiltration of the synovium by lymphocytes and plasma cells, and increased vascularity. Leukocytes move from the circulation through the synovium and into the joint cavity. More immune cells are recruited by complement activation and by cytokines released from activated macrophages and lymphocytes (see Chapters 25 and 27). Increased synovial permeability causes a joint effusion. Local cytokine production also causes juxta-articular osteoporosis, the first sign apart from soft tissue swelling to be seen on X-ray. The proliferating, inflamed synovium spreads out to cover the surface of the hyaline cartilage to form a so-called 'pannus', which alters

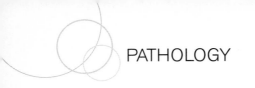
cartilage metabolism by blocking its normal nutrition and also damages cartilage by the local production of cytokines that affect the chondrocytes. Gradually the cartilage becomes thin. Eventually this shows as a reduction of the space between the bone ends on X-ray (joint space narrowing). The cartilage surface is no longer smooth and grating or crepitus during movement develops.

The inflamed synovium also infiltrates the bone from the margins, starting where the synovium joins the periosteum. This causes periarticular bone changes (known as erosions when seen on X-ray) (Figure 39.4). Erosions lead to irreversible bone damage and eventual joint deformity. Bone sclerosis and osteophyte formation only occur if secondary OA develops.

CLINICAL FEATURES

The most common pattern of onset of RA is a slowly progressive, peripheral polyarthritis, developing over a few weeks or months. It causes painful swelling and stiffness of the small joints of the hands and toes and commonly also affects the wrists, elbows, shoulders, knees, and ankles. The hips are generally affected in late disease. The pain and stiffness are worse in the morning, and the patient feels tired and unwell. This type of RA is often associated with a high RF titre in the serum. A stable genetic marker, part of the human leukocyte antigen (HLA) DR-beta-1 gene, may be a better predictor of a poor prognosis than the detection of RF, but this is not yet used widely in normal clinical practice.

Seronegative (RF negative), limited-distribution synovitis is also called seronegative rheumatoid arthritis. The wrists are often the worst affected joints. This group of patients usually has a more limited, less symmetrical pattern of arthritis, and the joint damage is not as severe and therefore less disabling.

Palindromic rheumatism causes short-lived and reversible swelling, pain, and redness of one joint at a time. In about 50 per cent of cases it develops into RA.

Joint damage in the hand caused by RA leads to typical deformities, including ulnar drift, and an almost diagnostic appearance of established RA within the metacarpophalangeal joints of the hand (Figure 39.5).

Wrist involvement may lead to carpal tunnel syndrome – the patient wakens with numb, tingling, and painful index finger, middle finger, and thumb. This is due to compression of the median nerve at the wrist; it is usually helped by a night splint to hold the wrist in slight dorsiflexion. A corticosteroid injection into the carpal tunnel or surgery are occasionally needed.

Painful swelling of the metatarsophalangeal joints causes the foot to broaden. Deformities in the foot are very much analogous to those seen in the hands, and they cause pain, callous formation and ulceration in the ball of the foot.

The knee may be affected, with marked swelling due to synovitis and an effusion. Occasionally, a swelling at the back of the knee (a Baker's cyst) develops. If such a cyst ruptures, it causes pain and swelling in the calf and may be mistaken for a deep venous thrombosis.

Index   Middle   Ring

Figure 39.4 Juxta-articular osteoporosis. This X-ray of three proximal interphalangeal joints shows juxta-articular osteoporosis in the ring finger. In the middle finger, classic erosions (arrows) and narrowing of the joint space can be seen.

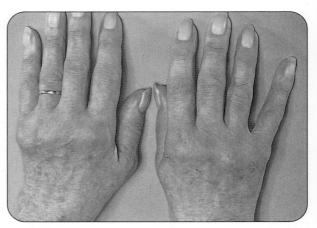

Figure 39.5 Typical features of rheumatoid arthritis affecting the hands. There is marked swelling of all the metacarpophalangeal joints, which the patient is unable to straighten fully. The proximal interphalangeal joints are also swollen. The right little finger shows early ulnar shift.

An important risk in severe RA is the development of an unstable atlantoaxial joint in the neck, which causes neck and occipital pain and may lead to spinal cord damage. Great care is taken with the neck of all patients with RA before they go for surgery to ensure that it is not damaged during intubation for anaesthesia. Patients are sent to theatre in a collar as a reminder to the anaesthetist to be careful.

RA relapses and remits either spontaneously or because of drug treatment. Disability in early disease is caused by synovitis but, as the disease progresses, joint destruction and deformity also cause pain, stiffness, and joint instability. This progressive damage may be slowed or halted by antirheumatic drugs.

Patients with active synovitis also develop systemic symptoms, such as malaise and tiredness, and a normochromic, normocytic anaemia.

Rheumatoid nodules develop subcutaneously over the elbows and other pressure points. Their histology resembles rheumatoid synovitis but they contain a necrotic centre.

Other systemic effects include Raynaud's phenomenon, vasculitis, and dry mouth and eyes (sicca syndrome or Sjögren's disease; see Chapter 27).

TREATMENT

Non-Steroidal Anti-Inflammatory Drugs and Analgesics

A wide variety of NSAIDs is available to control pain and stiffness in RA, although they do not reduce the underlying inflammation or reduce the acute phase reactants. Slow-release preparations in the evening or a suppository at bed time prevent morning pain and stiffness. Most patients with RA need NSAIDs, despite their potential side-effects, and many also require simple or compound analgesics.

Disease-Modifying Drugs

No curative agent is available for RA, but drugs may be prescribed to reduce the chronic inflammation and the levels of acute phase reactants. These drugs potentially reduce the risk of developing joint erosions and irreversible joint damage but are unpredictable in their benefit and side-effects. However, they do not work immediately since they need to accumulate in the body; this is why they are also called slow-acting agents.

Patients require regular monitoring, looking for benefit and side-effects, and these drugs are usually administered under the care of a rheumatologist. Such drugs include hydroxychloroquine, sulphasalazine, gold salts, D-penicillamine, methotrexate, and azathioprine.

Corticosteroids

Corticosteroids in RA are most commonly given by intra-articular injection. Intramuscular depot injections rapidly help severe flares. They may be given just before a holiday to help enjoyment by reducing the pain and increasing mobility, but they are best used infrequently. Low oral doses of 5 mg prednisolone daily are sometimes used in early disease to prevent erosions from developing but their long-term benefit remains to be established; this is a controversial topic.

Physical Exercise

Exercise is essential. Advice and support are obtained from a physiotherapist about how to adapt to the disease but still remain fit, active, and effective in society by using a combination of rest and exercise to maintain muscle power and range of joint movement. Exercise in a hydrotherapy pool is helpful and soothing when the joints are stiff and painful.

Advice about activities of daily living and about gadgets, suitable furniture, and structural changes in the home or at work is obtained from an occupational therapist.

Surgery

In early disease, referral to a surgeon with an interest in RA surgery for synovectomy (removal of the synovium) may help to reduce the inflamed synovium and prevent damage. Later, the removal of part or the whole of a joint (excision arthroplasty), joint fusion (arthrodesis), or – the most important surgical advance – total replacement of a joint (replacement arthroplasty) may be appropriate. All surgical interventions need careful discussion, planning and preparation.

POST-VIRAL ARTHRITIS

A transient polyarthritis may develop after an acute viral illness, such as rubella (German measles), parvovirus ('slapped cheek' disease) and hepatitis B. It may also occur after rubella vaccination. The arthritis is similar to acute RA and is treated with NSAIDs and rest. Viral arthritis does not persist beyond 6–12 weeks or cause long-term damage.

ERYTHEMA NODOSUM

Acutely tender, red skin nodules on the legs which resolve to a bruise are sometimes associated with a transient lower limb arthritis. It may be triggered by

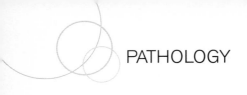

infections, drugs, or sarcoidosis. This is treated with NSAIDs or a short course of corticosteroids.

SERONEGATIVE SPONDARTHRITIS AND REACTIVE ARTHRITIS

Seronegative spondarthritis is a group of conditions affecting the spine and peripheral joints (Box 39.2). These conditions show familial clustering and are linked with HLA class I (see also Chapter 24). The arthritis is more asymmetrical and affects fewer joints than in RA. The synovitis is histologically similar to RA, except that RF are not produced in the joint or detected in the serum; hence the term 'seronegative'.

Reactive arthritis occurs when there is a precipitating infection. Compared with the general population, seronegative spondarthritis is associated with an increased incidence of sacroiliitis (morning buttock pain) and an increased frequency of HLA-B27. A strong association with HLA-B27 has been known for 25 years, but its role in causing the disease remains unclear. It is possible that there is a more important linked gene close by on the same chromosome (see also Chapter 7).

The immune systems of the gut and genitourinary mucous membranes appear to be important, possibly stimulated by an infective trigger. A variety of non-articular problems are seen in seronegative spondarthritis – uveitis (inflammation of the iris of the eye) occurs in all types, for example. Skin lesions include keratoderma blenorrhagica in reactive arthritis, which is histologically identical to pustular psoriasis and psoriasis itself. Nail dystrophy is seen in psoriasis and reactive arthritis.

ANKYLOSING SPONDYLITIS

Anklylosing spondylitis starts in the late teenage years or the early 20s with sacroiliitis and spinal stiffness that are improved by regular exercise. The diagnosis may be delayed for several years until the typical sacroiliitis appears on X-ray or a bout of iritis develops. Inflammation at the insertion of the intervertebral ligaments around the vertebrae causes spinal pain. Anterior chest pain is due to costochondral junction inflammation. Eventually, bony bridges (syndesmophytes) develop across the otherwise normal disc and the sacroiliac joints and costovertebral joints fuse, the latter causing reduced chest expansion. Failure to control pain or to do regular spinal and chest exercises leads to poor posture, a severe dorsal kyphosis, and wasting of the paraspinal muscles.

Peripheral arthritis occurs occasionally, most commonly in the hips or knees. Iritis (acute anterior uveitis) causes severe eye pain, blurred vision, and photophobia and the cornea around the iris turns dusky red, owing to inflammation.

Urgent specialist advice is essential for pain relief and to prevent permanent eye damage and later glaucoma. Topical or subconjunctival corticosteroids are used and the pupil is dilated using atropine to reduce pain and prevent adhesions forming to the anterior surface of the lens. Patients with ankylosing spondylitis are asked to report eye pain and redness immediately.

Treatment

Exercises each morning should become a way of life to prevent irreversible spinal stiffening and reduced chest expansion. NSAIDs, usually given as an evening dose of a slow-release or suppository preparation, control pain and so increase compliance with a morning exercise regime. Sulphasalazine or methotrexate may help the peripheral arthritis.

PSORIATIC ARTHRITIS

Arthritis is seen in people with psoriasis or with a family history of psoriasis. About 8 per cent of people with psoriasis develop arthritis either before or after the onset of the skin or nail lesions (Box 39.3). Psoriatic arthritis has a more limited distribution than RA. Common diseases, such as RA and nodular OA, may co-exist with psoriasis.

ENTEROPATHIC ARTHRITIS

Enteropathic arthritis may occur in Crohn's disease or ulcerative colitis. An asymmetrical arthritis in the lower limbs may precede or occur with the bowel disease. Selective intestinal mucosal leakiness caused by the inflammation permits antigens to cross into the blood and possibly triggers the synovitis. Remission of ulcerative colitis or total colectomy leads to remission of the arthritis.

BOX 39.2 TYPES OF SERONEGATIVE SPONDARTHRITIS

- ankylosing spondylitis
- psoriatic arthritis
- arthritis associated with ulcerative colitis and Crohn's disease (enteropathic arthritis)
- reactive arthritis
  sexually acquired arthritis (Reiter's disease)
  post-dysenteric arthritis

BOX 39.3 SUBTYPES OF PSORIATIC ARTHRITIS

- distal interphalangeal joint arthritis with adjacent nail dystrophy
- asymmetrical monoarticular or pauciarticular arthritis
- seronegative rheumatoid-like arthritis
- psoriatic arthritis mutilans or periarticular osteolysis ('telescopic' fingers)
- psoriatic sacroiliitis or spondylitis

Crohn's disease is more difficult to treat. Sulphasalazine is used in both conditions (see also Chapter 34).

REACTIVE ARTHRITIS

Reactive arthritis is the term given to a sterile, acute, asymmetrical arthritis in the lower limbs that occurs a few days or weeks after an infection such as dysentery, sexually acquired non-specific urethritis, or cervicitis. Organisms that may trigger reactive arthritis include some strains of *Salmonella* or *Shigella* (causing dysentery), *Yersinia enterocolitica* (causing diarrhoea), and *Chlamydia* or *Ureaplasma* species (causing urethritis) (see Chapters 16 and 17). The triad of urethritis, arthritis and conjunctivitis is called Reiter's disease.

Early treatment of the infection probably prevents the arthritis. There may be plantar fasciitis or Achilles tendinitis and psoriasis-like lesions on the soles and palms (keratoderma blenorrhagica). A single attack of arthritis is usual, and it settles after a few weeks. A disabling, chronic, relapsing and remitting form may occur, but it is rare.

In 50 per cent of patients with non-specific urethritis, *Chlamydia* or *Ureaplasma* organisms are cultured from the genital tract or there is a rising titre of specific serum antibodies. Molecules derived from *Chlamydia*, *Yersinia*, *Shigella*, and *Salmonella* species may trigger the inflammation; these may be identified in the synovium by using special staining techniques (see also Chapter 17).

TREATMENT OF SERONEGATIVE SPONDARTHRITIS

NSAIDs and other analgesics on a 'when necessary' basis control pain and stiffness. Local synovitis responds to an intra-articular corticosteroid injection. Methotrexate or cyclosporin control psoriatic skin and joint disease but are only used in severe disease.

Sulphasalazine helps ulcerative colitis or Crohn's disease and also enteropathic arthritis. Antibiotics probably do not alter the outcome of reactive arthritis once it has started, but are usually prescribed.

CRYSTAL ARTHRITIS

Sodium urate and calcium pyrophosphate can be found in the joint during acute gout and pseudogout. They appear under the microscope as crystals, and they can be distinguished from each other by their different shapes and properties under polarized light and using a red filter. Leukocytes ingest the crystals and, in so doing, release inflammatory enzymes from their phagosomes. This triggers activation of complement and attracts more neutrophils to the area (see Chapter 25).

GOUT AND HYPERURICAEMIA

In humans, uric acid is the end-product of the breakdown of endogenous purines (70 per cent) and dietary purines (30 per cent). It is excreted by the kidneys (70 per cent) and by the gut (30 per cent). Blood concentration of uric acid depends on:

- dietary intake;
- the enzymes that produce it; and
- renal excretion.

The renal handling mechanism is complex, but renal excretion of uric acid is reduced in renal failure and by most diuretics. There is a normal (bell-shaped) distribution of serum urate concentration in the population but with a skew at the upper end of the range. Levels are higher in men than in women. Although most people with hyperuricaemia are asymptomatic, hyperuricaemia may cause acute urate synovitis – gout.

In gout, there is a sudden onset of agonizing pain, swelling, and redness of a joint (often the first metatarsophalangeal joint). An alcoholic binge, dehydration, starvation prior to surgery or starting a diuretic may be the immediate cause. There is often a family history of gout, and finding a raised urate in the blood or urate crystals in the joint is diagnostic. Untreated attacks last a few days. The pain is agonizing but responds quickly to a high dose of an NSAID, such as naproxen (750 mg immediately, then 500 mg every 8–12 hours) or diclofenac (75–100 mg immediately, then 50 mg every 6–8 hours). Colchicine (1000 mcg immediately, then 500 mcg every 6–12 hours) is used if the patient has a history of peptic ulcers. A reduction in alcohol intake and other dietary advice are important – diet sheets are available.

In patients with a history of recurrent attacks or attacks that are difficult to control and in those who have side-effects with NSAIDs, the best treatment is allopurinol. This drug blocks the formation of urate from xanthine by inhibiting the metabolic enzyme, xanthine oxidase. Accordingly, there is a rapid fall in serum urate levels with allopurinol, but it may precipitate an acute attack when first prescribed. The most probable reason for this is because urate is highly insoluble and remains at high levels in the tissues, even after the serum level has fallen. Therefore, it is important that allopurinol is not prescribed during an acute attack of gout or too soon after one. In the first month of treatment, it is given in combination with a regular dose of an NSAID or colchicine. Allopurinol is excreted by the kidneys and therefore it must be used in lower doses in renal failure in order to prevent toxicity.

Uricosuric agents increase urate excretion and are sometimes given with allopurinol for tophaceous gout or if patients have developed an allergy to allopurinol (see also Chapters 13 and 26).

Chronic Tophaceous Gout

Chronic tophaceous gout is associated with sodium urate deposited as white smooth lumps (tophi) in people with a very high level of serum urate. Tophaceous gout occurs in patients on long-term diuretic treatment and in renal impairment. The diuretics are stopped if possible.

Renal stones may form in chronic hyperuricaemia and may lead to renal damage (see Chapter 36).

ACUTE PSEUDOGOUT

Calcium pyrophosphate deposits in hyaline and fibrocartilage are seen as chondrocalcinosis on X-ray. If these crystals are shed into the joint they cause an acute arthritis, especially in older adults. Men and women are equally affected, and the joints most commonly involved are the knees and wrists.

The diagnosis is made by finding crystals of calcium pyrophosphate in the joint fluid or chondrocalcinosis on X-ray. The patient may be febrile and joint fluid should always be sent for microbiological investigation. In young people, chondrocalcinosis is occasionally caused by hyperparathyroidism or haemochromatosis.

Treatment.

Removing the crystals by aspiration dramatically reduces the pain, especially when the knee is affected. A corticosteroid injection may be used if infection has been excluded. NSAIDs or colchicine are used, as for gout. Allopurinol and uricosuric agents have no role in the treatment of acute pseudogout.

SEPTIC ARTHRITIS

Joint infection rarely occurs from direct injury. It usually develops from bacteria spreading via the blood from an infected skin lesion or other site. The risk of septic arthritis is increased in people with chronically inflamed joints (especially older adults) and in immunosuppressed people. Infection of joint replacements is an important complication of joint replacement surgery and is difficult to treat.

Suspected septic arthritis is a medical emergency and must always be referred to a hospital.

The infected joint is agonizingly painful and hot, red, and swollen. The patient is febrile. However, these symptoms and signs are often less dramatic in older adults and immunosuppressed patients (see Chapters 23 and 28). Septic arthritis is diagnosed by aspiration of the joint fluid and examination of it by Gram staining and by culture. A combination of two antibiotics to which the organism is sensitive is given, first intravenously then orally for 6–12 weeks.

LYME ARTHRITIS

Lyme disease develops in people who have been in heathlands infested with ticks of the *Ixodes* genus that are infected with *Borrelia burgdorferi* (a spirochaete). Fever and headache and an expanding, erythematous rash (erythema migrans) may be followed by neurological or cardiac complications, and 25 per cent of people with Lyme disease develop an acute pauciarticular arthritis. IgM anti-*Borrelia* antibodies are diagnostic, and the disorder is treated with penicillin.

POLYMYALGIA RHEUMATICA AND GIANT CELL ARTERITIS

Polymyalgia rheumatica causes severe morning pain and stiffness of the neck, lumbar spine, and proximal limbs in people aged over 50 years. Patients feel ill, lose weight, and become depressed. The cause is unknown, and occasionally polymyalgia rheumatica is mistaken for late-onset RA. There are no specific tests, but the ESR or CRP are always raised. It is necessary to exclude other diseases such as RA or a malignancy.

Giant cell arteritis (also known as temporal arteritis) is an inflammatory, granulomatous arteritis that is sometimes seen with polymyalgia rheumatica. It causes severe, temporal or occipital headaches as well as tenderness and swelling of a temporal or occipital artery. An arterial biopsy is the diagnostic procedure of choice. The ESR and CRP are very high. Arteritis may also affect the ophthalmic artery and lead to blindness, although this can be prevented by early recognition of giant cell arteritis and treatment with high doses of corticosteroids.

TREATMENT

Corticosteroids are essential and they are rapidly effective. Starting doses are 10–15 mg prednisolone for polymyalgia rheumatica and 60–100 mg prednisolone for giant cell arteritis. These doses are reduced gradually over at least 12 months, often longer. The use of drugs to reduce the risk of secondary osteoporosis should be considered (see below).

DRUGS USED IN THE TREATMENT OF ARTHRITIS

Analgesics and NSAIDs are used to relieve pain and stiffness. NSAIDs, colchicine (in crystal synovitis), and specific anti-rheumatic drugs relieve inflammation. Specific anti-rheumatic drugs and immunosuppressant agents alter the immune events that cause inflammation in RA and seronegative spondarthritis. It is always necessary to weigh up the risks and benefits of therapy and the appropriateness of the drugs being used should be constantly reviewed, especially in older adults in whom the risk of serious side-effects is greater (see Chapter 12).

Analgesics (paracetamol, codeine compounds, and combinations of these) are available without prescription. They are safe and effective for mild pain. Stronger analgesic compounds (dihydrocodeine or tramadol) are sometimes prescribed. NSAIDs (ibuprofen, diclofenac, and naproxen are common examples) are also analgesic agents, but they are best reserved for use in inflammatory arthritis, when they are often essential to maintain normal function. Because of their greater risk of side-effects, they are used with care in older adults. The most common side-effect is indigestion, but peptic ulceration may also occur; this can lead to serious and occasionally life-threatening gastrointestinal bleeding without any warning symptoms of indigestion (see Chapters 10 and 14).

Corticosteroid drugs are sometimes life saving in autoimmune rheumatic diseases (see Chapter 29), but they should be used with caution in RA and other forms of inflammatory arthritis. Intra-articular or intramuscular injections help control localized flares or cope with acute flares, but these are best used infrequently. Corticosteroids are a vital part of the treatment of polymyalgia rheumatica and temporal arteritis.

BONE DISEASES

NORMAL BONE STRUCTURE AND FORMATION

The skeleton provides a rigid structure for the body and is the site of attachment of muscles. Bone comprises an extracellular collagenous matrix (predominantly type I collagen and proteoglycans) and is constantly being formed by osteoblasts. Another bone cell type, the osteoclast, is responsible for bone resorption (dissolving), which is a very necessary mechanism for bone remodelling in growth and repair (e.g. during childhood and adolescence or following a fracture). The processes of bone formation and resorption are normally in balance, and they are maintained by an elaborate array of factors including mechanical stress, systemic hormones, and local cytokines. Parathyroid hormone is a powerful stimulant of bone resorption. The organic matrix of bone is impregnated with mineral salts (mainly calcium hydroxyapatite) and this confers both rigidity and hardness. Bone contains about 99 per cent of total body calcium and phosphate, and is essential to maintaining a steady level of these minerals in the blood. Vitamin D has a direct effect on osteoblasts and affects the absorption of calcium from the gut and its resorption in the kidney (see Box 39.4).

Compact or cortical bone forms the shafts of long bones and the surfaces of flat bones; it represents about 90 per cent of the skeleton. It is laid down concentrically around a central (haversian) canal. Trabecular or cancellous bone is found at the ends of long bones and inside the flat bones. It comprises interconnecting bars and plates, which surround fatty or haematopoietic bone marrow (see Chapters 23 and 31).

OSTEOPOROSIS

Primary osteoporosis occurs in women after the menopause, when it is due to the fall in oestrogen levels. Oestrogen stimulates osteoblast cell activities (i.e. bone production). There is marked loss of bone density during the 5–10 years after the menopause. Younger women with eating disorders and amenorrhoea may also become osteoporotic. Other risk factors include lack of exercise, severe inflammatory or disabling disease, or the long-term use of corticosteroids. There also appears to be a higher incidence in patients with a family history of osteoporosis. Caucasian and Asian women are more prone to the disorder than Afro-Caribbean women. Osteoporosis is less common in men, whose most important risk factors are alcoholism, smoking, and poor nutrition.

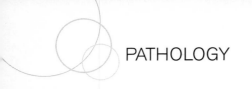

PATHOLOGY

> ## BOX 39.4 VITAMIN D
>
> **Vitamin D is central to bone and calcium metabolism in that:**
> it affects calcium absorption from the gut and resorption in the kidney
> it has a direct effect on osteoblast activities
>
> **Vitamin D is derived from:**
> diet (e.g. eggs, liver, oily fish, fortified fat spread)
> endogenous production (it is produced in the skin under the influence of ultraviolet light)

Screening

Risk factors for osteoporosis include a family history of osteoporosis or fractures, an early menopause, a diet poor in calcium, heavy smoking, and heavy alcohol consumption. Economically, screening is best focused on those at risk. The bone density at the femoral neck and in the lumbar spine may be compared either with that of a large number of women of the same age and weight (Z score) or with young adult peak bone mass, matched for sex and race (T score). Normal bone density is not more than one standard deviation below the young adult mean (T > –1.0). Osteopenia is defined as bone mass of 1–2.5 standard deviations below the young adult mean (–1.0 < T > –2.5). Osteoporosis is present at T < – 2.5; established osteoporosis is defined as being osteoporosis in which a fracture has occurred. The threshold for fracture appears to be T < –2.0. For women over the age of 75 years of age it is best to use the Z score.

Peak bone mass is reached during early adulthood, but everyone, irrespective of sex or race, loses bone mass with age. However, there is individual variation in the amount and the rate of bone loss. Osteoporosis is a failure to maintain bone of normal thickness (i.e. bone resorption is more rapid than bone formation), which leads to a net loss of bone density. The cortices of long bones become gradually thinner after the age of 40 years in both men and women. However, the major impact of postmenopausal osteoporosis is on trabecular bone, which forms a high proportion of the bone mass in the vertebrae, the ribs, and the pelvis. The trabeculae become fewer and thinner than normal, resulting in increased bone fragility (see also Chapter 40).

Osteoporosis does not cause symptoms itself but leads to an increased risk of fracture of peripheral bones (classically the neck of femur and wrist) and of crush fractures of the thoracic or lumbar spine. There is a high morbidity and mortality from femoral neck fractures in older adults. Vertebral fractures develop with or without trauma and may be painless or severely painful. A kyphosis or acute angulation of the spine may develop. On X-ray the vertebral bone looks demineralized and there is a wedge-shaped collapse of vertebrae. Osteoporosis is confirmed by bone densitometry (DEXA). In crush fractures, it is essential to exclude a pathological fracture caused by a malignant deposit in the bone. Severe pain is treated with bed rest and analgesia, when constipation is a possible problem (see Chapter 14). Intravenous parmidronate or subcutaneous calcitonin are also used to control the pain of acute vertebral crush fractures.

Preventative Therapy

The aim of preventative treatment is to reduce the risk of developing osteoporosis and therefore of fractures in old age. A risk of fracture still exists, however, even after effective preventative treatment (see Chapter 37).

Preventative therapy for those with osteopenia includes a calcium-rich diet, education about avoiding falls and taking regular weight-bearing exercise, giving up smoking, and reducing alcohol intake. Drug measures include supplements of calcium and vitamin D as well as hormone replacement therapy for 10 years after the menopause. It is essential to use cyclical oestrogen and progesterone replacement if the woman still has her uterus, but this may result in persistence or recurrence of periods. Unopposed oestrogen is acceptable after a hysterectomy. The benefits of hormone therapy greatly outweigh the risks, although there is a very slightly increased incidence of breast cancer. Bisphosphonate drugs, which inhibit bone resorption, may also be used.

OSTEOGENESIS IMPERFECTA

Osteogenesis imperfecta is also known as 'brittle bone disease'. It is an hereditary disorder associated with abnormalities of type I collagen. There is marked osteoporosis and a greatly increased risk of fractures. The skin is thin and there is generally increased hypermobility of the joints. Another typical feature is bluish discoloration of the cornea of the eye. The presentation and symptoms of the disease are extremely variable, but in severe cases it is fatal *in utero* or in childhood. Some patients live to adulthood and require genetic counselling about having children.

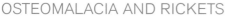

OSTEOMALACIA AND RICKETS

In osteomalacia there are increased amounts of unmineralized bone matrix and the normal coupling of bone matrix deposition and mineralization is disrupted. Rickets is the form of the disease that is seen in childhood before the epiphyseal plates have closed. The cause is an abnormality of osteoblast function resulting from vitamin D deficiency or occasionally from phosphate deficiency. Vitamin D deficiency may be due to decreased absorption of vitamin D from the gut (e.g. in poor diet or fat malabsorption states) or to abnormal metabolism of vitamin D (e.g. with certain drugs or in chronic renal failure). In northern Europe, Asian girls and young women who wear a veil (and so are rarely exposed to the sun) and have a calcium-depleted diet are especially at risk. In developed countries, many foods contain vitamin D supplements (e.g. fortified margarines).

Osteomalacia produces bone pain, fractures and skeletal deformity. Muscle weakness may be severe, resulting in a waddling gait. The picture is often subtle in adults, however, and diagnosis may be delayed. Children with rickets are short and have abnormal epiphyseal plates, leading to swollen joints and periarticular pain.

The serum alkaline phosphatase is raised and there may be evidence of renal failure (raised urea and creatinine). In adults the classical X-ray appearance is of linear areas of demineralization perpendicular to the bone surface, called 'Looser's zones'. These are pseudofractures of the cortex and are most commonly seen in the long bones, the pubic rami, and the ribs. They contain fibrous, immature bone.

Treatment is with vitamin D supplements and dietary advice. Vitamin D must be metabolized into its active form $1,25(OH)_2$-vitamin D in the kidney. However, in patients with renal failure this does not occur; therefore they require treatment with $1,25(OH)_2$-vitamin D to prevent renal osteodystrophy (see Chapter 36).

PATHOLOGY

- The chronic course of many of the locomotor diseases means that healthcare professionals who deal with such patients must be skilled in caring and communication. Furthermore, they must be able to interpret the symptoms and signs and know when the patients needs to be referred on.
- Laboratory investigations are used as diagnostic indicators and to monitor the progress of the disease. Investigations include full blood count, ESR, and CRP; biochemical estimations (e.g. serum urate and alkaline phosphatase); and immune profile of autoantibodies.
- Imaging techniques (e.g. X-rays, magnetic resonance imaging, and ultrasound scans) can provide details of bony anatomy and certain soft tissues.
- Joints may be aspirated and synovial fluids examined (e.g. for colour and the presence of crystals and infection).
- Osteoarthritis is the most prevalent form of arthritis. There is a genetic predisposition, but a combination of the ageing processes, including abnormal attempts to repair damaged cartilage and bone, are its causes.
- Rheumatoid arthritis is an autoimmune disorder in which the disease process is associated with autoantibodies, abnormal cytokine production and increased immune cells in the synovium. Although the main impact is on the joints, other organs are also affected.
- Seronegative spondarthritis is a group of disorders affecting the spine and peripheral joints in which serum rheumatoid factors are not detected. If the joint disorder is precipitated by an infection (e.g. with *Salmonella* species), it is called reactive arthritis. It is important to distinguish this from a true septic arthritis, which requires specific antibiotic treatment.
- Treatments for arthritis depend on the cause, and treatment may include one or more of the following: analgesics, anti-inflammatory drugs, corticosteroids (oral or injectable), and occasionally antibiotics.
- If the arthritis is associated with crystal formation (e.g. uric acid crystals), anti-inflammatory drugs and allopurinol (to reduce serum urate levels) may be given.
- Osteoporosis is a failure to maintain bone of normal thickness (i.e. bone resorption is more rapid than bone formation). People at risk include postmenopausal women, younger women with amenorrhoea or eating disorders, alcohol misusers, and those who have been on long-term corticosteroid therapy.
- Screening for osteoporosis involves the evaluation of the bone density of the femoral neck and the lumbar spine. The disorder is treated with weight-bearing exercises and calcium and vitamin D supplements; bisphosphonate drugs may be used to reduce bone resorption.
- Osteogenesis imperfecta is an inherited 'brittle bone disease' caused by an abnormality of type I collagen. Patients have a greatly increased risk of fractures, and those who live to adulthood require genetic counselling.
- Osteomalacia and rickets are generally caused by an abnormality resulting from vitamin D deficiency. Insufficient active vitamin D may be the result of an inadequate intake, decreased synthesis in the skin, or renal impairment.

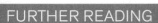

FURTHER READING

Caldwell JR (1996) Intra-articular corticosteroids. Guide to selection and indications for use. Drugs 52:507–14.

Dearborn JT, Jergesen HE (1996) The evaluation and initial management of arthritis. Prim Care 23:215–40.

Grahame R, West J (1996) The role of the rheumatology nurse practitioner in primary care: an experiment in the further education of the practice nurse. Br J Rheumatol 35(6):581–8.

Goldenberg DL (1998) Septic arthritis. Lancet 351:197–202.

Hedstrom SA (1996) Septic bone and joint infections. Curr Opin Rheumatol 8:322–6.

Hill J (1997) Patient satisfaction in a nurse-led rheumatology clinic. J Adv Nurs 25:347–54.

Hudgins TH, Brander VA, Chang RW (1997) Rehabilitation advances in the treatment of arthritis and musculoskeletal disease. Curr Opin Rheumatol 9:112–17.

Keefe FJ, Caldwell DS (1997) Cognitive behavioral control of arthritis pain. Med Clin North Am 81:277–90.

Maddison PJ, Isenberg D, Woo P, Glass DN (1998) Oxford Textbook of Rheumatology, 2nd edition. Oxford University Press, Oxford.

Newbold D (1996) Coping with rheumatoid arthritis. How can specialist nurses influence it and promote better outcomes? J Clin Nurs 5:373–80.

Oen KG, Cheang M (1996) Epidemiology of chronic arthritis in childhood. Semin Arthritis Rheum 26:575–91.

Peterfy CG (1996) MR imaging. Baillieres Clin Rheumatol 10:635–78.

Raff ML, Byers PH (1996) Joint hypermobility syndromes. Curr Opin Rheumatol 8:459–66.

Ryan S (1997) Nurse-led drug monitoring in the rheumatology clinic. Nurs Stand 11:24 45–7

Shipley M, Newman SP (1993) Psychological aspects of rheumatic diseases. Baillieres Clin Rheumatol 7:215–19.

Shipley M (1993) A Colour Atlas of Rheumatology, 3rd edition. Mosby–Year Book, London.

Shipley M (1995) ABC of Rheumatology. Pain in the hand and wrist. BMJ 310:239–43.

Sigal LH (1997) Lyme disease: a review of aspects of its immunology and immunopathogenesis. Ann Rev Immunol 15:63–92.

Smith R (1995) Osteogenesis imperfecta, non-accidental injury, and temporary brittle bone disease. Arch Dis Child 72:169–71.

Snaith ML (ed) (1995) ABC of Rheumatology. BMJ Books, London.

Sowers M (1997) Clinical epidemiology and osteoporosis. Measures and their interpretation. Endocrinol Metab Clin North Am 26:219–31.

Swannel AJ (1997) Polymyalgia rheumatica and temporal arteritis: diagnosis and management. BMJ 314:1329–32.

Walgenbach AW (1996) The knee joint: evaluation and treatment. Nurse Pract Forum 7:112–19.

DISEASES OF OLDER ADULTS

8

LEARNING OBJECTIVES

After studying this chapter students should have a clearer understanding of:
- the concept of the ageing process associated with specific diseases
- when and how age can affect the presentation and management of disease

---

Before reading this chapter, it is expected that you will have read the previous chapters concerning pathologies of specific systems.

INTRODUCTION

Human beings, in common with all other animals, have a fixed biological life span. Development from childhood into adulthood has well-characterized phases of maturation through puberty, but the onset of 'old age' is much less clearly defined. Senescence has been described as a phase of mammalian life when the body's maintenance and repair mechanisms become less effective and cells die and organ function diminishes. The ageing process may be compounded by disease or injury, and the two can be very difficult to dissociate.

Although there is a fixed life span, life expectancy has increased steadily through the 20th century. This is mainly a result of improvements in child health and survival so that more children grow old, which are due more to social and economic improvements than medical interventions. The average life expectancy in the UK is 74 years for a baby boy and 80 years for a baby girl, according to *Social Trends* published by the Office for National Statistics in 1996. The increase in population in developing countries is predominantly in children and young adults; in the Western world, the proportion of older adults is set to increase dramatically over the next 30 years (Table 40.1).

THE AGEING PROCESS

Cells appear to age in different ways depending on the tissue type they form. Non-dividing cells, such as specialized cells in nervous tissue, diminish in number over time as the cells die, and with this cell loss comes functional decline. Cells that are able to replicate by mitosis and cell division can replace themselves, but there is a deterioration in function over the life span (see Chapter 4).

At a cellular level, both the replication of DNA and the transcription of RNA in the process of protein synthesis may be impaired. Chromosomal aberrations are seen in ageing cells and damaged DNA function may explain some of the features of ageing (see also Chapters 1, 3 and 7).

Another marker of the ageing system, is an impaired immune system. Immunosurveillance is thought to be an important mechanism whereby aberrant molecules and cells are recognized as alien by the immune system and dealt with. Cellular immunity as seen on skin prick testing is impaired in older adults, and autoantibodies – antibodies against normal human cells – are found in increasing levels as people age (see Chapter 27).

There is also a genetic component to ageing, in that longevity appears to be hereditary and is sex-linked in favour of females.

Other explanations of the ageing process have focused more on hormone levels, which decline through life, particularly the levels of those produced by the

557

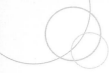

Population Projections for the Year 2000 in the UK, the USA, and Nigeria						
	Total population (millions)		Population >70 years (millions)		Population >80 years (millions)	
	1980	2000	1980	2000	1980	2000
UK	55.9	55.2	5.4	6.0	1.4	1.8
USA	223.2	263.8	15.6	20.6	4.4	5.8
Nigeria	77.1	150	1.0	2.2	0.2	0.4

Table 40.1 Population projection: UK, USA and Nigeria for the year 2000.

pituitary. There has been a resurgence of interest in this in the USA with the use of growth hormone in older adult patients, which is said to improve overall function.

In clinical practice, ageing may be summed up as the older person having reduced physiological reserves and impaired homeostasis, which can be compounded by supervening events such as injury or illness.

Pain thresholds may be altered with age, and a myocardial infarction may go almost unnoticed. Conversely, older patients are more likely to suffer from post-herpetic neuralgia after shingles, where the nerve supply to the skin is particularly sensitized, often for years after the original infection.

PRESENTATIONS OF DISEASE IN OLD AGE

In youth it is unusual for more than one disease to be present, but in old age it is common for several different conditions to co-exist, although symptoms may only be due to one particular disease at any one time. This can make diagnosis difficult and sometimes quite vague, since different disease processes interact. For example, elderly patients with non-insulin-dependent diabetes mellitus usually also have hyperlipidaemia, impaired renal function, ischaemic heart disease, and hypertension, to name but a few (Figure 40.1).

Furthermore, many diseases present very slowly and insidiously, and often it is only when a new doctor or nurse sees a patient that the problem becomes obvious. Hypothyroidism is a classic example of this (see Chapter 35); parkinsonism, which may present as slowness or unsteadiness, may be written off as 'old age'.

Reduced physiological reserves mean that illnesses present in different ways. Impaired temperature regulation means that the person may not develop a fever in response to infection, so a normal temperature may be falsely reassuring. This also means that older patients are prone to hypothermia, which is compounded by physical inactivity. Fluid balance is also often impaired, which may lead to dehydration and constipation. Elderly people themselves may contribute to this if they suffer from incontinence, since they may cut back on their fluid intake in order to control their bladder problem.

MRS. PETERS' DRUG CHART - AGE 66

Mrs Peters has been diabetic for 8 years and was started on insulin 3 years ago after her blood sugar failed to be controlled on oral hypoglycaemic drugs. She had a myocardial infarction 2 years ago. She is obese and has osteoarthritis of the knees, and a hiatus hernia which causes reflux oesophagitis.

1) Mixtard insulin 20 iu bd
2) Needles, syringes, blood monitoring test strips, needle clipper
3) Isosorbide mononitrate 20mg bd - ischaemic heart disease
4) Glyceryl trinitrate spray PRN - angina
5) Captopril 25mg bd - hypertension + protective effect on diabetic nephropathy
6) Simvastatin 20mg od - for hypercholesterolaemia
7) Timoptol 0.5% eye drops - for glaucoma
8) Aspirin 150mg od - for ischaemic heart disease
9) Paracetamol tabs 500mg - 2 tablets upto 4 x daily - for osteoarthritis
10) Omeprazole 10mg od - for reflux oesophagitis

Figure 40.1 Multiple drug prescriptions.

Recovery from illness may be slower, and healing times of wounds may be longer. Older patients are particularly prone to pressure sores if bed-bound for even short periods of time, and these may be very slow to heal (see Chapter 4).

THE NERVOUS SYSTEM

Between the ages of 30 and 70 years, the brain loses 10 per cent of its weight owing to cerebral atrophy. Histologically, the changes of ageing include the reduction of synaptic connections of neurones and atheroma of the cerebral blood vessels. The autonomic nervous system controlling reflex activity in muscles, gut, and other organs also shows degenerative changes, causing symptoms such as postural hypotension (low blood pressure on standing, leading to dizziness and faints) and poor balance.

DEMENTIA

In the UK, approximately 5–7 per cent of the population over the age of 65 years have dementia, and about 20 per cent of people over the age of 80 are affected. Dementia is not a diagnosis in its own right and has many different causes (see Box 40.1). It can be defined as sustained intellectual deterioration with mental, behavioural and motor changes. The diagnosis of dementia is based on the demonstration of impaired memory and intellect. The Abbreviated Mental Test (Box 40.2) or a similar one may be used as part of the examination. A score of 7 or below suggests intellectual impairment. It is sometimes described as 'chronic brain failure' and can be sub-divided into two groups, vascular and non-vascular.

VASCULAR CAUSES OF DEMENTIA

Multi-Infarct Dementia

Dementia caused by vascular disease is sometimes called multi-infarct dementia, and patients usually have evidence of vascular disease elsewhere in the body. They may have peripheral vascular disease or ischaemic heart disease with a history of myocardial infarction. The patient may suffer a series of minor strokes, with intellectual function diminishing after each one, or a more major stroke may be followed by intellectual dysfunction. Emotional instability is a frequent element of this type of dementia, with the patient bursting into tears for no apparent reason, which can be very upsetting for carers.

BOX 40.1 CAUSES OF DEMENTIA

Degenerative disorders
Alzheimer's disease
Huntingdon's disease
Parkinson's disease

Vascular disorders
Multi-infarct dementia

Toxic substances
alcohol
lead

Drugs
(e.g. barbiturates, neuroleptics)

Trauma
head injury

Neoplasms
frontal brain tumour
cerebral metastases

Infections
syphilis
tuberculous meningitis
acquired immunodeficiency syndrome (AIDS)
Creutzfeld–Jakob disease

Metabolic disorders
hypothyroidism
uraemia
hepatic failure
vitamin B12 deficiency

NON-VASCULAR CAUSES OF DEMENTIA

Non-vascular causes include dementia caused by progressive Parkinson's disease. A rarer cause is Huntingdon's disease, which is an inherited dementia that normally presents in middle age rather than old age.

Creutzfeldt–Jakob disease is a dementia seen in younger patients; it is transmitted by an infectious agent, not yet specifically identified (see Chapter 38). It has been transmitted from human to human through pituitary extract and corneal grafts. New variant Creutzfeldt–Jakob disease (nvCJD) is associated with bovine spongiform encephalopathy.

Toxins such as alcohol and lead, as well as hormonal and nutritional deficiencies can also present with dementia.

PATHOLOGY

> ## BOX 40.2 ABBREVIATED MENTAL TEST
>
> 1. Age
> 2. Time (to nearest hour)
> 3. Address for recall at end (e.g. 42 West Street)
> 4. What year is it?
> 5. Name of institution
> 6. Recognition of two persons
> 7. Date of birth
> 8. Year of First World War
> 9. Name of present monarch
> 10. Backwards counting from 20 to 1
>
> Each correct answer scores 1 mark
> Total of 7 or less suggests intellectual impairment

Alzheimer's disease

The most common type of non-vascular dementia is Alzheimer's disease, for which there is no specific diagnostic test; rather, it is a diagnosis made when other causes have been excluded. This is very important because treatable causes, such as hypothyroidism and vitamin B12 deficiency, may cause dementing symptoms that are reversible on treatment. Another important differential diagnosis is depression, which may co-exist with dementia but which may cause dementing symptoms in its own right. Treatment with antidepressants can be very effective.

There are histological changes in the brain on post-mortem examination, which make up the picture of Alzheimer's disease but none of these changes is unique. Evidence is growing of a genetic predisposition to the disease associated with the gene for apolipoprotein E, which is one of the circulating proteins for transporting lipids.

The main clinical features are the inexorable decline of global brain function with loss of memory, particularly recent and short-term memory, and personality and behavioural changes. Physical motor retardation usually follows later.

There is no curative treatment for Alzheimer's disease. Some drugs, such as tacrine, have been on trial, but there is no clear-cut benefit in their use owing to the many side-effects. Donepezil is newly licensed and on the market in the UK; it increases the levels of acetylcholine (a neurotransmitter) by inhibiting acetylcholinesterase, the enzyme that breaks it down. In preliminary trials, cognitive testing has shown some benefit from the drug but the use of this expensive drug is so far limited to patients in ongoing trials.

Patients with dementia require increasing levels of care as the condition deteriorates. They decline physically and mentally until they become bed-bound, and they eventually die from their disease or because of intercurrent infection from immobility.

ACUTE BRAIN FAILURE

Acute brain failure has many other names, such as acute confusional state and delirium. It presents with a sudden onset of clouding of consciousness and a fluctuating level of awareness. The patient may have hallucinations and memory disturbances. There are many causes; infection is a common one. A simple urinary tract or chest infection may precipitate an acute confusional state. The patient may not be able to give any useful history and the diagnosis depends on careful examination and investigations of common causes. Another frequent trigger to confusional states is the use of some drugs, in particular sleeping pills and tranquillizers. Many causes of acute brain failure are treatable and the confusion reversible, so hunting for the cause is very worthwhile.

STROKE

Although the frequency and severity of cerebrovascular disease has decreased over the last 20 years, it is still a major problem. The risk rises with age, and about 75 per cent of all strokes occur in people over the age of 65 years. Common risk factors include hypertension, atherosclerosis, and diabetes mellitus. At particular risk are patients with atrial fibrillation, a cardiac arrhythmia in which small emboli may detach from thrombus in the atrium and travel into the cerebral circulation and occlude a small vessel. There is good evidence that these patients should be anticoagulated with warfarin to reduce their risk of stroke (see Chapter 38 for the clinical presentation of strokes).

Treatment of a stroke is focused on supportive medical care in the initial phases. This may mean initial catheterization and intravenous hydration followed by an active rehabilitation programme to improve function. It is important to remember that recovery expectations are based on previous function, so that, for example, a patient who was disabled by arthritis before the stroke will have more mobility problems afterwards because of the combined effects of the two conditions.

Mental impairment is common and, although it may be subtle and difficult to detect, it can have a profound effect on recovery. In particular, depression is very common, for understandable reasons. If left untreated, the depression may slow the recovery process or prevent it altogether if the patient gives up, and effective antidepressants can make a huge difference.

CAUSES OF FALLS

One of the characteristics of disease in older adults is the difficulty of making a single diagnosis. Often the presenting symptoms may result from a variety of contributing causes, and managing the combination can be challenging. Falls come into this category. Falls are very common in older adults and they are a major cause of morbidity since they often result in fractures requiring admission to hospital (see Person-Centred Study: The Social and Health Problems of an Older Adult). There are a number of common causes of falls.

Postural Hypotension

In postural hypertension, there is a failure of the compensatory mechanism to maintain the blood pressure in the brain when the patient stands up, and so the patient faints. Postural hypotension may result from myocardial ischaemia or follow a stroke. Another very common cause of the problem is medication (e.g.

antihypertensive drugs). The autonomic nervous system is less effective in older adults and this also impairs the normal feedback mechanisms for maintaining blood pressure on standing.

Gait and Posture Disturbance

There is an age-related decline in the control of posture, balance, and gait. It is thought that this may be due to neuronal loss, particularly in the cerebellum and brain stem, and to cerebral ischaemia.

Sensory Impairment

Poor vision, parkinsonism, and sensory inattention can all contribute to older adult patients not noticing potential hazards and therefore tripping up.

Arrhythmias

Although less common as a cause of falls, arrhythmias that lead to sudden interruption of the cerebral blood flow can cause faints. They can often be treated. A Stokes–Adams attack is a temporary asystole which can be demonstrated on 24-hour electrocardiographic monitoring or event recording. It can be treated with a pacemaker or drugs.

PERSON-CENTRED STUDY: THE SOCIAL AND HEALTH PROBLEMS OF AN OLDER ADULT.

One Sunday afternoon, there is a phone call to the duty doctor from Mrs Archer's daughter. 'Something's got to be done about my mother,' she demands. 'I've come to visit her today, and the place is in a mess, there's food lying around, and the house is freezing cold. She should be in a home.' A visit to the house reveals that Mrs Archer is mildly confused but adamant that she does not want to leave her home. There is no evidence that things have markedly deteriorated, but her daughter only visits once a month and is unable to provide any support.

The following day, the general practitioner arranges for the Health Visitor for older adults to do a home visit to assess the situation. He had already done the baseline investigations, such as a full blood count, urinalysis, and thyroid function test, when he had previously seen Mrs Archer for a blood pressure check, and noticed that she was not as well as usual. No treatable causes have been discovered and a tentative diagnosis of early Alzheimer's disease has been made. The Health Visitor arranges Social Services

support and helps Mrs Archer to apply for her entitled benefits so that she can pay for some extra help. She also arranges for her to attend a day centre twice a week and organizes Meals on Wheels.

Another few weeks go by, and Mrs Archer's daughter comes to visit again one Sunday. She requests that the Health Visitor go to see her mother, saying that she should not be living on her own and that she wants something sorted out. However, Mrs Archer is still firm in her resolve that she wants to continue to live in her own home and the situation is unchanged.

The problem continues to rumble on until one morning, Mrs Archer is found on the floor by her Home Care assistant. She is admitted to hospital with a fractured neck of femur. She undergoes surgery and rehabilitation but having been in hospital for 4 weeks, she has lost her confidence and agrees to her daughter's request that she should move into a residential home. Sadly, 3 months later she dies.

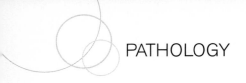
DEPRESSION

Depression is a common condition affecting people of all ages. In older adults, it may occur in isolation but it is often present with physical diseases such as strokes. It tends to present with withdrawal and apathy, and often patients have physical symptoms of depression, such as disturbed sleep patterns, weight loss, and somatic pains (e.g. headaches). In surveys using specific depression rating scales, many older adult people have unrecognized depression, which will often respond to treatment and is therefore a diagnosis well worth making.

Treatment involves correcting, if possible, any physical symptoms that may be aggravating the depression, such as chronic pain from arthritis, and also using antidepressant therapy in effective doses. Other input, such as day centres and social contacts, may also be therapeutic if loneliness and bereavement are contributing to the depression.

THE SENSORY ORGANS

As people age, they expect to experience problems with vision and hearing to the point that this is perceived as the normal ageing process. Other conditions commonly affect the older adult population but are not an inevitable consequence of ageing.

VISION

As a person ages, the pupils tend to be smaller and to be slower to react to light and accommodation, causing focusing problems. Dilatation of the pupil in darkness is reduced, which may cause problems with night vision and driving. The lens becomes less elastic, and focusing on print is increasingly difficult (presbyopia), meaning that the majority of people require magnifying lenses for reading as they age.

In the UK, about 1 per cent of the population over the age of 65 years is registered as partially sighted, which is about 70 000 people in total, and there are many more with impaired vision who are not registered. In the majority of these people, the visual problem is due to senile macular degeneration; the next most common cause is cataracts, with glaucoma and diabetic eye disease forming a sizeable minority.

Cataracts

Cataracts are opacities of the normally transparent lens. They are irreversible. The lens is an avascular structure and the cells cannot divide to repair themselves. Cataracts are uncommon under the age of 60 years, though they may develop as a response to injury

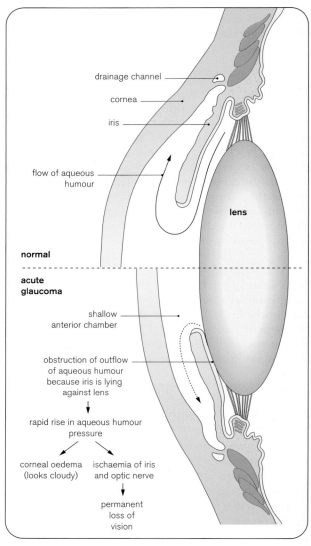

Figure 40.2 Changes caused by acute glaucoma. This diagram demonstrates the normal structure of the anterior chamber of the eye, and the obstruction of the flow of aqueous humour that leads to acute glaucoma. The rise in intraocular pressure can cause ischaemia of the optic nerve and permanent loss of vision.

or as a result of drugs such as topical steroids. Cataracts may also be congenital and this is important to diagnose early in the newborn, since the lack of stimulation to the brain visual cortex may lead to irreversible visual loss (cortical blindness) even if the cataract is removed later on.

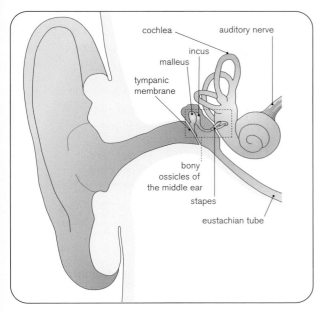

Figure 40.3 Schematic diagram of the normal ear.

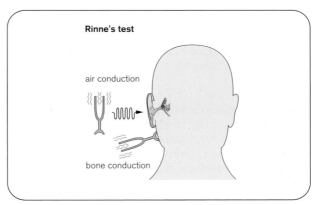

Figure 40.4 Rinne's test. Normally, air conduction of sound is better than bone conduction. The tuning fork is struck and held close to the ear until the patient can no longer hear it; it is then placed on the mastoid bone. If there is still no sound, the deafness is likely to be due to neural (nerve) damage, but if the patient can hear the sound again through bone conduction, the deafness is probably conductive (e.g. caused by damaged ossicles or ear wax).

As the lens opacifies, the person gradually notices a loss of visual acuity, usually asymmetrically. Removal of the damaged lens and replacement with a synthetic substitute is quick and extremely effective at restoring useful vision.

Glaucoma

Glaucoma is a condition in which the internal pressure within the eye is raised, causing damage to the retinal cells and optic nerve fibres and leading to visual loss. It may occur very suddenly with a blockage to the drainage channels. An acute glaucoma attack is extremely painful and can cause vomiting as well as a red eye with loss of vision. This is an emergency requiring treatment in hospital, where the pressure is reduced with drug therapy and sometimes surgery in the hope of saving the vision.

Much more commonly, the rise in pressure is insidious (chronic open-angle glaucoma) and the patient may not notice any problems until there is irretrievable damage. Peripheral vision is lost first and the end result can be 'tunnel vision' with only the central field preserved. Regular eye checks can detect rises in pressure and the condition can be controlled with eye drops and sometimes laser treatment to reduce the intraocular pressure and preserve vision (Figure 40.2).

Senile Macular Degeneration

This is a condition of unknown aetiology in which the macula, the most sensitive portion of the retina, degenerates. This results in loss of the central vision, which is extremely disabling. There is no effective treatment and patients rely on magnifying aids and bright lighting to get by.

HEARING

As people age, they will often notice loss of hearing for high-frequency noise (presbycusis) as well as difficulty in hearing when there is background noise. Another common cause of hearing difficulty is thick impacted ear wax. Approximately 60 per cent of people over the age of 70 years have impaired hearing (Figure 40.3).

Hearing loss can be divided into two categories:

- nerve deafness, in which there is dysfunction of the auditory neural pathways (e.g. presbycusis or nerve compression); and
- conductive deafness, in which there is interference with the conduction of sound from the ear drum through the ossicles – this may be due to diseases, such as otosclerosis, or to damage to the drum from infection or injury.

Audiometry testing can differentiate between the two categories of hearing loss, and on this basis hearing aids may be appropriate (Figure 40.4). Surgery may occasionally be helpful in conductive deafness.

Tinnitus

Tinnitus is a sensation of noise, buzzing, hissing, or ringing in the ears. Although some ear diseases are accompanied by tinnitus, there is usually no

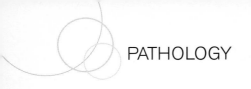

associated disease and it is often considered to be degenerative. It can be intolerable to live with and patients will resort to extreme measures to try and blot out the sound.

Ménière's Disease

Ménière's disease is a triad of acute vertigo (often with nausea and vomiting), deafness, and tinnitus. It is more common in men and usually starts between the ages of 40 and 60 years. Only one side is usually affected, although it may become bilateral. The underlying cause is not known but there seems to be an increase in the pressure of the endolymph within the labyrinth. The disease progresses until hearing is completely lost, at which time the attacks of vertigo stop. Surgery to destroy the labyrinth is sometimes used to stop the incapacitating vertigo, but as there is a chance of bilateral disease, this can be a risky manoeuvre.

THE MUSCULOSKELETAL SYSTEM

OSTEOPOROSIS

Osteoporosis denotes loss of bone mass when the bone composition is normal. This contrasts with osteomalacia (vitamin D deficiency), in which there is deficient calcification of normal amounts of bone osteoid. Bone loss from the skeleton starts to occur from around the age of 35 years, and it is difficult to define the difference between 'age-related osteoporosis' and 'pathological osteoporosis'.

Clinical Features

Osteoporosis is much more common in women than men, partly because men achieve a greater bone mass in youth and therefore have more bone mass to lose before the risk of fracture increases. Approximately 25 per cent of women over 65 are osteoporotic compared with about 5 per cent of men (Box 40.3). <5>By the age of 70, many women are left with only half their peak bone mass.

Oestrogen plays a very important role in the preservation of bone mass in women, and the most dramatic rate of bone loss is seen around the time of the menopause and in the 10 years following it. Another important hormonal influence arises from glucocorticosteroid effects. Patients who are on long-term steroid therapy (used in a variety of diseases, such as rheumatoid arthritis and asthma) are also at increased risk of developing osteoporosis. Hyperthyroidism also seems to accelerate the rate of bone loss. Other risk factors include smoking, low body weight, lack of dietary calcium, and physical inactivity.

> ### BOX 40.3 APPROXIMATE INCIDENCE ON X-RAY OF VERTEBRAL CRUSH FRACTURE
>
> | | |
> |---|---|
> | Women over 60 years | 25 per cent |
> | Men over 60 years | 5 per cent |
> | | |
> | Women over 80 years | 45 per cent |
> | Men over 80 years | 25 per cent |

Osteoporosis is usually asymptomatic until the patient suffers a fracture. This is commonly a crush fracture of a vertebral body, reducing the bone to a wedge shape and causing sudden acute back pain. If the process continues, the spine becomes kyphotic (curved), creating the characteristic appearance of the 'dowager's hump'. Other common fracture sites are the neck of the femur and the wrist. The cost of fractured necks of femur to the National Health Service runs into millions of pounds, and prevention can be very cost-effective. Sadly, admission with a fracture often signals the end of an independent life for an older adult patient, since many fail to regain full mobility, so the ongoing costs may include residential care or home support services.

The diagnosis can be made from an ordinary X-ray if the disease is advanced – the bone appears thinned and there may be evidence of old healed vertebral crush fractures. Bone density scanning may be done in order to pick up the disease at an earlier stage so that treatment can be started. However, at the moment, there is no objective evidence to support the introduction of screening on a national scale, but doctors are encouraged to seek out the 'at-risk' population for treatment (see Chapter 39).

Treatment

For women, the most effective preventative treatment is hormone replacement therapy, in which oestrogen is the bone-preserving element. Recently introduced non-hormonal treatments, such as etidronate and alendronate, appear to halt the loss of bone and in some cases partly restore the bone mass. Other important treatments include ensuring the person is taking adequate quantities of dietary calcium and is exercising regularly to maintain bone mass.

ARTHRITIC DISORDERS

Arthritic disorders can occur an any age, but they are frequently present in older adults and represent a significant part of the workload of health professionals involved in primary care. The clinical signs and symptoms of arthritic diseases and their treatments are discussed in Chapter 39; also included there are the diagnostic features of polymyalgia rheumatica and giant cell arteritis.

THE GASTROINTESTINAL SYSTEM

Older adults are often quite focused on the function of the gut, particularly the regularity of the bowel. Their diet is often limited, sometimes for financial reasons but often because of habit and routine.

CONSTIPATION

Normal transit times of food vary enormously from person to person, but an average transit time is 3–6 hours through the small intestine and about 36–72 hours through the large intestine. An overall time of about 5 days is usually accepted as the upper limit of normal. Constipation can be defined as the infrequent passage of hard stools. The urge to have a bowel movement is often suppressed either because there is no convenient toilet or the person needs assistance that is not instantly available. This sometimes leads to faecal matter building up in the gut, and if this continues, the faeces can become impacted. In turn this can cause spurious diarrhoea, when more liquid stool following behind leaks around the faecal mass with no control. If this is misdiagnosed and treated as diarrhoea, the problem is compounded.

Many drugs are potent causes of constipation, in particular analgesics of the codeine and opiate groups and tricyclic antidepressants. Some diseases, such as hypothyroidism, also lead to constipation, so a search should be made for treatable causes.

The treatment requires co-operation from the patient. Dietary fibre and fluid intake should be increased, as should physical activity, which stimulates gut activity. Patients should be encouraged to respond to the impulse to open the bowels and not to suppress it. Laxatives fall in to three main categories:

- osmotic laxatives (e.g. lactulose), which have a high concentration of sugar to draw fluid into the gut, thereby softening the stool;
- bulking agents (e.g. ispaghula husk), which are dehydrated granules taken with copious fluids – the granules swell in the gut, creating a softer, bulkier stool, which stimulates gut peristalsis
- stimulant purgatives (e.g. senna), which stimulate gut contraction but sometimes lead to pain, cramping, and diarrhoea.

MALNUTRITION

Nutrient requirements are less in older adults; for a sedentary lifestyle, the average recommended intake for women over 75 is 1810 kcal and for men, 2100 kcal. Many factors contribute to malnutrition, and many of them are social factors. Not surprisingly, in surveys of diets, men aged over 75 years who live alone have the poorest diets and were found to be deficient in a variety of nutrients. Particularly lacking were protein and some of the vitamins.

Vitamin C Deficiency

The 'tea and toast' diet is an obvious example of a diet with so little vitamin C in it that patients can develop scurvy. This causes clotting abnormalities, with gum bleeding and skin bruising, as well as poor skin healing.

Vitamin D Deficiency

Osteomalacia (vitamin D deficiency) may also develop. Dietary vitamin D comes from dairy products; sunlight is also required for adequate levels of vitamin D. Vitamin D is essential for the absorption and metabolism of calcium, and reduced levels lead to uncalcified osteoid tissue, which weakens and softens the bony structure. This may contribute to fractures, and it may co-exist with osteoporosis (see above).

Thiamine Deficiency

Alcohol misuse is not uncommon in older adults and will take a different pattern from that seen in younger patients. It tends to take the form of regular excessive intake rather than binge drinking to the point of being obviously drunk. However, over the long term this may have serious detrimental effects on liver function and nutrition. Deficiency of thiamine (vitamin B1) is common in alcoholics. Wernicke–Korsakoff syndrome, is an acute form of this deficiency, in which patients become very confused and may develop postural hypotension and visual disturbances. High doses of parenteral thiamine may reverse some of the changes but the intellectual impairment may be irreversible.

Vitamin B12 Deficiency

Vitamin B12 deficiency is a result of malabsorption of the vitamin rather than a lack of dietary intake in most cases. In order to be absorbed, the vitamin is bound to intrinsic factor, which is secreted by the parietal cells in the gastric mucosa. The vitamin B12–intrinsic factor complex is then absorbed in the terminal ileum in the small intestine. Vitamin B12 is obtained from animal products, and humans store large quantities of vitamin B12 in the liver. In pernicious anaemia, patients develop autoantibodies against their own gastric parietal cells, which block the secretion of intrinsic factor and hydrochloric acid; without intrinsic factor vitamin B12 cannot be absorbed in the ileum (see Chapter 27). Diseases of the ileum, such as Crohn's disease, may also lead to vitamin B12 deficiency, since the area of absorption of the vitamin B12–intrinsic factor complex is quite localized. In order to overcome this malabsorption of vitamin B12, it can be administered by injection to correct the deficiency.

Clinical Features of Malabsorption

Diseases causing malabsorption can lead to malnutrition either globally or for specific nutrients such as vitamins as in pernicious anaemia. The clinical sign that is most often connected with malabsorption is steatorrhoea. This is a description of the stool which has an excess of fat and is pale, frothy, floats and is difficult to flush away. The patient often has loose motions rather than frank diarrhoea and may develop symptoms related to other deficiencies. (Box 40.4) (see Chapters 6 and 34).

THE SKIN

The skin is the most obvious marker of the ageing process and some people will go to any lengths to disguise the effects. Much of the damage is related as much to ultraviolet exposure from the sun as to the passage of time, and this can be exemplified by comparing the skin of the buttocks with that of the face – they are the same age, but usually the buttock skin has not been much exposed to ultraviolet light and is less wrinkled and pigmented.

Certain skin lesions are markers of ageing, such as seborrhoeic keratoses, the rough brown warty marks that most people develop on their trunk. Also characteristic are Campbell de Morgan spots, bright red, slightly raised spots that are little haemangiomas (dilated superficial capillaries). With age, the skin becomes thinner and the underlying dermis loses some of its elastic fibres and collagen, leading to wrinkling.

The ability of the skin to heal reduces with age, making older adult people more vulnerable to ulceration such as venous ulcers and pressure sores.

VENOUS ULCERS

Venous ulcers are typically found on the lower leg and are usually associated with varicose veins. Incompetent vein valves cause back pressure and ankle oedema, making the skin less likely to heal after a trivial injury. Many patients are able to date their ulcer back to a minor

> **BOX 40.4 CONSEQUENCES OF MALABSORPTION**
>
> Iron and folate
> anaemia
> angular cheilitis (cracking of mouth angles)
>
> Protein
> oedema
>
> Fat
> weight loss
> steatorrhoea
>
> Carbohydrate
> weight loss
>
> Vitamin K
> abnormal clotting & bruising
>
> Vitamin B12
> pernicious anaemia
>
> Vitamin C
> scurvy
>
> Calcium and vitamin D
> osteomalacia, malaise, muscle weakness
>
> Vitamin A
> reduced light adaptation – night blindness

knock on a chair leg or a similar episode. The ulcer may inexorably spread, and it may require dressings for years.

Treatment involves trying to reduce local swelling by elevation and compression bandaging and encouraging calf muscle exercise to pump the blood flow back to the pelvic veins.

PRESSURE SORES

Pressure sores form as a result of immobility when there is local ischaemia, particularly on the buttocks and heels, and the skin breaks down. Healing times may be very prolonged, and the most important element is prevention. This requires meticulous skin care as well as special low-pressure mattresses and regular turning and changes of pressure areas (see Chapter 4).

SHINGLES

Shingles (herpes zoster) is more common in older patients. It occurs when the chickenpox virus has lain dormant in the nerve roots and then erupts in the distribution of one or two nerve roots. This commonly occurs on the face, in one of the three divisions of the trigeminal nerve. If the ophthalmic division is affected, the eye may be damaged by the infection. Prompt treatment with antiviral agents such as acyclovir can reduce the eruption and may protect the eye.

Older patients who suffer from shingles are also more likely to suffer from post-herpetic neuralgia, in which there is persistent sensory abnormality long after the blisters have gone. This can be very painful, with burning, soreness, or deep aching pain in the line of the nerve. It may be difficult to treat.

MALIGNANCIES

Skin malignancies are very common with increasing age, in particular the non-melanoma types, basal cell and squamous cell carcinomas. These tend to be found incidentally on routine examinations, though the patient may complain of a 'spot that just won't heal'. Basal cell carcinomas can be dealt with by local excision, since they virtually never metastasize. Squamous cell carcinomas, however, do have the potential for metastasis, and in the head and neck region they have a relatively high recurrence rate and mortality. Pipe and cigarette smokers are vulnerable to developing them on the lip, which does not have a good prognosis.

Malignant melanomas may develop at any age. They are an increasing problem, particularly in older men. They are often on the back where the patients cannot see them, and may be related to repeated sun exposure. Men who have worked outside without shirts have been exposed to high levels of ultraviolet radiation. Today's older population also includes a generation of men who served overseas in the World Wars, and they too had high levels of prolonged sun exposure (Figure 40.5). Unless melanomas are detected early when they are still thin (superficial spreading), they rapidly become deeply invasive (nodular) with a high mortality. The death rate from melanoma now exceeds that of cancer of the cervix in the UK (see Chapters 3 and 5).

MALIGNANT DISEASE

In the UK, cancer is the second most common cause of death after cardiovascular disease in people over the age of 65. At all ages, cancers in four sites account for 60 per cent of cancer mortality, and all of these are frequently encountered in older patients; lung, breast, colorectal, and stomach cancers. The increase in incidence of malignant disease in older adults has been explained in various ways:

- increasing age means longer exposure to environmental influences, such as ultraviolet radiation, diet, and cigarette smoke;
- 'immunological surveillance', the destruction of random abnormal cells with malignant potential, becomes less efficient with age; and

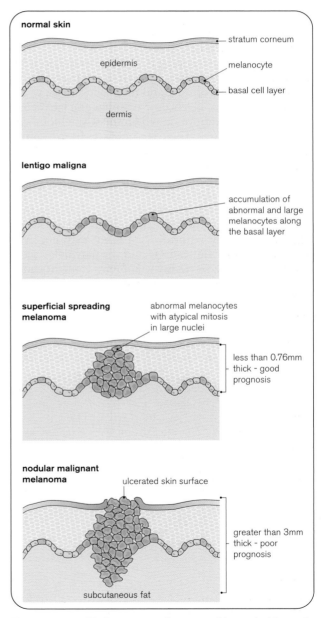

Figure 40.5 Malignant melanoma. Normal skin and three types of malignant melanoma are shown.

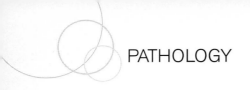

- changes in hormonal balance may predispose to increased vulnerability to such hormone-dependent malignancies as cancer of the breast and cancer of the prostate.

In addition to these factors, the influence of genetic predisposition probably plays a part.

RESPONSE TO TREATMENT

Most of the individual cancers are covered within specific chapters. However, some general principles apply to the treatment and prognosis of malignant disease in the older patient.

Because life expectancy is shorter overall, control of the disease rather than aggressive attempts at cure may be more appropriate and more acceptable to the patient. For example, chronic lymphocytic leukaemia is an indolent condition in which the white blood cell count gradually rises. There is a predisposition to infection and general malaise. However, the older adult patient is much more likely to die of another disease before the leukaemia kills him, and so aggressive chemotherapy is not appropriate.

Comparing survival rates also depends on the time of diagnosis, and in the older adult this is often delayed. The older woman with a breast lump may not even notice it until it is quite large, and she may delay seeking treatment if she is frightened of what it might entail. She will not fall within the mammographic screening programme, in which tiny non-palpable lesions are being detected, and so comparing survival rates of older and younger women is not very useful.

Age also seems sometimes to moderate the disease process. It is not uncommon for an older woman with a large breast cancer to have a prolonged survival on tamoxifen treatment alone, without evidence of metastatic spread. Likewise, in men, the incidence of prostate cancer at routine post-mortem is very much higher than the incidence presented during life. This suggests that case-finding and screening may not change the individual's life expectancy and may increase morbidity from worry and any treatment related effects.

Reactions to Radiotherapy and Chemotherapy

Radiotherapy and chemotherapy exert the same toxic effects on the tumour as in younger patients, but older patients are more susceptible to the side-effects. They may have impaired renal function, which means that doses of the chemotherapy have to be adjusted, and they may not tolerate the gastrointestinal effects of nausea, vomiting, and diarrhoea as well as younger patients. Associated diseases, such as heart disease, may also mean some drugs (e.g. daunorubicin) are unsuitable for use in older adults. Palliative radiotherapy for localized bone pain caused by metastases may be very effective in relieving the pain with minimal side-effects (see also Chapters 12 and 14).

SUMMARY

This chapter has given a brief view of the difference that the age of the patient can make to both the diagnosis and management of disease. It can be a great challenge to sort out the treatable from the untreatable, but at the same time maintain the patient's quality of life and not strive to prolong a life of pain and distress at all costs.

KEY POINTS

- In old age, multiple pathologies are common and disease processes interact with each other.
- Dementia is a description of a set of symptoms and signs and has many different causes, some of which are reversible. Alzheimer's disease is irreversible and is the most frequent cause of dementia in the UK.
- Strokes can be prevented in a significant number of people by treating hypertension and anticoagulating patients with atrial fibrillation.
- Coronary heart disease causes most deaths over the age of 65, followed by cancers of the lung, breast, colon, and stomach.

- Osteoporosis describes a loss of bone mass in which the bone composition is normal, whereas osteomalacia occurs when there is a normal amount of osteoid bone but it is not calcified owing to abnormalities of calcium and vitamin D metabolism. Osteoporosis can be partly prevented by use of oestrogen in menopausal women.
- Glaucoma, senile macular degeneration, and cataracts are responsible for the majority of cases of partial and complete visual loss in the UK.

FURTHER READING

Allen SC (1998) Medicine in Old Age, 4th edition. Churchill Livingstone, London.

Audit Commission (1995) United They Stand. Co-ordinating Care for Elderly People with Hip Fractures. Her Majesty's Stationery Office, London.

Benbow SJ, Walsh A, Gill GV (1997) Diabetes in institutionalised elderly people: a forgotten population? BMJ 314:1868–9.

Boutsen Y, Devogelaer JP, Malghem J, Noel H, Nagant de Deuxchaisnes C (1996) Antacid-induced osteomalacia. Clin Rheumatol 15:75–80.

Caris-Verhallen WM, Kerkstra A, Bensing JM (1997) The role of communication in nursing care for elderly people: a review of the literature. J Adv Nurs 25:915–33.

Compston JE (1997) Prevention and management of osteoporosis. Current trends and future prospects. Drugs 53:727–35.

Coni N, Davison W, Webster S (1991) Lecture Notes on Geriatrics, 4th edition. Blackwell Science, Oxford.

Curl PE, Warren JJ (1997) Nutritional screening for the elderly: a CNS role. Clin Nurse Spec 11:153–8.

Daly GM, Mitchell RD (1996) Case management in the community setting. Nurs Clin North Am 31:527–34.

Esser K, Martin GM (eds) (1995) Molecular Aspects of Aging. J Wiley and Sons, Chichester.

Gage BF, Cardinalli AB, Albers GW, Owens DK (1995) Cost-effectiveness of warfarin and aspirin for prophylaxis of stroke in patients with nonvalvular atrial fibrillation. JAMA 274:1839–45.

Hodkinson HM (1972) Evaluation of a mental test score for the assessment of mental impairment in the elderly. Age Ageing 1:233–8.

Khaw KT (1997) Healthy aging. BMJ 315:1090–6.

Monane M, Avorn J (1996) Medications and falls. Causation, correlation, and prevention [Review]. Clin Geriatr Med 12:847–58.

National Institute for Aging – Alzheimer's Association Working Group (1996) Apolipoprotein E genotyping in Alzheimer's disease. Lancet 347:1091–5.

Pahor M, Applegate WB (1997) Geriatric medicine. BMJ 315:1071–4.

Report of Health and Social Subjects 41: Dietary reference values for food energy and nutrients for the UK. Report of the Panel on Dietary Reference Values of the Committee on Medical Aspects of Food Policy (1991) Her Majesty's Stationery Office, London.

Thomas RJ (1997) Seizures and epilepsy in the elderly. Arch Intern Med 157:605–17.

APPENDIX 1
VITAMINS, MINERALS AND THEIR SOURCES

VITAMIN B1 (THIAMINE)

An important coenzyme; essential for acetylcholine synthesis; thiamine triphosphate is found in peripheral nerve endings. Deficiency affects neurological function; conditions associated include beri-beri, peripheral neuropathy, and Wernicke–Korsakoff syndrome in alcoholics.

Sources: meat, eggs, grains, green vegetables, nuts.

VITAMIN B2 (RIBOFLAVIN)

Found in the coenzymes FMN and FAD. Deficiency inhibits cellular respiration and is associated with dermatitis and capillary growth in the cornea of alcoholics.

Sources: meat, milk cheese, grains, gut flora.

NIACIN (NICOTINIC ACID)

Can be synthesized very inefficiently from tryptophan. Forms the active part of the coenzymes NAD and NADP. Deficiency causes pellagra (dermatitis, diarrhoea and dementia). Deficiency is common in maize-based diets because high leucine levels inhibit its synthesis from tryptophan.

Sources: meat, fish, grains, legumes.

VITAMIN B6 (PYRIDOXINE)

Cofactor for transamination enzymes; required for glycogen breakdown and synthesis of serotonin, noradrenalin, and myelin. Deficiency and high doses affect neurological function. The use of oral contraceptives may increase dietary requirements.

Sources: meat, fish, grains, yeast, yoghurt, gut flora; destroyed by food processing.

VITAMIN B12 (CYANOCOBALAMIN)

Some similarities to haemoglobin, but contains cobalt rather than iron. Absorption requires intrinsic factor secreted by the gastric parietal cells. Lack of intrinsic factor causes pernicious anaemia. Required for synthesis of methionine (with folate) and fatty acids. Deficiency leads to pernicious anaemia, loss of myelin from nerves, and disruption of cell membranes.

Sources: meat, liver, fish, eggs, milk, cheese.

BIOTIN

Forms a prosthetic group in enzymes that transfer carbon dioxide. Deficiency is rare but is associated with prolonged antibiotic use (which destroys gut bacteria) and a high consumption of raw eggs (which contain a binding-protein, avidin).

Sources: eggs, liver, yeast, gut flora.

FOLIC ACID (FOLATE)

Required for DNA, choline, and amino acid synthesis. Deficiency very common world-wide as a result of poor diet or heavy demand on the body caused by infections (malaria), haemorrhage, pregnancy, and drug interactions; also associated with alcoholism (megaloblastic anaemia). The use of oral contraceptives decreases folate absorption and increases its metabolism.

Sources: green vegetables, grains, legumes, liver; degraded by boiling for only 10 minutes. Supplementation is given during the first 12 weeks of pregnancy and recommended preconceptually to reduce the risk of neural tube defect.

PANTOTHENIC ACID

A component of acetyl coenzyme A; deficiency very rare.

Sources: fish, grains, legumes, meat, vegetables, gut flora.

VITAMIN C (ASCORBIC ACID)

Required for collagen synthesis and as an antioxidant (protects vitamin A, E, and some of the B vitamins); may reduce cancer incidence. Deficiency slows wound healing and impairs maintenance of connective tissues and bone; scurvy may result. High doses are claimed to prevent the common cold (though this is controversial) but may also cause kidney stones and scurvy if suddenly withdrawn. Smokers metabolize and excrete vitamin C rapidly.

Sources: citrus fruits, peppers, tomatoes, potatoes. Oxidized by overcooking and degraded during prolonged food storage.

FAT-SOLUBLE VITAMINS

VITAMIN A (RETINOL)

Retinol is the active part of the visual pigment rhodopsin and is essential for normal development of mucous-secreting cells. Deficiency causes night blindness, loss of mucous secretion, and serious eye disorders. The anti-oxidant effects of vitamin A may protect against cancers, and derivatives are used in the treatment of psoriasis and acne. It may be teratogenic. Excessive intake is associated with liver damage and abnormal bone growth in children, but the dangers are well recognized.

Sources: eggs, liver, milk, yellow and green vegetables, stores in liver.

VITAMIN D (CHOLECALCIFEROL)

A group of cholesterol-like compounds; synthesized by the action of ultraviolet light on the skin. Essential for calcium and phosphorus homoeostasis in the body. Deficiency characterized by rickets in children and osteomalacia in adults; may be precipitated by migration from sunny to low-sun countries. Overdoses also lead to calcium loss from bone.

Sources: eggs, fish oils, fortified dairy products, cereals, ultraviolet on skin.

VITAMIN E (TOCOPHEROL)

A group of antioxidants (tocopherols), which scavenge toxic free radicals and oxygen in the body, protecting membranes and fats. Alpha-tocopherol is a permitted antioxidant in baby foods.

Sources: nuts, seed oils, stores in liver and fat.

VITAMIN K

Cofactor for the synthesis of blood clotting factors. Deficiency increases clotting times; most common in neonates and the elderly with poor fat absorption. Routine supplementation for neonates to prevent haemorrhagic disease of the newborn.

Sources: liver, spinach (K1), cabbage (K2), gut flora (K2), stores in liver. Also available as a synthetic derivative (K3).

MINERALS

CALCIUM

The most common element in the body. Hydroxyapatite (a complex form of calcium phosphate) is the main constituent of the hard component of bones and teeth. Important for muscular contraction, blood clotting, and as an enzyme cofactor and a second messenger. A calcium-rich diet, exercise, adequate vitamin D, and trace element intake throughout life optimizes bone mass Postmenopausal osteoporosis results from a reduction in oestrogen, which promotes bone deposition. Hormone-replacement therapy therefore assists in maintaining bone mass.

Sources: milk, cheese, yoghurt, green vegetables, endogenous stores in bones; fibre and plant phytic acids reduce gut absorption; caffeine increases excretion of calcium in the kidney.

CHLORINE

Chloride is the most common anion in the extracellular fluid. Important ion in the maintenance of osmotic balance in body fluids and in the transport of carbon dioxide in the blood (chloride shift mechanism). Hydrochloric acid is secreted in the stomach.

Sources: cooking salt, table salt.

COBALT

Trace element; essential constituent of vitamin B12
Sources: fish, liver, meat.

COPPER

Trace element; cofactor for enzymes such as ferrooxidase, which oxidizes iron to the ferric form for blood transport. Transported by the protein ceruloplasmin in the blood. Deficiency leads to anaemia, hypercholesterolaemia, bone demineralization, and weakening of blood vessels.

Sources: grains, legumes, nuts, liver, seafood, stores in liver.

FLUORINE

Common in the body (2.6 g in total) but regarded as an important rather than an essential dietary component. Fluoride ions influences the crystalline structure of tooth enamel and, at a concentration of 1 mg/l in drinking water (Royal College of Physicians recommendation) minimizes the incidence of dental caries. Mottling of tooth enamel and increase bone deposition associated with excessive intake. Fluoride is also an enzyme cofactor.

Sources: drinking water (natural or added), fluoride toothpaste, most foods.

IODINE

Component of thyroid hormones; deficiency causes goitre (enlarged thyroid) and is rare. Oral iodide or iodate used to protect the thyroid from radioactive forms of iodine released in nuclear accidents.

Sources: sea salt, supplement in table salt, seafood.

IRON

Essential constituent (in the ferrous form) of the oxygen carriers myoglobin and haemoglobin and of the cytochromes, which are enzymes or electron carriers. Iron is a constituent of the enzyme monoamine oxidase, which is involved in neurotransmitter synthesis. Total body content 4.2 g. Iron is toxic in its free form as and is therefore always bound to proteins (transferrin) for transport and storage as ferritin and lactoferrin. Most body iron is recycled but menstruation significantly increases losses (an additional 9 mmol/day above normal losses of 20 mmol/day). White blood cells use iron to generate free radicals to attack microbes. Iron-deficiency anaemia is one of the commonest nutritional deficiencies world-wide (affecting two-thirds of women and children in developing countries). Deficiency reduces the capacity for physical activity and impairs immune function. Permanent loss of learning abilities and abnormal behaviours may occur in children. Iron supplements are a common cause of poisoning in children. Iron overload can also result from repeated blood transfusions and the use of iron cooking vessels.

Sources: liver, meat, shellfish, dried apricots, stores in liver. Haem iron most readily absorbed. Added to bread flour and found in eggs and vegetables but only 5 per cent is absorbed from these sources.

MAGNESIUM

Required as an enzyme cofactor (ATPases), for bone formation, and for neuromuscular transmission, which is impaired when levels are low or excessive.

Sources: green vegetables, legumes, milk, seafood; stores in liver.

MANGANESE

Trace element essential for bone metabolism and as an enzyme cofactor; required for synthesis of urea, fatty acids, and cholesterol.

Sources: green vegetables, grains, nuts, legumes, stores in liver.

PHOSPHORUS

Hydroxyapatite (a complex form of calcium phosphate) is the main constituent of the hard component of bones and teeth. Phosphates are common throughout metabolism (in DNA and RNA, sugar phosphates, etc) and act as buffers in body fluids. Phosphorus and calcium are metabolism closely linked.

Sources: cheese, fish, milk, meat; stores in bones; vitamin D required for absorption.

SODIUM AND POTASSIUM

Sodium and potassium are the most common extracellular and intracellular metal ions respectively; they have key role in the transmission of nerve impulses where the sodium–potassium balance is critical. Hypokalaemia (low serum potassium) is commonly associated with starvation, diseases of the gastrointestinal tract, diabetic coma and alkalosis. It is a side effect of many drugs. Hyperkalaemia is rare and results from excessive potassium intake or acidosis. Both conditions impair neuromuscular transmission.

Sources: most foods plus added cooking salt and table salt.

SULPHUR

Found in thiamine, biotin, and the amino acids cysteine and methionine. Required for the synthesis of peptides and proteins such as insulin and keratin.

Sources: eggs, meat.

ZINC

Trace element but common in the body (2.6 g in total). Important enzyme cofactor (notably for carbonic anhydrase); essential for normal protein and membrane metabolism, taste bud development, and for DNA and RNA synthesis. Deficiency is rare; characterized by rashes, dermatitis, anorexia, and growth retardation; may occur with prolonged parenteral feeding.

Sources: grains, legumes, meat, seafood.

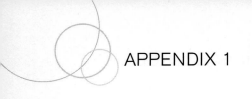

APPENDIX 1

APPENDIX 2
REFERENCE RANGES

INVESTIGATIONS PERFORMED BY CLINICAL PATHOLOGY LABORATORIES

Note: These reference ranges apply locally to St. George's Hospital, London, and may differ slightly between laboratories. Therefore it is advisable to check before interpreting individual results.

CLINICAL CHEMISTRY: BLOOD TESTS

Test	Reference Range
UREA AND ELECTROLYTE PROFILE	
Sodium	135–145 mmol/L
Potassium	3.5–4.7 mmol/L
Urea	2.5–8.0 mmol/L
Creatinine	60–110 µmol/L
Chloride	98–109 mmol/L
Bicarbonate	22–28 mmol/L

Test	Reference Range
LIVER PROFILE	
Bilirubin (total)	<17 mmol/L
Alkaline phosphatase	30–100 U/L
Albumin	38–48 g/L
Alanine aminotransferase (ALT)	5–40 U/L
Gamma glutamyl trans-peptidase (γGT)	<60 U/L (males)
	<30 U/L (females)
Total protein	60–80 g/L

Test	Reference Range
BONE PROFILE	
Calcium (total)	2.15–2.55 mmol/L
Phosphate	0.75–1.50 mmol/L
Albumin	38–48 g/L
Alkaline phosphatase	30–100 U/L

Test	Reference Range
ACTH	<50 ng/L (0900)
Aldosterone	100–450 pmol/L
	(Overnight recumbency)
Ammonia	<50 µmol/L
Amylase	20–80 U/L
Androstenedione:	
adult	4–11 nmol/L
child	<3.6 nmol/L
Angiotensin-converting enzyme	25–105 U/L
Aspartate aminotransferase (ALT)	10–35 U/L
Bilirubin (total)	<17 µmol/L
Bilirubin (conjugated)	<9 µmol/L
C-reactive protein	<8 mg/L
Caeruloplasmin	0.24–0.63 g/L
Calcitonin	<0.08 µg/L
Carotene	<0.35 mg/L
Catecholamines:	
Noradrenaline	<5 nmol/L
Adrenaline	<1 nmol/L
Cholesterol	3.3–7.3 mmol/L
desirable:	<5.2 mmol/L
Copper	14–23 µmol/L
Cortisol (total)	
0900	150–650 nmol/L
midnight	30–250 nmol/L
Creatine kinase (CK)	30–250 U/L (males)
	30–180 U/L females
Creatine kinase (CK-MB)	<5 µg/L
Dehydroepiandrosterone sulphate	0.7–11.5 µmol/L
Ferritin:	
males	15–300 µg/L
females	15–200 µg/L

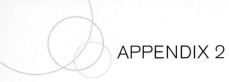

APPENDIX 2

Test	Reference Range
Follicle stimulating hormone (FSH):	
males	1–10 IU/L
follicular/luteal	1–10/2–9 IU/L:
mid-cycle peak	5–27 IU/L:
post-menopausal	>30 IU/L
Gastrin	<40 pmol/L
Glucose	
fasting	<6.0 mmol/L
2 h post 75g glucose	<8.0 mmol/L
Growth hormone	<10 MU/L
Haemoglobin A,C	3.5–5.5%
HDL cholesterol:	
males	0.9–1.9 mmol/L
females	1.1–2.6 mmol/L
17-Hydroxyprogesterone	<20 nmol/L
25-Hydroxycholecalciferol	8–75 nmol/L
Iron	14–30 µmol/L
Lactate	0.6–2.4 mmol/L
Lactate dehydrogenase (LDH)	100–200 U/L
LDL cholesterol	<3.5 mmol/L (desirable)
Lead (adults)	<1.4 µmol/L
(children)	<0.5 µmol/L
Lipoprotein (a)	>300 mg/L associated with increased risk of IHD
Luteinising hormone (LH)	
males:	1–9 IU/L
follicular/luteal:	2–9/1–13 IU/L:
mid-cycle peak:	14–90 IU/L
post-menopausal:	>15 IU/L
Magnesium	0.70–0.95 mmol/L
Oestradiol:	
early follicular:	110–183 pmol/L
preovulatory	550–1650 pmol/L
luteal	550–845 pmol/L
post-menopausal	<90 pmol/L
males	<130 pmol/L
Osmolality (serum)	280–300 mmol/kg
Parathyroid hormone	1–6.9 pmol/L
Phenylalanine	0.18–0.48 mmol/L (*Treatment range*)
Progesterone:	
follicular phase	<3 nmol/L
luteal phase	10–80 nmol/L

Test	Reference Range
Prolactin	<480 mU/L
Pyruvate	<80 µmol/L
Sex hormone binding globulin	
(SHBG) female	20–120 nmol/L
male	15–75 nmol/L
Testosterone:	
males	9–24 nmol/L
females	0.5–2.5 nmol/L
prepubertal	<1.1 nmol/L
Testosterone/SHBG ratio:	
females	<4
males	20–100
Thyroxine (free T4) (adults)	11–23 pmol/L
Thyroid-stimulating hormone (TSH)	0.5–4.0 mU/L
Triglyceride (fasting)	0.8–2.0 mmol/L
Triiodothyronine (adults) (free T3)	4.0–8.0 pmol/L
Troponin T	<0.2 µg/L
Urate	0.15–0.42 mmol/L
Vitamin A	0.4–1.1 mg/L
Vitamin D (25-OH cholecalciferol)	8–75 nmol/L
Vitamin E	5.3–16.3 mg/L
Zinc	11–24 µmol/L

CLINICAL CHEMISTRY: URINE TESTS

Test	Reference Range
Bilirubin (ictotest) [random urine]	Not detected
Calcium (total) [24h urine (U)]	2.5–7.5 mmol/24h
Catecholamines:	
Noradrenaline	<500 nmol/24h
Adrenaline [24 h urine (U~HCL~)]	<100 nmol/24h
Cortisol [24h urine]	60–260 nmol/24h
Creatinine clearance	80–140 ml/min
Cystine/homocystine [random urine]	Trace present (*qualitative*)
Electrolyte profile:	
Sodium [24 h urine (U)	40–220 mmol/24h
Potassium or random urine	40–90 mmol/24h
Urea (Na/K)]	250–500 mmol/24h
Creatinine (male)	10–18 mmol/24h
(female)	8–16 mmol/24h
Osmolality [random urine]	100–1400 mmol/kg

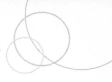

AMNIOTIC FLUIDS

Alpha-fetoprotein	Depends on gestational age

CEREBROSPINAL FLUID

Glucose	Related to plasma glucose (normal = 2/3 value)

FAECES

Fat (faecal)	<18 mmol/24h
Occult blood	Not detected
Porphyrins (qualitative)	Not detected

SWEAT

Sodium	<70 mmol/L

HAEMATOLOGY

Adult Reference Range

White cell count (WBC)	$4.0 –11.0 \times 10^9$/L	
Red cell count (RBC)	$4.5–6.0 \times 10^{12}$/L	(male)
	$3.8–5.2 \times 10^{12}$/L	(female)
Haemoglobin	13.0–17.0 g/dl	(male)
	12.0–16.0 g/dl	(female)
Packed cell volume/	0.40–0.52 l/l	(male)
haematocrit	0.37–0.47 l/l	(female)
Mean cell volume (MCV)	78–97fl	
Mean cell haemoglobin (MCH)	27 – 32 pg	
Platelets	$150–400 \times 10^9$/L	
Reticulocytes	0.2 – 2.0%	
	$20 – 100 \times 10^9$/L	
Erythrocyte sedimentation rate (ESR)		
<50 years	1–10 mm/hr	
>50 years	<20 mm/hr	
Plasma viscosity	1.1–1.35 mPa.s	
Differential WBC		
Neutrophils	$1.6 – 7.5 \times 10^9$/L	
Eosinophils	0.04 –0.45	
Basophils	<0.1	
Lymphocytes	1.5–4.0	
Monocytes	0.1–0.8	
Vitamin B12	150–1000 ng/L	
Red cell folate	150–750 µg/L	
Schilling Test	10–35% in 24 hours	
Haemoglobin A2	1–3.5%	
Haemoglobin F	<1.0%	
G6PD	Reported as normal or reduced-assay will then be performed.	
Red cell volume	30 ± 5 ml/kg (male)	
	25 ± 5 ml/kg (female)	
Plasma volume	45 ± 5ml/kg	

Total blood volume	70 ± 10 ml/kg

Coagulation:

Screening Tests

Prothrombin time	11–15 secs
Activated partial thromboplastin time	34–47 secs
Thrombin time	11–15 secs
Reptilase time	control + 4 secs
Fibrinogen	2–4 g/L
Fibrin(ogen) degradation products (FDP)	<8 mg/L
D-dimers	<0.5mg/L

Anticoagulant Control Values

INR (Warfarin)	0.8–1.1
APTT (Heparin iv)	60–140 sec
Anti-Xa (Heparin sc)	0.0 –0.15 u/ml

Thrombophilia screening

Lupus inhibitor	Written comment
Antithrombin III	70–150 iu/dl
Protein S	70 – 150% of normal control plasma
Protein C	70–150 iu/dl
Activated Protein C Resistance	ratio > 2.0

BLOOD TRANSFUSION

For blood grouping, antibody screening and cross-matching, provide 6 ml in special red cap EDTA tube.

HLA (Tissue) typing	20 ml EDTA anticoagulated blood
Cold Agglutinin Titre	Discuss with laboratory. 5 ml clotted blood which must be kept at 37ºC.

IMMUNOLOGY

References ranges taken from: PRU Handbook of Clinical Immunochemistry (5th edition). PRU publications; 1996. By kind permission of editors: A. Milford Ward, Pamela G. Riches, R. Fifield & A.M. Smith

ALBUMIN

Hospital patients (a.m. sample)	30–42 g/L	male
	27–42 g/L	female
Healthy ambulant individuals	35–47 g/L	male
	33–47 g/L	female

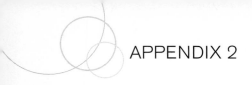

APPENDIX 2

α1ANTITRYPSIN

Age	5th	50th	95th centile
		(values in g/L)	
Birth	0.9	1.6	2.2
6 months	0.8	1.2	1.8
1 year	1.1	1.5	2.0
5 years	1.1	1.5	2.2
10 years	1.4	1.7	2.3
15 years	1.2	1.6	2.0
Adult	1.1	1.6	2.1

α1MICROGLOBULIN

Normal adult urine   less than 15 mg/L

or 1.3 mg/mmol creatinine

α2HS GLYCOPROTEIN

Adults   0.4–0.9 g/L

α2MACROGLOBULIN

	male	female
Birth – 15 years	2.8–6.7 g/L	2.8–6.7 g/L
16 – 30 years	2.0–4.5 g/L	2.2–5.0 g/L
31 – 45 years	1.6–4.0 g/L	1.8–4.5 g/L
over 45 years	1.3–3.5 g/L	1.4–4.0 g/L

ANTITHROMBIN III

antigenic (g/L)	male	female
newborn	0.11–0.18	0.11–0.18
1–35 years	0.21–0.36	0.21–0.36
36–55 years	0.20–0.33	0.19–0.32
over 55 years	0.18–0.30	0.21–0.34
functional (kU/L)		
newborn	0.4–0.6	0.4–0.6
1–35 years	0.8–1.2	0.8–1.2
36–55 years	0.7–1.1	0.6–1.1
over 55 years	0.6–1.0	0.8–1.2

ALPHA-FETOPROTEIN

All values in relation to BS 72/227

Serum Birth	50–150 MU/L
1–5 weeks	5–30 kU/L
over 2 months	<10 kU/L
50 – 70 years	<15 kU/L
70 – 90 years	< 20 kU/L

Maternal serum weeks gestation	values in kU/L with body weight correction		
	10th	50th	95th centile
14	<10	19	50
15	<10	24	60
16	10	31	69
17	11	37	81
18	13	43	98
19	15	50	115
20	18	60	123
21	21	67	142

Amniotic fluid weeks gestation	values in MU/L	
	50th centile	Discriminant value
13	21.9	65.7
14	18.1	54.3
15	15.0	45.0
16	11.9	41.7
17	10.0	35.0
18	8.8	30.8
19	6.9	27.6
20	5.6	22.4
21	5.0	20.0
22	4.4	17.6

β2MICROGLOBULIN

Serum 1.2–2.4 mg/L

CSF   0.1–2.8 mg/L

Urine <300 μg/L

CA-125

mean	7.8 kU/L
99th centile	30 kU/L

CA-153

mean	13 kU/L
99th centile	30 kU/L

CA-199

mean	16 kU/L
99th centile	35 kU/L

CEA

Non smokers   less than 2.5 μg/L

CERULOPLASMIN

values in g/L

	5th	95th centile
<4 months	0.08	0.23
to 1 year	0.12	0.35
1–10 years	0.20	0.40
10–13 years	0.15	0.23
adult	0.20	0.60

COMPLEMENT

values in g/L

	5th	95th centile
C3	0.75	1.65
C4	0.14	0.54
C5	0.08	0.12
C1 INH	0.15	0.35
C1 INH-functional	75%	125%
C4-binding protein	0.14	0.22

COMPLEMENT ACTIVATION PRODUCTS

C3a	10–570 µg/L
C3d	<150 mg/L
C4a	102–212 µg/L
C5a	<10 µg/L

CORTISOL-BINDING GLOBULIN

normal adults	20–50 mg/L

CRP

normal adults	less than 10 mg/L

CSF PROTEINS

50th centile values

Age	Albumin g/L	IgG g/L
<30 years	0.17	0.017
31–40 years	0.18	0.021
41–50 years	0.20	0.024
51–60 years	0.24	0.027
61–77 years	0.24	0.026
CSF/serum IgG–Albumin Index		<0.7
IgG - Total protein		<10%
Tau - asialotransferrin		3–5 mg/L

HAPTOGLOBIN

0.5–2.0 g/L	male
0.4–1.6 g/L	female

HUMAN CHORIONIC GONADOTROPHIN (BETA-HCG)

Male and non-pregnant female	less than 2 IU/L
free beta chain	
Male and non-pregnant female	less than 0.1 µg/L

IMMUNOGLOBULINS IgG, IgA and IgM

Age	IgG g/L	IgA g/L	IgM g/L
Cord	5.2–18.0	<0.02	0.02–0.2
Weeks			
0–2	5.0–17.0	0.01–0.08	0.05–0.2
2–6	3.9–13.0	0.02–0.15	0.08–0.4
6–12	2.1–7.7	0.05–0.4	0.15–0.7
Months			
3–6	2.4–8.8	0.10–0.5	0.2–1.0
6–9	3.0–9.0	0.15–0.7	0.4–1.6
9–12	3.0–10.9	0.20–0.7	0.6–2.1
Years			
1–2	3.1–13.8	0.3–1.2	0.5–2.2
2–3	3.7–15.8	0.3–1.3	0.5–2.2
3–6	4.9–16.1	0.4–2.0	0.5–2.0
6–9	5.4–16.1	0.5–2.4	0.5–1.8
9–12	5.4–16.1	0.7–2.5	0.5–1.8
12–15	5.4–16.1	0.8–2.8	0.5–1.9
15–45	6.0–16.0	0.8–2.8	0.5–1.9
over 45	6.0–16.0	0.8–4.0	0.5–2.0

IgG SUBCLASSES

	IgG1	IgG2	IgG3	IgG4
Cord blood	3.6–8.4	1.2–4.0	0.3–1.5	<0.5
–6 months	1.5–3.0	0.3–0.5	0.1–0.6	<0.5
–2 years	2.3–5.8	0.3–2.9	0.1–0.8	<0.5
–5 years	2.3–6.4	0.7–4.5	0.1–1.1	<0.8
–10 years	3.6–7.3	1.4–4.5	0.3–1.1	<1.0
–15 years	3.8–7.7	1.3–4.6	0.2–1.2	<1.1
Adult	3.2–10.2	1.2–6.6	0.2–1.9	<1.3

IgA SUBCLASSES

Normal adult values	IgA1	0.7–2.3 g/L
	IgA2	0.1–0.5 g/L

IMMUNOGLOBULIN LIGHT CHAINS

Serum kappa		5.0–13.0 g/L
lamda		3.0–6.0 g/L
kappa:lambda ratio		1.0–2.7

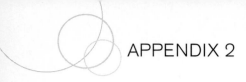

APPENDIX 2

IgE

values in kU/L WHO 75/502

	median	+1 SD
Newborn	0.5	5
–3 months	3	11
–1 year	8	29
–5 years	15	52
–10 years	18	63
–15 years	22	75
Adult	26	81

Racial factors may be important.

ALLERGEN SPECIFIC IgE

Grade	Units	Interpretation
0	<0.35	Negative
1	0.35–0.7	Weak positive
2	0.7–3.5	Positive
3	3.5–17.5	Positive
4	17.5–52.5	Strong positive
5	52.5–100	Strong positive
6	>100	Strong positive

PROSTATE SPECIFIC ANTIGEN

Normal males	values in µg/L
– 49 yrs	0.1–2.5
50–59	0.1–3.5
60–69	0.1–4.5
70–79	0.1–6.5

TAU PROTEIN

Tau -	asialotransferin	3–5 mg/L lumbar CSF
Tau -	Alzheimer's disease associated	
	Tau	55–285 ng/L
	PHF-tau	140–1140 ng/L

PROTEINS IN URINE

Total Protein		**less than 150 mg/day**
Albumin	day or 24 hr	less than 20 mg/24h
		or 14 µg/min
		or 2 mg/mmol creatinine
	overnight	less than 10 µg/min
		or 1.5 mg/mmol creatinine
α1microglobulin		less than 15 mg/L
		or 1.3 mg/mmol creatinine
β2microglobulin		less than 300 µg/L
		or 25 µg/mmol creatinine
Retinol-binding protein		less than 15 µg/mmol
		creatinine
IgG-Albumin clearance ratio		
	selective	<0.16
	moderately selective	0.16–0.30
	non selective	>0.3

GLOSSARY

Ablate To remove (e.g. by excision, amputation, cytotoxicity)

Acellular vaccine Vaccine made of soluble products of an organism and free of whole cells

Acetylation An important route of drug metabolism, which is genetically controlled

Achlorhydria Lack of hydrochloric acid in the stomach

Acquired immunodeficiency syndrome (AIDS) A syndrome where there is progressive immunodeficiency caused by the human immunodeficiency virus (HIV) infection of CD4+ cells (e.g. T helper cells, macrophages)

Activated immune cell An immune cell active in the immune response (e.g. having made contact with an antigen or in response to cytokine stimulation)

Adverse drug reaction (ADR) An unwanted drug reaction that does the patient harm

Aerobic Refers to energy-generating metabolic reactions that require oxygen

Agglutination Clumping together

Agonist A drug or other substance that mimics the action of a naturally occurring chemical substance at a receptor site

Albumin A major binding-protein for many natural substances and drugs

Alkylating agent Used with respect to cytotoxic drugs, such as cyclophosphamide, that interfere with mitosis in rapidly dividing cells by replacing a hydrogen atom on DNA with an alkyl group; as a result the DNA can not be effectively copied

Allergen An antigen that elicits an IgE antibody response, causing a hypersensitivity type I (allergic) reaction

Allogeneic graft donation Graft donation in which the donor is genetically unrelated to the recipient

Alternative pathway A complement pathway which is set off by the presence of lipopolysaccharide and involves C3, factors B and D, and properdin

Anaerobic organisms Bacteria that fail to grow in the presence of oxygen; some may be extremely fastidious and die in the presence of trace of oxygen

Analgesic A drug that relieves pain

Anaphylaxis Induced hypersensitivity of tissues to a specific antigen (e.g. a drug), resulting in release of histamine and other cell constituents. Symptoms include wheezing, chest tightness, abdominal pain, nausea and vomiting, and circulatory and respiratory collapse

Antagonist A substance or drug that blocks or opposes the action of an agonist

Antibody A protein (immunoglobulin) produced by a B lymphocyte or plasma cell that specifically binds to part of an antigen that prompted its secretion

Antibody-dependent cytotoxicity (ADCC) Cells bearing Fc receptors, which are a point of contact for exerting a cytotoxic effect on antibody-coated cells

Antigen Any substance that the body regards as foreign and against which the immune system mounts a response (e.g. an antibody)

Antigen processing The intracellular processes required for an antigen to be displayed on the cells surface in the groove of HLA class I or class II for recognition by T lymphocytes

Aortic stenosis Obstruction of blood supply from the left ventricle of the heart into the aorta. Characteristic features include angina, faint pulse, systolic murmur, and exercise intolerance

Aplasia Failure of the bone marrow to produce blood cells

Apoptosis Programmed cell death

Apparent Volume of Distribution (Vd) The apparent volume in which a drug is distributed in the body

Arthus reaction Manifestation of hypersensitivity type III reaction; it is an inflammatory skin response that arises within hours of injection with an antigen

Ascites Accumulation of fluid in the intraperitoneal cavity that leads to abdominal swelling. It occurs in conditions such as congestive cardiac failure, liver disease, and certain malignancies. It is treated with diet and diuretic therapy

Asplenia The absence of a spleen

Atherosclerosis A disorder of blood vessels characterized by the presence of plaques (made up of lipid, cholesterol, cellular debris, platelets) in blood vessels wall. These plaques can become calcified and fibrous and cause narrowing of the lumen, restricting the blood supply to the organs and tissues the blood vessels serves

Atopy Term used to characterize people within a population who suffer from allergies

Atrophy Shrinkage in the size of a cell, tissue, or organ

Attenuation A process by which a virulent microbe is transformed to become avirulent. This can be achieved by repeatedly subculturing a microbe in artificial environment (e.g. subculturing *Mycobacterium bovis*, more than 100 times, which results in the transformation of this virulent organism into avirulent BCG culture, which is used for vaccination against tuberculosis)

Autoantibody An antibody raised against an autoantigen. This arises when the immunological tolerance breaks down and an attacks is made against one of the body's own components (e.g. antithyroid antibodies detected in Hashimoto's thyroiditis)

Autoantigens Antigens that are present on the surface or parts of body tissues or that are naturally occurring in body fluids

Autocrine Used with respect to the ability of a cytokine or hormone to act on the cell that synthesized and secreted it

Autologous graft donation Donation of the patient' own cells (e.g. skin grafted from the thigh to the face)

Autosomal chromosomes All of the chromosomes (1–22) other than the sex chromosomes

β2-microglobulin One of the proteins that constitutes the HLA class I molecule

Basophil A granulocyte that possesses cell surface receptors for IgE antibodies and generally represents about 1 per cent of the leukocyte population in peripheral blood in healthy adults

B lymphocytes A population of lymphocytes that synthesize and display membrane-bound immunoglobulins on their cells surface

bd (bis die) Used with respect to a drug – to be taken twice a day

Bence Jones proteins Immunoglobulin light chains, which are excreted in the urine (e.g. in patients with multiple myeloma)

Bioavailability The overall proportion of a drug that passes into the systemic circulation after administration by mouth. It takes into account both the absorption and local metabolic breakdown of the drug

Biliary colic Visceral pain associated with the passage of a gallstone down the bile duct

Bradykinesis Characteristics include slowed speech and voluntary movements (e.g. a feature presented with certain tranquillizers and in Parkinson's disease)

Bronchopneumonic consolidation Inflammation of bronchus and alveolus and collection of exudate leading to patchy consolidation

Bronchoalveolar lavage (BAL) A procedure that involves washing bronchial and alveolar walls with isotonic saline. A bronchoscope is used to introduce the isotonic saline which may then be aspirated and examined. This procedure is useful for obtaining good specimens for microscopy and culture

Bursa of Fabricius Organ found in the end of the gut of birds, which is the site of immunoglobulin production

Calculi Abnormal formation of stones in a body tissue or organ that results from the accumulation of mineral salts (e.g. gallstone, renal stone)

Capsular polysaccharide Some bacteria are enclosed by a thick layer (capsule) of polysaccharide or mucopolysaccharide. These substances are antigenically active and evoke immune response. They also can protect those organisms from phagocytosis

Carbuncle Fusion of several small abscesses of the hair follicles leading to a large area of pyogenic lesion

Carcinogen A substance that is responsible for causing cancer

Catabolism Metabolic reactions where energy is released e.g. heat

Cellulitis Infection of the soft tissue under the skin with swelling and often redness

Chemotaxis Chemical attraction that promotes the migration of cells into a site of injury or infection

Cholangitis Inflammation of bile ducts

Classical pathway A complement pathway triggered by IgM or IgG immune complexes and involving complement proteins, C1, C2, and C4 in order to generate a C3 convertase enzyme

Class switch A property of B lymphocytes whereby, during the maturation of the immune response, they produce a different isotype of immunoglobulin (e.g. IgM in the primary immune response, then IgG, IgA, or IgE in the secondary immune response)

Clone Cells that arise from cell division which are identical to the original progenitor cell

Colonized Pathogenic organisms establishing multiplication on the body surface (skin or mucosal) of a host but without causing harm to the host

Commensal Generally used for microbes that inhabit on the external surface or in the host without harming the host

Complement A series of proteins that are found in body fluids and are synthesized and released by the liver and macrophages. They assist the humoral arm of immunity

Congenital Defective features present at birth but not inherited

Constant region Used with respect to lymphocyte receptors, these are parts of the receptor that are not variable (whereas the site for antigen-binding is variable)

Contagious Infection that can be transferred from host to host by contacts and other methods such as aerial transmission

Controlled drugs (CDs) Drugs to which legal restrictions imposed by the Misuse of Drug Regulations 1985 apply

Cowpox Poxvirus of cows, also known as the vaccinia virus, non-pathogenic for humans

Consolidation Lungs full of exudate giving the appearance of solid white shadow on X-ray

Cross-match Test performed prior to transplantation or blood transfusion: cells of the donor are mixed with the serum of the potential recipient to assess whether antibodies are present that could recognize and respond to the donor cells

Cyanosis Blue discoloration of skin and mucosal tissue owing to presence of deoxygenate haemoglobin

Cyanotic heart disease A congenital defect in which venous and arterial blood mix and cause cyanosis

Cytokines Substances produced by immune cells (e.g. macrophages and lymphocytes) that control the immune system and are responsible for producing some of the symptoms and signs of disease (e.g. fever, rash). Examples include tumour necrosis factor-alpha, interleukin-1 and interferon-gamma

Cytotoxic Substances that are toxic to cells

Cytotoxic T lymphocyte A subpopulation of T lymphocytes that respond to antigen bound to HLA class I and kill their target cell by lysis

Dedifferentiation The changing of a cell back to its precursor cell type; it is abnormal in humans and appears to occur in certain tumours

Degranulation The release of the contents of cytoplasmic granules by exocytosis e.g. histamine released by mast cells

Dendritic cells Cells present in tissues that engulf and process antigens for presentation to T lymphocytes in the spleen and lymph nodes

Dermatome Segment of skin that developed from a embryological segment of the body

Dermatophytes A group of fungi that cause infections of the skin

Determined cell A cell that has differentiated to the point where the process can no longer be reversed, so it is committed to becoming a specialized cell type

Dialysis A technique that involves removal of toxic material from body fluid or blood (haemodialysis) by passing through a selectively permeable membrane

Differentiation The process that gives rise to the various different specialized cell types in a multicellular organism

Dimerization The formation of a compound from the uniting to two molecules or free radicals

Disseminated infection Infection spreading throughout the body

Dissolution The physical change from a solid state to a solution

Drug clearance The volume of blood or plasma from which a drug is cleared in a unit of time (e.g. ml/minute)

Dysplasia Deranged development which may lead to changes in the architecture of tissues. It is a phenomenon generally associated with epithelial or parenchymal cells that have undergone hyperplasia, which then led to the formation of daughter cells with abnormal characteristics (e.g. shape, size)

Dyspnoea Severe difficulty in breathing

Desquamate Skin surfaces are lined by epithelial cells which are regularly replaced by new cells. The ageing cells fall off (desquamate) as tiny scales, carrying with them a large number of surface (usually non-pathogenic) organisms

Efficacy The ability of a drug to produce a therapeutic effect

Efflux system A mechanism in the bacterial cell membrane that confers tetracycline resistance by repelling the drug from entering the cell

Endarterectomy Surgical removal of the intimal lining of an artery

Endemic An infection that is present in a community or an area, and continues to spread sporadically

Endotoxin Lipopolysaccharide, which is a component of Gram-negative bacterial walls that can stimulate macrophages and B lymphocytes

Enteropathogenic Isolates which cause pathogenic effect on the intestine

Enzyme-linked immunosorbent assay (ELISA) A method for detecting and estimating the levels of an antigen or component of a body fluids. It utilizes a specific antibody and a detectable enzyme with a colour change measured in the assay fluid

Eosinophil A granulocyte involved in anti-parasitic immune response and allergic reactions

Epidemic An infection that spreads to a large number of people involving a large area

Epitope Part of an antigen which is recognized by a lymphocyte receptor

Erythema nodosum A raised red nodular skin rash, which is generally a manifestation of a hypersensitivity reaction

Eukaryotic cell Cell that possesses a nucleus, e.g. genetic material bound by a nuclear membrane

Eustachian tube Also called the pharyngotympanic tube, it connects pharynx to the middle ear

Exfoliation The sloughing off of cells (e.g. occurs in the skin but may be exaggerated in certain pathological conditions)

Exudate Fluid that leaks through capillaries at the site of injury or infection and contains plasma proteins and electrolytes

Fab region Part of the immunoglobulin molecule and involved an antigen-binding and consists of heavy and light chains

Fc region Part of the immunoglobulin molecule which bears the binding-site for attachment to Fc receptors present on immune cells and the C1 molecule of complement

Fibronectin A glycoprotein detected in cells at mucosal surfaces and connective tissues

First-pass effect The rapid metabolism of drugs as they pass through the liver prior to entering the systemic circulation

Fistula An abnormal opening between an hollow organ (e.g. intestine) and either another organ or the skin

Foci Sites of (for example) infection or pain

Follicular dendritic cells Cells that engulf antigens and present them to lymphocytes in the lymphoid organs

Fontanelles Skull bones are not well formed in the neonates. With age the bones expand and cover the whole skull area. Therefore in the newborn infant there are gaps under the scalp skin, the fontanelles, which feel soft and may even be pulsatile. If there is increased pressure within the cerebrospinal space around the brain, either owing to infection or bleeding in this space, there may be bulging of the fontanelles. Cerebrospinal fluid (CSF) is sometimes collected in the newborn infant by aspiration with a needle through the fontanelles

Fluorescent microscopy An ordinary microscope uses a simple light source such as a light bulb (or a more sophisticated version of that). An ultraviolet light source is used for fluorescence microscopy, and the object to be examined is stained with a special fluorescent dye. This allows visualization of the object fluorescing in a dark background. It is commonly used for rapid diagnosis of various infections (e.g. *Mycobacterium* species, viruses)

Free radicals Extremely energetic and reactive molecular species with single unpaired electrons in their outer orbitals. Free radicals have been implicated in diseases such as atherosclerosis and cancer by causing damage to cell membranes and DNA

Fungal hyphae Most fungi display the presence of filamentous elements in the skin scrapings as well as in the culture – fungal hyphae

Gamma irradiation Short-wave electromagnetic radiation which is damaging to the genetic material of bacteria. This method is used for disinfection of sophisticated electronic equipment

Gene Information found in DNA is organized into discrete sections called genes

Generic name The non-trade, universally accepted pharmaceutical name of the drug

Giant cells Large multinucleated cells that are present in granulomas and result from the fusion of two or more macrophages

Glomerular filtration rate A measurement of renal function with respect to the rate of filtration of plasma within a fixed time interval

Glomerulonephritis Inflammation of the glomerulus in the kidneys

Graft-versus-host disease (GvHD) A complication of transplantation in which immune cells of the donor present in the graft emerge and attack the tissues of the recipient. The gut and skin are particularly affected and if it occurs there is a possible risk of mortality

Gram stain Bacteria may be seen using ordinary microscopes, either unstained or by staining with appropriate stains. Gram stain is the most common variety of bacterial stains and allows preliminary identification of bacteria. Some of these appear dark violet (Gram positive) while others take the counterstain (second stain) and appear red (Gram negative)

Granulocytes Neutrophils, eosinophils, and basophils

Granuloma A mass of cells, such as macrophages, T lymphocytes, giant cells, which occurs in some chronic inflammatory reactions (e.g. hypersensitivity type IV)

Grey baby syndrome A toxic syndrome in neonates and preterm infants which is the reaction to the drug, chloramphenicol. Characteristic features include grey cyanosis, respiratory distress, hypothermia, abdominal distension, vomiting, and vascular collapse

Haematopoietic system System involved in the production of blood cells

Haemoglobinopathies Collective term for diseases that result form a mutation or absence of one or more haemoglobin genes (e.g. sickle cell disease, beta-thalassaemia)

Haemolysis Breakdown of red blood cells with the subsequent release of haemoglobin

Haemolytic anaemia Premature red blood cell destruction which may be associated with certain infections, drug therapies, or autoimmune haemolytic disorders

Half-life The time taken for the plasma concentration of a drug to fall by half

HEPA filter High-efficiency filters that may be incorporated into masks; it filters out many pathogenic particles, including most bacteria and fungal spores

Hepatotoxic A drug or chemical that is toxic to the liver is said to be hepatotoxic

Heterozygous A diploid cell that contains different alleles of a same gene at a specific locus

High endothelial venule Part of the venule, which allows the migration of lymphocytes into the lymph node

High extraction ratio A characteristic possessed by drugs which are rapidly cleared by the liver

Histamine A chemical mediator of inflammation produced by basophils and mast cells. It is found in nearly all tissues of the body

HLA See human leukocyte antigen

Homozygous A diploid cell that contains identical alleles of a same gene at a specific locus

Horner's syndrome A neurological disorder of sympathetic nerve fibres supplying an eye. Characteristic features include: constriction of the pupil, ptosis (drooping eyelids), and facial anhydrosis (lack of sweating) on the side of the face affected. Syndrome results from a spinal cord lesion with cervical nerve damage

Host Person (or animal) in whom a micro-organism establishes as a commensal or pathogen

Hydrocephalus Blockage of cerebrospinal fluid (CSF) circulation results in increase in the intracranial pressure leading to bulging of the head in the infants. If the pressure is not relieved by shunting this may result in pressure damage to the brain

Human leukocyte antigen (HLA) The human equivalent of major histocompatibility complex. These cell surface molecules act as signboards and signal the presence of antigen to the T lymphocytes

Humoral immunity Immunity conveyed by immunoglobulins (antibodies)

Hypnotic A drug that depresses brain function and thereby induces sleep

Hypercalcaemia Raised serum calcium level above the normal range

Hypercholesterolaemia Raised serum cholesterol level above the normal range

Hyperkalaemia Raised serum potassium level above the normal range

Hypernatraemia Raised serum sodium level above the normal range

Hyperplasia Increase in the number of cells within a tissue or organ, which leads to an enlarged volume of that tissue or organ

Hypersensitivity reaction Exaggerated or inappropriate activities mounted by the immune system against an antigen

Hypertension High blood pressure

Hypertrophy An adaptive response to a changed environment in which the size of cells is increased

Hypervariable region Areas of the lymphocyte receptor involved in antigen binding which have been encoded by the V, D, and J genes

Hypocalcaemia Low serum calcium level below the normal range

Hypokalaemia Low serum potassium level below the normal range

Hyponatraemia Low serum sodium level below the normal range

Hypotension Low blood pressure

Hypoxia Reduced tissue oxygenation, which may be caused by inadequate blood circulation to the tissue or organ; anaemia, in which there is a limited capacity of the blood to transport oxygen; diseases of respiratory system; insufficient oxygen supply in the inhaled air; or inability of the cell to utilize oxygen (e.g. following cyanide poisoning)

Iatrogenic infections Infections inadvertently transmitted by health-care workers (doctors, nurses, and other staff)

Immune complex Formed by the binding of antibody and antigen, and may also contain complement proteins

Immunogenic Antigen with the ability to produce a specific immune response

Immunoglobulins Another name for antibodies

Immunosuppressive Agents or compounds that suppresses the immune system (either humoral or cellular, or both) and are used during transplantation to prevent rejection of transplanted tissues

Induced sputum A method of obtaining sputum samples by spraying sterile distilled water in the throat, thereby inducing cough reflex

Inflammation A sequence of events that results in immune cell migration into an area of injury or infection and where there has been vasodilatation and vascular permeability

Interferons A group of cytokines that are involved in antiviral and anticancer immune activities

Interleukins Cytokines that have a signalling role and are involved in the control of the immune response

Intubation The introduction of a flexible tube in the airways to maintain respiration

In vivo Mechanisms within or experiments carried out on an intact body

In vitro **cell line** An immortalized collection of cells grown in culture medium in the laboratory

Ionization The separation of a molecule into its positively and negatively charged components

Isotype Immunoglobulins may be subdivided into five smaller classes or isotypes by classifying them according to their overall structure (IgG, IgA, IgM, IgE, and IgD)

Karyotype Structure and size of the chromosomes within a cell

Keratoconjunctivitis Inflammation of cornea and conjunctiva

Laminin A protein that is a component of the basal lamina

Langerhans' cell Antigen-presenting cell found in skin that engulfs and presents antigen to T lymphocytes in lymphoid tissues (e.g. lymph nodes)

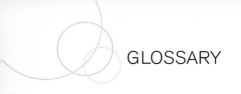

Large granular lymphocytes Another name for natural killer cells

Ligand The component of a structure that binds to a receptor or enzyme binding-site

Lipid-soluble drugs Drugs which are soluble in fatty tissues

Lipofuscin A pigment that accumulates in cells. It is thought to contribute to the ageing process

Lipopolysaccharide (LPS) A component of the cell wall of Gram-negative bacteria (also known as endotoxin)

Loading dose An initial dose which will achieve a desired drug concentration almost immediately

Low extraction ratio drugs Drugs that are not rapidly cleared by the liver

Lymph node Organs that are spread throughout the lymphatic system (e.g. groin, arm pit). They are sites where lymphocytes and antigen-presenting cells make contact with antigens, and a location for memory cells

Lyophylized Freeze dried

Lysozyme An enzyme found in body fluids (e.g. tears, sweat) that breaks down proteoglycan, a component of some microbes (e.g. staphylococci and streptococci)

Macrophage A monocyte that has migrated into a tissue from the bloodstream

Macular rash A small flat plaque of discoloration on skin

Maculopapular rash As above but mixed with slightly raised papules (solid swellings)

Major histocompatibility complex See HLA

Malaise General feeling of being unwell, weak, and lethargic

Mast cell Basophil that migrates into a tissue which possess cytoplasmic granules containing chemical mediators of inflammation

Membrane attack pathway Pathway of complement that utilizes proteins (C5b, C6, C7, C8, and C9) that are fragments that aggregate on the surface of cells to puncture hole and evoke its demise by osmotic lysis

Metabolism The chemical transformations that occur within the body

Metastatic Transfer of disease from one part of the body to another

Memory cell A long-living lymphocyte, which was previously generated following the first encounter with an antigen that remembers and responds rapidly to a subsequent encounter

Metaplasia The replacement of an epithelial or mesenchymal cells with another cell type. Metaplasia is an adaptive response to a stressful stimulus

Monoclonal antibody An antibody synthesized by one cell. In the context of monoclonal antibody preparation, one cell has been immortalized *in vitro* ('locked in time') and upon cell division, identical clones are produced. The antibodies they synthesize are specific for the same antigenic epitope, and never switch immunoglobulin isotype

Monocyte A mononuclear leukocyte present in blood; it becomes a macrophage when it enters a tissue

Mononuclear phagocytic system Cells such as monocytes and macrophages, which are involved in phagocytosis

Morbidity Damaging effect of disease

Morphology The appearance of a cell, tissue, or organism (i.e. size, shape, colour)

MRSA Methicillin-resistant *Staphylococcus aureus*, also called multiple-resistant *Staphylococcus aureus*; very common agent in hospital cross-infection in high intensity areas of a hospital (e.g. intensive therapy and surgical units). They usually cause surface colonization of patients but have also been involved in deeper infections

Mucopurulent Mixed with mucus and pus

Myeloma A tumour that has arisen from a mutation of bone marrow cells

Nasopharyngeal aspirate In newborn infants and very small children, it may be difficult to obtain a good specimen from the throat for culturing. A thin plastic tube is passed through the nose to the posterior pharyngeal space and the collection aspirated for culture

Natural immunity (innate immunity) The immune mechanisms of the host that protect against infections but that are not specific for the antigen (e.g. phagocytic cells, complement)

Natural killer cell Also known as a large granular lymphocyte, it is part of the natural immune response. It has cytotoxic properties and is able to destroy some tumours and virus-infected cells

Necrotizing injury Injury with major tissue damage leading to reduced blood circulation of the affected site and further tissue or cell death

Negative-pressure isolation Isolation of patients in a room, air supply of which is maintained at a lower atmospheric pressure than its surrounding. This is to prevent air borne infective particles escaping from the room and contaminating the surrounding environment and putting other patients and health-care workers at risk

Neoplasm Tumour

Nephrotoxic A drug or other substance which is toxic to the kidney is said to be nephrotoxic

Neurone (nerve cell) A cell with the specialized function of transmitting nerve impulses

Neuralgia Pain that distributes along a nerve or nerve pathway

Neurotransmitter A chemical substance that transmits nerve impulses

Neutropenic Reduction of neutrophil numbers in blood

Neutrophil The most abundant leukocyte in peripheral blood of healthy people; it is phagocytic and sometimes referred to as an inflammatory cell

od (omne die) Used with respect to a drug – to be taken once a day (every day)

Oedema Swelling due to inflammation

Oncogene A gene that, when activated in a cell, is identified with malignant changes

Opportunistic pathogens Some commensals may have minimal virulence, which under normal circumstances will not be adequate to establish an infection. In a patient who is compromised with regards to his normal immunological resistance, such an organism may establish an infection (i.e. an opportunistic infection, such as yeast (candidal) infection in an immunocompromised patient)

Opsonin Complement, immunoglobulins, or acute phase proteins that bind to an antigen to facilitate phagocytosis

Opsonization A process whereby phagocytosis of an antigen facilitated once it has been coated with an opsonin

Osmotic lysis To puncture a cell membrane or wall and allow the influx of water that causes the cell to burst

Osteoblast Cell involved in the formation of bone whose activities are stimulated by oestrogen

Osteoclast Cell involved in bone resorption and necessary for the remodelling and repair of bone

Palliation Therapy that offers temporary relief rather than a cure

Pandemic An infection when the spread occurs to very large areas sometime involving many countries (e.g. influenza pandemics)

Para- Abnormal, beside

Paracrine With respect to a cytokine or hormone – upon its release it produces a response by a distinct cell nearby

Paraquat poisoning Toxicity caused by ingestion of paraquat dichloride, a chemical found in weed-killer. Characteristic features include mouth and oesophageal ulceration, epistaxis, vomiting, diarrhoea, respiratory failure, renal failure, and pulmonary oedema. Could possibly occur accidentally if a person smoked paraquat-contaminated marijuana, but most often follows occupational exposure

Pathogens Organisms that are harmful to the host

PCR test Polymerase chain reaction, a method of amplifying small amounts of DNA in order to obtain larger quantities for investigation

Perforin A molecule hat has a cytotoxic effect by puncturing holes in a cell membrane so that it is killed by osmotic lysis

Pernicious anaemia An autoimmune disorder that results in malabsorption of vitamin B12 and thus a nutritional deficiency. It is characterized by a macrocytic anaemia, muscle weakness, and neurological disturbances

Phagocytosis Process performed by distinct cells types (e.g. neutrophils, macrophages) whereby antigens are engulfed and digested

Phantom pain A sensation of pain that seems to come from a part of the body that has been amputated (e.g. an arm or a leg)

Pharmacodynamics Explains the way in which a drug acts within the body and how it alters the body's processes to bring about its effects

Pharmacokinetics Describes what effect the body has on a drug. It encompasses the way in which the drug is absorbed, distributed, metabolized, and finally excreted from the body

Placebo A 'dummy' drug made from an inactive substance

Plasma cell Cells that are differentiated B lymphocytes that synthesize and secrete immunoglobulins

Plasmids Small amounts of nuclear material (genetic sequence) found free in the cytoplasm. These may contain genes encoding different genetic messages (e.g. antibiotic resistance, enzyme induction)

Polymorphism Used with respect to genes or proteins such as HLA – existing in many different forms

Positive pressure ventilation Enforced ventilation of lung to present oxygen under positive pressure

Porin Protein channels in the outer membrane of Gram-negative bacteria. The porins allow nutrients and antibiotics to pass from outside the cell to the periplasmic space (i.e. a space between the outer membrane and the cell membrane of these bacteria)

Potency The amount (weight) of a drug in relation to its effect

Prevalent pneumococcal types *Streptococcus pneumoniae* or pneumococcus are classified into over 70 different types on the basis of their capsular polysaccharide. Only a small number of types have been found to be associated with pneumococcal disease. Pneumococcal vaccine contains polysaccharide antigens from these types and the other types that are prevalent in a community at a particular time

Primary immune response Immune response of the first encounter with an antigen

Primary immunodeficiency Immunodeficiency due to an inherited defect of part of the immune system

Primary lymphoid organs Site of immune cell production and maturation (i.e. bone marrow, thymus)

prn (pro re nata) Used with respect to a drug – to be taken as necessary

Prodromal Initial symptoms that develop while the patient is incubating the infection

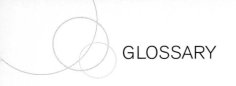

GLOSSARY

Pro-drugs Drugs that need to be converted to an active drug by the body

Prokaryotic cell A cell that lacks a nucleus but possesses a single chromosome

Proliferate To rapidly divide and thus increase cell numbers

Proprietary name A drug name that is restricted in use by virtue of being a trade name

Prostaglandin A substance synthesized from arachidonic acid that can alter the immune response, and may also be a mediator of pain and fever

Prosthetic valve Artificial heart valve, either mechanical or made from human and animal material

Proteinuria Abnormally large quantities of protein in the urine

Proto-oncogene Gene present in normal cells which when altered (e.g. as a result of the action of a carcinogen), can develop into an oncogene

Purulent Mixed with pus

Pustular rash A vesicular rash containing pus instead of watery exudate, often caused by secondary infection of a vesicle with *Staphylococcus aureus*

Pyaemic emboli A clot consisting of blood cells and pus, which often obstructs a small blood vessel

Pyogenic An infection in which there is accumulation of dead white blood cells and other necrotic tissue material giving the appearance of thick white exudative material – pus

Quiescent Dormant, inactive

Radioimmunoassay A method of detecting and measuring an antigen or component of a body fluids which utilized a specific antibody and a radiolabelled antigen

Receptor A molecule that may be present on the cell surface, in the cytoplasm, or the nucleus. When it binds to its specific ligand, a sequence of events or changes in the cell's activities occurs

Recombinant protein Used with respect to a human protein; it is a protein whose genetic sequence has been cloned into a microbe for it to be synthesized using the microbe's intracellular machinery. The protein may be purified from this non-human source, thus obviating the risk of blood-borne infections

Referred pain Pain felt in a part of the body other than where it should be expected (e.g. pain felt in the shoulder following upper abdominal surgery)

Refractory Used with respect to a micro-organism – not affected by an antibiotic; may either be due to resistance (as discussed in Chapter 19) or naturally unaffected by an antibiotic

Respiratory burst Metabolic changes that occurs during phagocytosis that requires oxygen

Resuscitation Reviving a patient who has developed sudden failure of respiratory, cardiac, and other systemic functions

Reticuloendothelial system Term previously used when referring to the mononuclear phagocytic system

Reye's syndrome Clinical manifestation include encephalopathy, hypoglycaemia, and fatty infiltration of the liver, which generally presents in susceptible children and has been associated with certain viral infection (e.g. chickenpox, influenza A) and with aspirin therapy

Rheumatoid factors Autoantibodies whose antigenic target is the Fc region of IgG molecules; detectable in the serum of patients with autoimmune disorders such as rheumatoid arthritis and systemic lupus erythematosus

Ribosomes Organelles in the cytoplasm of a cell where proteins are synthesized

Saprophytes Microbes found in the environment that are harmless to man and animal

Sarcoidosis A chronic condition of unknown aetiology where there is tubercle formation at sites such as the spleen liver, lungs, lymph nodes, and salivary glands

Scarlet fever Disease, usually of children, caused by streptococci, and manifested by red skin rashes caused by a streptococcal toxin called erythrogenic toxin

Sclerosis Hardening of tissue (e.g. due to deposition of mineral salts, inflammation, infiltration of connective tissue)

Secondary immune response Immune response of the second or subsequent encounter with an antigen

Secondary immunodeficiency Immunodeficiency that is the result of an external factor (e.g. infection, diet, drugs) and that compromises the function of an otherwise normal immune system

Senescence Ageing; growing old

Septicaemia Invasion by bacteria of the blood stream with large-scale multiplication. This leads to severe manifestation with high fever, toxic changes, fall of blood pressure, and involvement of a number of different systems of the body

Seroconversion Used with respect to human immunodeficiency virus (HIV) infection, when HIV antibodies have been detected in body fluids

Serological tests Evidence of infection can be confirmed either by isolation of the pathogenic agent from the infected host or by demonstration of the presence of products of immune response against these agents

Serotype On contact with host immune system, many of the microbial products act as antigens and evoke an immune response with the production of antibodies or stimulation of cellular immune system. Depending on the antigen, bacteria may be classified according to the antisera (antibodies in serum) that they bind with

Shunt There is continuous production and circulation of fluid within the cerebrospinal space and the ventricles of the brain – the cerebrospinal fluid (CSF). If there is a blockage in the circulation, the CSF may accumulate and cause increased pressure on the brain tissue. To relieve this pressure, the CSF is drained through an external shunt (for urgent relief) or a shunt is introduced to allow the excess CSF to drain into internal cavities such as peritoneal cavity (a ventricular–peritoneal shunt)

Seronegative Negative antibody test

Seropositive Positive antibody test

Somatic hypermutation A process that occurs on B lymphocytes during the immune response, which modifies the antigen-binding ability of the immunoglobulin molecules it produces

Southern blot Technique used for the analysis of stretches of DNA sequence

Spleen A secondary lymphoid organ which has two main tissue types – red pulp, the site of red blood cell destruction, and white pulp, where there are designated areas of lymphocyte activities that deal with blood-borne antigens

Sterilization A process that results in destruction of all living organisms and spores

Stigmata Physical characteristics of a disease

Stomatitis Inflammation of the mouth, e.g. as a result of infection, drugs, chemical or a vitamin deficiency

Stratum A uniform layer of cells that is in association with other cell layers (e.g. stratum basale of the epidermis)

Stridor Acute obstruction of breathing caused by constriction of the larynx

Stroma Connective tissue and blood supply that supports parenchymal cells

Sty Pyogenic infection of hair follicles of the eyelid leading to a small abscess with redness and swelling of the eyelids

Suprapubic aspiration Used to collect urine specimens from a distended bladder (e.g. in an infants) by introducing a long sterile needle above the pubis and collecting urine aseptically in a sterile container

Surveillance Regular observation and follow up

Syngeneic graft donation Graft donated by a genetically identical sibling

Synergistic Two components (e.g. drugs, cytokines) assisting each other, with the result that their joint effect is more remarkable

tds or tid Used with respect to a drug – to be taken three times a day

Terminal differentiation In the process of differentiation, some cell types still retain the ability to divide. However, in terminal differentiation, the cells do not have the ability to divide

Terminal disinfection Used to indicate making a facility (such as an isolation room) safe after a source of infection (e.g. an infected patient) has vacated the area

T helper cell A subpopulation of T lymphocytes that respond to antigens bound to HLA class II and work with other immune cells to promote the immune response (e.g. cytotoxic T lymphocytes to generate a cell mediated immune response, B lymphocytes to produce immunoglobulin)

Therapeutic index The balance between desired and unwanted drug effects achieved when prescribing a drug

Thymus A site of T lymphocyte maturation, which is located in the thoracic cavity

Tolerance Used with respect to immunity, it is a specific unresponsiveness to an antigen by lymphocytes

Toxins Poisonous substances produced by a number of pathogenic microbes. These are either actively produced (exotoxins) or released when the microbes die and disintegrate (endotoxins)

Toxoid A toxin that has been treated either with a chemical or heat in order to diminish its toxicity. As a result it may be used as a vaccine to stimulate an immune response without causing harm

Tracheostomy Emergency incision of the trachea to allow the breathing to continue

Transcription To make a single strand copy of messenger RNA from the DNA template

Transdifferentiation Generally demonstrated in *in-vitro* cell culture within the laboratory, where one cell type differentiates into another. One such example is the culture of an embryonic eye in the laboratory – if the lens is experimentally removed, then some of the pigmented retina cells may differentiate into lens cells

Transfection The transfer of genetic material (e.g. plasmid, recombinant DNA) into a cells for the synthesis of recombinant proteins by the cell

Transgenic animal An animal that has been genetically manipulated to possess genes it would not naturally have acquired from its parents

Transient colonization Pathogenic organisms established in a host either producing manifestations of infection or surviving by colonizing different body surfaces and deriving nutrition from the host but not causing any pathogenic effect. Generally this is a short-term phenomenon and the pathogens eventually disappear

T suppressor cells A subpopulation of T lymphocytes that regulate the immune response

Tubercle A small nodular lesion, single or multiple, characteristic of tuberculosis of lung

Tumour marker Molecules that can be detected in body fluids which can aid the diagnosis of certain tumours

Tympanic membrane Membrane that separates external ear from the middle ear

Unbound drug Free and therefore pharmacologically active fraction of a drug, not bound to tissues or plasma proteins

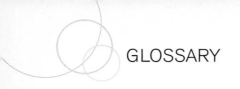

Unsaturated fatty acids A fatty acid where its molecular structure contains one or more carbon–carbon double bonds

Uraemia The accumulation of urea and other toxic nitrogenous waste products in blood, which may arise because of renal insufficiency

Urothelium Epithelial cells in the bladder

Vaccine Antigenic material that has been commercially prepared for inducing immunity to a disease

Varicella pneumonitis Inflammation of the alveoli of the lung with little or no exudate in the alveoli (in contrast to pneumonia, in which there is extensive exudation in the alveoli, leading to consolidation). This is produced more often by viral infections such as varicella infection

Vasculitis Inflammation of blood vessels

Ventricular fibrillation A cardiac arrhythmia in which there is a rapid and irregular ventricular activation; it is characterized by a loss of pulse and blood pressure; respiration stops and the patients becomes unconscious. Defibrillation and ventilation is must be commenced immediately to prevent death

Vesicular fluid Vesicles are small swellings in the skin containing a watery fluid. Many virus infections give rise to vesicular eruptions on the skin. These can sometimes be infected with common bacteria such as Staphylococcus aureus, which replaces the watery fluid with pus – the pustules. Such vesicles may be punctured with a needle to obtain the vesicular fluid

Vesicular rash A rash of small raised spots on the skin, like a small blister, filled with watery (serous) exudate

Western blot A laboratory technique that uses antibodies to identify the presence of a protein

Xenogeneic graft donation Used with respect to humans, the donation of an organ or tissue which has been acquired from a non-human source

INDEX

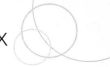

INDEX

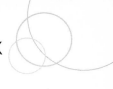

INDEX

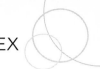

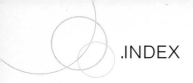

DATE DE RETOUR **A.-Taché**
